PARAMEDIC CARE: Principles & Practice

MEDICAL EMERGENCIES

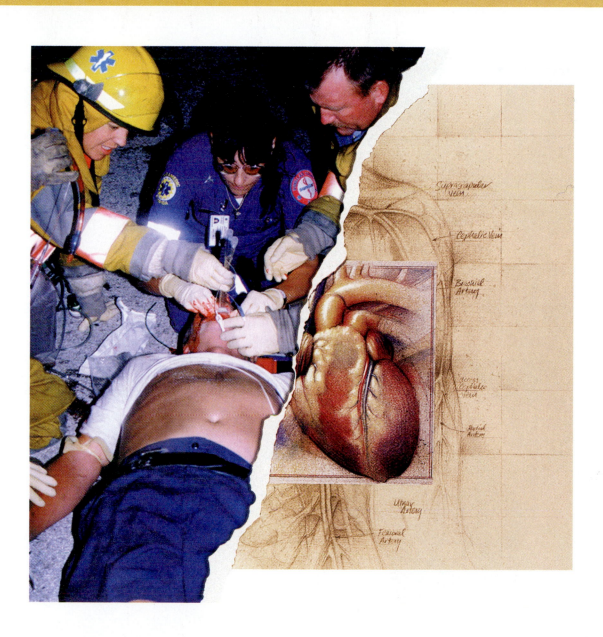

Suprascapular Vein

Cephalic Vein

Brachial Artery

access Cephalic Vein

Radial Artery

Ulnar Artery

Femoral Artery

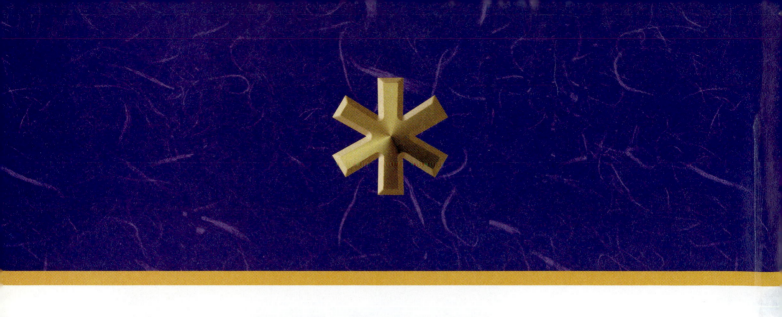

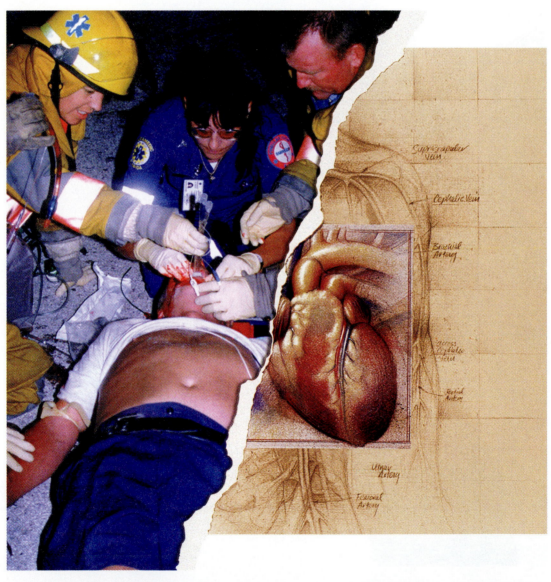

PARAMEDIC CARE: Principles & Practice

MEDICAL EMERGENCIES

BRYAN E. BLEDSOE, D.O., F.A.C.E.P., F.A.A.E.M., F.A.E.P., EMT-P

Emergency Department Staff Physician
Baylor Medical Center—Ellis County
Waxahachie, Texas
and
Clinical Associate Professor of Emergency Medicine
University of North Texas Health Sciences Center
Fort Worth, Texas

ROBERT S. PORTER, M.A., NREMT-P

Senior Advanced Life Support Educator
Madison County Emergency Medical Services
Canastota, New York
and
Flight Paramedic
AirOne, Onondaga County Sheriff's Department
Syracuse, New York

RICHARD A. CHERRY, M.S., NREMT-P

Clinical Assistant Professor of Emergency Medicine
Director of Paramedic Training
SUNY Upstate Medical University
Syracuse, New York

Prentice Hall

Brady
Prentice Hall Health
Upper Saddle River, NJ 07458

Library of Congress Cataloging-in-Publication Data

Bledsoe, Bryan E., 1955-
    Paramedic care: principles & practice / Bryan E. Bledsoe, Robert S. Porter,
Richard A. Cherry
        p. ; cm.
    Includes bibliographical references and index.
    Contents: vol. 3. Medical Emergencies
    ISBN 0-13-021598-8 (alk. paper)
        1. Emergency medicine. 2. Emergency medical technicians. I. Porter,
Robert S., 1950-   II. Title.

Art Acknowledgments

Rolin Graphics, Plymouth, Minnesota

Photo Acknowledgments

All photographs not credited adjacent to the
photograph were photographed on assignment
for Brady/Prentice Hall Pearson Education.

Publisher: Julie Alexander
Acquisitions editor: Laura Edwards
Managing development editor: Lois Berlowitz
Development editors: Sandra Breuer, John Joerschke,
    Terse Stamos
Managing production editor: Patrick Walsh
Editorial/production supervision: Larry Hayden IV
Senior production manager: Ilene Sanford
Marketing manager: Tiffany Price
Marketing coordinator: Cindy Frederick
Interior design: Jill Yutkowitz
Cover design: Rob Richman
Cover photography: Eddie Sperling Photography
Cover illustration: Malcolm Farley
Managing photography editor: Michal Heron
Assistant photography editor: Suzanne Mapes
Interior photographers: Michael Gallitelli, Michal Heron,
    Richard Logan
Page makeup: Carlisle Communications, Inc.

©2001 by Prentice-Hall, Inc.
Upper Saddle River, New Jersey 07458

Printed in the United States of America
10 9 8 7 6 5 4 3 2 1

ISBN   0-13-021598-8

Prentice-Hall International (UK) Limited, *London*
Prentice-Hall of Australia Pty. Limited, *Sydney*
Prentice-Hall Canada Inc., *Toronto*
Prentice-Hall Hispanoamericana, S.A., *Mexico*
Prentice-Hall of India Private Limited, *New Delhi*
Prentice-Hall of Japan, Inc., *Tokyo*
Prentice-Hall (Singapore) Pte Ltd
Editora Prentice-Hall do Brasil, Ltda., *Rio de Janeiro*

SPECIAL NOTES

This book is respectfully dedicated to the EMTs and paramedics who toil each day in an environment that is unpredictable, often dangerous, and constantly changing. They risk their lives to aid the sick and the injured, driven only by their love of humanity and their devotion to this profession we call emergency medical services.

B.E.B.

To those who answer the call to care on cold, dark, and rainy nights.

R.S.P.

"At one time or another in everyone's lives the inner fire goes out. Then it is burst into flame by an encounter with another human being." Rudyard Kipling just described what my wife Sue has meant to me.

R.A.C.

Content Overview

Below is a brief content description of each chapter in *Medical Emergencies*.

CHAPTER 1   PULMONOLOGY   2

* Discusses respiratory system anatomy, physiology, and pathophysiology
* Discusses respiratory system emergencies
* Emphasizes recognition and treatment of reactive airway diseases such as asthma

CHAPTER 2   CARDIOLOGY   62

* Discusses cardiovascular anatomy, physiology, and pathophysiology
* Presents material crucial to advanced prehospital cardiac care
* Is presented in three parts: Part 1—essential cardiac anatomy, physiology, and electrophysiology; Part 2—cardiac and peripheral vascular system emergencies; and Part 3—12-lead ECG monitoring and interpretation

CHAPTER 3   NEUROLOGY   260

* Discusses nervous system anatomy, physiology, and pathophysiology
* Discusses recognition and management of neurological emergencies

CHAPTER 4   ENDOCRINOLOGY   312

* Discusses endocrine system anatomy, physiology, and pathophysiology
* Discusses recognition and management of endocrine emergencies, with emphasis on diabetic emergencies

CHAPTER 5   ALLERGIES AND ANAPHYLAXIS   344

* Reviews the immune system and the pathophysiology of allergic and anaphylactic reactions
* Discusses recognition and treatment of allergic reactions, with emphasis on anaphylactic reactions

CHAPTER 6   GASTROENTEROLOGY   360

* Discusses gastrointestinal system anatomy, physiology, and pathophysiology
* Discusses recognition and management of gastrointestinal emergencies

CHAPTER 7   UROLOGY AND NEPHROLOGY   392

* Discusses genitourinary system anatomy, physiology, and pathophysiology
* Discusses recognition and management of urinary system emergencies in males and females and male reproductive system emergencies

CHAPTER 8   TOXICOLOGY AND SUBSTANCE ABUSE   426

* Discusses basic toxicology and both common and uncommon causes of poisoning
* Discusses overdose and substance abuse, including drug and alcohol abuse
* Discusses recognition and management of poisoning, overdose, and substance abuse emergencies

CHAPTER 9   HEMATOLOGY   470

* Discusses the anatomy, physiology, and pathophysiology of the blood, blood-forming organs, and the reticuloendothelial system
* Discusses recognition and management of hematological emergencies

CHAPTER 10   ENVIRONMENTAL EMERGENCIES   502

* Details the impact of the environment on the body, emphasizing physical, chemical, and biological aspects
* Discusses recognition and management of heat disorders, cold disorders, drowning and near-drowning emergencies, diving emergencies, high altitude emergencies, and radiation emergencies

CHAPTER 11   INFECTIOUS DISEASE   546

* Addresses specific infectious diseases and modes of transmission
* Emphasizes prevention of disease transmission, especially the protection of prehospital personnel
* Discusses recognition and management of specific infectious diseases

CHAPTER 12   PSYCHIATRIC AND BEHAVIORAL EMERGENCIES   606

* Presents an overview of psychiatric disorders and behavioral problems
* Discusses recognition and management of psychiatric and behavioral emergencies

CHAPTER 13   GYNECOLOGY   634

* Discusses female reproductive system anatomy, physiology, and pathophysiology
* Discusses recognition and management of gynecological emergencies

CHAPTER 14   OBSTETRICS   654

* Discusses the anatomy and physiology of pregnancy
* Discusses how to assist a normal delivery
* Discusses recognition and management of complications of pregnancy and delivery

Detailed Contents

SERIES PREFACE   xvii

PREFACE TO VOLUME 3   xix

ACKNOWLEDGMENTS   xxi

ABOUT THE AUTHORS   xxv

NOTICES   xxvii

PRECAUTIONS ON BLOODBORNE PATHOGENS AND INFECTIOUS DISEASES   xxviii

---

CHAPTER 1   PULMONOLOGY   2

Introduction   4

Review of Respiratory Anatomy and Physiology   5
Upper Airway Anatomy 5 ✳ Lower Airway Anatomy 8 ✳ Physiological Processes 11

Pathophysiology   18
Disruption in Ventilation 19 ✳ Disruption in Diffusion 21 ✳ Disruption in Perfusion 21

Assessment of the Respiratory System   22
Initial Assessment 22 ✳ Focused History and Physical Examination 25

Management of Respiratory Disorders   34
Management Principles 35

Specific Upper Respiratory Diseases   35
Upper-Airway Obstruction 35 ✳ Non-cardiogenic Pulmonary Edema/Adult Respiratory Distress Syndrome 36 ✳ Obstructive Lung Disease 38 ✳ Emphysema 39 ✳ Chronic Bronchitis 41 ✳ Asthma 43 ✳ Upper Respiratory Infection (URI) 48 ✳ Pneumonia 49 ✳ Lung Cancer 51 ✳ Toxic Inhalation 52 ✳ Carbon Monoxide Inhalation 53 ✳ Pulmonary Embolism 54 ✳ Spontaneous Pneumothorax 56 ✳ Hyperventilation Syndrome 57 ✳ Central Nervous System Dysfunction 58 ✳ Dysfunction of the Spinal Cord, Nerves, or Respiratory Muscles 59

CHAPTER 2   CARDIOLOGY   62

Introduction   68

PART 1:   CARDIOVASCULAR ANATOMY AND PHYSIOLOGY, ECG MONITORING, AND DYSRHYTHMIA ANALYSIS   69

Cardiovascular Anatomy   70
Anatomy of the Heart 70 ✳ Anatomy of the Peripheral Vascular Circulation 76

Cardiac Physiology   77
The Cardiac Cycle 77 ✳ Nervous Control of the Heart 78 ✳ Electrophysiology 80

Electrocardiographic Monitoring   84
The Electrocardiogram 84 ✻ Relationship of the ECG to Electrical Events in the Heart 88 ✻ Interpretation of Rhythm Strips 95

Dysrhythmias   97
Mechanism of Impulse Formation 98 ✻ Classification of Dysrhythmias 98 ✻ Dysrhythmias Originating in the SA Node 99 ✻ Dysrhythmias Originating in the Atria 109 ✻ Dysrhythmias Originating within the AV Junction (AV Blocks) 122 ✻ Dysrhythmias Sustained or Originating in the AV Junction 132 ✻ Dysrhythmias Originating in the Ventricles 140 ✻ Pulseless Electrical Activity 154 ✻ Dysrhythmias Resulting from Disorders of Conduction 154 ✻ ECG Changes Due to Electrolyte Abnormalities and Hypothermia 157

PART 2: ASSESSMENT AND MANAGEMENT OF THE CARDIOVASCULAR PATIENT   158

Assessment of the Cardiovascular Patient   160
Scene Size-up and Initial Assessment 161 ✻ Focused History 162 ✻ Physical Examination 166

Management of Cardiovascular Emergencies   170
Basic Life Support 170 ✻ Advanced Life Support 170 ✻ Monitoring ECG in the Field 171 ✻ Vagal Maneuvers 174 ✻ Precordial Thump 175 ✻ Pharmacological Management 175 ✻ Defibrillation 180 ✻ Emergency Synchronized Cardioversion 183 ✻ Transcutaneous Cardiac Pacing 186 ✻ Carotid Sinus Massage 190 ✻ Support and Communication 190

Managing Specific Cardiovascular Emergencies   191
Angina Pectoris 191 ✻ Myocardial Infarction 196 ✻ Heart Failure 202 ✻ Cardiac Tamponade 206 ✻ Hypertensive Emergencies 208 ✻ Cardiogenic Shock 209 ✻ Cardiac Arrest 212 ✻ Peripheral Vascular and Other Cardiovascular Emergencies 217

PART 3: 12-LEAD ECG MONITORING AND INTERPRETATION   221

Reviewing the Cardiac Conductive System   222

ECG Recording   222

ECG Leads   224
Bipolar Limb Leads 226 ✻ Unipolar or Augmented Limb Leads 226 ✻ Precordial Leads 228

Mean QRS Axis Determination   228

Axis Deviation   229

The Normal 12-Lead ECG   231

Disease Findings   232
Evolution of Acute Myocardial Infarction 235 ✻ Localization of Acute Myocardial Infarction 235

Conduction Abnormalities   240
AV Blocks 241 * Bundle Branch Blocks 245 * Chamber
Enlargement 249

Prehospital ECG Monitoring   255
Prehospital 12-Lead ECG Monitoring 255

CHAPTER 3   NEUROLOGY   260

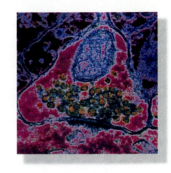

Introduction   262

Anatomy and Physiology   262
The Central Nervous System 264 * The Peripheral Nervous
System 273 * The Autonomic Nervous System 275

Pathophysiology   275
Alteration in Cognitive Systems 275 * Central Nervous System
Disorders 275 * Cerebral Homeostasis 276 * Peripheral
Nervous System Disorders 276

General Assessment Findings   277
Scene Size-up and Initial Assessment 277 * Focused History
and Physical Exam 279 * Ongoing Assessment 286

Management of Nervous System Emergencies   286
Altered Mental Status 287 * Stroke and Intracranial
Hemorrhage 289 * Seizures and Epilepsy 294 *
Syncope 299 * Headache 300 * "Weak and Dizzy" 301 *
Neoplasms 302 * Brain Abscess 304 * Degenerative
Neurological Disorders 304 * Back Pain and Nontraumatic
Spinal Disorders 307

CHAPTER 4   ENDOCRINOLOGY   312

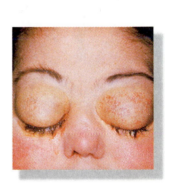

Introduction   315

Anatomy and Physiology   316
Hypothalamus 317 * Pituitary Gland 317 * Thyroid
Gland 321 * Parathyroid Glands 322 * Thymus
Gland 322 * Pancreas 322 * Adrenal Glands 324 *
Gonads 325 * Pineal Gland 325 * Other Organs with
Endocrine Activity 326

Endocrine Disorders and Emergencies   326
Disorders of the Pancreas 326 * Disorders of the Thyroid
Gland 336 * Disorders of the Adrenal Glands 339

CHAPTER 5   ALLERGIES AND ANAPHYLAXIS   344

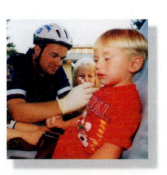

Introduction   346

Pathophysiology   347
The Immune System 347 * Allergies 349 * Anaphylaxis 351

Assessment Findings in Anaphylaxis   352

Management of Anaphylaxis   354
Protect the Airway 354 ✻ Administer Medications 354 ✻
Offer Psychological Support 356

Assessment Findings in Allergic Reaction   356

Management of Allergic Reactions   357

Patient Education   357

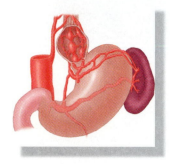

CHAPTER 6   GASTROENTEROLOGY   360

Introduction   363

General Pathophysiology, Assessment, and Treatment   363
General Pathophysiology 363 ✻ General Assessment 365 ✻
General Treatment 367

Specific Illnesses   368
Upper Gastrointestinal Diseases 368 ✻ Lower Gastrointestinal
Diseases 376 ✻ Accessory Organ Diseases 385

CHAPTER 7   UROLOGY AND NEPHROLOGY   392

Introduction   395

Anatomy and Physiology   396
Kidneys 396 ✻ Ureters 401 ✻ Urinary Bladder 402 ✻
Urethra 402 ✻ Testes 402 ✻ Epididymis and Vas
Deferens 404 ✻ Prostate Gland 404 ✻ Penis 404

General Mechanisms of Nontraumatic Tissue Problems   404

General Pathophysiology, Assessment, and Management   404
Pathophysiologic Basis of Pain 404 ✻ Assessment and
Management 404

Renal and Urologic Emergencies   409
Acute Renal Failure 409 ✻ Chronic Renal Failure 413 ✻
Renal Calculi 419 ✻ Urinary Tract Infection 421

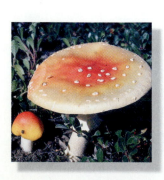

CHAPTER 8   TOXICOLOGY AND SUBSTANCE ABUSE   426

Introduction   428

Epidemiology   429

Poison Control Centers   429

Routes of Toxic Exposure   430
Ingestion 430 * Inhalation 430 * Surface Absorption 431 *
Injection 431

General Principles of Toxicologic Assessment and Management   431
Scene Size-up 431 * Initial Assessment 432 * History, Physical
Exam, and Ongoing Assessment 432 * Treatment 432 *
Suicidal Patients and Protective Custody 434

Ingested Toxins   434

Inhaled Toxins   437

Surface-Absorbed Toxins   437

Specific Toxins   438
Cyanide 438 * Carbon Monoxide 439 * Cardiac
Medications 442 * Caustic Substances 443 * Hydrofluoric
Acid 444 * Alcohol 444 * Hydrocarbons 444 * Tricyclic
Antidepressants 445 * MAO Inhibitors 446 * Newer
Antidepressants 447 * Lithium 447 * Salicylates 448 *
Acetaminophen 449 * Other Non-prescription Pain
Medications 449 * Theophylline 450 * Metals 450 *
Contaminated Food 451 * Poisonous Plants and Mushrooms 452

Injected Toxins   453
General Principles of Management 453 * Insect Bites and
Stings 454 * Snakebites 457 * Marine Animal Injection 461

Substance Abuse and Overdose   461
Drugs of Abuse 462

Alcohol Abuse   463
Physiological Effects 463 * General Alcoholic Profile 466 *
Consequences of Chronic Alcohol Ingestion 466

CHAPTER 9   HEMATOLOGY   470

Introduction   472

Anatomy, Physiology, and Pathophysiology   473
Components of Blood 473 * Hemostasis 481 * Blood
Products and Blood Typing 484 * Transfusion Reactions 485

General Assessment and Management   486
Scene Size-up 487 * Initial Assessment 487 * Focused
History and Physical Exam 487 * General Management of
Hematopoietic Emergencies 491

Managing Specific Patient Problems   492
Diseases of the Red Blood Cells 492 * Diseases of the White
Blood Cells 495 * Diseases of the Platelets/Blood Clotting
Abnormalities 497 * Other Hematopoietic Disorders 499

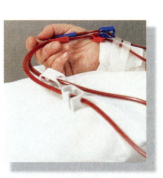

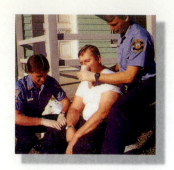

CHAPTER 10 ENVIRONMENTAL EMERGENCIES
502

Introduction   505

Homeostasis   505

Pathophysiology of Heat and Cold Disorders   506
Mechanisms of Heat Gain and Loss 506 ✳ Thermogenesis (Heat Generation) 506 ✳ Thermolysis (Heat Loss) 506 ✳ Thermoregulation 507

Heat Disorders   510
Hyperthermia 510 ✳ Predisposing Factors 510 ✳ Preventive Measures 511 ✳ Specific Heat Disorders 511 ✳ Role of Dehydration in Heat Disorders 515 ✳ Fever (Pyrexia) 516

Cold Disorders   516
Hypothermia 517 ✳ Mechanisms of Heat Conservation and Loss 517 ✳ Predisposing Factors 517 ✳ Preventive Measures 518 ✳ Degrees of Hypothermia 518 ✳ Frostbite 523 ✳ Trench Foot 524

Near-Drowning and Drowning   525
Pathophysiology of Drowning and Near-Drowning 525 ✳ Treatment for Near-Drowning 527

Diving Emergencies   528
The Effects of Air Pressure on Gases 528 ✳ Pathophysiology of Diving Emergencies 530 ✳ Classification of Diving Injuries 530 ✳ General Assessment of Diving Emergencies 531 ✳ Pressure Disorders 532 ✳ Other Diving-Related Illnesses 535 ✳ Divers Alert Network (DAN) 535

High Altitude Illness   536
Prevention 536 ✳ Types of High Altitude Illness 538

Nuclear Radiation   539
Basic Nuclear Physics 539 ✳ Effects of Radiation on the Body 541 ✳ Principles of Safety 542 ✳ Management 543

CHAPTER 11 INFECTIOUS DISEASE
546

Introduction   549

Public Health Principles   549

Public Health Agencies   550

Microorganisms   550
Bacteria 551 ✳ Viruses 552 ✳ Other Microorganisms 553

Contraction, Transmission, and Stages of Disease   555
Phases of the Infectious Process 557

The Body's Defenses against Disease   557
The Immune System 558 ✳ The Complement System 559 ✳ The Lymphatic System 559 ✳ Individual Host Immunity 560

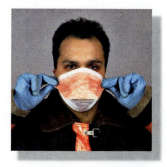

Infection Control in Prehospital Care   561
Preparation for Response 561 * Response 562 * Patient
Contact 562 * Recovery 564 * Infectious Disease Exposures 567

Assessment of the Patient with Infectious Disease   568
Past Medical History 568 * The Physical Examination 569

Selected Infectious Diseases   569
Diseases of Immediate Concern to EMS Providers 570 * Other
Infectious Conditions of the Respiratory System 588 * GI System
Infections 590 * Nervous System Infections 592 * Sexually
Transmitted Diseases 596 * Diseases of the Skin 599 *
Nosocomial Infections 601

Patient Education   602

Preventing Disease Transmission   602

CHAPTER 12   PSYCHIATRIC AND BEHAVIORAL DISORDERS   606

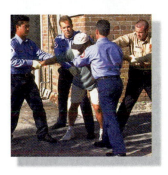

Introduction   608

Behavioral Emergencies   608

Pathophysiology of Psychiatric Disorders   609
Biological 609 * Psychological 610 * Sociocultural 610

Assessment of Behavioral Emergency Patients   610
Scene Size-up 610 * Initial Assessment 611 * Focused
History and Physical Examination 611 * Mental Status
Examination 613 * Psychiatric Medications 614

Specific Psychiatric Disorders   614
Cognitive Disorders 614 * Schizophrenia 615 * Anxiety
and Related Disorders 616 * Mood Disorders 617 * Substance
Related Disorders 620 * Somatoform Disorders 620 * Factitious
Disorders 620 * Dissociative Disorders 621 * Eating
Disorders 621 * Personality Disorders 623 * Impulse Control
Disorders 623 * Suicide 623 * Age-Related Conditions 624

Management of Behavioral Emergencies   625
Medical 626 * Psychological 626

Violent Patients and Restraint   627
Methods of Restraint 628 * Positioning and Restraining Patients for
Transport 630 * Chemical Restraint 631

CHAPTER 13   GYNECOLOGY   634

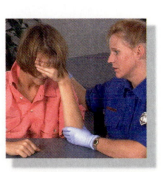

Introduction   637

Anatomy and Physiology   637
Female Reproductive Organs 637

The Menstrual Cycle   **641**
The Proliferative Phase 642 ✳ The Secretory Phase 642 ✳
The Ischemic Phase 642 ✳ The Menstrual Phase 642

Assessment of the Gynecological Patient   **643**
History 643 ✳ Physical Exam 645

Management of Gynecological Emergencies   **646**

Specific Gynecological Emergencies   **647**
Medical Gynecological Emergencies 647 ✳ Traumatic
Gynecological Emergencies 650

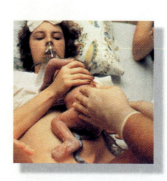

CHAPTER 14 OBSTETRICS   654

Introduction   **656**

The Prenatal Period   **656**
Anatomy and Physiology of the Obstetric Patient 656 ✳ Fetal
Development 661 ✳ Fetal Circulation 662

General Assessment of the Obstetric Patient   **664**
Initial Assessment 664 ✳ History 664 ✳ Physical
Examination 666

General Management of the Obstetric Patient   **667**

Complications of Pregnancy   **668**
Trauma 668 ✳ Medical Conditions 669 ✳ Bleeding in
Pregnancy 669 ✳ Medical Complications of Pregnancy 674 ✳
Braxton-Hicks Contractions 678 ✳ Preterm Labor 678

The Puerperium   **679**
Labor 680 ✳ Management of a Patient in Labor 681 ✳ Field
Delivery 683 ✳ Neonatal Care 686

Abnormal Delivery Situations   **689**

Other Delivery Complications   **693**

Maternal Complications of Labor and Delivery   **694**

**SUGGESTED RESPONSES TO "YOU MAKE
THE CALL"**   **698**

GLOSSARY   **706**

INDEX   **722**

Series Preface

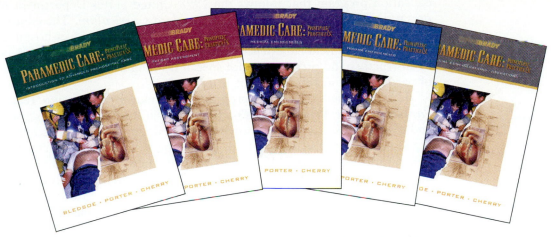

Congratulations on your decision to further your EMS career by undertaking the course of education required for certification as an Emergency Medical Technician-Paramedic! The world of paramedic emergency care is one that you will find both challenging and rewarding. Whether you will be working as a volunteer or paid paramedic, you will find the field of advanced prehospital care very interesting.

This textbook program will serve as your guide and reference to advanced out-of-hospital care. It is based upon the 1998 United States Department of Transportation *EMT-Paramedic: National Standard Curriculum* and is divided into five volumes. The first volume is entitled *Introduction to Advanced Prehospital Care* and addresses the fundamentals of paramedic practice, including pathophysiology, pharmacology, medication administration and advanced airway management. The second volume, *Patient Assessment,* builds on the assessment skills of the basic EMT with special emphasis on advanced patient assessment at the scene. The third volume of the series, *Medical Emergencies,* is the most extensive and addresses paramedic level care of medical emergencies. Particular emphasis is placed upon the most common medical problems as well as serious emergencies, such as respiratory and cardiovascular emergencies. *Trauma Emergencies,* the fourth volume of the text, discusses advanced prehospital care from the mechanism of injury analysis to shock/trauma resuscitation. The last volume in the series addresses *Special Considerations/Operations* including neonatal, pediatric, geriatric, home health care, and specially challenged patients, and incident command, ambulance service, rescue, hazardous material, and crime scene operations. These five volumes will help prepare you for the challenges of prehospital care.

SKILLS

The psychomotor skills of fluid and medication administration, advanced airway care, ECG monitoring and defibrillation, and advanced medical and trauma patient care are best learned in the classroom, skills laboratory, and then the clinical and field setting. Common advanced prehospital skills are discussed in the text as well as outlined in the accompanying procedure sheets. Review these before and while practicing the skill. It is important to point out that this or any other text cannot teach skills. Care skills are only learned under the watchful eye of a paramedic instructor and perfected during your clinical and field internship.

HOW TO USE THIS TEXTBOOK

Paramedic Care: Principles & Practice is designed to accompany a paramedic education program that follows the 1998 United States Department of Transportation *EMT-Paramedic: National Standard Curriculum.* The education program should include ample classroom, practical laboratory, in-hospital clinical, and prehospital field experience. These educational experiences must be guided by instructors and preceptors with special training and experience in their areas of participation in your program.

It is intended that your program coordinator will assign reading from *Paramedic Care: Principles & Practice* in preparation for each classroom lecture and discussion section. The knowledge gained from reading this text will form the foundation of the information you will need in order to function effectively as a paramedic in your EMS system. Your instructors will build upon this information to strengthen your knowledge and understanding of advanced prehospital care so that you may apply it in your practice. The in-hospital clinical and prehospital field experiences will further refine your knowledge and skills under the watchful eyes of your preceptors.

In preparing for each classroom session, read the assigned chapter carefully. First, review the chapter objectives. They will identify important concepts to be learned from the reading. Read the Case Study to get a feeling of why a chapter is important and how the knowledge it contains can be applied in the field. Read the chapter content carefully, while keeping the chapter objectives in mind. Read the You Make the Call feature and answer the questions to assure you understand the application of the knowledge presented in the chapter. Last, re-read the chapter objectives and be sure that you are able to answer each one completely. If you cannot, reread the section of the chapter to which the objective relates. If you still do not understand the objective or any portion of what you have read, ask your instructor to explain it at your next class session.

Ideally, you should read this entire text series at least three times. The volume chapter should be read in preparation for the class session, the entire volume should be read before the division or course test, and the entire text series should be reread before the program final exam and/or certification testing. While this might seem like a lot of reading, it will improve your classroom performance, your knowledge of emergency care, and ultimately, the care you provide to emergency patients.

The workbook that accompanies this text can also assist in improving classroom performance. It contains information, sample test questions, and exercises designed to assist learning. Its use can be very helpful in identifying the important elements of paramedic education, in exercising the knowledge of prehospital care, and in helping you self-test your knowledge.

Paramedic Care: Principles & Practice presents the knowledge of emergency care in as accurate, standardized, and clear a manner as is possible. However, each EMS system is uniquely different, and it is beyond the scope of this text to address all differences. You must count heavily on your instructors, the program coordinator, and ultimately the program medical director to identify how specific emergency care procedures are applied in your system.

Advanced life support (ALS) and paramedic care were initially developed to treat cardiac problems in the field, specifically sudden death. Many people were suffering acute coronary events and dying before reaching the hospital. Physicians with foresight believed that rapid prehospital intervention could mean the difference between life and death for many people. The earliest origins of EMS were this early emphasis on prehospital cardiac care, which developed simultaneously with the early advances in trauma care. Over the years, EMS proved effective in treating different types of cardiac emergencies. As EMS evolved, prehospital care was expanded to many other types of medical emergencies, including diabetic emergencies and respiratory emergencies.

Now, with the advent of the 1998 U.S. DOT *EMT-Paramedic National Standard Curriculum,* paramedics are responsible for a much more detailed understanding of medical emergencies. The new curriculum, upon which this book is based, now addresses in detail the various types of medical emergencies. Cardiac emergencies still represent the most common reason EMS is summoned, and the discussion of cardiac emergencies remains the most comprehensive in the text. However, paramedics are expected to have a high level of understanding of emergencies involving other body systems. In this book, we will briefly review important anatomy and physiology as it applies to the emergency in question. This is followed by discussion of the relevant pathophysiology. Finally, focused prehospital assessment and treatment for each type of medical emergency is presented. With *Paramedic Care: Principles and Practice,* Volume 3, *Medical Emergencies,* we have followed the U.S. DOT curriculum and provided a detailed discussion of virtually all types of medical emergencies likely to be encountered in the prehospital setting.

This book follows a systems approach that also parallels the various subspecialties of internal medicine.

Chapter 1 "Pulmonology" introduces the paramedic student to commonly encountered respiratory system emergencies. Emphasis is on the recognition and treatment of reactive airway diseases such as asthma.

Chapter 2 "Cardiology" presents the material crucial to advanced prehospital cardiac care. The first part of the chapter reviews essential anatomy and physiology and introduces the student to electrophysiology. The second part of the chapter deals with cardiac emergencies and peripheral vascular system emergencies. Finally, the third division addresses 12-lead ECG interpretation and prehospital application of 12-lead ECG diagnostics and monitoring.

Chapter 3 "Neurology" reviews the anatomy and physiology of the central and peripheral nervous system. This is followed by a detailed discussion of neurological emergencies.

Chapter 4 "Endocrinology" is a detailed discussion of the endocrine system, which is an alternate control system for the body. Emphasis is placed on diabetic emergencies, as they are by far the most common endocrine emergency encountered by paramedics.

Chapter 5 "Allergies and Anaphylaxis" reviews the immune system, with particular emphasis on hypersensitivity reactions (allergic reactions). The chapter emphasizes prehospital recognition and treatment of allergic reactions, particularly anaphylaxis.

Chapter 6 "Gastroenterology" is a detailed discussion of emergencies arising within the gastrointestinal system. The chapter initially reviews the relevant anatomy and physiology of the gastrointestinal system and follows this with a discussion of assessment and treatment of gastroenterological emergencies.

Chapter 7 "Urology and Nephrology" presents an overview of emergencies that arise from the genitourinary system and the male reproductive system. This includes a discussion of infectious emergencies, renal failure, and other problems.

Chapter 8 "Toxicology and Substance Abuse" provides a detailed description of basic toxicology as it applies to prehospital care. The chapter reviews both common and uncommon causes of poisoning. In addition to accidental poisoning, there is a detailed discussion of the various drugs of abuse that are frequently seen in prehospital care.

Chapter 9 "Hematology" is a comprehensive chapter covering the blood and the reticuloendothelial system. The initial part of the chapter provides a detailed discussion of the blood and blood-forming organs. This is followed by a discussion of hematological emergencies seen in emergency care.

Chapter 10 "Environmental Emergencies" details the impact of the environment on the body. A review of relevant physics, chemistry, and biology is followed by a discussion of environmental emergencies.

Chapter 11 "Infectious Disease" addresses an important but often overlooked aspect of prehospital care. Infectious diseases pose a risk to both the paramedic and the patient. This chapter reviews the basics of infectious disease, including disease transmission. This is followed by a discussion of infectious diseases likely to be encountered in prehospital care.

Chapter 12 "Psychiatric and Behavioral Disorders" provides an overview of psychiatric and behavioral problems. Paramedics are often the first members of the health care profession that a patient with a psychiatric disorder encounters. Because of this, paramedics must be ready to recognize and manage these emergencies appropriately.

Chapter 13 "Gynecology" is a chapter devoted to the recognition and treatment of emergencies arising from the female reproductive system. The chapter provides an overview of female reproductive anatomy and physiology. This is followed by a discussion of common gynecological emergencies.

Chapter 14 "Obstetrics" pertains to the reproduction of the organism. Although a normal process, paramedics are called upon to treat various emergencies arising from pregnancy. Following a review of the anatomical and physiological changes that arise from pregnancy, this chapter addresses emergencies that arise before, during, or after childbirth.

This volume, *Medical Emergencies,* details the basic medical knowledge and skills expected of twenty-first century paramedics. This material should be mastered before undertaking actual patient care.

Brady's *Paramedic Care: Principles & Practice,* is a five-volume series designed to provide educational enrichment as prescribed by the 1998 U.S. D.O.T. *EMT–Paramedic: National Standard Curriculum.* Volume 1, *Introduction to Advanced Prehospital Care* presents the foundations of paramedic practice as well as an introduction to pathophysiology, pharmacology, medication administration, and airway management and ventilation. Volume 2, *Patient Assessment* adds the cognitive and psychomotor skills of patient assessment, communications, and documentation. This knowledge base expands as the series applies it to the medical patient in Volume 3, *Medical Emergencies* and to the trauma patient in Volume 4, *Trauma Emergencies.* Volume 5, *Special Considerations/Operations* enriches these general patient care concepts and principles with applications to special patients and circumstances we commonly see as paramedics. The product of this complete and integrated series is a set of principles of paramedic care you will be required to practice in the twenty-first century.

Acknowledgments

CHAPTER CONTRIBUTORS

We wish to acknowledge the remarkable talents and efforts of the following people who contributed to this volume of *Paramedic Care: Principles & Practice*. Individually, they worked with extraordinary commitment on this new program. Together, they form a team of highly dedicated professionals who have upheld the highest standards of EMS instruction.

Chapter 1 Pulmonology
Howard A. Werman, M.D., F.A.C.E.P., Associate Professor of Clinical Emergency Medicine, The Ohio State University College of Medicine and Public Health, Columbus, Ohio; Medical Director, MedFlight of Ohio

Chapter 2 Cardiology
Lawrence C. Brilliant, M.D., F.A.C.E.P., Clinical Assistant Professor, Department of Primary Care Education and Community Services, Hahnemann University; Emergency Physician, Doylestown Hospital, Doylestown, Pennsylvania.
Kevin Waddington, MedStar, Forth Worth, Texas

Chapter 3 Neurology
Eric W. Heckerson, R.N., M.A., NREMT-P, EMS Coordinator, Mesa Fire Department, Mesa, Arizona

Chapter 4 Endocrinology
Beth Lothrop Adams, M.A., R.N., NREMT-P, ALS Coordinator, EHS Programs, Adjunct Assistant Professor, Emergency Medicine, The George Washington University
Elizabeth Coolidge-Stolz, M.D., Medical Writer, Health Educator, North Reading, Massachusetts

Chapter 5 Allergies and Anaphylaxis
Bryan E. Bledsoe, D.O., F.A.C.E.P., F.A.A.E.M., F.A.E.P, EMT-P, Emergency Department Staff Physician, Baylor Medical Center—Ellis County, Waxahachie, Texas; Clinical Associate Professor of Emergency Medicine, University of North Texas Health Sciences Center, Fort Worth, Texas

Chapter 6 Gastroenterology
Elizabeth Coolidge-Stolz, M.D., Medical Writer, Health Educator, North Reading, Massachusetts
Matthew S. Zavarella, B.S.A.S., REMT-P, CCTEMT-P, Instructor, Department of Emergency Medical Technology, School of Health Related Professions, University of Mississippi Medical Center, Jackson, Mississippi

Chapter 7 Urology and Nephrology
Elizabeth Coolidge-Stolz, M.D., Medical Writer, Health Educator, North Reading, Massachusetts

Chapter 8 Toxicology
John M. Saad, M.D., Medical Director of Emergency Services, Navarro Regional Hospital, Corsicana, Texas; Medical Director of Emergency Services, Medical Center at Terrell, Terrell, Texas

Chapter 9 Hematology
Bryan E. Bledsoe, D.O., F.A.C.E.P., F.A.A.E.M., F.A.E.P, EMT-P, Emergency Department Staff Physician, Baylor Medical Center—Ellis County, Waxahachie, Texas; Clinical Associate Professor of Emergency Medicine, University of North Texas Health Sciences Center, Fort Worth, Texas

Deborah Kufs, R.N., B.S., C.C.R.N., C.E.N., NREMT-P, Clinical Instructor, Hudson Valley Community College, Institute for Prehospital Emergency Medicine, Troy, New York

Craig A. Soltis, M.D., F.A.C.E.P., Assistant Professor of Clinical Emergency Medicine, Northeastern Ohio Universities College of Medicine; Chairman, Department of Emergency Medicine, Forum Health, Youngstown, Ohio

Chapter 10 Environmental Emergencies
John M. Saad, M.D., Medical Director of Emergency Services, Navarro Regional Hospital, Corsicana, Texas; Medical Director of Emergency Services, Medical Center at Terrell, Terrell, Texas

Jo Anne Schultz, B. A., NREMT-P, Paramedic, Lifestar Ambulance, Inc., Salisbury, Maryland; Level II Emergency Medical Services Instructor, Maryland Fire and Rescue Institute, University of Maryland; Paramedic Instructor, Maryland Institute of Emergency Medical Services Systems, University of Maryland; ACLS, BTLS, and PALS instructor

Chapter 11 Infectious and Communicable Diseases
Clyde Deschamp, M.Ed., NREMT-P, Chairman and Assistant Professor, Department of Emergency Medical Technology, Director, Helicopter Transport, University of Mississippi Medical Center

Eric W. Heckerson, R.N., M.A., NREMT-P, EMS Coordinator, Mesa Fire Department, Mesa, Arizona

John S. Saito, M.P.H., EMT-P, Director, EMS/Paramedic Education, Assistant Professor, Oregon Health Sciences University, School of Medicine, Department of Emergency Medicine, Portland, Oregon

Chapter 12 Behavioral and Psychiatric Disorders
Daniel Limmer, EMT-P, Frederick Maryland

Eric W. Heckerson, R.N., M.A., NREMT-P, EMS Coordinator, Mesa Fire Department, Mesa, Arizona

Chapter 13 Gynecology
Beth Lothrop Adams, M.A., R.N., NREMT-P, ALS Coordinator, EHS Programs, Adjunct Assistant Professor, Emergency Medicine, The George Washington University

Chapter 14 Obstetrics
Beth Lothrop Adams, M.A., R.N., NREMT-P, ALS Coordinator, EHS Programs, Adjunct Assistant Professor, Emergency Medicine, The George Washington University

DEVELOPMENT AND PRODUCTION

The task of writing, editing, reviewing, and producing a textbook the size of *Paramedic Care: Principles & Practice* is complex. Many talented people at Brady have been involved in developing and producing this new program.

First, the authors would like to acknowledge the support of Julie Alexander and Laura Edwards. Their belief in us and support of EMS has allowed us to assure that *Paramedic Care: Principles & Practice* will be in the forefront of paramedic education. Special thanks go to Sandra Breuer, who served as Project Coordinator for this new paramedic series and Development Editor for this volume, and John Joerschke and Terse Stamos, who also contributed as Development Editors for this volume. The extraordinary efforts of these exceptionally dedicated editors are deeply appreciated.

The challenges of production were in the very capable hands of Patrick Walsh and Larry Hayden, who skillfully supervised all production stages to create the final product you now hold. In developing our art and photo program we were fortunate to work with yet additional talent, leaders within their professions. Most of the staged photographs are by Michal Heron of New York City, whose commitment to excellence never falters. The new art was drafted by Rolin Graphics of Plymouth, Minnesota.

REVIEW BOARDS

Our special thanks to Brenda Beasley, RN, BS, EMT-P, EMS Program Director at Calhoun College in Decatur, Alabama, for her review of material in *Medical Emergencies*. Her experience and high standards proved to be significant contributions to text development. Our special thanks also to Robert A. De Lorenzo, MD, FACEP; Major, Medical Corps, US Army; Associate Clinical Professor of Military and Emergency Medicine; Uniformed Services University of the Health Sciences. Dr. De Lorenzo's reviews were carefully prepared, and we appreciate the thoughtful advice and keen insight he shared with us.

INSTRUCTOR REVIEWERS

The reviewers of *Paramedic Care: Principles & Practice* have provided many excellent suggestions and ideas for improving the text. The quality of the reviews has been outstanding, and the reviews have been a major aid in the preparation and revision of the manuscript. The assistance provided by these EMS experts is deeply appreciated.

Mike Coakley
EMS Director
Alabama Fire College
Program in Emergency Medicine
Tuscaloosa, AL

Janice Dorcy, RN, BS
EMS Coordinator, Education
Christ Hospital and Medical Center
Oaklawn, IL

Darren K. Ellenburg, B.S., EMT-P
Assistant Professor, Paramedic
   Education
Northeast State Technical Community
   College
Blountville, TN

Joseph P. Funk, MD, FACEP
Emory University
Department of Emergency
   Medicine
Atlanta, GA

Mary Gillespie, RN, EMT-P, I/C
Allied Health Division Chair
Davenport College
Grand Rapids, MI

Blaine Griffiths, BSAS, RN, NREMT-P
Youngstown State University
Paramedic Program
Youngstown, OH

J. Scott Hartley, NREMT-P, EMS-I
A.L.S. Affiliates
Omaha, NE

Larry Impson, AS, NREMT-P
Dean of Prehospital Education
METS. Inc.
Lodi, CA

Kevin McCoy, CCEMT-P
EMS Administrator/Paramedic
    Instructor
Cherokee Nation EMS
Tahlequah, OK

Robert G. Nixon, BA, EMT-P
Lifecare Medical Training
Walnut Creek, CA

Robert C. Rajsky, MSEd, NREMT-P
Manager of the Department of EMS
    Education
Chair-Southern Tier Regional EMS
    Council
Education Supervisor Erway
    Ambulance
President-Southern Tier ALS

Andria Savary, RN, MSN, ANP, EMT-P
Assistant Director
Institute for Emergency Medical
    Services
Northeastern University
Boston, MA
Andrew Stern, NREMT-P, MPA, MA
Senior Medic/Flightmedic
Town of Colonie Emergency Medical
    Services
Colonie, NY

Dave Tauber, NREMT-P I/C
Executive Director Advanced Life
    Support Institute
Paramedic/Firefighter
Conway, NH

Timothy Walsh, RN, ANP, NREMT-P
Assistant Professor
Community College of Rhode Island
Lincoln, RI

Steve Weinman, RN, BSN, CEN
Emergency Department Instructor
New York Hospital—Cornell Medical
    Center
New York, NY

Gail Weinstein
Paramedic Instructor
SUNY Health Science Center
Department of Emergency Medicine
Syracuse, NY

Paul A. Werfel, NREMT-P
Director Paramedic Program SUNY
Stony Brook, NY

About the Authors

BRYAN E. BLEDSOE, D.O., F.A.C.E.P., F.A.A.E.M., F.A.E.P., EMT-P

Dr. Bryan Bledsoe is an emergency physician with special interest in prehospital care. He received his B.S. degree from the University of Texas at Arlington and received his medical degree from the University of North Texas Health Sciences Center / Texas College of Osteopathic Medicine. He completed his internship at Texas Tech University and residency training at Scott and White Memorial Hospital / Texas A&M College of Medicine. Dr. Bledsoe is board-certified in emergency medicine and family practice. He is presently a Ph.D. candidate at Charles Sturt University at Wagga Wagga, New South Wales, Australia.

Prior to attending medical school, Dr. Bledsoe worked as an EMT, paramedic, and paramedic instructor. He completed EMT training in 1974 and paramedic training in 1976, and worked for 6 years as a field paramedic in Fort Worth, Texas. In 1979, he joined the faculty of the University of North Texas Health Sciences Center and served as coordinator of EMT and paramedic education programs at the university. Dr. Bledsoe is active in emergency medicine and serves as medical director for several EMS agencies and educational programs.

Dr. Bledsoe has authored several EMS books published by Brady including *Paramedic Emergency Care, Intermediate Emergency Care, Atlas of Paramedic Skills, Prehospital Emergency Pharmacology,* and *Pocket Reference for EMTs and Paramedics.* He is married to Emma Bledsoe. They have two children, Bryan and Andrea, and live in Midlothian, Texas, a suburb of Dallas. He enjoys saltwater fishing and listening to Jimmy Buffett.

ROBERT S. PORTER, M.A., NREMT-P

Robert Porter has been teaching in Emergency Medical Services for 25 years and currently serves as the Senior Advanced Life Support Educator for Madison County, New York, and as a Flight Paramedic with the Onondaga County Sheriff's Department helicopter service, AirOne. Mr. Porter is a Wisconsin native and received his Bachelor's degree in education from the University of Wisconsin. He completed his Paramedic training at Northeast Wisconsin Technical Institute in 1978 and earned a Master's Degree in Health Education at Central Michigan University in 1990.

Mr. Porter has been an EMT and EMS educator and administrator since 1973 and obtained his National Registration as an EMT-Paramedic in 1978. He has taught both basic and advanced level EMS courses in the states of Wisconsin, Michigan, Louisiana, Pennsylvania, and New York. Mr. Porter served for more than ten years as a paramedic program accreditation-site evaluator for the American Medical Association and is a past chair of the National Society of EMT Instructor/Coordinators. He has published numerous articles in EMS periodicals and has authored Brady's *Paramedic Emergency Care, Intermediate Emergency Care, Tactical Emergency Care,* and *Weapons of Mass Destruction: Emergency Care* as well as the workbooks accompanying this text, *Paramedic Emergency Care,* and *Intermediate Emergency Care.* When not writing or teaching, Mr. Porter enjoys offshore sailboat racing, historic home restoration, and listening to Dr. Bryan Bledsoe complain about the Texas heat.

RICHARD A. CHERRY, M.S., NREMT-P

Richard Cherry is Clinical Assistant Professor of Emergency Medicine and Director of Paramedic Training at SUNY Upstate Medical University in Syracuse, NY. His experience includes years of classroom teaching and emergency field work. A native of Buffalo, Mr. Cherry earned his Bachelor's degree and teaching certificate at nearby St. Bonaventure University in 1972. He taught high school for the next 10 years while he earned his Master's degree in Education from Oswego State University in 1977. He holds a permanent teaching license in New York State.

Mr. Cherry entered the emergency medical services field in 1974 with the De-Witt Volunteer Fire Department where he served his community as a firefighter and EMS provider for over 15 years. He took his first EMT course in 1977 and became an ALS provider two years later. He earned his paramedic certificate in 1985 as a member of the area's first paramedic class. He still answers emergency calls for Brewerton Ambulance.

Mr. Cherry has authored several books for Brady. Most notable is *EMT Teaching: A Common Sense Approach*. He has made presentations at many state, national, and international EMS conferences on a variety of teaching topics. In addition to his paramedic teaching, he is course director, instructor, and instructor trainer for ACLS, PALS, and PHTLS courses conducted for physicians, residents, nurses, medical students, and other house staff. He lives in Parish, New York with his wife Sue, a paramedic with Rural-Metro Medical Services, their children, and many pets.

Notices

It is the intent of the authors and publishers that this textbook be used as part of a formal paramedic education program taught by a qualified instructor and supervised by a licensed physician. The care procedures presented here represent accepted practices in the United States. They are not offered as a standard of care. Paramedic-level emergency care is to be performed only under the authority and guidance of a licensed physician. It is the reader's responsibility to know and follow local care protocols as provided by medical advisors directing the system to which he or she belongs. Also, it is the reader's responsibility to stay informed of emergency care procedure changes.

NOTICE ON DRUGS AND DRUG DOSAGES

Every effort has been made to ensure that the drug dosages presented in this textbook are in accordance with nationally accepted standards. When applicable, the dosages and routes are taken from the American Heart Association's Advanced Cardiac Life Support Guidelines. The American Medical Association's publication *Drug Evaluations,* the *Physician's Desk Reference,* and the Appleton & Lange *Health Professionals Drug Guide 2000* are followed with regard to drug dosages not covered by the American Heart Association's guidelines. It is the responsibility of the reader to be familiar with the drugs used in his or her system, as well as the dosages specified by the medical director. The drugs presented in this book should only be administered by direct order, whether verbally or through accepted standing orders, of a licensed physician.

NOTICE ON GENDER USAGE

The English language has historically given preference to the male gender. Among many words, the pronouns "he" and "his" are commonly used to describe both genders. Society evolves faster than language and the male pronouns still predominate in our speech. The authors have made great effort to treat the two genders equally, recognizing that a significant percentage of paramedics and patients are female. However, in some instances, male pronouns may be used to describe both male and female paramedics and patients solely for the purpose of brevity. This is not intended to offend any readers of the female gender.

NOTICE ON PHOTOGRAPHS

Please note that many of the photographs contained in this book are taken of actual emergency situations. As such, it is possible that they may not accurately depict current, appropriate, or advisable practices of emergency medical care. They have been included for the sole purpose of giving general insight into real-life emergency settings.

NOTICE ON CASE STUDIES

The names used and situations depicted in the case studies throughout this program are fictitious.

Prehospital emergency personnel, like all health care workers, are at risk for exposure to bloodborne pathogens and infectious diseases. In emergency situations it is often difficult to take or enforce proper infection control measures. However, as a paramedic, you must recognize your high-risk status. Study the following information on infection control before turning to the main portion of this book.

Infection control is designed to protect emergency personnel, their families, and their patients from unnecessary exposure to communicable diseases.

Laws, regulations, and standards regarding infection control include:

* *Centers for Disease Control (CDC) Guidelines.* The CDC has published extensive guidelines regarding infection control. Proper equipment and techniques that should be used by emergency response personnel to prevent or minimize risk of exposure are defined.

* *The Ryan White Act.* The Ryan White Act of 1990 allows emergency personnel to find out if they were exposed to an infectious disease while rendering patient care. Employers are required to name a "designated officer" to coordinate communications with the treating hospital.

* *Americans with Disabilities Act.* This act prohibits discrimination against individuals with disabilities including those with contagious diseases. It guarantees equal employment opportunities and job protection if the infected individual can perform essential job functions and does not pose a threat to the safety and health of patients and coworkers.

* *Occupational Safety and Health Administration (OSHA) Regulations.* OSHA recently enacted a regulation entitled Occupational Exposure to Bloodborne Pathogens that classifies emergency response personnel as being at the greatest risk of occupational exposure to communicable diseases. This regulation requires employers to provide hepatitis B (HBV) vaccinations free of charge, maintain a written exposure control plan, and provide personal protective equipment (PPE). These requirements primarily apply to private employers. Applicability to local and state governmental employees varies by locality. Many states have developed their own OSHA plans.

* *National Fire Protection Association (NFPA) Guidelines.* This is a national organization that has established specific guidelines and requirements regarding infection control for emergency response agencies, particularly fire departments and EMS services.

BODY SUBSTANCE ISOLATION PRECAUTIONS AND PERSONAL PROTECTIVE EQUIPMENT

Emergency response personnel should practice *Body Substance Isolation (BSI)*, a strategy that considers ALL body substances potentially infectious. To achieve this, all emergency personnel should utilize *Personal Protective Equipment (PPE)*.

Appropriate PPE should be available on every emergency vehicle. The minimum recommended PPE includes the following:

* *Gloves.* Disposable gloves should be donned by all emergency response personnel BEFORE initiating any emergency care. When an emergency incident involves more than one patient, you should attempt to change gloves between patients. When gloves have been contaminated, they should be removed as soon as possible. To remove gloves, first hook the gloved fingers of one hand under the cuff of the other glove. Then pull that glove off without letting your gloved fingers come in contact with bare skin. Then slide the fingers of the ungloved hand under the remaining glove's cuff. Push that glove off, being careful not to touch the glove's exterior with your bare hand. Always wash hands after gloves are removed, even when the gloves appear intact.

* *Masks and Protective Eyewear.* Masks and protective equipment should be present on all emergency vehicles and used in accordance with the level of exposure encountered. Proper eyewear and masks prevent a patient's blood and body fluids from spraying into your eyes, nose, and mouth. Masks and protective eyewear should be worn together whenever blood spatter is likely to occur, such as arterial bleeding, childbirth, endotracheal intubation, invasive procedures, oral suctioning, and clean-up of equipment that requires heavy scrubbing or brushing. Both you and the patient should wear masks whenever the potential for airborne transmission of disease exists.

* *HEPA Respirators.* Due to the resurgence of tuberculosis (TB), prehospital personnel should protect themselves from TB infection through use of a high-efficiency particulate air (HEPA) respirator, a design approved by the National Institute of Occupational Safety and Health (NIOSH). It should fit snugly and be capable of filtering out the tuberculosis bacillus. The HEPA respirator should be worn when caring for patients with confirmed or suspected TB. This is especially true when performing "high hazard" procedures such as administration of nebulized medications, endotracheal intubation, or suctioning on such a patient.

* *Gowns.* Gowns protect clothing from blood splashes. If large splashes of blood are expected, such as with childbirth, wear impervious gowns.

* *Resuscitation Equipment.* Disposable resuscitation equipment should be the primary means of artificial ventilation in emergency care. Such items should be used once, then disposed of.

Remember, the proper use of personal protective equipment ensures effective infection control and minimizes risk. Use ALL protective equipment recommended for any particular situation to ensure maximum protection.

Consider ALL body substances potentially infectious and ALWAYS practice body substance isolation.

HANDLING CONTAMINATED MATERIAL

Many of the materials associated with the emergency response become contaminated with possibly infectious body fluids and substances. These include soiled linen, patient clothing, and dressings, and used care equipment, including intravenous needles. It is important that you collect these materials at the scene and dispose of them appropriately to assure your safety as well as that of your patients, their family members, bystanders, and fellow care-givers. Properly dispose of any contaminated materials according to the recommendations outlined below.

* Handle contaminated materials only while wearing the appropriate personal protective equipment.

* Place all blood- or body-fluid-contaminated clothing, linen, dressings and patient care equipment and supplies in properly marked biological hazard bags and assure they are disposed of properly.
* Assure all used needles, scalpels and other contaminated objects that have the potential to puncture the skin are properly secured in a puncture-resistant and clearly-marked sharps container.
* Do not recap a needle after use, stick it into a seat cushion or other object, or leave it lying on the ground. This increases the risk of an accidental needle stick.
* Always scan the scene before leaving to assure all equipment has been retrieved and all potentially infectious material has been bagged and removed.
* Should you be exposed to an infectious disease, have contact with body substances with a route for system entry (such as an open wound on your hand when a glove tears while moving a soiled patient), or receive a needle stick with a used needle, alert the receiving hospital and contact your service's infection control officer immediately.

Following these recommendations will help protect you and the people you care for from the dangers of disease transmission.

Welcome to Paramedic Care

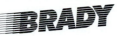

ONE LAKE STREET
UPPER SADDLE RIVER, NJ 07458

Dear Paramedic Instructor,

Brady, Your Partner in Education, is pleased to present *Paramedic Care: Principles & Practice*—a comprehensive series developed specifically to meet the new U.S. DOT National Standard Curriculum for EMT-Paramedics.

We recognize that for many of you the new curriculum represents a dramatic change in the way your paramedic course will be taught. *Paramedic Care: Principles & Practice* was developed specifically to help both you and your students succeed. Written in a student-friendly, easy-to-understand style, our new series consists of five volumes:

- Volume 1: *Introduction to Advanced Prehospital Care*
- Volume 2: *Patient Assessment*
- Volume 3: *Medical Emergencies*
- Volume 4: *Trauma Emergencies*
- Volume 5: *Special Considerations/Operations*.

The texts in this series are designed to work in tandem to cover all the objectives in the eight modules of the new U.S. DOT curriculum. However, each volume may also be used individually to help you tailor your course to state and local protocols.

Our high-quality instructor materials provide everything you need to help get your new curriculum course up and running. The Instructor's Resource Manual will contain lecture outlines and lesson plans that cover the new curriculum, along with student handouts and suggestions for class activities.

The *Paramedic Care* series also offers the latest multimedia technology to enhance and enrich your students' classroom experiences and to help you manage your classes more efficiently. The series' accompanying Companion Website contains chapter-by-chapter interactive student quizzes and links to related EMS sites for students. The Companion Website also offers downloadable instructor resources, teaching tips, links to curriculum-related websites, and an online syllabus builder. Our partnership with Victory Technology brings you *MedMedic*, an interactive CD-ROM tied chapter by chapter to each of the books. These new CDs include video, interactive student quizzes, and animations.

We wish you the best of luck as you transition to the new paramedic curriculum.

Sincerely,

Julie Levin Alexander
Vice President and Publisher

BRADY
Your Partner in Education

EMPHASIZING PRINCIPLES

Chapter Objectives with Page References

Each chapter begins with clearly stated **Objectives** that follow the new DOT Paramedic curriculum. Students can refer to these objectives while studying to make sure they understand the material fully. Page references after each objective indicate where relevant content is covered in the chapter.

Content Review

Content Review summarizes important content and gives students a format for quick review.

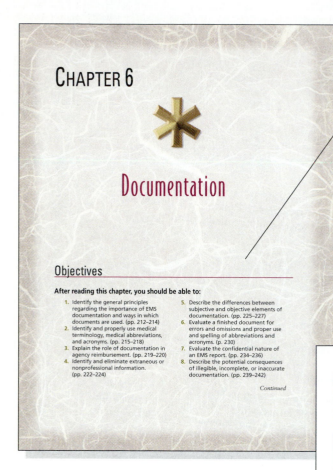

CHAPTER 6

Documentation

Objectives

After reading this chapter, you should be able to:

1. Identify the general principles regarding the importance of EMS documentation and ways in which documents are used. (pp. 212–214)
2. Identify and properly use medical terminology, medical abbreviations, and acronyms. (pp. 215–218)
3. Explain the role of documentation in agency reimbursement. (pp. 219–220)
4. Identify and eliminate extraneous or nonprofessional information. (pp. 222–224)
5. Describe the differences between subjective and objective elements of documentation. (pp. 225–227)
6. Evaluate a finished document for errors and omissions and proper use and spelling of abbreviations and acronyms. (p. 230)
7. Evaluate the confidential nature of an EMS report. (pp. 234–236)
8. Describe the potential consequences of illegible, incomplete, or inaccurate documentation. (pp. 239–242)

Continued

Content Review

FACILITATING BEHAVIORS
- Stay calm
- Plan for the worst
- Work systematically
- Remain adaptable

Be like the duck—cool and calm on the water's surface, while paddling feverishly underneath.

Except for safety concerns, never allow anything to distract you from your most important job—assessing and caring for your patient.

✱ reflective acting thoughtfully, deliberately, and analytically.

✱ impulsive acting instinctively without stopping to think.

✱ divergent taking into account all aspects of a complex situation.

USEFUL THINKING STYLES

As a paramedic, you will face confusing emergencies that would challenge even the most knowledgeable, analytical care provider. You must be able to stay calm and not panic. Your self-control in the face of extreme chaos will set the example for other team members to follow. Even when you are struggling to maintain your composure—especially then—never let others know. The key is focusing on the task and blocking out the distractions. Be like the duck—cool and calm on the water's surface, while paddling feverishly underneath.

Assume and plan for the worst, and always err on the side of benefiting your patient. For example, if you are deliberating whether to immobilize your patient, initiate advanced life support procedures, or administer oxygen, just do it! It is better to err by providing care than by withholding it. Be pessimistic! Anticipate all potential bad side effects of your treatments and prepare "plan B." For example, as you deliver a bronchodilating drug to your severe asthmatic patient, anticipate that it will not work and mentally prepare to intubate him and perform positive pressure ventilation. Or while you are administering atropine to your patient with symptomatic bradycardia, plan ahead for external cardiac pacing and dopamine, if atropine therapy fails to restore adequate circulation.

Establish and maintain a systematic assessment pattern. Practice your assessments until they become second nature, and you will avoid skipping and missing steps. Be disciplined and stay focused, especially when you are confronted with a complex emergency scene. For example, your patient lies moaning on the ground in a pool of blood. Bystanders are screaming at you to help him; others are trying to tell you what happened. The police are gathering the story and trying unsuccessfully to talk with your patient. You must gain control of this scene. You do so by focusing on your patient and performing a systematic assessment. Use common acronyms (MS-ABC, OPQRST, SAMPLE) or make up your own to help you remember the key elements of your assessment. Except for safety concerns, never allow anything to distract you from your most important job—assessing and caring for your patient.

The different situations you encounter will require a variety of management styles. Adapting your styles of situation analysis (reflective vs. impulsive), data processing (convergent vs. divergent), and decision making (anticipatory vs. reactive) to each situation will enable you to provide the best possible care in every case.

Reflective vs. Impulsive Some situations call for you to be **reflective**, take your time, and figure out what is wrong with your patient. You have a patient who complains of "not feeling well." She has a long history of cardiac, renal, respiratory, and diabetic problems. Since she is in no real distress and is hemodynamically stable, you can take your time to determine her primary problem. Other situations call for immediate action. They require you to make an instinctive, **impulsive** decision and manage your patient's life-threatening condition. For example, if your patient presents apneic and pulseless, you will immediately begin CPR and prepare for rapid defibrillation. If he presents with a spurting artery, you will at once take measures to control the hemorrhage. If he is choking and has a weak, ineffective cough, you will quickly perform the Heimlich maneuver. You have to think fast in these situations.

Divergent vs. Convergent To process the data you receive from your patient and the scene, you can use either a divergent approach or a convergent approach. The **divergent** approach considers all aspects of a situation before arriving at a solution. It is insightful and works well when you are confronted with complex

4 CHAPTER 1 *The History*

Key Points

Key Points in the margins help students identify and learn the fundamental principles of paramedic practice.

Key Terms

Reinforcement of **Key Terms** helps students master new terminology.

communicating with other
emergency care professionals.

...story ha... ...own t... ...adio
...e 5-1). These wo... ...horten air time and transmit thoughts and
ideas quickly. For exampl... Copy, 10-4, and roger mean "I heard you and I understand what you said." Using industry terminology appropriately is an important part of effective communication. It provides a common means of communicating with other emergency care professionals.

Table 5-1	COMMON RADIO TERMINOLOGY
Term	**Meaning**
Copy, 10-4, roger	I understand
Affirmative	Yes
Negative	No
Stand by	Please wait
Repeat	Please repeat what you said
Land-line	Telephone communications
Rendezvous	Meet with
LZ	Landing zone (helicopter)
ETA	Estimated time of arrival
Over	I am finished with my transmission
Mobile status	On the air, driving around
Stage	Wait before entering a scene
Clear	End of transmission
Unfounded	We cannot find the incident/patient
Be advised	Listen carefully to this

Tables and Illustrations

Tables and **illustrations** offer visual support to enhance students' understanding of paramedic principles and practice.

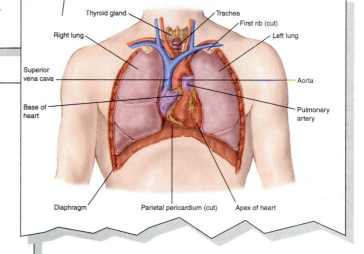

Thyroid gland
Trachea
First rib (cut)
Right lung
Left lung
Superior vena cava
Aorta
Base of heart
Pulmonary artery
Diaphragm
Parietal pericardium (cut)
Apex of heart

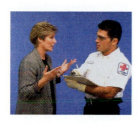

FIGURE 1-3 If the patient cannot provide useful information, gather it from family members or bystanders.

BLINDNESS

Blind patients present special problems. They need you to identify yourself immediately, since they cannot see your uniform. Always announce yourself and explain
who you are and why you are there. If possible, take your patient's hand to establish a personal contact and to show him where you are. Remember that nonverbal
communication such as hand gestures, facial expressions, and body language, are
useless in these cases. Your voice is your only tool for effective communication.

TALKING WITH FAMILIES OR FRIENDS

You will often encounter patients who cannot give you any useful information. In
these cases, find a third party who can augment the patient history and offer a useful adjunct to the patient's answers (Figure 1-3). The typical case is the postictal
patient who cannot describe his seizure activity to you. Another example is learning from his friend that your patient's wife died in an automobile accident just three
weeks ago. Now you better understand why your patient appears depressed and
suicidal. Make sure that patient confidentiality is a priority when you accept personal information from a family member, friend, or bystander.

SUMMARY

This chapter dealt with taking a good history. While it presented the patient
history in its entirety, common sense will determine which parts are appropriate for a given situation. Most of a paramedic's work is patient contact. It
is making a connection with people in crisis. Patients most often comment on
the attitudes of their paramedics. How well did they relate to them? Did they
make them feel at ease? Did they care for them? Patients rarely comment on
a paramedic's technical skills. Top-notch paramedics are technically skillful
and treat all their patients with dignity and compassion. This begins with the
history.

Good patient interaction can lead to good patient outcomes, improved patient satisfaction, and better adherence to treatment. As a paramedic you have

Summar...

End-of-Chapter Summary

Each end-of-chapter **Summary** reviews the main topics covered.

c) Past Hi...
c) Current He...
d) Review of Systems

FURTHER READING

Bates, Barbara, Lynn S. Bickley, and Robert A. Hoekelman. *A Guide to Physical Examination and History Taking.* 6th ed. Philadelphia: J.B. Lippincott, 1995.
Coulehan, John L. and Marian R. Block. *The Medical Interview: Mastering Skills for Clinical Practice.* 3rd ed. Philadelphia: F.A. Davis, 1997.
Epstein, Owen, et al. *Clinical Examination.* St. Louis: Mosby, 1997.
Lipkin, Mack Jr., Samuel M. Putnam, and Aaron Lazare. *The Medical Interview: Clinical Care, Education, and Research.* New York: Springer, 1994.
Seidel Henry M. *Mosby's Guide to Physical Examination.* 3rd ed. St. Louis: Mosby, 1994.
Willms, Janice L., Henry Schniederman, and Paula S. Algranati. *Physical Diag-nosis: Bedside Evaluation of Diagnosis and Function.* Baltimore: Williams & Wilkins, 1994.

ON THE WEB

Visit Brady's Paramedic Website through www.brady books.com/paramedic.

Further Reading and On the Web

Each chapter ends with recommendations for books and journal articles. Links to relevant websites plus a link to the text's Companion Website can be found at **www.bradybooks.com/paramedic.**

EMPHASIZING PRACTICE

Case Study

Case Studies draw students into the reading and create a link between text content and real-life situations and experiences.

Objectives Continued

8. Identify and differentiate among the following communications systems:
   - Simplex (pp. 101–102)
   - Multiplex (pp. 102–103)
   - Duplex (p. 104)
   - Trunked (pp. 104–106)
   - Digital communications (pp. 110–113)
   - Cellular telephone (p. 114)
   - Facsimile (pp. 114–115)
   - Computer (pp. 116–118)
9. Describe the functions and responsibilities of the Federal Communications Commission. (pp. 120–122)
10. Describe the role of emergency medical dispatch and the importance of prearrival instructions in a typical EMS response. (pp. 122–124)
11. List appropriate caller information gathered by the emergency medical dispatcher. (pp. 124–125)
12. Describe the structure and importance of verbal patient information communication to the hospital and medical direction. (pp. 128–131)
13. Diagram a basic communications system. (pp. 130–133)
14. Given several narrative patient scenarios, organize a verbal radio report for electronic transmission to medical direction. (pp. 138–142)

CASE STUDY

On a dry, warm Sunday afternoon, a 31-year-old male loses control of his motorcycle and strikes a highway sign. Several people witness the incident. The first bystander to reach the patient rushes to his automobile to dial 911 on his cellular telephone. Emergency medical dispatcher Vern Holland takes the necessary information and dispatches a basic life support engine company and an advanced life support ambulance. As Holland dispatches the emergency units, his partner, paramedic dispatcher Fred Hughes, instructs the caller in basic emergency care. The units receive the call via a computer printout of essential information.

They quickly arrive at the scene and initiate the appropriate care. Because the patient has a severe head injury, the paramedic performs only a limited assessment and immediately initiates transport. As the ambulance departs, he relays the following to Dr. Doyle, the medical direction physician:

Paramedic: Depew Ambulance to Mercy Hospital.

Dr. Doyle: Go ahead, Depew.

Paramedic: We are leaving the scene of a motorcycle accident on I-90. We have one patient, a male who is in his 30s, the rider of a motorcycle that went off the roadway and struck a sign. He responds to pain only, with obvious facial and chest

Documentation

Covered thoroughly throughout the text, **proper documentation techniques** are critical to ensuring provider protection on the job as well as patient safety during the transition of care.

of injury may also help rehabilitation provide better therapy. Your PCR becomes an important document that helps ensure your patient's continuous effective care.

Prehospital Care Report

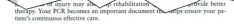

FIGURE 6-1 The run data in a prehospital care report is vital to your agency's efforts to improve patient care.

Uses for Documentation 12

You Make the Call

Promoting critical thinking skills, each **You Make the Call** presents a hypothetical situation that requires students to apply principles to actual practice. Suggested responses are found at the back of the text.

YOU MAKE THE CALL

A call comes into your unit for a "possible heart attack" on State Route 11. You and your partner climb into Palermo Rescue, a nontransport first-response vehicle. Your response time is about ten minutes. Upon arrival, a family member meets you. He leads you into the den of a small farm house. Here you see your patient sitting in an overstuffed chair. You note that your patient is a 69-year-old male in obvious distress.

You begin questioning your patient to develop a history. As he speaks, you immediately notice that he has difficulty breathing. He complains of severe chest pain, which began about 30 minutes ago. With his hand, he indicates that the pain is pressure-like and substernal. He also indicates that it radiates to his left arm and jaw. He describes a history of heart disease, including two prior heart attacks. Three years ago, he had cardiac bypass surgery. He currently takes Lanoxin, Lasix, Capoten, and an aspirin a day. He is allergic to Mellaril.

You and your partner complete your assessment. Your patient says he weighs about 250 pounds. He is alert, but anxious. He exhibits jugular venous distention and bibasilar crackles. His abdomen is nontender. His distal pulses are good. Vital signs include: blood pressure 210/110 mmHg, pulse of 70 per minute and regular, and respirations of 20 breaths per minute and mildly labored. Pulse oximetry is 93% on supplemental oxygen. During your assessment, your patient becomes progressively more dyspneic. The transporting ambulance arrives and the paramedic asks you to give a radio report to the receiving hospital based on your assessment while she prepares her patient for transport.

- Based on the information above, organize and prepare your radio report to inform the receiving hospital of your patient's condition.

See Suggested Responses at the back of this book.

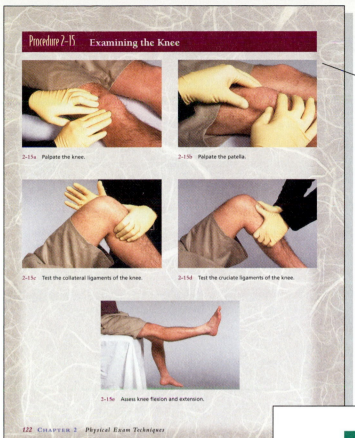

Procedure 2-15   Examining the Knee

2-15a Palpate the knee.

2-15b Palpate the patella.

2-15c Test the collateral ligaments of the knee.

2-15d Test the cruciate ligaments of the knee.

2-15e Assess knee flexion and extension.

Procedure Scans

Newly photographed **Procedure Scans** provide step-by-step visual support on how to perform skills included in the DOT curriculum.

Patient Care Algorithms

Clearly presented **algorithms** provide graphic "pathways" that integrate assessment and care for medical or trauma emergencies. These visual summaries give students a step-by-step flow of assessment and emergency care procedures.

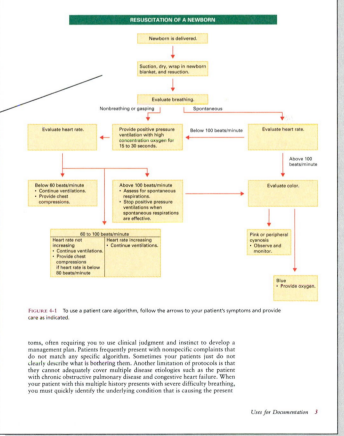

FIGURE 4-1 To use a patient care algorithm, follow the arrows to your patient's symptoms and provide care as indicated.

toms, often requiring you to use clinical judgment and instinct to develop a management plan. Patients frequently present with nonspecific complaints that do not match any specific algorithm. Sometimes your patients just do not clearly describe what is bothering them. Another limitation of protocols is that they cannot adequately cover multiple disease etiologies such as the patient with chronic obstructive pulmonary disease and congestive heart failure. When your patient with this multiple history presents with severe difficulty breathing, you must quickly identify the underlying condition that is causing the present

Uses for Documentation 3

TEACHING & LEARNING PACKAGE

FOR THE INSTRUCTOR

Instructor's Resource Manual

The Instructor's Resource Manual for each volume contains everything needed to teach the 1998 U.S. DOT National Standard Curriculum for Paramedics. It fully covers the DOT curriculum with:

- time estimates for various topics
- listing of additional resources
- lecture outlines
- student activities handouts
- answers to student review questions
- case study discussion questions.

The manual is also available on disk so instructors can customize resources to their individual needs.

PowerPoint® Presentations on CD-ROM

This CD-ROM offers PowerPoint® presentations that contain word slides and images organized by chapter. The entire presentation is fully customizable.

Computerized Test Bank

The Computerized Test Bank contains textbook-based questions in a format that enables instructors to select questions based on topic area and degree of difficulty.

FOR THE STUDENT

Student Workbook

A student workbook with review and practice activities accompanies each volume of the *Paramedic Care* series. The workbooks include multiple-choice questions, fill-in-the-blank questions, labeling exercises, case studies, and special projects, along with an answer key with text page references.

ONLINE RESOURCES

Paramedic Care Companion Website: www.bradybooks.com/paramedic

This free site, tied chapter-by-chapter to the five texts, reinforces student learning through interactive online study guides, quizzes based on the new curriculum, and case studies, as well as links to important EMS-related Internet resources. The *Paramedic Care* Companion Website also includes instructor resources, such as a bridge guide to help instructors transition to the new curriculum, links to EMS-related sites (including a site to download the new curriculum), and teaching tips. Instructors can also use the site to create a customized syllabus.

EMS Supersite: www.bradybooks.com/ems

Brady's EMS Supersite is a free, one-stop Web resource for both students and instructors offering:

- Online Brady catalog
- Links to all Brady Companion Websites
- Interactive case studies
- Case Study of the Month
- Useful EMS-related links
- Games, puzzles, and activities
- Test-taking tips
- Test writing and teaching tips
- Sample chapters and multimedia demos.

**For information on additional media to support the series, please contact your Brady representative:
1-800-638-0220**

OTHER TITLES OF INTEREST

ANATOMY & PHYSIOLOGY

GUY, Learning Human Anatomy, Second Edition (0-8385-5657-4)

Organized by body regions, this popular text helps students learn human anatomy. Its outline format and easy-to-remember illustrations make it ideal for review and a perfect introductory gross anatomy text.

MARTINI et al., Essentials of Anatomy and Physiology, Second Edition (0-13-082192-6)

A one-semester/one-quarter anatomy and physiology text for students in allied health, physical education, and other programs requiring an overview of the human body's systems. An extensive instructor support package is available.

CARDIAC/EKG

BEASLEY, Understanding EKGs (0-8359-8571-7)

This text is a direct, basic approach to EKG interpretation that presents all the essential concepts for mastering the basics of this challenging field, while assuming no prior knowledge of EKGs.

BEASLEY, Understanding 12-Lead EKGs (0-13-027281-7)

This comprehensive, reader-friendly text teaches beginning students basic 12-lead EKG interpretation.

MISTOVICH et al., Advanced Cardiac Life Support (0-8359-5050-6)

Straightforward and easy to follow, this text offers clear explanations, a colorful design, and covers all of the core concepts covered in an advanced cardiac life support course.

PAGE, 12-Lead ECG for the Acute Care Provider (0-13-022460-X)

This full-color text presents EKG interpretation in a practical, easy-to-understand and user-friendly manner. Practice cases are included throughout the text.

For a complete listing of additional Brady titles, visit us on the Web: www.bradybooks.com

WALRAVEN, Basic Arrhythmias, Fifth Edition (0-8359-5305-X)

This classic bestseller covers all the basics of EKG and includes appendices on Clinical Implications of Arrhythmias, Cardiac Anatomy & Physiology, 12-Lead EKG, Basic 12-Lead Interpretation and Pacemakers.

MATHEMATICS

BENJAMIN-CHUNG, Math Principles and Practice: Preparing for Health Career Success (0-8359-5272-X)

This easy-to-follow text provides basic math skills for students or practicing health care professionals. It employs a common sense approach that builds on basic math skills to facilitate the understanding of more complex math calculations.

TIGER, Mathematical Concepts for Clinical Sciences (0-13-011549-5)

This book is geared for all entry-level clinical science curricula and presents material in a step-by-step approach that emphasizes the understanding of concepts, not the memorization of numbers and formulas.

MEDICAL

DALTON et al., Advanced Medical Life Support (0-8359-5179-0)

This groundbreaking text offers a practical approach to adult medical emergencies. Each chapter discusses realistic methods that a seasoned EMS practitioner would use.

MEDICAL TERMINOLOGY

FREMGEN, Medical Terminology: An Anatomy & Physiology Systems Approach (0-8359-4991-5)

In this full-color text-workbook, Bonnie F. Fremgen uses an integrated body systems approach and reader-friendly writing style to teach medical terminology.

LILLIS, A Concise Introduction to Medical Terminology (0-8385-4321-9)

A basic introduction to over 700 commonly used medical terms and word elements to help students learn the terminology they need to succeed.

(continued on next page)

OTHER TITLES OF INTEREST

MEDICAL TERMINOLOGY *(continued)*

RICE, Medical Terminology with Human Anatomy, Fourth Edition (0-8385-6274-4)

Providing comprehensive coverage of all aspects of medical terminology, the Fourth Edition of this popular text is arranged by body systems and specialty areas. Rice makes learning easy and interesting by presenting important prefixes, roots, and suffixes as they relate to each specialty or system.

RICE, The Terminology of Health and Medicine (0-8385-6260-4)

This self-study text presents learning concepts in numbered frames—with a series of statements on the right side of the page and the answers provided in a column on the outside. Terms are arranged by body system.

PATHOPHYSIOLOGY

BURNS, Pathophysiology (0-8385-8084-X)

Students will master the basics of general disease processes—as well as major diseases of the body system—by using the only pathophysiology text that offers a programmed approach with questions within each frame that test comprehension, and self-tests at the end of each section.

KENT/HART, Introduction to Human Disease, Fourth Edition (0-8385-4070-8)

This is the perfect text for any student seeking a reliable and concise overview of human disease. Each chapter contains most frequently encountered and serious problems, symptoms, signs and tests, specific diseases, and review questions.

MULVIHILL, Human Disease, Fourth Edition (0-8385-3928-9)

This popular book comprehensively covers mechanisms of disease and health problems, as well as commonly occurring diseases. Normal anatomy and physiology is reviewed at the beginning of each chapter.

For a complete listing of additional Brady titles, visit us on the Web: www.bradybooks.com

PEDIATRICS

EICHELBERGER, Pediatric Emergencies, Second Edition (0-8359-5123-5)

This text was developed to provide a standard of prehospital pediatric emergency care for both basic and advanced providers.

MARKENSON et al., Pediatric Prehospital Care (0-13-022618-1)

Written for all levels of EMS providers, this text presents a physiological approach to rapid and accurate pediatric assessment, identification of potential problems, establishing treatment priorities with effective on-going assessment, and rapid and safe transport.

PHARMACOLOGY

GRAJEDA-HIGLEY, Pharmacology (0-8385-8136-6)

This pharmacology handbook combines a systems approach with cartoon-type illustrations for a unique and user-friendly physiological presentation of pharmacological concepts.

MIKOLAJ, Drug Dosage Calculations (0-8359-4994-X)

This practical volume gives readers all the tools needed to solve virtually every type of dosage and calculation problem they will encounter in the workplace.

SHANNON, The Health Professional's Drug Guide 2000 (0-8385-0424-8)

This drug guide provides health care professionals with accurate, easily accessible information about their patients' medications. Comprehensive yet user-friendly, this handy resource includes important clinical implications for hundreds of drugs, including adverse reactions, interactions and side effects.

TRAUMA

CAMPBELL, Basic Trauma Life Support for Paramedics and Advanced Providers, Fourth Edition (0-13-084584-1)

Brady's best selling BTLS text provides a complete course that covers all the skills necessary for rapid assessment, resuscitation, stabilization and transportation of the trauma patient.

PARAMEDIC CARE: Principles & Practice

MEDICAL EMERGENCIES

CHAPTER 1

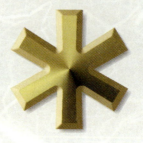

Pulmonology

Objectives

After reading this chapter, you should be able to:

1. Discuss the epidemiology of pulmonary diseases and pulmonary conditions. (p. 4)
2. Identify and describe the function of the structures located in the upper and lower airway. (pp. 5–11)
3. Discuss the physiology of ventilation and respiration. (pp. 11–18)
4. Identify common pathological events that affect the pulmonary system. (pp. 18–21)

5. Compare various airway and ventilation techniques used in the management of pulmonary diseases. (p. 36)
6. Review the use of equipment utilized during the physical examination of patients with complaints associated with respiratory diseases and conditions. (pp. 29–30, 32–34)
7. Identify the epidemiology, anatomy, physiology, pathophysiology, assess-

Continued

Objectives Continued

ment findings, and management (including prehospital medications) for the following respiratory diseases and conditions:

a. Adult respiratory distress syndrome (pp. 36-38)
b. Bronchial asthma (pp. 38–39, 43–48)
c. Chronic bronchitis (pp. 38–39, 41–43)
d. Emphysema (pp. 38-43)
e. Pneumonia (pp. 49–51)
f. Pulmonary edema (pp. 36–38)
g. Pulmonary thromboembolism (pp. 54–56)

h. Neoplasms of the lung (pp. 51–52)
i. Upper respiratory infections (pp. 48–49)
j. Spontaneous pneumothorax (pp. 56–57)
k. Hyperventilation syndrome (pp. 57–58)

8. Given several preprogrammed patients with non-traumatic pulmonary problems, provide the appropriate assessment, prehospital care, and transport. (pp. 4–59)

CASE STUDY

Paramedics Tony Alvarez and Lee Smith are just finishing their barbecue lunch when they are toned out for a "medical emergency." They quickly go to the ambulance for the rest of the dispatch information. The emergency communications center dispatches them to 423 Black Champ Road where a male patient is reportedly having difficulty breathing. The dispatcher also informs the crew that First Responders from the Maypearl Fire Department are already en route. The paramedics are familiar with this area. It is a rural part of the county with mainly cotton farms. The response time is approximately 12 minutes. Upon arrival at the farmhouse, the paramedics are met by Alice Swenson, a First Responder from the Maypearl Volunteer Fire Department. Alice reports they have a 55-year-old white male who is having difficulty breathing. She further states that oxygen is already being administered.

The paramedics grab the drug box, monitor/defibrillator, airway kit, and stretcher. They then enter the small farmhouse. A quick scene size-up reveals that there are no immediate dangers. Tony and Lee find the patient seated at the kitchen table, obviously short of breath. They quickly perform an initial assessment. The airway is clear, the patient is moving little air, and has a strong pulse. Tony replaces the nasal cannula placed by the First Responders with a

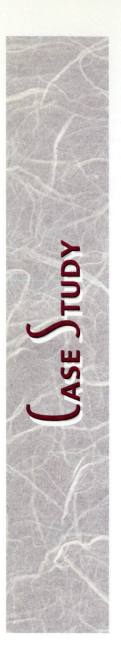

nonrebreather mask. Lee and Tony then complete a focused history and physical exam. The patient has diminished breath sounds, occasional rhonchi, and is using the accessory muscles of respiration. There is a hint of cyanosis around the mouth.

The team learns that, several years ago, doctors at the Veterans Administration (VA) Hospital diagnosed the patient as having emphysema. Over the last 24 hours, he has had progressive dyspnea and didn't sleep at all the previous night. His wife reports that he paced the floor and repeatedly opened and closed windows. Vital signs reveal a blood pressure of 140/78 mmHg, a pulse of 96 beats per minute, and a respiratory rate of 28 breaths per minute. The monitor shows a sinus rhythm. Pulse oximetry reveals an oxygen saturation of 90 percent while receiving supplemental oxygen. The patient is mentally alert but slightly anxious. His current medications include an albuterol (Ventolin) metered dose inhaler, theophylline (Slow-Bid), and amoxicillin (Amoxil). He still smokes a pack and a-half of cigarettes per day and has done so for 40 years accumulating a 60 pack/year history.

The patient wants to be transported to the VA Hospital. Lee contacts medical direction and provides a brief patient report. Medical direction approves transport to the VA Hospital, as it is only 5 miles farther than the nearest hospital. The transport time will be approximately 40 minutes. Medical direction orders the placement of an IV of 0.9% sodium chloride (normal saline) at a "to keep open" rate. In addition, they order a nebulizer treatment with 0.5 milliliters of albuterol (Ventolin) placed in 3 milliliters of normal saline. Because of the long transport time, medical direction also orders the administration of 125 milligrams of methylprednisolone (Solu-Medrol) by IV push.

Halfway through the nebulizer treatment, the patient shows marked improvement. His respiratory rate slows to 20 breaths per minute, and his oxygen saturation reading increases to 94 percent. Transport to the VA hospital is uneventful. He remains at the VA Hospital for two days and is discharged.

INTRODUCTION

The respiratory system is a vital body system responsible for providing oxygen to the tissues, at the same time removing the metabolic waste-product, carbon dioxide. Oxygen is required for the conversion of essential nutrients into energy and must be constantly available to all body tissues.

Respiratory emergencies are among the most common emergencies EMS personnel are called upon to treat. In fact, according to a U.S. study of over 2.5 million EMS calls, respiratory complaints accounted for 28 percent of all calls. Over 200,000 people die each year as the result of respiratory emergencies. As a paramedic, you must promptly recognize and treat respiratory problems appropriately in order to reduce mortality and morbidity.

Several risk factors increase the likelihood of developing respiratory disease. *Intrinsic risk factors* are those that are influenced by or are from within the patient. The most important intrinsic risk factor is genetic predisposition. The likelihood of developing respiratory disease, such as bronchial asthma, **chronic obstructive pulmonary disease (COPD)**, and lung carcinoma (cancer), is increased in patients who have family members with these diseases.

Certain respiratory conditions are increased in patients who have underlying cardiac or circulatory problems. For example, patients with cardiac conditions that result in ineffective pumping of blood are prone to the development of pulmonary edema. Also, both cardiac and circulatory disease may allow blood to pool in the large veins of the pelvis and lower extremities, leading to the development of pulmonary emboli. Both pulmonary edema and pulmonary emboli often present with a respiratory complaint as the primary complaint. Finally, the patient's level of stress may increase the severity of any respiratory complaint. Also remember that stress can actually precipitate acute episodes of asthma or COPD.

Extrinsic risk factors, those that are external to the patient, are also important in increasing the likelihood of developing respiratory disease. The most important of these is cigarette smoking. There is a strong link between cigarette smoking and the development of pulmonary diseases such as lung carcinoma and COPD. Additionally, diseases such as pneumonia and pulmonary emboli are more likely in patients who smoke. Finally, cigarette smoking has been implicated as a risk factor in the development of cardiac disease that may lead to the development of pulmonary edema. In any case, underlying lung damage caused by cigarette smoke causes virtually all lung disorders to be worse in smokers.

Another important extrinsic risk factor is environmental pollutants. Patients who live in highly industrialized areas, particularly where there is little movement of air, are at particular risk for respiratory problems. The prevalence of patients with COPD is markedly increased in areas with high environmental pollutants. The number and severity of acute attacks of both asthma and COPD are also worse under these conditions.

This chapter will help you to develop an understanding of the pathophysiology of respiratory disease, then to integrate this knowledge with your assessment findings to develop a field impression and manage the patient with respiratory problems. (Before continuing with this chapter, you may want to review Volume 1, Chapter 13 "Airway Management and Ventilation.")

REVIEW OF RESPIRATORY ANATOMY AND PHYSIOLOGY

As you may recall, the airway is divided anatomically into the upper airway and the lower airway (Figure 1-1).

UPPER AIRWAY ANATOMY

The upper airway (Figure 1-2) is responsible for warming and humidifying incoming air. It is also very effective in air purification. Each day, approximately 10,000 liters of air are filtered, warmed, humidified, and exchanged by the adult respiratory system.

Nasal Cavity

Air enters the upper airway through the nose. It initially passes through the external nares, or nostrils, and enters the nasal cavity. The nasal cavity is divided

The most important intrinsic factor in the development of respiratory disorders is genetic predisposition. The most important extrinsic factor is smoking.

* **chronic obstructive pulmonary disease (COPD)** a disease characterized by a decreased ability of the lungs to perform the function of ventilation.

Content Review

THE UPPER AIRWAY
Nasal cavity
Pharynx
Larynx

FIGURE 1-1 Overview of the upper and lower airways.

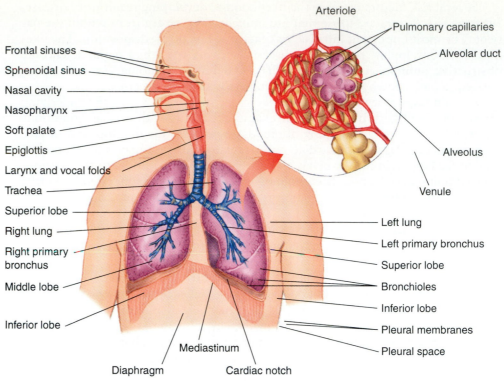

Arteriole
Pulmonary capillaries
Alveolar duct

Frontal sinuses
Sphenoidal sinus
Nasal cavity
Nasopharynx
Soft palate
Epiglottis
Larynx and vocal folds
Trachea
Superior lobe
Right lung
Right primary bronchus
Middle lobe

Inferior lobe

Alveolus

Venule

Left lung
Left primary bronchus
Superior lobe
Bronchioles
Inferior lobe
Pleural membranes
Pleural space

Diaphragm   Mediastinum   Cardiac notch

FIGURE 1-2 Anatomy of the upper airway.

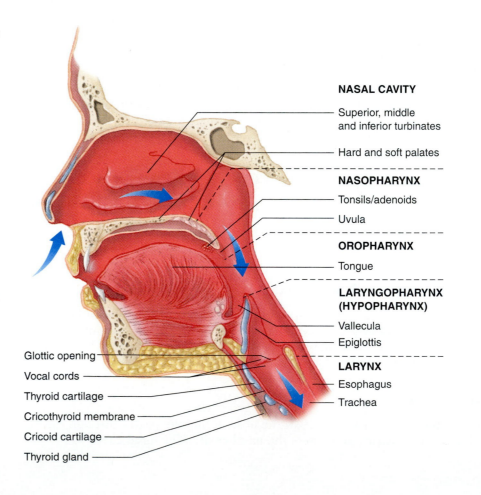

NASAL CAVITY

Superior, middle and inferior turbinates

Hard and soft palates

NASOPHARYNX

Tonsils/adenoids

Uvula

OROPHARYNX

Tongue

LARYNGOPHARYNX (HYPOPHARYNX)

Vallecula

Epiglottis

LARYNX

Glottic opening
Vocal cords
Thyroid cartilage
Cricothyroid membrane
Cricoid cartilage
Thyroid gland

Esophagus

Trachea

into two chambers (right and left) by the nasal septum. In the anterior portion of the nose, there are many hair follicles that help trap large dust particles. The lateral wall of the nasal cavity is marked by three bony prominences called the *turbinates*. Between each set of turbinates is a passageway, or *meatus,* that leads to the *paranasal sinuses* (Figure 1-3). The turbinates cause turbulence in the incoming air flow. This facilitates the entrapment and removal of any inhaled foreign particles, such as dust.

As air passes posteriorly, any small inhaled particles not filtered by the hair follicles are trapped by the thin layer of mucus that lines the nose. This mucus is constantly produced by goblet cells found in the mucous membrane. Some of the cells lining the respiratory tract have *cilia*. Cilia are thin, fingerlike projections that have the ability to contract in a single direction. In the nose, the cilia move in a manner that produces a steady posterior flow of mucus, at the same time removing any entrapped particles. Once the mucus and any entrapped particles reach the posterior part of the nasopharynx, they are swallowed and removed from the body via the digestive tract.

There is a rich supply of blood vessels in the nasal septum that warms the inspired air. These functions of filtering and warming are also supported by the paranasal sinuses, which are air cavities in the frontal, ethmoid, sphenoid, and maxillary portions of the skull. All are connected to the nasal cavity. The superior portion of the nose contains nerve fibers that are important to our sense of smell (olfactory sense). These fibers, derived from the first cranial nerve (CN I, the Olfactory Nerve), pass through the thin cribriform plate that separates the nasal cavity from the cranial cavity.

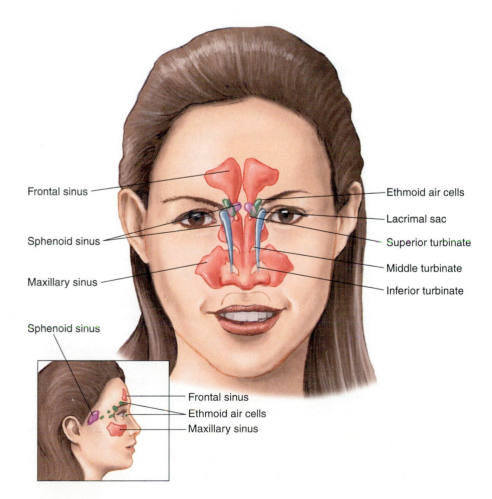

FIGURE 1-3 Paranasal sinuses.

Frontal sinus

Sphenoid sinus

Maxillary sinus

Sphenoid sinus

Ethmoid air cells

Lacrimal sac

Superior turbinate

Middle turbinate

Inferior turbinate

Frontal sinus
Ethmoid air cells
Maxillary sinus

Pharynx

The *pharynx* is a funnel-shaped structure that connects the nose and mouth to the larynx. It has three divisions: the nasopharynx, the oropharynx, and the laryngopharynx. The *nasopharynx* is the portion of the pharynx that is posterior to the nose and is the most superior aspect of the pharynx. Filtering, humidification, and warming of inspired air continue in the nasopharynx. Both food and air are conducted through the lower divisions of the pharynx, the *oropharynx* and the *laryngopharynx.* The tonsils are nodules of lymphatic tissue that are located in the posterior pharynx. There are three types of tonsils. The pharyngeal tonsils, also called the adenoids, are found in the nasopharynx. The palatine tonsils and lingual tonsils are located in the oropharynx.

Larynx

In addition to its role in speech, the larynx serves as a filtering device for the digestive and respiratory tracts. Externally, you can locate the larynx by feeling the thyroid cartilage, or Adam's apple. The larynx is composed of three pairs of cartilage (arytenoid, corniculate, and cuneiform), the thyroid cartilage, the cricoid cartilage, and the epiglottis. The larynx also possesses two pairs of folds that are derived from the internal lining of the larynx. The upper lining forms a pair of folds called the *vestibule,* or false vocal cords. The lower pair forms the true vocal cords. The vocal cords and the space in between them are referred to as the *glottic opening.* During inspiration, the three paired cartilages remain widely separated and the epiglottis sits upright so that air can freely enter the trachea. With swallowing, the epiglottis tips backward and the cartilage pairs close, diverting food to the esophagus.

LOWER AIRWAY ANATOMY

Trachea

During inspiration, air exits the upper airway and passes through the larynx into the *trachea* (Figure 1-4). The trachea is approximately 11 cm in length and is composed of a series of C-shaped cartilaginous rings. It is lined with the same kind of cells that line the nares. Mucus produced by these cells continues to trap air contaminants, and the cilia propel the mucus toward the pharynx. Additionally, stimulation of the trachea by food or other ingested products triggers a coughing response that helps keep the airway free of foreign material. Cigarette smoking ultimately leads to destruction of the cilia, leaving the cough reflex as the only protective mechanism.

Bronchi

At the **carina,** the trachea divides into the right and the left mainstem bronchi. The carina has many nerve endings and stimulation of this area produces violent coughing. The right mainstem bronchus is almost a straight continuation of the trachea, whereas the left mainstem bronchus angles more acutely to the left. This anatomical difference between the two mainstem bronchi helps to explain why gastric contents or other aspirated material tend to pass down the right mainstem bronchus into the lungs. It also explains why pneumonia that results from aspiration occurs more commonly in the right lung. Additionally, this is why, in most instances, an endotracheal tube advanced too far into the trachea will pass into the right mainstem bronchus.

The mainstem bronchi divide into the secondary (lobar) bronchi. These secondary bronchi divide into tertiary (segmental) bronchi, which ultimately divide

---

Content Review

THE LOWER AIRWAY

Trachea
Bronchi
Alveoli
Lungs

---

* **carina** the point at which the trachea bifurcates into the right and left mainstem bronchi.

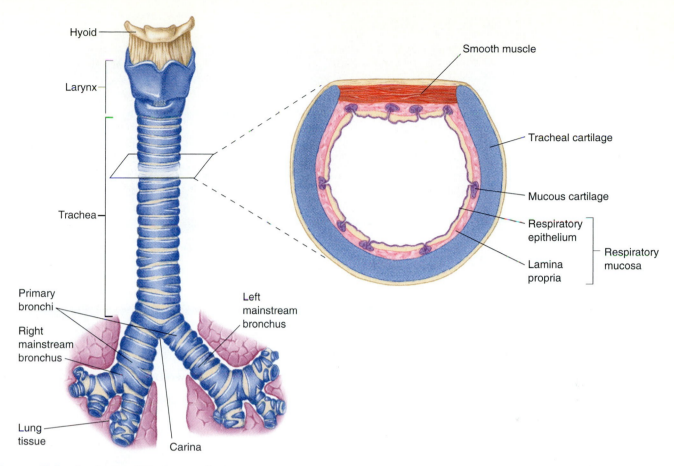

Labels on figure:
- Hyoid
- Larynx
- Trachea
- Primary bronchi
- Right mainstream bronchus
- Lung tissue
- Left mainstream bronchus
- Carina
- Smooth muscle
- Tracheal cartilage
- Mucous cartilage
- Respiratory epithelium
- Lamina propria
- Respiratory mucosa

FIGURE 1-4   Anatomy of the lower airway.

into the bronchioles, or the small airways. The bronchioles are approximately 1 mm thick and contain smooth muscle that can contract, thus reducing the diameter of the airway.

The conduit system, from the trachea to the terminal bronchioles, must be intact for air to enter the lungs. Both the upper airway and lower airway must be patent so that air may pass through the bronchial system into the alveoli. The upper airway is the gateway to the body's respiratory system, and occlusion by the patient's tongue or a foreign body prevents air from reaching the alveoli. Lower airway disease such as bronchial asthma can have the same result. You can see, therefore, how important it is to maintain a patent airway as you attempt to resuscitate a patient.

After approximately 22 divisions, the bronchioles become terminal bronchioles. The terminal bronchioles divide into the respiratory bronchioles, and it is at this point that the airway shifts from being a conduit for air to an organ of gas exchange. The respiratory bronchioles contain mostly smooth muscle and have limited gas exchange ability.

The conduit system, from the trachea to the terminal bronchioles, must be intact for air to enter the lungs. Maintaining an open airway is critical.

Alveoli

The respiratory bronchioles divide into the alveolar ducts. These terminate in the alveolar sacs, or alveoli. It is estimated that there may be 300 million alveoli in the lungs. Most of the gas exchange (exchange of oxygen and carbon dioxide)

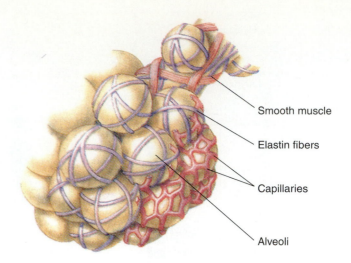

Smooth muscle

Elastin fibers

Capillaries

Alveoli

FIGURE 1-5a   The alveoli and the pulmonary capillaries.

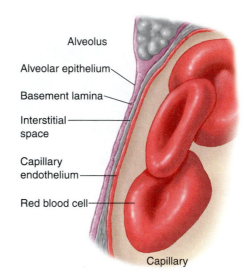

Alveolus

Alveolar epithelium

Basement lamina

Interstitial space

Capillary endothelium

Red blood cell

Capillary

FIGURE 1-5b   Supportive tissue contained in the interstitial space that separates capillaries from the alveolar surface.

takes place in the alveoli (Figure 1-5a), although limited gas exchange may occur in the alveolar ducts and respiratory bronchioles.

The alveolar wall consists of a thin layer of cells (type I cells) that line the lung surface. In close proximity to the alveoli are the pulmonary capillaries. These capillaries carry carbon dioxide-rich blood from the heart into the lungs and oxygen-rich blood away from the lungs for return to the heart. A small amount of supportive tissue contained in the interstitial space separates the capillaries from the alveolar surface (Figure 1-5b).

The alveolar lining, supportive tissue, and capillaries make up the *respiratory membrane*. This gas exchange surface measures approximately 70 m². Diseases such as emphysema destroy the walls between the alveoli and reduce the total surface area available for gas exchange. When this surface area is reduced by more than two-thirds, oxygen diffusion will be unable to meet the needs of the resting patient.

The alveoli are moistened and kept open because of the presence of an important chemical called **surfactant** that is secreted by type II cells found on the alveolar surface. Surfactant tends to decrease the surface tension of the alveoli, thus keeping them open for gas exchange. The alveolar macrophages are another

✳ **surfactant** a compound secreted by the lungs that contributes to the elastic properties of the pulmonary tissues.

type of cell found within the alveoli. These cells are part of the body's immune system and function to digest particles, bacteria, and other foreign material.

Remember that, in a normal patient, not all of the alveoli remain patent during gas exchange. This means that a small percentage of blood will pass through the alveoli without exchanging oxygen and carbon dioxide. This is referred to as *physiologic shunt* and affects approximately 2 percent of the total blood flow to the lungs.

Lungs

The lungs are the main organs of respiration. The right lung contains three main divisions or *lobes*, whereas the left lung has only two lobes. The lungs are covered by connective tissue called *pleura*. Unattached to the lung, except at the *hilum* (the point at which the bronchi and blood vessels enter the lungs), the pleura consists of two layers, visceral and parietal. The *visceral pleura* covers the lungs and does not contain nerve fibers. In contrast, the *parietal pleura* lines the thoracic cavity and does contain nerve fibers. A small amount of pleural fluid is usually found in the pleural space, a potential space between the two layers of pleura. This fluid serves as a lubricant for lung movement during respiration. The surface tension maintains the contact between the lungs and chest wall (similar to the attractive force that is generated when you place water in between two glass slides).

Pulmonary and Bronchial Vessels

Blood is supplied to the lungs through two systems: the pulmonary vessels and the bronchial vessels. The pulmonary arteries transport deoxygenated, carbon-dioxide rich blood from the heart and present it to the lungs for oxygenation. The pulmonary veins then transport the oxygenated blood from the lungs back to the heart. The lung tissue itself receives little of its blood supply from the pulmonary arteries and veins. Instead, bronchial arteries that branch from the aorta provide most of the blood supply to the lungs. Bronchial veins return blood from the lungs to the superior vena cava.

PHYSIOLOGICAL PROCESSES

The major function of the respiratory system is to exchange gases with the environment. Oxygen is taken in while carbon dioxide is eliminated, a process known as gas exchange.

Oxygen is vital to our bodies, allowing us to generate the energy that drives our many body functions. Oxygen from the atmosphere diffuses into the bloodstream through the lungs. Oxygen is then available for use in cellular metabolism by the body's 100 trillion cells. Waste products, including carbon dioxide, produced by cellular metabolism, must be eliminated from the body. In the lungs, carbon dioxide is exchanged for oxygen and the carbon dioxide is excreted from the lungs.

Three important processes allow gas exchange to occur:

- Ventilation
- Diffusion
- Perfusion

Ventilation

Ventilation is the mechanical process of moving air in and out of the lungs. In order for ventilation to occur, several body structures must be intact, including the chest wall, the nerve pathways, the diaphragm, the pleural cavity, and the brainstem.

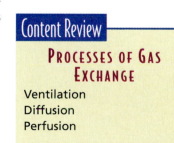

Content Review

PROCESSES OF GAS EXCHANGE

Ventilation
Diffusion
Perfusion

✱ **ventilation** the mechanical process of moving air in and out of the lungs.

FIGURE 1-6 The intercostal
vessels and nerves are located at
the inferior borders of the ribs.

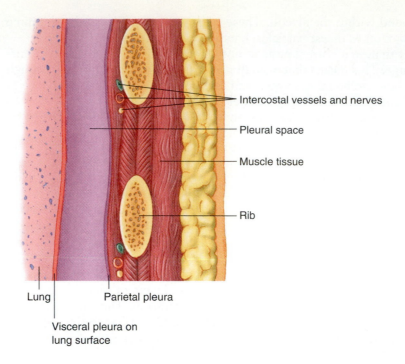

Intercostal vessels and nerves

Pleural space

Muscle tissue

Rib

Lung

Parietal pleura

Visceral pleura on
lung surface

The chest wall is made up of a series of ribs that are supported posteriorly by the thoracic spine and anteriorly by the sternum and costal cartilages. Each set of ribs is connected by a thick array of muscles called the *intercostal muscles*. These muscles are nourished by a paired artery and vein, the intercostal vessels, and they receive their nerve supply from the intercostal nerve. The nerve and blood vessels lie along the lower edge of each rib in a groove on the posterior surface (Figure 1-6). The chest wall is an important component of ventilation and also serves to protect the heart, lungs, and other organs of the thorax.

The *diaphragm*, a dome-shaped muscle separates the thorax and abdomen. Nerve impulses from the phrenic nerve, which begins in the region of the cervical portion of the spinal cord and travels through the chest cavity, stimulate the diaphragm to contract. Several traumatic, infectious, and even neoplastic conditions (cancer, tumors) can interrupt the nerve supply to the diaphragm.

Inspiration and Expiration Ventilation is divided into two phases: inspiration and expiration. During inspiration, air is drawn into the lungs. During expiration, air leaves the lungs. These phases of ventilation depend on changes in the volume of the thoracic cavity.

As inspiration begins, the diaphragm contracts and thus flattens. In addition, the intercostal muscles contract, producing an expansion in both the anteroposterior and lateral diameter of the chest cavity (Figure 1-7a). These two actions result in an expansion in the chest volume, which produces a decrease in the air pressure inside the chest cavity. This decrease to approximately 1 to 2 mmHg *below* atmospheric pressure causes air outside the body to be drawn through the trachea into the lungs. During periods of heavy respiratory demand, the accessory muscles of the neck (primarily the sternocleidomastoid and scalene muscles) and abdominal wall are recruited to assist in increasing the chest wall volume. Inspiration is always an active process, requiring energy.

Inspiration is dependent not only on an intact chest wall but on an intact pleural cavity as well. The pleural space has a pressure between 4 and 8 mmHg less than atmospheric pressure. This pressure difference between the lung and pleural

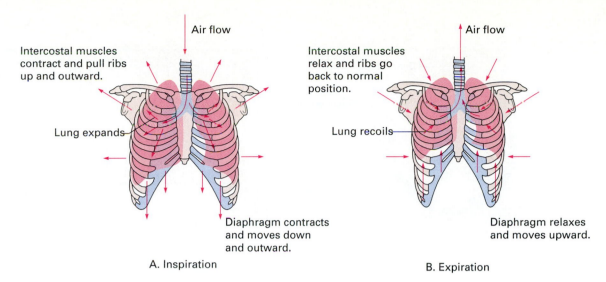

Intercostal muscles contract and pull ribs up and outward.

Air flow

Lung expands

Diaphragm contracts and moves down and outward.

A. Inspiration

Intercostal muscles relax and ribs go back to normal position.

Air flow

Lung recoils

Diaphragm relaxes and moves upward.

B. Expiration

FIGURE 1-7   The phases of respiration: (a) inspiration; (b) expiration.

space, as well as the surface tension of the pleural fluid, assures that the lungs will move in concert with the chest wall. You can see how an opening into the pleural cavity from a knife or gunshot wound would severely disrupt the normal ventilatory mechanism. A wound opening would eliminate the negative pressure that exists in the pleural space that causes the lungs to expand with the chest wall.

During expiration, both the chest wall and diaphragm recoil to their normal resting state, which increases the pressure inside the chest to approximately 1 to 2 mmHg *above* atmospheric pressure (Figure 1-7b). This drives air out of the lungs. Expiration is generally a passive process that does not require energy. In some disease states such as emphysema, however, the normal elasticity of the lungs is lost. Additionally, during heavy exercise, use of expiratory muscles (such as the rectus muscle and some of the intercostal muscles) is required to generate a larger expiratory effort. In either of these situations, expiration of air becomes an active process, requiring energy.

Airway Resistance and Lung Compliance The amount of air flow into the lungs (ventilation) is dependent not only on the difference between the pressure in the atmosphere and that inside the chest cavity but also on two additional factors: airway resistance and lung compliance.

The more *airway resistance* (or drag to the flow of air), the less air flowing into the chest cavity. Of the passages that conduct air into the alveoli, the medium-sized bronchi offer the greatest resistance to air flow. In patients who have asthma, the smooth muscle within these structures is stimulated by environmental allergens, cold weather, infection, and other factors. This stimulation leads to *bronchospasm* (widespread constriction of the bronchial smooth muscle) and increased resistance to air flow. This makes breathing more strenuous for the patient. The bronchi contain smooth muscle that is also very sensitive to input from the sympathetic nervous system. This is why sympathetic stimulants such as epinephrine, or parasympathetic blocking agents such as atropine or ipratropium bromide (Atrovent), are useful in the treatment of asthma.

Another factor that influences air flow into the lungs is *lung compliance*. Simply stated, compliance refers to the ease with which the chest expands. More specifically, it is defined as the change in volume of the chest cavity that results from a specific change in pressure within the chest cavity. The more the chest wall expands as the result of a change in pressure, the greater the lung compliance.

Airway resistance and lung compliance govern the amount of air that flows into the lungs.

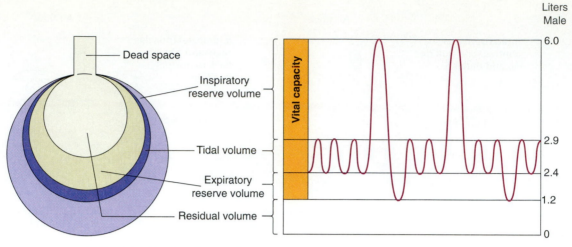

FIGURE 1-8 The lung volumes.

One natural change that occurs with aging is a decrease in lung compliance. This is caused by a loss of elasticity in the muscles, ribs, and cartilage that forms the chest wall, which results in a shrinking of the chest wall. The reverse is true with emphysema patients. Because elastic tissue is destroyed in these patients, their lung compliance is abnormally high, so that small changes in pressure result in large expansion of lung volume.

Lung Volumes The volume of air entering the lungs varies based on the metabolic needs of the patient. Several important lung volumes can be measured (Figure 1-8). Factors such as age, sex, physical conditioning, and medical illness will alter these volumes. During quiet respiration, approximately 500 ml of air move in and out of the lungs of a 70-kg adult. This is referred to as the *tidal volume*. The lungs are capable of drawing in an additional volume of air beyond the volume inspired during quiet respiration. This is referred to as the *inspiratory reserve volume*. In an adult male, this volume is approximately 3000 ml. Similarly, the amount of air that can be forcibly expired out of the lung after a normal breath is referred to as the *expiratory reserve volume* and measures approximately 1200 ml. An additional 1200 ml of air remains in the lungs at all times and is important in maintaining the patency of the alveoli. This is called the *residual volume*.

There are several calculated volumes that can be derived from these volumes that we have already discussed. Such derived volumes are referred to as *lung capacities*. The *inspiratory capacity* is the sum of the tidal volume and inspiratory reserve volume. This is approximately 3600 ml in adult males. The sum of the expiratory reserve volume and the residual volume is the *functional residual capacity*, which measures approximately 2400 ml. The *vital capacity* is the amount of air that is measured from a full inspiration to a full expiration. This is the sum of the inspiratory reserve volume, tidal volume, and expiratory reserve volume and measures 4800 ml. The total volume of air in the lungs, called the *total lung capacity*, measures approximately 6000 ml in an adult male (Table 1-1).

There are several measures of pulmonary function that you may come across in caring for patients with respiratory disorders. These measurements reflect the dynamic nature of air movement in and out of the lungs. The *minute respiratory volume* is the amount of air moved in and out of the lungs during a minute. It is calculated by multiplying the tidal volume and the respiratory rate. For an adult

Table 1-1	LUNG VOLUMES IN HEALTHY RESTING ADULT MALE

Capacity/Volumes (Male, in ml)	
Total Lung Capacity	6000
Vital capacity	4800
Inspiratory reserve	3000
Tidal volume	500
Expiratory volume	1200
Residual volume	1200

male, the typical minute respiratory volume is approximately 6 L (or 500 ml $\times$ 12 breaths per minute). Similarly, the *minute alveolar volume* is the volume of air moving through the alveoli in one minute. It is calculated by subtracting the dead space (approximately 150 ml—see explanation below) from the tidal volume and multiplying by the respiratory rate.

The *forced expiratory volume (FEV)* is the volume of air exhaled over a measured period of time. Most commonly the FEV_1 measures the volume of air expelled during the first second of a forced expiration. Similarly a *peak flow* measures the maximum rate of air flow during a forced expiration. This is measured in liters of air expiration per minute. Both of these measurements are commonly used in the assessment of patients with lung diseases such as asthma or COPD where the expiration of gases may be impaired.

Remember that when a patient breathes in a tidal volume of 500 ml, some of that air rests in the trachea, mainstem bronchi, and bronchioles and is unavailable for gas exchange. This is called the *anatomical dead space* and is approximately 150 ml. You should also remember that under certain conditions, some alveoli may be unavailable for gas exchange (because they are collapsed or are filled with fluid). This is referred to *alveolar dead space*. This volume varies depending on the degree of alveolar collapse.

Regulation of Ventilation The lower portions of the brainstem, specifically the *medulla*, control ventilation. This area of the brain sends a constant, repetitive signal to the lungs to initiate inspiration. The medulla contains both an inspiratory and an expiratory center. However, since expiration is generally a passive process, the inspiratory center plays a more active role in the rhythm of breathing. The resting rate of respiration varies between 12 and 20 breaths per minute in an adult.

The medullary signal is transmitted through the phrenic and intercostal nerves to the primary muscles of ventilation, that is, to the diaphragm and the intercostal muscles, respectively. The medullary signal can be modified by input from voluntary centers in the cerebral cortex, from other centers in the hypothalamus and brainstem (pons), and from other areas of the medulla. Other receptors throughout the body also provide input to the respiratory center. This allows tight control of ventilation in response to the body's physiologic needs.

One important body structure that provides input to the medulla's respiratory center are *stretch receptors* located on the visceral pleura and on the walls of the bronchi and bronchioles. As the patient continues to inhale, signals from these receptors become stronger until they completely inhibit impulses transmitted from the medulla. As the lungs begin to recoil, the signals become less intense, allowing the medulla to begin another inspiratory phase. This mechanism prevents overinflation of the lungs and is called the *Hering-Breuer reflex*. The medulla also receives input to increase the ventilatory rate from receptors that are stimulated by irritants in the lung and bronchial tree and, additionally, from receptors that detect increased activity in muscles and joints.

The most important determinant of the ventilatory rate is the arterial PCO_2. An increase in the patient's arterial PCO_2 results in a decrease in the **pH** of the blood. An increase of carbon dioxide in the blood also results in an increase in carbon dioxide in *cerebrospinal fluid* (the fluid that bathes the brain and spinal cord). Carbon dioxide and water combine to produce an acid, resulting in a lowering of the pH (increasing the concentration of hydrogen ions) in the cerebrospinal fluid. Chemical receptors in the area of the medulla detect this decrease in the pH, which produces an increase in the ventilatory rate, which helps the body eliminate excess CO_2 and return the pH to a normal level. There are also chemical receptors in the carotid artery and aorta that are directly sensitive to the arterial PCO_2. Stimulation of these receptors by an increase in arterial PCO_2 will also stimulate respiration. Remember that there is instantaneous feedback through these chemical receptors to the medulla so that once changes in cerebrospinal fluid pH and arterial PCO_2 are corrected, the stimulus to increase respiration ceases.

Unfortunately, regulation of ventilation in patients with COPD does not take place as described above. In patients with this disorder, the body becomes less responsive to changes in arterial PCO_2. Instead, the major stimulus to breathing comes from the level of oxygen detected in arterial blood by receptors in the aortic arch. As a result, patients with COPD will achieve a delicate balance in the PO_2, with the level being low enough to continually stimulate the medulla's respiratory center while having enough oxygen to maintain normal body functions. Measured PO_2 levels of between 50 and 60 mmHg are not uncommon in this patient population.

Diffusion

Diffusion is the process by which gases move between the alveoli and the pulmonary capillaries. Remember that gases tend to flow from areas in which there is a high concentration of gas into an area of low concentration. The normal concentration of oxygen in the alveoli is 104 mmHg as opposed to a concentration of 40 mmHg in the pulmonary arterial circulation. Therefore, oxygen will move from the oxygen-rich alveoli into the oxygen-poor capillaries in response to the gradient that exists in the concentration of gases. As the red blood cells move through the pulmonary capillaries, they become enriched with oxygen. Less oxygen will pass into the bloodstream as the gradient between alveolar and capillary oxygen concentration decreases.

Similarly, carbon dioxide passes out of the blood in response to a gradient that exists between the concentration of carbon dioxide in the blood in the pulmonary capillaries (45 mmHg) and in the alveoli (40 mmHg). By the time blood leaves the pulmonary capillaries, it has a dissolved concentration of oxygen of 104 mmHg and a carbon dioxide concentration of 40 mmHg.

The respiratory membrane, which normally measures 0.5 to 1.0 micrometer in thickness, must remain intact for gas exchange to occur. Any disorder that damages the alveoli or allows them to collapse will impede oxygen from entering the body and will reduce carbon dioxide elimination. Changes in the respiratory membrane or any increase in the interstitial space will also impede the process of diffusion. For example, fluid accumulation in the interstitial space as the result of pulmonary edema or pneumonia will prevent proper diffusion of gases. Finally the endothelial lining of the capillaries must be intact for exchange of oxygen and carbon dioxide to occur. Diseases that produce thickening of the endothelial lining will also interfere with the process of diffusion.

There are certain measures that you can take to address problems with lung diffusion. Providing the patient with high concentrations of oxygen is one simple step that can be utilized. Remember that the concentration gradient provides the driving force in moving oxygen into the capillaries. Therefore, the larger the difference between the concentration of oxygen in the alveoli and the capillaries, the greater the diffusion of oxygen into the bloodstream. Similarly, when fluid accumulation or inflammation is the underlying cause of the thickening of the interstitial space within the alveoli, medications such as diuretic agents or anti-inflammatory drugs (corticosteroids, antibiotics) are given to reduce fluid and inflammation.

Provide oxygen to a patient with a lung diffusion problem to increase the concentration gradient that drives oxygen into the capillaries. When fluid accumulation or inflammation is present, consider administering diuretics or antiinflammatory drugs.

Perfusion

One additional process that occurs in the lungs is **perfusion.** Lung perfusion is the circulation of blood through the lungs or, more specifically, the pulmonary capillaries. Lung perfusion is dependent on three conditions:

* Adequate blood volume
* Intact pulmonary capillaries
* Efficient pumping of blood by the heart

✱ perfusion the circulation of blood through the capillaries.

For perfusion to proceed effectively, there must be an adequate volume of blood in the bloodstream. Equally important is the concentration of **hemoglobin,** which is the transport protein that carries oxygen in the blood. Remember that oxygen is transported in the bloodstream in one of two ways: bound to hemoglobin or dissolved in the plasma. Under normal conditions, less than 2 percent of all oxygen is transported dissolved in plasma (this is what is measured by the PO_2), whereas more than 98 percent is carried by hemoglobin.

Hemoglobin has some unique properties. It is made up four iron-containing heme molecules and a protein-containing globin portion. Oxygen molecules bind to the heme portion of the hemoglobin molecule. As oxygen binds to hemoglobin, its structure changes so that it more readily binds additional oxygen molecules. Similarly, as fully oxygen-bound hemoglobin begins to release oxygen, it more readily sheds additional oxygen. The relationship is described by the *oxygen dissociation curve* (Figure 1-9). You can see that with between 10 and 50 mmHg, there is a marked increase in the saturation of hemoglobin. However, as the PO_2 increases above 70 mmHg, there is only a small change in the saturation of hemoglobin which is already near 100 percent.

✱ hemoglobin the transport protein that carries oxygen in the blood.

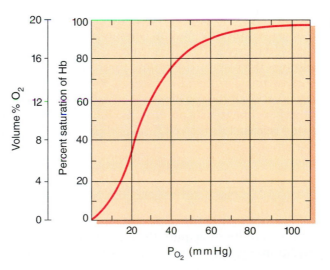

FIGURE 1-9 Oxygen dissociation curve.

Changes in the body temperature, the blood pH, and the PCO_2 can all alter the oxygen dissociation curve. Within the tissues, as hemoglobin becomes bound with carbon dioxide, it loses its affinity for oxygen. As a result, more oxygen is released and is thus available to cells for metabolism (called the Bohr effect).

Carbon dioxide is transported from the cells to the lungs in one of three ways:

- As bicarbonate ion
- Bound to the globin portion of the hemoglobin molecule
- Dissolved in plasma (measured as PCO_2)

The greatest portion of CO_2 produced during metabolism in cells is converted into bicarbonate ion. As the CO_2 is released into the capillaries, it enters the red blood cell where an enzyme (carbonic anhydrase) combines carbon dioxide with water to form two ions, hydrogen (H^+) and bicarbonate (HCO_3^-). Bicarbonate is then released from the red blood cell and transported in plasma. In the lungs, the reverse process takes place, producing water and carbon dioxide. The carbon dioxide then diffuses into the alveoli where it is eliminated during exhalation.

The carbon dioxide that is bound to hemoglobin is released in the lung because of the lower concentration of this gas in the alveoli. Additionally, as the heme portion of the hemoglobin molecule becomes saturated with oxygen, more carbon dioxide is released (called the Haldane effect). Finally, the approximately 10 percent of carbon dioxide that is dissolved in the plasma flows into the alveoli due to the gradient that exists between the concentration of gases (PCO_2 of 45 mmHg in pulmonary artery versus 40 mmHg in the alveoli).

For perfusion to take place, in addition to having adequate blood volume, the pulmonary capillaries must be able to transport blood through all portions of the lung tissue. These vessels must be open and not occluded, or blocked. For example, a pulmonary embolism will occlude the pulmonary artery in which it lodges, making that artery unavailable for perfusion of the portion of the lung it usually supplies with blood. Finally, the heart must pump efficiently in order to push blood effectively through the pulmonary capillaries to perfuse the lung tissues.

In order to maintain perfusion, ensure that the patient has an adequate circulating blood volume. Also, take all necessary steps to improve the pumping action of the heart.

In order to maintain perfusion, you must ensure that the patient has an adequate circulating blood volume. In addition, take all the necessary steps to improve the pumping action of the heart. For example, in patients with acute pulmonary edema the use of diuretic agents reduces the blood return (preload) to an ineffectively pumping heart and improves cardiac efficiency.

The entire system we have just discussed provides for **respiration,** which is the exchange of gases between a living organism and its environment. Pulmonary respiration occurs in the lungs when the respiratory gases are exchanged between the alveoli and the red blood cells in the pulmonary capillaries through the respiratory membranes. Cellular respiration, on the other hand, occurs in the peripheral capillaries. It involves the exchange of the respiratory gases between the red blood cells and the various tissues. Many of the principles of gas exchange that occur in the lungs are reversed in the tissues, with oxygen being released to the cells and carbon dioxide accumulating in the plasma and red blood cells.

* **respiration** the exchange of gases between a living organism and its environment.

PATHOPHYSIOLOGY

Remember that many disease states affect the pulmonary system and interfere with its ability to acquire the oxygen required for normal cellular metabolism. Additionally, respiratory diseases limit the body's ability to get rid of waste products such as carbon dioxide. Your understanding of normal anatomy and physiology—ventilation, diffusion, and perfusion—will aid in understanding the mechanism of each disease process and will direct you toward the appropriate corrective actions. Ultimately, any disease process that impairs the pulmonary system will result in a derangement in ventilation, diffusion, perfusion, or a combination of these processes.

DISRUPTION IN VENTILATION

Diseases that affect ventilation will result in obstruction of the normal conducting pathways of the upper or lower respiratory tract, impairment of the normal function of the chest wall, or abnormalities involving the nervous system's control of ventilation.

Upper and Lower Respiratory Tracts

Disease states that affect the upper respiratory tract will result in obstruction of air flow to the lower structures. Upper airway trauma, for example, produces both significant hemorrhage and swelling. Infections of the upper airway structures, including epiglottitis, soft tissue infections of the neck, tonsillitis, and abscess formation within the pharynx (peritonsillar abscess and retropharyngeal abscess), can all obstruct air flow. Similarly, lower airway obstruction may be produced by trauma, foreign body aspiration, mucus accumulation (as in asthmatics), smooth muscle constriction (in asthma and COPD), and airway edema produced by infection or burns.

Chest Wall and Diaphragm

As you read earlier, the chest wall and diaphragm are mechanical components that are essential for normal ventilation. Traumatic injuries to these areas will disrupt the normal mechanics causing loss of negative pressure within the pleural space. This occurs in patients with **pneumothorax,** including open pneumothorax, tension pneumothorax, or **hemothorax.** Infectious processes such as empyema (pus accumulation in the pleural space) or inflammatory conditions produce similar effects. Chest wall injuries including rib fractures or **flail chest** and diaphragmatic rupture limit the patient's ability to expand the thoracic cavity. Certain neuromuscular diseases, such as muscular dystrophy, multiple sclerosis, or amyotrophic lateral sclerosis (ALS or Lou Gehrig's Disease), impair muscular function so as to limit the ability to generate a negative pressure within the chest cavity.

Nervous System

Finally, any disease process that impairs the nervous system's regulation of breathing may also alter ventilation. Central nervous system depressants such as alcohol, benzodiazepines, or barbiturates, alone or in combination, can alter the brain's response to important signals such as rising PCO_2. Similarly, stroke, diseases, or injuries that involve the respiratory centers within the central nervous system can change the normal ventilatory pattern. In fact, certain abnormal respiratory patterns are produced by specific brain injury (Figure 1-10).

- *Cheyne-Stokes respirations* describes a ventilatory pattern with progressively increasing tidal volume, followed by a declining volume,

* **pneumothorax** a collection of air in the pleural space, causing a loss of the negative pressure that binds the lung to the chest wall. In an *open pneumothorax,* air enters the pleural space through an injury to the chest wall. In a *closed pneumothorax,* air enters the pleural space through an opening in the pleura that covers the lung. A *tension pneumothorax* develops when air in the pleural space cannot escape, causing a build-up of pressure and collapse of the lung.

* **hemothorax** a collection of blood in the pleural space.

* **flail chest** one or more ribs fractured in two or more places, creating an unattached rib segment.

FIGURE 1-10 Abnormal
respiratory patterns.

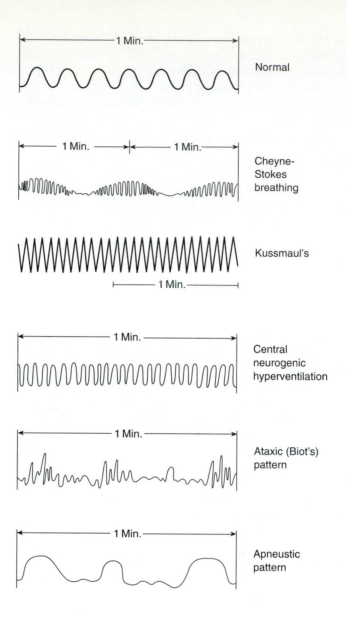

Normal

Cheyne-
Stokes
breathing

Kussmaul's

Central
neurogenic
hyperventilation

Ataxic (Biot's)
pattern

Apneustic
pattern

✱ **apnea** absence of breathing.

separated by periods of **apnea** at the end of expiration. This pattern
is typically seen in older patients with terminal illness or brain injury.

- *Kussmaul's respirations* are deep, rapid breaths that result as a
  corrective measure against conditions such as diabetic ketoacidosis
  that produce metabolic acidosis.
- *Central neurogenic hyperventilation* also produces deep, rapid
  respirations that are caused by strokes or injury to the brainstem. In
  this case, there is loss of normal regulation of ventilatory controls
  and respiratory alkalosis is often seen.
- *Ataxic (Biot's) respirations* are characterized by repeated episodes of
  gasping ventilations separated by periods of apnea. This pattern is
  seen in patients with increased intracranial pressure.
- *Apneustic respiration* is characterized by long, deep breaths that are
  stopped during the inspiratory phase and separated by periods of
  apnea. This pattern is a result of stroke or severe central nervous
  system disease.

Also remember that damage to the major peripheral nerves that supply the diaphragm and intercostal muscles, the phrenic nerve, and intercostal nerves will also affect normal ventilatory mechanics. Traumatic disruption of the phrenic nerve during chest surgery, with penetrating trauma, or by neoplastic (cancerous, tumorous) invasion of the nerve can paralyze the diaphragm on the side of involvement.

DISRUPTION IN DIFFUSION

Other disease states can disrupt the diffusion of gases. Any change in the concentration of oxygen in the alveoli, such as occurs when a person ascends to high altitudes, can limit the diffusion of oxygen and produce **hypoxia.** Similarly, any disease that alters the structure or patency of the alveoli will limit diffusion. Destruction of alveoli by certain environmental pathogens such as asbestos or coal (black lung disease), in patients with COPD, or with inhalation injury reduces the capacity of the lungs to diffuse gases.

✱ **hypoxia** state in which insufficient oxygen is available to meet the oxygen requirements of the cells.

Finally, disease states that alter the thickness of the respiratory membrane will limit the diffusion of gases. The most common cause of this alteration is accumulation of fluid and inflammatory cells in the interstitial space. Fluid can accumulate in the interstitial space if high pressure within the pulmonary capillaries forces fluid out of the circulatory system. This is seen in patients with left-sided heart failure (cardiogenic causes) and is due to increased venous pressure as a result of poor functioning of the left ventricle. Patients with pulmonary hypertension have high resting pressures in the pulmonary circulation which ultimately leads to fluid accumulation in the interstitial space, causing right heart failure.

Similar effects can be produced by changes in the permeability (or leakiness) of the pulmonary capillaries (non-cardiogenic causes). Permeability can be affected by adult respiratory distress syndrome, asbestosis and other environmental pathogens, near-drowning, prolonged hypoxia, and inhalation injury. Also remember that disease states that alter the pulmonary capillary endothelial lining, such as advanced atherosclerosis or vascular inflammatory states, can affect diffusion.

DISRUPTION IN PERFUSION

As detailed earlier, any alteration in appropriate blood flow through the pulmonary capillaries will limit normal gas exchange in the lungs. Any disease state that reduces the normal circulating blood volume, such as trauma, hemorrhage, dehydration, shock or other causes of hypovolemia, will limit normal perfusion of the lungs. Remember that hemoglobin is the major transport protein for oxygen and plays a significant role in the elimination of carbon dioxide. Therefore, any reduction in the normal circulating hemoglobin will also affect perfusion. All causes of anemia, a condition in which the number of red blood cells or amount of hemoglobin in them is below normal, must be considered. Such causes include acute blood loss, iron or vitamin deficiency, malnutrition, and anemia from chronic disease states.

Remember that blood must be available to all of the lung segments for maximum gas exchange to occur. When an area of lung tissue is appropriately ventilated but no capillary perfusion occurs, available oxygen is not moved into the circulatory system. This is referred to as a *pulmonary shunting*. In patients with pulmonary embolism, a blockage of a division of the pulmonary artery by a clot prevents perfusion of the lung segments supplied by that branch of the artery. As a result, there may be significant shunt with return of unoxygenated blood to the pulmonary venous circulation.

ASSESSMENT OF THE RESPIRATORY SYSTEM

Assessment of the respiratory system is a vital aspect of prehospital care. You must quickly assess the airway and ventilation status during the initial assessment. If the patient's complaints suggest that the respiratory system is involved in the patient's problem, the focused history and physical examination should be directed to this aspect of the assessment.

If the patient's complaints suggest respiratory system involvement, direct the focused history and physical examination to this aspect.

When you approach the scene, consider: (1) Is the scene safe? and (2) Are there visual cues to the patient's medical complaint?

SCENE SIZE-UP

When you approach the scene, you should consider two major questions: (1) Is the scene safe to approach the patient? and (2) Are there visual clues that might provide information regarding the patient's medical complaint?

Remember that there are several hazards that may result in respiratory complaints by the patient that are also potentially dangerous for emergency care providers. Certain gases and toxic products that are causing respiratory complaints from your patient may also present a significant risk to you. Carbon monoxide, for example, is a colorless and odorless gas that may be present in quantities enough to overcome unsuspecting emergency care personnel. Other toxins from incomplete combustion produced in fires or industrial processes pose a similar risk. Recent incidents involving chemical agents such as saran gas or biologic agents like anthrax highlight the need for emergency care providers to be aware of hazards to themselves as well as to their patient.

You should also be aware that there are certain rescue environments in which the concentration of available oxygen is significantly reduced. This would include areas such as grain silos, enclosed storage containers, or any enclosed space in which there is an active fire. You must take the appropriate precautions before entering such environments, including the use of your own supplemental oxygen supply.

In any situation where you believe there is a hazard to you as a care provider, make sure that the scene is appropriately secured before you enter. If specific protective items such as hazardous materials suits, self-contained breathing apparatus, or supplemental oxygen are needed, make sure they are available before you attempt to care for your patient. Similarly, if other personnel such as fire suppression units or hazmat teams are required, contact dispatch and have them available on scene before putting yourself at risk.

Once it is safe to enter the scene, look for clues that will provide information regarding the patient's complaints. Do you see evidence of cigarette packs or ashtrays to suggest that the patient or family members are smokers? Look for any home nebulizer machines or supplemental oxygen tanks that may suggest a patient with underlying COPD or asthma. If the patient is a small child, look for small items lying around the house that could suggest potential ingested foreign bodies. Using your eyes, ears, and nose can lead you to several important clues that are useful as you begin your assessment of the patient.

INITIAL ASSESSMENT

General Impression

Take the following considerations and steps to help form your initial impression of the patient's respiratory status:

- *Position.* Consider the patient's position. Patients with respiratory diseases tend to tolerate an upright posture better than lying flat. In-

Content Review

GENERAL IMPRESSION OF RESPIRATORY STATUS

Position
Color
Mental status
Ability to speak
Respiratory effort

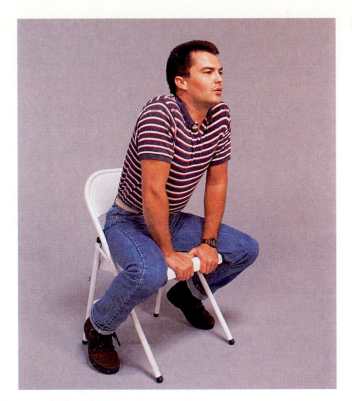

FIGURE 1-11 Tripod position.

dications of severe respiratory distress include a patient who is sitting upright with feet dangling over the side of the bed. In the most severe cases, the patient will assume the "tripod" position in which the patient leans forward and supports his weight with the arms extended (Figure 1-11).

- *Color.* Patients with severe respiratory distress display **pallor** and **diaphoresis. Cyanosis** is a late finding and may be absent even with significant hypoxia. Peripheral cyanosis (bluish discoloration involving only the distal extremities) is not a specific finding and is also found in patients with poor circulation. Peripheral cyanosis reflects the slowing of blood flow and increased extraction of oxygen from red blood cells. Central cyanosis (involving the lips, tongue, and truncal skin) is a more ominous finding seen in hypoxia.

- *Mental Status.* Briefly assess the patient's mental status. The hypoxic patient will become restless and agitated. Confusion is seen with both hypoxia (deficiency of oxygen) and hypercarbia (excess of carbon dioxide). When respiratory failure is imminent, the patient will appear severely lethargic and somnolent. The eyelids will begin to droop and the head will bob with each respiratory effort.

- *Ability to Speak.* Assess the patient's ability to speak in full, coherent sentences. Determine the ease with which the patient can discuss symptoms. Patients with respiratory distress will be able to speak only 1 to 2 words before they need to pause to catch their breath. Rambling, incoherent speech indicates fear, anxiety, or hypoxia.

- *Respiratory Effort.* As we have already described, normal ventilation is an active process. However, the use of accessory muscles in the neck (scalenes and sternocleidomastoids) and visible contractions of the intercostal muscles indicate significant breathing effort.

✱ **pallor** paleness.

✱ **diaphoresis** sweatiness.

✱ **cyanosis** bluish discoloration of the skin due to an increase in reduced hemoglobin in the blood. The condition is directly related to poor ventilation.

As you form your general impression, also make specific note of any of the following signs of respiratory distress

* nasal flaring excessive widening of the nares with respiration.

- **Nasal flaring**
- Intercostal muscle retraction
- Use of the accessory respiratory muscles
- Cyanosis
- Pursed lips
- **Tracheal tugging**

* tracheal tugging retraction of the tissues of the neck due to airway obstruction or dyspnea.

Your initial assessment of the patient is directed at identification of any life-threatening conditions resulting from compromise of airway, breathing, or circulation (the ABCs). Because this chapter concerns the respiratory system, we will focus here on assessment of airway and breathing.

Airway

Any significant abnormality in the respiratory tract must be viewed as potentially life threatening.

Remember that oxygen is one of the most basic necessities for life, and the respiratory system is responsible for supplying it to the body tissues. As a result, any significant abnormality in the respiratory tract must be viewed as potentially life threatening.

After quickly forming your general impression, immediately focus on the patient's airway. When assessing the airway, keep these principles in mind:

- Noisy breathing nearly always means partial airway obstruction.
- Obstructed breathing is not always noisy.
- The brain can survive only a few minutes in **asphyxia.**
- Artificial respiration is useless if the airway is blocked.
- A patent airway is useless if the patient is apneic.
- If you note airway obstruction, do not waste time looking for help or equipment. Act immediately.

* asphyxia a decrease in the amount of oxygen and an increase in the amount of carbon dioxide as a result of some interference with respiration.

If the airway is compromised, quickly institute basic airway management techniques. Once you have secured a patent airway, ensure that the patient has adequate ventilation.

If the airway is compromised, quickly institute basic airway management techniques. Once you have secured a patent airway, ensure that the patient has adequate ventilation. Your initial assessment of the respiratory system should be brief and directed. A more detailed examination should be conducted once you have been able to establish that an immediate threat to life does not exist.

Breathing

The following signs should suggest a possible life-threatening respiratory problem in adults. They are listed in order from most ominous to least severe.

- Alterations in mental status
- Severe central cyanosis
- Absent breath sounds
- Audible stridor
- 1-to-2-word **dyspnea** (need to breathe between every word or two)
- **Tachycardia** $\geq$ 130 beats per minute
- Pallor and diaphoresis

* dyspnea difficult or labored breathing; a sensation of "shortness of breath."

* tachycardia rapid heart rate.

- The presence of intercostal and sternocleidomastoid retractions
- Use of accessory muscles

If any of these signs are present, you should direct your efforts toward immediate resuscitation and transport of the patient to a medical facility.

FOCUSED HISTORY AND PHYSICAL EXAMINATION

History

The history and physical exam should be directed at problem areas as determined by the patient's chief complaint or primary problem. Patients with respiratory diseases will often present with a complaint of "shortness of breath" (dyspnea). Obtain a SAMPLE history. If the chief complaint suggests respiratory disease, ask the OPQRST questions including the following questions about the current symptoms. The answers to these or similar questions will provide you with a pertinent patient history.

> How long has the dyspnea been present?
>
> Was the onset gradual or abrupt?
>
> Is the dyspnea better or worse by position? Is there associated **orthopnea** or **paroxysmal nocturnal dyspnea?**
>
> Has the patient been coughing?
>
> > If so, is the cough productive?
> >
> > What is the character and color of the sputum?
> >
> > Is there any **hemoptysis** (coughing up of blood)?
>
> Is there any chest pain associated with the dyspnea?
>
> > If so, what is the location of the pain?
> >
> > Was the onset of pain sudden or slow?
> >
> > What was the duration of the pain?
> >
> > Does the pain radiate to any area?
> >
> > Does the pain increase with respiration?
>
> Are there associated symptoms of fever or chills?
>
> What is the patient's past medical history?
>
> Has the patient experienced wheezing?
>
> Is the patient or close family member a smoker?

It is also important to ask the patient if he has ever experienced similar symptoms in the past. Patients with chronic medical conditions such as COPD or asthma can usually relate the severity of their current presenting complaints to other episodes that they have experienced. Question the patient or family about prior hospitalizations for respiratory disease. In particular, you should try to determine whether the patient required care in the intensive care unit (ICU) for breathing problems. Ask if the patient has ever required endotracheal intubation and ventilatory support. Consider patients who have been previously intubated to be potentially seriously ill and approach them with great caution.

Similarly, it is important to ask the patient if he already has a known respiratory disease. The most common reason for a call to emergency care personnel is a worsening of an already present respiratory disease. This is very typical for patients with COPD, asthma, or lung cancer. If you are not familiar with the patient's

If a patient complains of dyspnea, obtain a SAMPLE history. If the chief complaint suggests respiratory disease, ask the OPQRST questions about current symptoms.

* **orthopnea** dyspnea while lying supine.

* **paroxysmal nocturnal dyspnea** short attacks of dyspnea that occur at night and interrupt sleep.

* **hemoptysis** expectoration of blood from the respiratory tree.

diagnosis (for example, alpha-2 anti-trypsin deficiency), try to determine if the disease is affecting the process of ventilation, diffusion, or perfusion.

Continue history taking by determining:

What current medications is the patient taking? (Pay particular attention to oxygen therapy, oral bronchodilators, corticosteroids, and antibiotics.)

Does the patient have any allergies?

A good history of medication use is essential and may provide useful clues to the diagnosis. If time permits, gather the patient's current medications and transport them with the patient. This is a great benefit to the Emergency Department personnel who will be evaluating the patient. Pay particular attention to any medications that suggest pulmonary disease. These would include inhaled or oral sympathomimetics such as albuterol and related agents that are used to treat diseases such as COPD or asthma. Also ask about steroid preparations, which are also used in these conditions. Other common medications used by patients with COPD or asthma include cromolyn sodium, methylxanthines like theophylline, and antibiotic agents.

Also ask about drugs used for cardiac conditions, since cardiac patients often present with dyspnea. Nitrates, calcium channel blockers, diuretic agents, digoxin, and anti-dysrhythmic agents are all commonly used by patients with cardiac disease.

Finally, inquire about medication allergies. This is important information, since it helps to avoid administering agents to which the patient is allergic. Also, it's possible that a specific medication may be the cause of an allergic reaction that has resulted in upper airway edema and respiratory complaints.

Physical Examination

First address the patient's head and neck. Look at the lips. Pursed lips indicate significant respiratory distress. This is the patient's way of maintaining positive pressure during expiration and preventing alveolar collapse. Also examine the nose, mouth, and throat for any signs of swelling or infection that might be causing upper airway obstruction.

Occasionally, the patient may also produce sputum, which can suggest an underlying cause of the patient's complaints. An increase in the amount of sputum produced suggests infection of the lungs or bronchial passages (bronchitis). Thick, green or brown sputum is characteristic of these infections. On the other hand, thin, yellow or pale-gray sputum is more typical of inflammation or an allergic cause. Pink, frothy sputum is a sign of severe pulmonary edema. Truly bloody sputum (hemoptysis) may be seen with cancer, tuberculosis, and bronchial infection.

Assess the neck for signs of swelling or infection. Remember to look at the jugular veins for evidence of distention (Figure 1-12). This occurs when the right side of the heart is not pumping blood effectively, causing a "back-up" in the venous circulation. Such findings are often accompanied by left-sided heart failure and pulmonary edema.

Physical examination of the respiratory system should follow the standard steps of patient assessment: *inspection, palpation, percussion,* and *auscultation.*

- *Inspection.* Inspection should include an examination of the anterior-posterior dimensions and general shape of the chest (Figure 1-13). An increased anterior-posterior diameter is suggestive

Content Review

PHYSICAL EXAM OF RESPIRATORY SYSTEM

Head
Neck
Chest
  Inspection
  Palpation
  Percussion
  Auscultation
Extremities

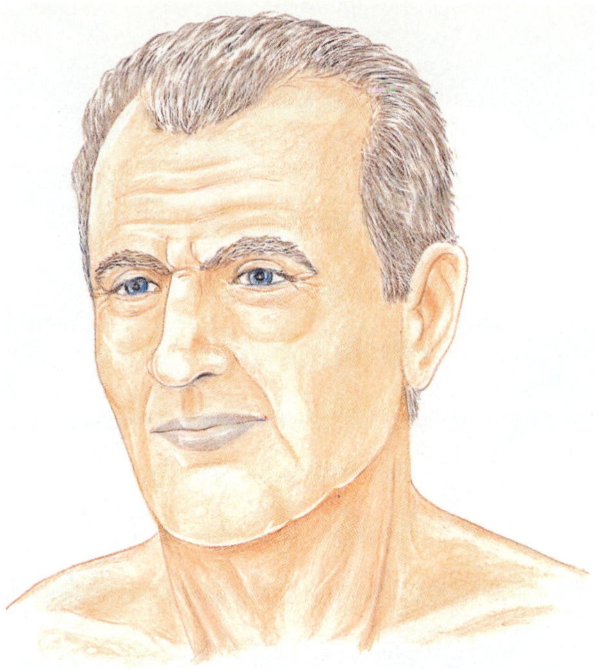

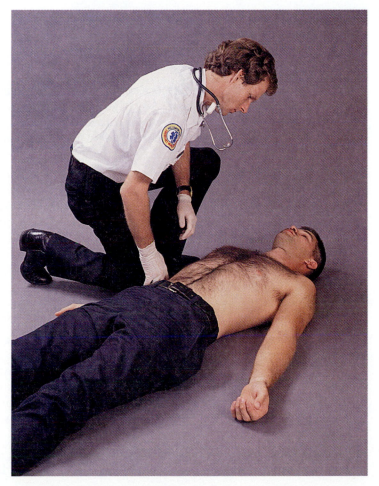

FIGURE 1-12   Jugular vein distention.

FIGURE 1-13   Inspection of the chest.

FIGURE 1-14   The chest should be palpated.

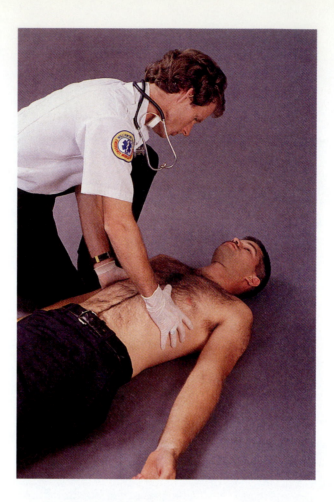

FIGURE 1-14   The chest should be palpated.

of chronic obstructive pulmonary disease (COPD). Inspect the chest for symmetrical movement. Any asymmetry may be suggestive of trauma. A paradoxical movement (moving in a fashion opposite to that expected) is suggestive of flail chest. Note any chest scars, lesions, wounds, or deformities.

* **Palpation.** Palpate the chest, both front and back, for any abnormalities (Figure 1-14). Note any tenderness, **crepitus,** or **subcutaneous emphysema.** Palpate the anterior chest first, then the posterior. Inspect your gloved hands for blood each time they are removed from behind the patient's chest. In some instances, it may be appropriate to evaluate **tactile fremitus,** the vibration felt in the chest during speaking. When evaluating tactile fremitus, compare one side of the chest with the other. Simultaneously, palpate the trachea for **tracheal deviation,** which is suggestive of a tension pneumothorax.

* **Percussion.** If indicated, quickly percuss the chest (Figure 1-15). Limit percussion to suspected cases of pneumothorax and pulmonary edema. A hollow sound on percussion is often indicative of pneumothorax or emphysema. In contrast, a dull sound is indicative of pulmonary edema, hemothorax, or pneumonia. Remember, however, that percussion may be of little value in the noisy environment typical of most emergency scenes.

* **Auscultation.** Auscultate the chest. Begin by listening to the patient without a stethoscope and from a distance. Note any loud stridor,

✱ **crepitus** crackling sounds.

✱ **subcutaneous emphysema** presence of air in the subcutaneous tissue.

✱ **tactile fremitus** vibratory tremors felt through the chest by palpation.

✱ **tracheal deviation** any position of the trachea other than midline.

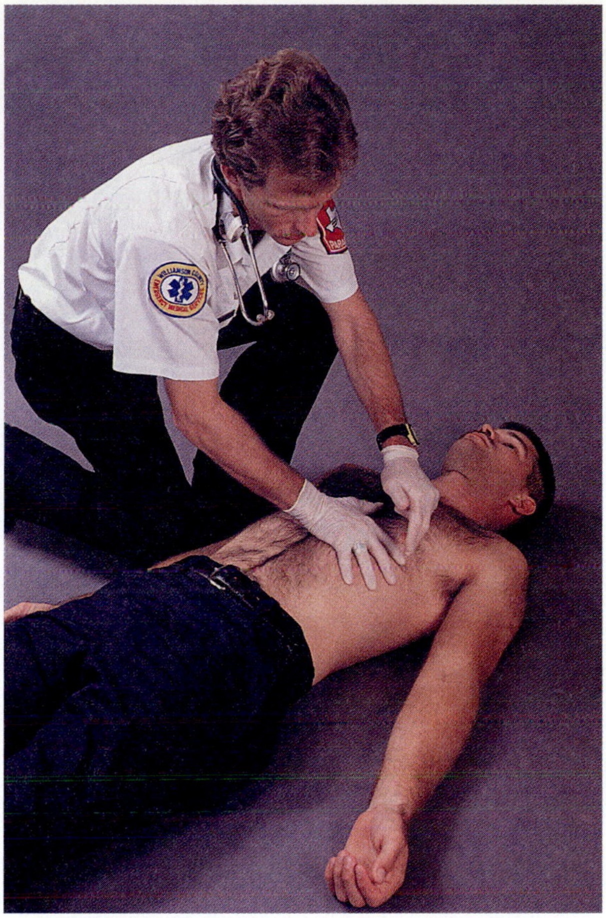

FIGURE 1-15 If indicated, the chest should be percussed.

wheezing, or cough. If possible, the patient should be in the sitting position and the chest auscultated in a symmetrical pattern. When the patient cannot sit up, auscultate the anterior and lateral parts of the chest (Figure 1-16). Each area should be auscultated for one respiratory cycle.

Normal breath sounds heard during auscultation can be characterized according to the following descriptions.

Normal Breath Sounds

- Bronchial (or tubular)
  - Loud, high-pitched breath sounds heard over the trachea
  - Expiratory phase lasts longer than inspiratory phase
- Bronchovesicular
  - Softer, medium-pitched breath sounds heard over the mainstem bronchi (below clavicles or between scapulae)
  - Expiratory phase and inspiratory phase equal
- Vesicular
  - Soft, low-pitched breath sounds heard in the lung periphery

While the patient breathes in and out deeply with the mouth open, note any abnormal breath sounds and their location. Many terms are used to describe abnormal breath sounds. The following list includes some of the more common terms.

FIGURE 1-16 The chest should be auscultated.

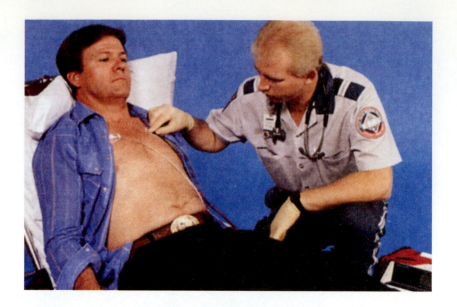

Abnormal Breath Sounds

- *Snoring.* Occurs when the upper airway is partially obstructed, usually by the tongue.
- *Stridor.* Harsh, high-pitched sound heard on inspiration and characteristic of an upper airway obstruction such as croup.
- *Wheezing.* Whistling sound due to narrowing of the airways by edema, bronchoconstriction, or foreign materials.
- *Rhonchi.* Rattling sounds in the larger airways associated with excessive mucus or other material.
- *Crackles* (also called *rales*). Fine, moist crackling sounds associated with fluid in the smaller airways.
- *Pleural Friction Rub.* Sounds like dried pieces of leather rubbing together; occurs when the pleura become inflamed, as in pleurisy.

Also examine the extremities. Look for peripheral cyanosis, which may indicate hypoxia. Examine the extremities for swelling, redness, and a hard, firm cord indicating a venous clot. This may suggest a possible cause for pulmonary embolism. Look for clubbing of the fingers (Figures 1-17a and 17b), suggesting long-standing hypoxemia. This is typical of patients with COPD or cyanotic heart disease. Finally, the patient may demonstrate *carpopedal spasm* in which the fingers and toes are contracted in flexion. This is found in patients with hyperventilation and is caused by transient shifts in the blood calcium concentration caused by changes in the serum CO_2 and pH levels.

Vital Signs

The patient's vital signs may also provide information regarding the severity of the respiratory complaints. In general, tachycardia (rapid heart rate) is a very nonspecific finding, seen with fear, anxiety, and fever. In patients with respiratory

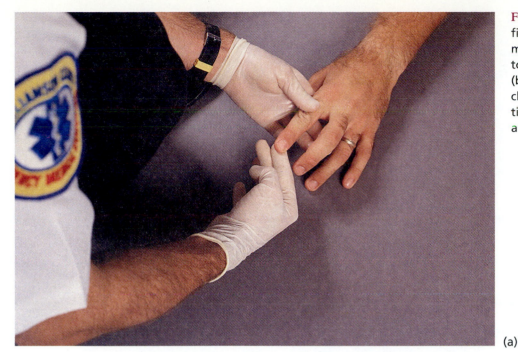

(a)

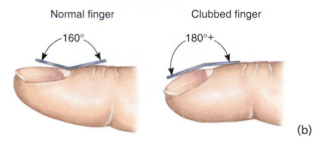

Normal finger   Clubbed finger

160°   180°+

(b)

FIGURE 1-17 (a) Inspect for finger clubbing. Any clubbing may indicate chronic respiratory or cardiac disease. (b) Characteristics of finger clubbing include large fingertips and a loss of the normal angle at the nail bed.

complaints, however, tachycardia may also indicate hypoxia. Remember that the patient may have recently used sympathomimetic drugs such as albuterol, which will accelerate the patient's heart rate. These same drugs will elevate the patient's blood pressure as well. During your assessment of the blood pressure, a patient will occasionally exhibit *pulsus paradoxus,* a drop in the systolic blood pressure of 10 mmHg or more with each respiratory cycle. Pulsus paradoxus is associated with chronic obstructive pulmonary disease (COPD) and cardiac tamponade. As a rule, however, you should not take the time to look for pulsus paradoxus.

A change in a patient's respiratory rate may be one of the earliest indicators of respiratory disease. The patient's respiratory rate can be influenced by several factors, including respiratory difficulty, fear, anxiety, fever, and underlying metabolic disease. Assume that an elevated respiratory rate in a patient with dyspnea is caused by hypoxia. Although fluctuations in the respiratory rate are common, a persistently *slow* rate indicates impending respiratory arrest.

Continually reassess the patient's respiratory rate during the time that you are caring for the patient. Trends in the respiratory rate (for example, an increasing rate) can give you an overall assessment of the effectiveness of any intervention

Assume that an elevated respiratory rate in a patient with dyspnea is caused by hypoxia. A persistently slow rate indicates impending respiratory arrest.

Constantly reassess the patient's respiratory rate and pattern.

you have made. Also assess the patient's respiratory pattern. The normal respiratory pattern (eupnea) is steady, even breaths occurring 12 to 20 times per minute with an expiratory phase that lasts between 3 to 4 times the inspiratory phase. **Tachypnea** describes a respiratory pattern with a rate that exceeds 20 breaths per minute. **Bradypnea** describes a respiratory pattern with a rate slower than 12 breaths per minute. Also, look for any abnormal respiratory patterns (e.g., Cheyne-Stokes, Kussmaul, or other) that were discussed earlier in the chapter.

* **tachypnea** rapid respiration.

* **bradypnea** slow respiration.

Diagnostic Testing

Three diagnostic measurements are of value in assessing the patient's respiratory status: *pulse oximetry, peak flow,* and *capnometry.*

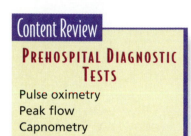

Content Review

PREHOSPITAL DIAGNOSTIC TESTS

Pulse oximetry
Peak flow
Capnometry

- *Pulse Oximetry.* Pulse oximetry offers a rapid and accurate means for assessing oxygen saturation. The pulse oximeter can be quickly applied to a finger or earlobe. The pulse rate and oxygen saturation can be continuously recorded. Use of the pulse oximeter, if available, is encouraged for any patient complaining of dyspnea or respiratory problems (Figure 1-18). Remember that the pulse oximetry reading may

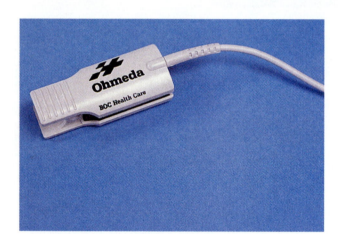

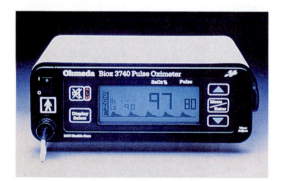

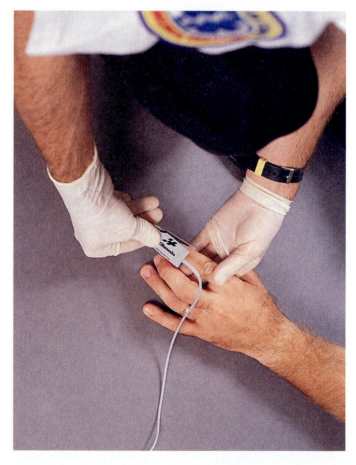

FIGURE 1-18 Sensing unit for pulse oximetry. This device transmits light through a vascular bed, such as in the finger, and can determine the oxygen saturation of red blood cells. To use the pulse oximeter, it is only necessary to turn the device on and attach the sensor to a finger. The desired graphic mode on the oximeter should be selected. The oxygen saturation and pulse rate can be continuously monitored.

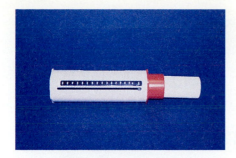

FIGURE 1-19 Wright Spirometer for determining Peak Expiratory Flow Rate (PEFR).

be difficult to obtain in a patient with peripheral vasoconstriction (as in sepsis or hypothermia). It may also be inaccurate under conditions in which an abnormal substance like carbon monoxide binds to hemoglobin, since the instrument measures the saturation of hemoglobin without indicating what substance has saturated it.

The oxygen saturation measurement obtained through pulse oximetry is abbreviated as SaO_2 (oxygen saturation). When pulse oximetry first came into use, some authors abbreviated the oxygen saturation measurement as SpO_2. However, this was sometimes confused with the PaO_2 obtained during blood gas measurement. Because of this, SaO_2 has become the preferred abbreviation.

- **Peak Flow.** Small portable hand-held devices are available for use in determining the patient's peak expiratory flow rate (PEFR). The normal expected peak flow rate is based on the patient's sex, age, and height. Remember that the measurement of the peak expiratory flow rate is somewhat effort dependent; you must have a cooperative patient who understands the use of the device in order to get an accurate reading.

  The PEFR is obtained using a Wright Spirometer (Figure 1-19), which is inexpensive and easy to use. Place the disposable mouth piece into the meter. First have the patient take in the deepest possible inspiration. Then encourage the patient to seal his lips around the device and forcibly exhale. The peak rate of exhaled gas is recorded in liters per minute. This should be repeated twice, with the highest reading recorded as the patient's PEFR (Table 1-2).

- **Capnometry.** Devices are now available that detect carbon dioxide at the end of the expiratory phase. If gases are sampled at the end of an endotracheal tube, the level of measured carbon dioxide is

Table 1-2	SPIROMETRY AND PEAK FLOW VALUES FOR ADULTS		
FEV₁ Severity	FEV₁ (Liters)	FVC (%)	Peak Flow (Liters/Min)
Normal	4.0–6.0 L	80–90%	550–650 (Male)
			400–500 (Female)
Mild	3.0 L	70%	300–400
Moderate	1.6 L	50%	200–300
Severe	0.6 L	40%	100

FIGURE 1-20 End-tidal CO_2
devices: (a) electronic
(b) colormetric.

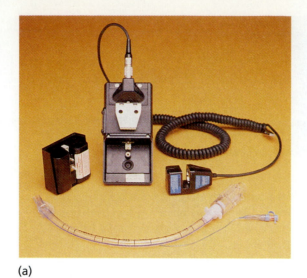
(a)

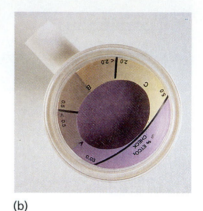
(b)

highest at the end of expiration. This is referred to as end-tidal CO_2 measurement. The fact that carbon dioxide is detected assumes that the metabolic processes of the body are active in producing CO_2 and that this gas is adequately exchanged in the lungs. Remember that almost no carbon dioxide is present in the esophagus and stomach. As a result, none would be detected by capnometry if the endotracheal tube is improperly placed into the esophagus. However, even a properly placed capnometry device will not detect CO_2 if the patient is in cardiac arrest.

Although several devices are available that measure the level of carbon dioxide during the entire ventilatory cycle (as a continuous waveform called *capnography*), most devices are used primarily in the out-of-hospital setting to assure the proper position of the endotracheal tube in the trachea. These devices, called end-tidal CO_2 detectors, focus only on the presence or absence of carbon dioxide in the sampled gas (*capnometry*). If the endotracheal tube becomes dislodged from its proper position, there is an almost immediate change in the readings from the end-tidal CO_2 device. This is in contrast to measurement of pulse oximetry which may take several minutes to reflect the hypoxia produced by tube dislodgement.

Two types of devices are commonly used for capnometry. The first device gives a numerical read-out of the level of carbon dioxide detected by the device (Figure 1-20a). The other device relies upon a color change produced by carbon dioxide to demonstrate the presence of the gas during exhalation (Figure 1-20b).

MANAGEMENT OF RESPIRATORY DISORDERS

The following sections will address the pathophysiology, assessment, and management of the more common respiratory disorders encountered in prehospital care. The discussion begins with a look at some general principles that can and should be applied to ALL respiratory emergencies.

MANAGEMENT PRINCIPLES

In cases of acute respiratory insufficiency, several principles should guide your actions in the prehospital setting. These include:

- The airway always has first priority. In trauma victims who may have associated cervical spine injuries, protect and maintain the airway without extending the neck.
- Any patient with respiratory distress should receive oxygen.
- Any patient whose illness or injury suggests the possibility of hypoxia should receive oxygen.
- If there is a question whether oxygen should be given, as in chronic obstructive pulmonary disease (COPD), administer it. *Oxygen should never be withheld from a patient suspected of suffering hypoxia.*

Keep these precautions in mind as you read through the descriptions of pathophysiology, assessment, and management of respiratory disorders frequently encountered in the field

Principles of management for respiratory disorders include (1) Give first priority to the airway, and (2) Always provide oxygen to patients with respiratory distress or the possibility of hypoxia, including patients with COPD.

SPECIFIC RESPIRATORY DISEASES

UPPER-AIRWAY OBSTRUCTION

The most common cause of upper-airway obstruction is the relaxed tongue. In an unconscious patient in the supine position, the tongue can fall into the back of the throat and obstruct the upper airway. Additionally, the upper airway can become obstructed by such common materials as food, dentures, or other foreign bodies. A typical example of upper-airway obstruction is the "cafe coronary," which tends to occur in middle-aged or elderly patients who wear dentures. These people often are unable to sense how well they have chewed their food. Thus, they accidentally inhale a large piece of food (often meat) that obstructs their airway. Concurrent alcohol consumption is often implicated in the "cafe coronary." Also, obstruction of the upper airway can be the result of facial or neck trauma, upper-airway burns, and allergic reactions. In addition, the upper airway can become blocked by an infection that causes swelling of the epiglottis (epiglottitis) or subglottic area (croup).

> **Content Review**
>
> **COMMON CAUSES OF AIRWAY OBSTRUCTION**
> Tongue
> Foreign matter
> Trauma
> Burns
> Allergic reaction
> Infection

Assessment

Assessment of the patient with an upper-airway obstruction varies, depending upon the cause of the obstruction and the history of the event. The unresponsive patient should be evaluated for snoring respirations, possibly indicating tongue or denture obstruction. If confronted by a patient suffering a "cafe coronary," determine whether the victim can speak. Speech indicates that, at present, the obstruction is incomplete. If the victim is unresponsive and has been eating, strongly suspect a food bolus lodged in the trachea. If a burn is present or suspected, assume laryngeal edema until proven otherwise.

Patients who may be having an allergic reaction to food or medications will often report an itching sensation in the palate followed by a "lump" in the throat. The situation may progress to hoarseness, inspiratory stridor, and complete obstruction. Pay particular attention to the presence of urticaria (hives). Intercostal muscle retraction and use of the strap muscles of the neck for breathing suggest attempts to ventilate against a partially closed airway.

Management

Management of the obstructed airway is based on the nature of the obstruction. Blockage by the tongue can be corrected by opening the airway, using either the head-tilt, chin-lift, the jaw-thrust, or the modified jaw-thrust maneuver. The airway can be maintained by employing either a nasopharyngeal or oropharyngeal airway. If possible, remove obstructing foreign bodies using the following basic airway maneuvers.

Conscious Adult In an adult patient who is conscious:

1. Determine if there is a complete obstruction or poor air exchange. Ask the patient: "Are you choking?" "Can you speak?" If the patient can speak, he should be asked to produce a forceful cough to expel the foreign body.
2. If the patient has complete obstruction or poor air exchange, provide up to five abdominal thrusts in rapid succession. If the thrusts prove unsuccessful, repeat until the obstruction is relieved or the patient becomes unconscious. In very obese or pregnant patients, use chest thrusts in lieu of abdominal thrusts.

Unconscious Adult If the patient is unconscious or loses consciousness:

1. Use the head-tilt, chin lift, the jaw-thrust, or the modified jaw-thrust maneuver in an attempt to open the airway.
2. Pinch the patient's nostrils and attempt to give two ventilations. If the attempts to ventilate fail, reposition the head and repeat attempt. If this fails . . .
3. Straddle the patient and administer up to five abdominal thrusts in quick succession. If this fails . . .
4. Try the tongue-jaw lift and, if the foreign body is seen, attempt finger sweeps. If successful, resume ventilation. If unsuccessful . . .
5. Continue the abdominal thrusts and finger sweeps, while preparing the laryngoscope and the Magill forceps. Visualize the airway with the laryngoscope. If the foreign body can be seen, grasp it with the Magill forceps and remove. Once removed, begin ventilation and administer supplemental oxygen.

In cases of airway obstruction caused by laryngeal edema (e.g., anaphylactic reactions, angioedema), establish the airway by the head-tilt, chin-lift, the jaw-thrust, or triple-airway maneuver. Then administer supplemental oxygen. Attempt bag-valve-mask ventilation. Often, air can be forced past the obstruction and the patient adequately ventilated using this technique. Next, start an IV with a crystalloid solution and administer subcutaneous epinephrine. Then administer diphenhydramine (Benadryl). Transtracheal ventilation may be required if the patient does not respond to the treatments described. See Volume 5, Chapter 2, for pediatric techniques.

NON-CARDIOGENIC PULMONARY EDEMA/ADULT RESPIRATORY DISTRESS SYNDROME

Adult respiratory distress syndrome (ARDS) is a form of pulmonary edema that is caused by fluid accumulation in the interstitial space within the lungs. Patients with *cardiogenic* pulmonary edema have a poorly functioning left ventricle. This leads to increases in hydrostatic pressure and fluid accumulation in the intersti-

* adult respiratory distress syndrome (ARDS) form of pulmonary edema that is caused by fluid accumulation in the interstitial space within the lungs.

tial space. In patients with ARDS, however, fluid accumulation occurs as the result of increased vascular permeability and decreased fluid removal from the lung tissue. This occurs in response to a wide variety of lung insults including:

- Sepsis, particularly with gram-negative organisms
- Aspiration
- Pneumonia or other respiratory infections
- Pulmonary injury
- Burns
- Inhalation injury
- Oxygen toxicity
- Drugs such as aspirin or opiates
- High altitude
- Hypothermia
- Near-drowning
- Head injury
- Emboli from blood clot, fat, or amniotic fluid
- Tumor destruction
- Pancreatitis
- Procedures such as cardiopulmonary bypass or hemodialysis
- Other insults such as hypoxia, hypotension, or cardiac arrest

The mortality in patients who develop ARDS is quite high, approaching 70 percent. While many patients die as the result of respiratory failure, many succumb to failure of several organ systems, including the liver and kidneys.

Pathophysiology

ARDS is a disorder of lung diffusion that results from increased fluid in the interstitial space. Each of the underlying conditions cited above results in the inability to maintain a proper fluid balance in the interstitial space. Severe hypotension, significant hypoxemia as the result of cardiac arrest, drowning, seizure activity or hypoventilation, high altitude exposure, environmental toxins and endotoxins released in septic shock—all can cause disruption of the alveolar-capillary membrane. Increases in pulmonary capillary permeability, destruction of the capillary lining, and increases in osmotic forces all act to draw fluid into the interstitial space and contribute to interstitial edema. This increases the thickness of the respiratory membrane and limits diffusion of oxygen. In advanced cases, fluid also accumulates in the alveoli, causing loss of surfactant, collapse of the alveolar sacs, and impaired gas exchange. This results in a significant amount of pulmonary shunting with unoxygenated blood returning to the circulation. The result is significant hypoxia.

Assessment

Specific clinical symptoms are related to the underlying cause of ARDS. For example, patients who develop ARDS as the result of sepsis will have symptoms related to their underlying infection. Determine if there is a history of prolonged hypoxia, head or chest trauma, inhalation of gases, or ascent to a high altitude without prior acclimation, all of which can suggest an underlying cause for the respiratory complaints.

With ARDS, symptoms are related to the underlying cause.

Patients with ARDS experience a gradual decline in their respiratory status. In rare cases, a seemingly healthy patient has a sudden onset of respiratory failure and hypoxia. Such a presentation is characteristic of patients with high altitude pulmonary edema (HAPE).

Dyspnea, confusion, and agitation are often found in patients with non-cardiogenic pulmonary edema. Patients may also report fatigue and reduced exercise ability. Symptoms such as orthopnea, paroxysmal nocturnal dyspnea, or sputum production are not commonly reported but may be seen.

The prominent physical findings are generally those associated with the underlying lung insult. Tachypnea and tachycardia are often found in association with ARDS. Crackles (rales) are audible in both lungs. Wheezing may also be heard if there is any element of bronchospasm. Severe tachypnea, central cyanosis, and signs of imminent respiratory failure are seen in severe cases. Pulse oximetry will demonstrate low oxygen saturations in those patients with advanced disease. In those patients requiring ventilatory support, a decreased lung compliance will be noted. (It will require more operator force to deliver an adequate lung volume.)

Management

Management of the patient's underlying medical condition is the hallmark of treatment for ARDS.

Oxygen supplementation is essential for all ARDS patients.

Specific management of the patient's underlying medical condition is the hallmark of treatment for this disorder. Treatment of gram negative sepsis with appropriate antibiotics, removal of the patient from any inciting toxin, or rapid descent to a lower altitude in patients with HAPE are the most important therapies for this condition. The patient will usually tolerate an upright position with the legs dangling off the cart.

Since the hypoxia seen in ARDS is the result of diffusion defects, oxygen supplementation is essential for all patients with this condition. Establish intravenous access, but provide fluids only if hypovolemia exists. Establish cardiac monitoring. Suctioning of lung secretions is often required to maintain airway patency.

Use positive pressure ventilation to support any ARDS patient who demonstrates signs of respiratory failure. Use bag-valve-mask ventilation for initial respiratory support but note that these patients generally require endotracheal intubation and support using a mechanical ventilator for early management. **Positive end expiratory pressure (PEEP)** is often required to maintain patency of the alveoli and adequate oxygenation. Diuretics and nitrates, which are used in patients with cardiogenic pulmonary edema, are usually not helpful in patients with ARDS. Your medical director may occasionally order corticosteroids for patients with ARDS/non-cardiogenic pulmonary edema. Corticosteroids are thought to stabilize the alveolar-capillary membrane, although clinical studies have not demonstrated any benefit to their use.

* **positive end-expiratory pressure (PEEP)** a method of holding the alveoli open by increasing expiratory pressure. Some bag-valve units used in EMS have PEEP attachments. Also EMS personnel sometimes transport patients who are on ventilators with PEEP attachments.

Maintain cardiac monitoring and pulse oximetry throughout transport of the patient. Transport patients to a facility capable of advanced hemodynamic monitoring (including Swan-Ganz catheter) and mechanical ventilation support.

OBSTRUCTIVE LUNG DISEASE

Obstructive lung disease is widespread in our society. The most common obstructive lung diseases encountered in prehospital care are asthma, emphysema, and chronic bronchitis (the last two are often discussed together as chronic obstructive pulmonary disease, or COPD). Asthma afflicts 4-5 percent of the U.S. population and COPD is found in 25 percent of all adults. Chronic bronchitis alone affects one in five adult males. Patients with COPD have a 50 percent mortality within 10 years of the diagnosis.

Content Review

OBSTRUCTIVE LUNG DISEASES
Emphysema
Chronic bronchitis
Asthma

Although asthma may have a genetic predisposition, COPD is known to be directly caused by cigarette smoking and environmental toxins. Other factors have been shown to precipitate symptoms in patients who already have obstructive airway disease. Intrinsic factors include stress, upper respiratory infections, and exercise. Extrinsic factors include tobacco smoke, drugs, occupational hazards (chemical fumes, dust, etc.), and allergens such as foods, animal danders, dusts, and molds.

Obstructive lung diseases all have abnormal ventilation as a common feature. This abnormal ventilation is a result of obstruction that occurs primarily in the bronchioles. Several changes occur within these air conduits. Bronchospasm (sustained smooth muscle contraction) occurs, which may be reversed by beta adrenergic receptor stimulation. Agents such as terbutaline, albuterol, and epinephrine are used to accomplish this stimulation. Increased mucus production by goblet cells that line the respiratory tree also contribute to obstruction. This effect may be worsened by the fact that in many patients, the cilia are destroyed, resulting in poor clearance of excess mucus. Finally, inflammation of the bronchial passages results in the accumulation of fluid and inflammatory cells. Depending on the underlying cause, some elements of bronchial obstruction are reversible, whereas others are not.

During inspiration, the bronchioles will naturally dilate, allowing air to be drawn into the alveoli. As the patient begins to exhale, the bronchioles constrict. When this natural constriction occurs—in addition to the underlying bronchospasm, increased mucus production, and inflammation that exist in patients with obstructive airway disease—the result is significant air trapping distal to the obstruction. This is one of the hallmarks of obstructive lung disease. This section will discuss each of these disease processes—emphysema, chronic bronchitis, and asthma—detailing the pathophysiology, assessment, and treatment.

EMPHYSEMA

Emphysema results from destruction of the alveolar walls distal to the terminal bronchioles. It is more common in men than in women. The major factor contributing to emphysema in our society is cigarette smoking. Significant exposure to environmental toxins is another contributing factor.

Pathophysiology

Continued exposure to noxious substances, such as cigarette smoke, results in the gradual destruction of the walls of the alveoli. This process decreases the alveolar membrane surface area, thus lessening the area available for gas exchange. The progressive loss of the respiratory membrane results in an increased ratio of air to lung tissue. The result is diffusion defects. Additionally, the number of pulmonary capillaries in the lung is decreased, thus increasing resistance to pulmonary blood flow. This condition ultimately causes pulmonary hypertension, which in turn may lead to right-heart failure, **cor pulmonale**, and death (Figure 1-21).

✱ **cor pulmonale** hypertrophy of the right ventricle resulting from disorders of the lung.

Emphysema also causes weakening of the walls of the small bronchioles. When the walls of the alveoli and small bronchioles are destroyed, the lungs lose their capacity to recoil and air becomes trapped in the lungs. Thus, residual volume increases while vital capacity remains relatively normal. The destroyed lung tissue (called *blebs*) results in alveolar collapse. To counteract this effect, patients tend to breathe through pursed lips. This creates continued positive pressure similar to PEEP (positive end-expiratory pressure) and prevents alveolar collapse.

As the disease progresses, the PaO$_2$ further decreases, which may lead to increased red blood cell production and **polycythemia** (an excess of red blood cells

✱ **polycythemia** an excess of red blood cells.

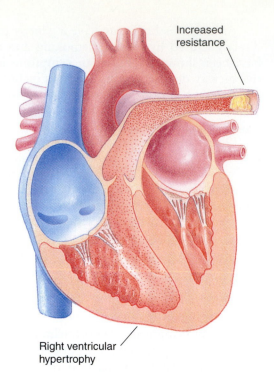

Increased resistance

Right ventricular hypertrophy

FIGURE 1-21 Chronic obstructive pulmonary disease of long standing can cause pulmonary hypertension, which in turn may lead to cor pulmonale.

resulting in an abnormally high hematocrit). The $PaCO_2$ also increases and becomes chronically elevated, forcing the body to depend upon hypoxic drive to control respirations. Finally, remember that emphysema is characterized by irreversible airway obstruction.

Patients with emphysema are more susceptible to acute respiratory infections, such as pneumonia, and to cardiac dysrhythmias. Chronic emphysema patients ultimately become dependent on bronchodilators, corticosteroids, and, in the final stages, supplemental oxygen.

Assessment

Emphysema is rarely associated with a cough except in the morning.

The patient with emphysema may report a history of recent weight loss, increased dyspnea on exertion, and progressive limitation of physical activity. Unlike chronic bronchitis, discussed in subsequent sections, emphysema is rarely associated with a cough, except in the morning. Question the patient about cigarette and tobacco usage. This is generally reported in pack/years. Ask the number of cigarette packs (20 cigarettes/pack) smoked per day and the number of years the patient has smoked. Multiply the number of packs smoked per day by the number of years. For example, a man who has smoked 2 packs per day for 15 years would have a 30 pack/year smoking history. Medical problems related to smoking, such as emphysema, chronic bronchitis, and lung cancer, usually begin after a patient surpasses a 20 pack/year history, although this can vary significantly.

Emphysema patients usually have a barrel chest, are often thin, and have a pink color ("pink puffers").

Physical exam of the emphysema patient usually reveals a barrel chest evidenced by an increase in the anterior/posterior chest diameter. You may also note decreased chest excursion with a prolonged expiratory phase and a rapid resting respiratory rate. Patients with emphysema are often thin since they must use a significant amount of their caloric intake for respiration. They tend to be pink in color due to polycythemia (excess of red blood cells) and are referred to as "pink puffers." Emphysema patients often have hypertrophy of the accessory respiratory muscles (Figure 1-22).

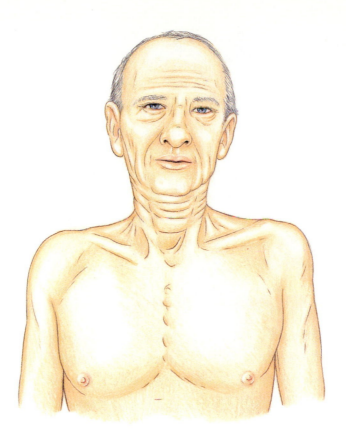

The patient will often involuntarily purse his lips to create continuous positive airway pressure. Clubbing of the fingers is common. Breath sounds are usually diminished. Wheezes and rhonchi may or may not be present, depending on the amount of obstruction to air flow. The patient may exhibit signs of right-heart failure as evidenced by jugular vein distention, peripheral edema, and hepatic congestion. Signs of severe respiratory impairment in all patients with obstructive lung disease include confusion, agitation, somnolence, 1-to-2-word dyspnea, and use of accessory muscles to assist ventilation.

Management

Although emphysema differs in the disease process from chronic bronchitis, the two respiratory disorders share several of the same symptoms and pathophysiology. As a result, you will treat the two disorders in a similar manner. The discussion of management of emphysema will be taken up with chronic bronchitis. (See next section.)

CHRONIC BRONCHITIS

Chronic bronchitis results from an increase in the number of the goblet (mucus-secreting) cells in the respiratory tree (Figure 1-23). It is characterized by the production of a large quantity of sputum. This often occurs after prolonged exposure to cigarette smoke.

Pathophysiology

Unlike emphysema, in chronic bronchitis the alveoli are not severely affected and diffusion remains normal. Gas exchange is decreased because there is lowered

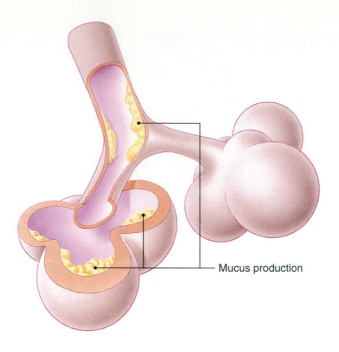

Mucus production

alveolar ventilation, which ultimately results in hypoxia and hypercarbia. Hypoxia may increase red blood cell production, which in turn leads to polycythemia (as occurs in emphysema). Increased $PaCO_2$ levels may lead to irritability, somnolence, decreased intellectual abilities, headaches, and personality changes. Physiologically, an increased $PaCO_2$ causes pulmonary vasoconstriction, resulting in pulmonary hypertension and, eventually, cor pulmonale. Unlike emphysema, the vital capacity is decreased, while the residual volume is normal or decreased.

Assessment

The patient with chronic bronchitis often will have a history of heavy cigarette smoking, but the disease may also occur in nonsmokers. There may also be a history of frequent respiratory infections. In addition, these patients usually produce considerable quantities of sputum daily. Clinically, the patient is described as having a productive cough for at least three months per year for two or more consecutive years.

Patients with chronic bronchitis tend to be overweight and can be cyanotic. Because of this, they are often referred to as "blue bloaters." This can be contrasted with the "pink puffer" image of emphysema patients described above. Auscultation of the thorax often will reveal rhonchi due to occlusion of the larger airways with mucus plugs. The patient may also exhibit signs and symptoms of right-heart failure such as jugular vein distention, ankle edema, and hepatic congestion.

Management

The primary goals in the emergency management of the patient with either emphysema or chronic bronchitis are to relieve hypoxia and reverse any bronchoconstriction that may be present. However, many of these patients are dependent upon hypoxic respiratory drive. As a result, the supplemental administration of oxygen may decrease respiratory drive and inhibit ventilation. You

Chronic bronchitis is usually associated with a productive cough and copious sputum production.

Chronic bronchitis patients tend to be overweight and are often cyanotic ("blue bloaters").

Content Review

EMPHYSEMA AND CHRONIC BRONCHITIS: MANAGEMENT GOALS
Relieve hypoxia
Reverse bronchoconstriction

must continually monitor the patient and be prepared to assist ventilations if signs of respiratory depression develop.

The first step in treating a patient suffering an exacerbation of emphysema or chronic bronchitis is to establish an airway. Then place the patient in a seated or semi-seated position to assist the accessory respiratory muscles. Apply a pulse oximeter and determine the blood oxygen saturation (SaO_2). Administer supplemental oxygen at a low flow rate while maintaining an oxygen saturation above 90 percent. A nasal cannula can often be used, but you must constantly monitor the respiratory rate and depth as well as oxygen saturation. Alternatively, you may use a Venturi mask at a low concentration (24–35 percent). If hypoxia or respiratory failure is evident, then increase the concentration of delivered oxygen. Be prepared to support the ventilation with bag-valve-mask assistance. Intubation may be required if respiratory failure is imminent.

Establish an intravenous line with lactated Ringer's or normal saline at a "to keep open" rate. More aggressive fluid administration is suggested if there are signs of dehydration present. This may also aid in loosening thick mucus secretions. Then, if ordered by medical direction, administer a bronchodilator medication, such as albuterol, metaproterenol or ipratropium bromide, through a small volume nebulizer or particle inhaler (Rotohaler). Corticosteriods are also commonly used in the early management of patients with COPD.

Administer oxygen to the COPD patient who needs it to relieve hypoxia. Since this may decrease the respiratory drive in the COPD patient, monitor the patient and be prepared to assist ventilations if necessary.

ASTHMA

Asthma is a common respiratory illness that affects many persons. Although deaths from other respiratory diseases are steadily declining, deaths from asthma have significantly increased during the last decade. Most of the increased asthma deaths have occurred in patients who are 45 years of age or older. In addition, the death rate for black asthmatics has been twice as high as for their white counterparts. Approximately 50 percent of patients who die from asthma do so before reaching the hospital. Thus, EMS personnel are frequently called upon to treat patients suffering an asthma attack. Prompt recognition followed by appropriate treatment can significantly improve the patient's condition and enhance his chance of survival.

Pathophysiology

Asthma is a chronic inflammatory disorder of the airways. In susceptible individuals, this inflammation causes symptoms usually associated with widespread but variable air flow obstruction. In addition to air flow obstruction, the airway becomes hyperresponsive. The air flow obstruction and hyperresponsiveness are often reversible with treatment. These conditions may also reverse spontaneously.

Asthma may be induced by one of many different factors. These factors, commonly referred to as "triggers" or "inducers," vary from one individual to the next. In allergic individuals, environmental allergens are a major cause of inflammation. These may occur both indoors and outdoors. In addition to allergens, asthma may be triggered by cold air, exercise, foods, irritants, stress, and certain medications. Often, a specific trigger cannot be identified. Extrinsic triggers tend predominantly to affect children, whereas intrinsic factors trigger asthma in adults.

Within minutes of exposure to the offending trigger, a two-phase reaction occurs. The first phase of the reaction is characterized by the release of chemical mediators such as histamine. These mediators cause contraction of the bronchial smooth muscle and leakage of fluid from peribronchial capillaries. This results in both bronchoconstriction and bronchial edema. These two factors can significantly decrease expiratory air flow causing the typical "asthma attack."

Often, the asthma attack will resolve spontaneously in 1–2 hours or may be aborted by the use of inhaled bronchodilator medications such as albuterol. However, within 6–8 hours after exposure to the trigger, a second reaction occurs. This late phase is characterized by inflammation of the bronchioles as cells of the immune system (eosinophils, neutrophils, and lymphocytes) invade the mucosa of the respiratory tract. This leads to additional edema and swelling of the bronchioles and a further decrease in expiratory air flow.

The second phase reaction will not typically respond to inhaled beta-agonist drugs such as metaproteranol or albuterol. Instead, anti-inflammatory agents such as corticosteroids are often required. It is important to point out that the severe inflammatory changes seen in an acute asthma attack do not develop over a few hours or even a few days. The inflammation will often begin several days or several weeks before the onset of the actual asthma attack.

Assessment

Begin the initial prehospital assessment of the asthmatic by considering immediate threats to the airway, breathing, or circulation. Then turn your attention to the focused history and physical examination.

The most common presenting symptoms of asthma are dyspnea, wheezing, and cough. Wheezing results from turbulent air flow through the inflamed and narrowed bronchioles. Many asthmatics will have a persistent cough. This is primarily due to hyperresponsiveness of the airway. It is important to point out that some asthmatics do not wheeze. Instead, their initial presentation may be a frequent and persistent cough. As asthma severity increases, the patient may exhibit hyperinflation of the chest due to trapping of air in the alveoli. In addition, tachypnea (rapid respiration) will occur. The patient may start to use accessory muscles to aid respiration.

Symptoms of a severe asthma attack include 1-to-2-word dyspnea (the inability to complete a phrase or sentence without having to stop to breathe), pulsus paradoxus (a drop of systolic blood pressure of 10 mmHg or more with inspiration), tachycardia, and decreased oxygen saturation on pulse oximetry. As hypoxia develops the patient may become agitated and anxious.

When conducting the focused history and physical examination, start by obtaining a brief patient history. Most asthmatics will report that they suffer from asthma. In addition, the patient's home medications may help confirm a history of asthma. Common asthma medications include inhaled beta-agonists (albuterol, metaproterenol), inhaled corticosteroids (betamethasone, beclomethasone), inhaled cromolyn sodium, and inhaled anticholinergics (ipratropium bromide). Often the patient will be taking oral bronchodilators such as theophylline or may be taking oral corticosteroids (prednisone).

Determine when symptoms started and what the patient has taken in an attempt to abort the attack. Also, find out whether the patient is allergic to any medications. Question the patient about hospitalizations for asthma. If the patient has been hospitalized, ask whether the patient has ever required intubation and mechanical ventilation. A prior history of intubation and mechanical ventilation should heighten your index of suspicion. Similarly, an asthmatic who is on continuous corticosteroid therapy is also a high-risk patient.

After you obtain the pertinent history, perform a brief physical examination. Place particular emphasis on the chest and neck. Examination of the chest should begin with inspection. Note any increase in the diameter of the chest that may indicate air trapping. Also, note the use of accessory muscles, including retraction of the intercostal muscles or use of the strap muscles of the neck. Following inspection, palpate the chest, noting any deformity, crepitus, or asymmetry. Next, auscultate the posterior chest. Note any abnormal breath sounds such as wheezing or rhonchi. Listen to the symmetry of breath sounds. Unilateral wheezing may indicate an aspirated foreign body or a pneumothorax.

Obtain accurate vital signs. One of the most important vital signs is the respiratory rate. An increase in the respiratory rate is one of the earliest symptoms of a respiratory problem. Many EMS personnel inaccurately measure the respiratory rate. The easiest method is to simply place your fingers on the patient's radial artery as if you were measuring the pulse rate. This will make the patient think you are obtaining the pulse rate, and he will not alter his breathing pattern. Measure the respiratory rate for at least 30 seconds. At the same time, note any alterations in the respiratory pattern. Pulse oximetry is an excellent adjunct to respiratory assessment. It will provide you with data regarding the oxygen saturation status (SaO_2) as well as an audible measure of the pulse rate.

EMS systems should be able to measure the Peak Expiratory Flow Rate (PEFR). (Review Figure 1-21 and Table 1-2.) The PEFR is a reliable indicator of air flow. If possible, measure peak flow rates to determine the severity of an asthma attack and the degree of response to treatment. The more severe the asthma attack, the lower will be the PEFR.

Management

Treatment of asthma is designed to correct hypoxia, reverse any bronchospasm, and treat the inflammatory changes associated with the disease. Administer oxygen at a high concentration (100 percent). Establish intravenous access and place the patient on an ECG monitor. Direct initial treatment at reversing any bronchospasm present. The most commonly used drugs are the inhaled beta-agonist preparations such as albuterol (Ventolin, Proventil) in conjunction with ipratropium bromide (Atrovent). These can be easily administered with a small volume, oxygen-powered nebulizer (Procedure 1-1). Monitor the patient's response to these medications by noting improvement in PEFR and pulse oximetry readings.

Many asthmatic patients will wait before summoning EMS. The longer the time interval from the onset of the asthma attack until treatment, the less likely it will be that bronchodilator medications will work. Often, after a prolonged asthma attack, the patient may become fatigued. A fatigued patient can quickly develop respiratory failure and subsequently require intubation and mechanical ventilation. Always be prepared to provide airway and respiratory support for the asthmatic.

Content Review

ASTHMA: MANAGEMENT GOALS
Correct hypoxia
Reverse bronchospasm
Reduce inflammation

Special Cases

While most cases of asthma conform to the preceding descriptions, you may run into several special cases in the field. Asthma conditions that require special concern include status asthmaticus and asthmatic attacks in children.

Status Asthmaticus *Status asthmaticus* is a severe, prolonged asthma attack that cannot be broken by repeated doses of bronchodilators. It is a serious medical emergency that requires prompt recognition, treatment, and transport. The patient suffering status asthmaticus frequently will have a greatly distended chest from continued air trapping. Breath sounds, and often wheezing, may be absent. The patient is usually exhausted, severely acidotic, and dehydrated. The management of status asthmaticus is basically the same as for asthma. *Recognize that respiratory arrest is imminent and be prepared for endotracheal intubation.* Transport immediately and continue aggressive treatment en route.

Asthma in Children Asthma in children is common. The pathophysiology and treatment are essentially the same as in adults, with altered medication dosages.

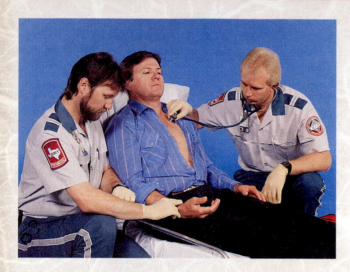

1-1a Complete the initial assessment.

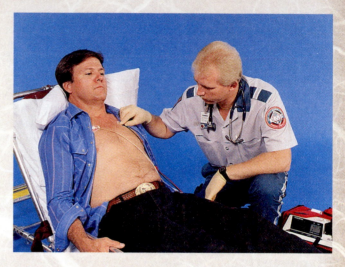

1-1b Place the patient on an ECG monitor.

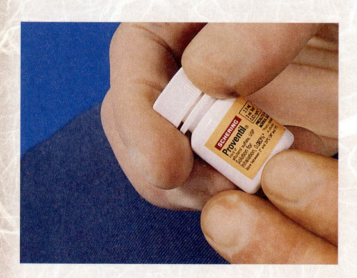

1-1c Select the desired medication.

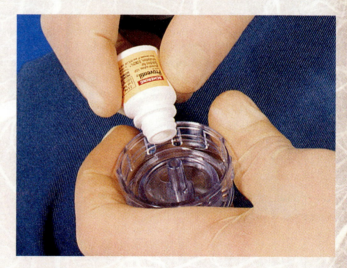

1-1d Add medication to the nebulizer.

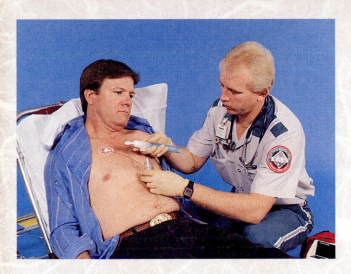

1-1e   Assemble the nebulizer and determine pre-treatment pulse rate.

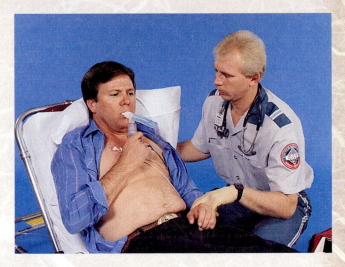

1-1f   Administer the medication.

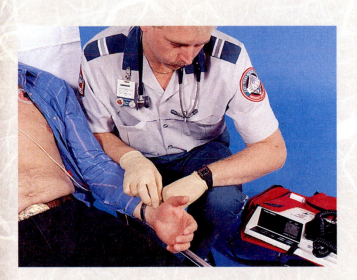

1-1g   Determine post-treatment pulse rate.

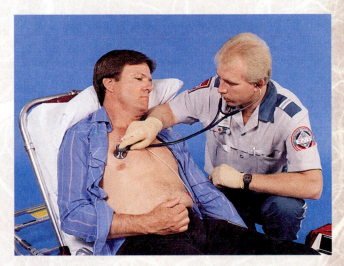

1-1h   Reassess breath sounds.

Several additional medications are used in the treatment of childhood asthma. (Asthma in children is discussed in greater detail in Volume 5, Chapter 2.)

UPPER RESPIRATORY INFECTION (URI)

Infections involving the upper airway and respiratory tract are among the most common infections for which patients seek medical attention. Although these conditions are rarely life-threatening, upper respiratory infections can make many existing pulmonary diseases worse or lead to direct pulmonary infection. The best defense against the spread of upper respiratory infection is common practices such as good hand washing and covering the mouth during coughing and sneezing. Attention to such details is important when caring for patients with underlying pulmonary disease or those who are immunosuppressed (HIV infection, cancer) because URIs are more severe in these populations. Because of the prevalence of such infections, complete protection is impossible.

Pathophysiology

Remember that the upper airway begins at the nose and mouth, passes through the pharynx and ends at the larynx. Other related structures are the paranasal sinuses and the eustachian tubes that connect the pharynx and the middle ear. In addition, several collections of lymphoid tissue found in the pharynx (palatine, pharyngeal, and lingual tonsils) produce antibodies and provide immune protection.

The vast majority of upper respiratory infections (URIs) are caused by viruses. A variety of bacteria may also produce infection of the upper respiratory tract. The most significant is Group A streptococcus, which is the causative organism in "strep throat" and accounts for up to 30 percent of URIs. This bacteria is also implicated in sinusitis and middle ear infections. Up to 50 percent of patients who have pharyngitis (inflammation of the pharynx) are not found to have a viral or bacterial cause. Fortunately, most URIs are self-limiting illnesses that resolve after several days of symptoms.

Assessment

The major symptoms of URI are dependent upon the portion of the upper respiratory tract that is predominantly affected (Table 1-3). Patients with URIs will often have accompanying symptoms such as fever, chills, myalgias (muscle pains), and fatigue.

Remember that any child with suspected epiglottitis (see Volume 5, Chapter 2) should be supported in a position of comfort. Do not attempt examination of the throat as this may produce severe laryngospasm. Adults do occasionally also develop epiglottitis, but this is generally a more benign condition.

Support the child with suspected epiglottitis in a position of comfort. Do not attempt examination of the throat, which may produce severe laryngospasm.

Management

In most cases, the diagnosis and treatment of upper respiratory conditions is based on the history and physical findings. Patients with pharyngitis are often diagnosed by obtaining a throat culture that confirms the presence of a bacterial cause of symptoms. A rapid test is also available. In patients with sinusitis and otitis media, treatment is based on a presumed bacterial cause.

As with other medical conditions, focus your attention on the patient's airway and ventilation. Generally, no intervention is required except in children with epiglottitis and in some complicated upper respiratory infections where a collection of pus may occlude the airway. Give oxygen supplementation to any patient who has underlying pulmonary disease.

In URI, as with other medical conditions, focus attention on the patient's airway and ventilation. Give supplemental oxygen to any patient with underlying pulmonary disease.

Table 1-3   LOCATIONS AND SIGNS AND SYMPTOMS OF UPPER RESPIRATORY INFECTIONS

Structure	Infection	Symptoms	Signs
Nose	Rhinitis	Runny nose, congestion, sneezing	Rhinorrhea
Pharynx	Pharyngitis	Sore throat, pain on swallowing	Erythematous pharynx, tonsil enlargement, pus on tonsils, cervical lymph node enlargement
Middle Ear	Otitis Media	Ear pain, decreased hearing	Red, bulging eardrum, pus behind ear drum, lymph node enlargement in front of or behind ear
Larynx	Laryngitis	Sore throat, hoarseness, pain on speaking	Red pharynx, hoarse quality to voice, cervical lymph node enlargement
Epiglottis	Epiglottitis	Sore throat, drooling, ill appearing	Upright position, drooling, ill appearing
Sinuses	Sinusitis	Headache, congestion	Tenderness over the sinuses, worsening of pain with leaning forward, yellow nasal discharge

Most upper respiratory infections are treated symptomatically. Acetaminophen or ibuprofen is prescribed for fever, headache, and myalgias. Encourage patients to drink plenty of fluids. Salt water gargles may be used for throat discomfort. Decongestants and antihistamines may be used to reduce mucus secretion. Encourage patients being treated with antibiotics for bacterial causes of URI to continue these agents.

In some patients with asthma or COPD, a URI may produce a worsening of their underlying medical condition. Use inhaled bronchodilators and corticosteroid agents according to local protocols or on advice of medical direction. Transport patients with underlying medical conditions to a health care facility capable of continued evaluation and management of the underlying condition. Continue appropriate monitoring with pulse oximetry and ECG during transport.

PNEUMONIA

Pneumonia is an infection of the lungs and a common medical problem, especially in the aged and those infected with the human immunodeficiency virus (HIV). In fact, pneumonia is one of the leading causes of death in both groups of patients and is the fifth leading overall cause of death in the U.S.

Patients with HIV infection and those on immune suppressive therapy (cancer patients) are at high risk of developing pneumonia. In addition, the very young and very old are at higher risk of acquiring pneumonia because of ineffective protective mechanisms. Other risk factors include a history of alcoholism, cigarette smoking, and exposure to cold temperatures.

Pathophysiology

Pneumonia is a collection of related respiratory diseases caused when a variety of infectious agents invade the lungs. Earlier in this chapter, you learned about the roles of mucus production and the action of respiratory tract cilia in protecting the body against bacterial invasion. When considering which patients are at risk, the unifying concept is that there is a defect in mucus production, ciliary action, or both.

Bacterial and viral pneumonias are the most frequent, although fungal and other forms of pneumonia do exist. More unusual forms of pneumonia are seen in those patients who are currently or recently have been hospitalized where they are exposed to a more unusual variety of microorganisms. This is referred to as hospital-acquired pneumonia. (Cases that develop in the out-of-hospital setting are described as community-acquired pneumonia.)

The infection begins in one part of the lung and often spreads to nearby alveoli. The infection may ultimately involve the entire lung. As the disease progresses, fluid and inflammatory cells collect in the alveoli, and alveolar collapse may occur. Pneumonia is primarily a ventilation disorder. Occasionally, the infection will extend beyond the lungs into the bloodstream and to more distant sites in the body. This systemic spread may lead to septic shock.

Assessment

A patient with pneumonia will generally appear ill. He may report a recent history of fever and chills. These chills are commonly described as "bed shaking." There is usually a generalized weakness and malaise. The patient will tend to complain of a deep, productive cough and may expel yellow to brown sputum, often streaked with blood. Many cases involve associated **pleuritic** chest pain. Therefore, pneumonia should be considered in any patient who presents complaining of chest pain, especially if accompanied by fever and/or chills. In pneumonia involving the lower lobes of the lungs, a patient may complain of nothing more than upper abdominal pain.

Physical examination will commonly reveal fever, tachypnea, tachycardia, and a cough. Respiratory distress may be present. Auscultation of the chest usually demonstrates crackles (rales) in the involved lung segment, although wheezes or rhonchi may be heard. There usually is decreased air movement in the areas filled with infection. Percussion of the chest may reveal dullness over these areas. *Egophony* (a change in the spoken "E" sound to an "A" sound on auscultation) may also be noted.

In the forms of pneumonia involving viral, fungal, and rare bacterial causes, the typical symptoms described above are not seen. Instead, these patients may report a non-productive cough with less prominent lung findings. Systemic symptoms such as headache, malaise, fatigue, muscle aches, sore throat, and abdominal complaints including nausea, vomiting, and diarrhea are more prominent. Fever and chills are not as impressive as in bacterial pneumonia.

Management

Pneumonia is generally diagnosed on the basis of physical examination, X-ray findings, and laboratory cultures. Therefore, diagnosis in the field is unlikely. The primary treatment is antibiotics to which the causative organism is susceptible. In the field, however, antibiotics are not indicated and treatment is purely supportive.

Place the patient in a comfortable position, and administer high-flow oxygen. Use pulse oximetry to assess the patient's oxygen requirements. In severe cases, ventilatory assistance is needed and endotracheal intubation may be required. Establish intravenous access and base fluid resuscitation on the patient's hydration status. Administering fluids for dehydration is appropriate, but over-hydration can also worsen the respiratory condition. Medical direction may

---

* pleuritic sharp or tearing, as a description of pain.

Consider pneumonia in any patient complaining of chest pain, especially if accompanied by fever and/or chills.

Field management of suspected pneumonia is purely supportive. Place the patient in a position of comfort and administer high-flow oxygen.

sometimes order a breathing treatment with a beta agonist, particularly if wheezing is present. Because patients with pneumonia often have some bronchospasm, these drugs will afford the patient some symptomatic relief. Give antipyretic agents such as acetaminophen or ibuprofen to reduce a high fever. Also, a cool, moistened wash cloth may soothe the patient.

Remember to be extremely careful when caring for the patient over age 65 with suspected pneumonia. These patients have high mortality and complication rates. Transport them to a facility capable of handling the significant complications associated with the disease for this population.

LUNG CANCER

Lung cancer (neoplasm) is the leading cause of cancer-related death in the U.S. in both men and women. Most patients with lung cancer are between the ages of 55 and 65 years. There is a high mortality rate for patients with lung cancer after only one year with the disease.

There are currently four major types of lung cancer based on the predominant cell type. Twenty percent of cases involve only the lung tissue. Another 35 percent involve spread to the lymphatic system, and 45 percent have distant metastases (cancer cells spreading to other tissues). In those cases where there is lung tissue invasion, the primary problem is disruption of diffusion. In some larger cancers, there may also be alterations in ventilation by obstruction of the conducting bronchioles.

Cigarette smoking has long been known to be a risk factor for development of lung cancer. Environmental exposure to asbestos, hydrocarbons, radiation, and fumes from metal production have also been identified as risk factors. Finally, home exposure to radon has been implicated in the development of lung cancer. Preventive strategies include educating teenagers about the dangers of cigarette smoking and encouraging current smokers to quit. Implementing environmental safety standards that reduce the risk of exposure to such substances as asbestos will also reduce the risk of lung cancer. Finally, cancer screening of populations at risk is encouraged.

Pathophysiology

Although cancers that start elsewhere in the body can spread to the lungs, the vast majority of lung cancers are caused by carcinogens (cancer-producing substances) from cigarette smoking. A small portion of lung cancers are caused by inhalation of occupational agents such as asbestos and arsenic. These substances irritate and adversely affect the various tissues of the lung, ultimately leading to the development of abnormal (cancerous) cells.

There are four major types of lung cancers depending upon the type of lung tissue involved. The most common type of lung cancer is referred to as *adenocarcinoma*. This cancer arises from glandular-type (i.e. mucus-producing) cells found in the lungs and bronchioles. The next most frequently encountered type of lung cancer is *small cell carcinoma* (also called "oat cell" carcinoma). Small cell carcinoma arises from bronchial tissues. The third type of lung cancer is referred to as *epidermoid carcinoma*. Finally, *large cell carcinoma* is the fourth major type of lung cancer. Like small cell carcinoma, epidermoid and large cell carcinomas typically arise from the bronchial tissues. Lung cancers generally have a bad prognosis with most patients dying within a year of the diagnosis.

Assessment

As with other respiratory diseases, your first priority is to address signs of severe respiratory distress. Look for altered mental status, 1-to-2-word dyspnea, cyanosis, hemoptysis, and hypoxia as documented by pulse oximeter. Severe uncontrolled hemoptysis can be a particularly life-threatening presentation.

Patients with lung cancer will present with a variety of complaints, depending on whether they are related to direct lung involvement, invasion of local structures, or metastatic spread. Patients with localized disease will present with cough, dyspnea, hoarseness, vague chest pain, and hemoptysis. Fever, chills, and pleuritic chest pain are seen in patients who develop pneumonia. Symptoms related to local invasion include pain on swallowing (dysphagia), weakness or numbness in the arm, and shoulder pain. Metastatic symptoms are related to the area of spread and include headache, seizures, bone pain, abdominal pain, nausea, and malaise.

Physical findings are non-specific. Patients with advanced disease have profound weight loss and cachexia (general physical wasting and malnutrition). Crackles (rales), rhonchi, wheezes, and diminished breath sounds may be heard in the affected lung. Venous distention in the arms and neck may be present if there is occlusion of the superior vena cava (called *superior vena cava syndrome*).

Management

Administer supplemental oxygen as needed based on the clinical status and pulse oximetry measurement. Support the patient's ventilation as needed and intubate as necessary. Be attentive, however, for any Do Not Resuscitate order or other advance directive, such as a living will, and follow your local protocol regarding these legal instruments. Consult medical direction if questions arise.

Initiate an IV of 0.9% normal saline and provide fluids if signs of dehydration are present. Follow your local protocol regarding the access of permanent indwelling catheters that many cancer victims have in place.

Out-of-hospital drug therapy consists of bronchodilator agents and corticosteroids when signs of obstructive lung disease are present. Continue any prescribed antibiotics. Transport the patient and monitor mental status, vital signs, and oxygen status, as appropriate. Be prepared to provide emotional support for both the patient and family during transport.

TOXIC INHALATION

Inhalation of toxic substances into the respiratory tract can cause pain, inflammation, or destruction of pulmonary tissues. Significant inhalations can affect the ability of the alveoli to exchange oxygen, thus resulting in hypoxemia.

Pathophysiology

The possibility of inhalation of products toxic to the respiratory system should be considered in any dyspneic patient. Causes of toxic inhalation include superheated air, toxic products of combustion, chemical irritants, and inhalation of steam. Each of these agents can result in upper airway obstruction due to edema and laryngospasm. In such cases, bronchospasm and lower-airway edema may additionally appear. In severe inhalations, disruption of the alveolar/capillary membranes may result in life-threatening pulmonary edema.

Assessment

When assessing the patient with possible toxic inhalation exposure, determine the nature of the inhalant or the combusted material. Several products can result in the formation of corrosive acids or alkalis that irritate and damage the airway. These include:

- Ammonia (ammonium hydroxide)
- Nitrogen oxide (nitric acid)
- Sulfur dioxide (sulphurous acid)
- Sulfur trioxide (sulfuric acid)
- Chlorine (hydrochloric acid)

It is also crucial to determine the duration of the exposure, whether the patient was in an enclosed area at the time of the exposure, or if he experienced a loss of consciousness. Loss of consciousness may cause the airway to became vulnerable as a result of the loss of airway protective mechanisms.

During physical examination, pay particular attention to the face, mouth, and throat. Note any burns or particulate matter. Next, auscultate the chest for the presence of any wheezes or crackles (rales). Wheezing may indicate bronchospasm, while crackles may suggest pulmonary edema.

Management

After assuring the safety of rescue personnel, remove the patient from the hazardous environment. Next, establish and maintain an open airway. Remember that the airway is often irritable and attempts at endotracheal intubation may result in laryngospasm, completely obstructing the airway. Laryngeal edema, as evidenced by hoarseness, brassy cough, and stridor is ominous and may require prompt endotracheal intubation. Administer humidified oxygen at high concentration. As a precaution, start an IV of a crystalloid solution to provide rapid venous access. Transport promptly.

CARBON MONOXIDE INHALATION

Carbon monoxide is an odorless, tasteless, colorless gas produced from the incomplete burning of fossil fuels and other carbon-containing compounds. Carbon monoxide can be encountered in industrial sites, such as mines and factories. It is present in the environment in various concentrations primarily because of automotive exhaust emissions. Most poisonings occur from automobile emissions and home-heating devices used in poorly ventilated areas. Carbon monoxide is often used in suicide attempts. In addition, it is a particular hazard for fire-fighters and rescue personnel.

Pathophysiology

Carbon monoxide exposure is potentially life-threatening because it easily binds to the hemoglobin molecule. It has an affinity for hemoglobin 200 times that of oxygen. Once bound, receptor sites on the hemoglobin can no longer transport oxygen to the peripheral tissues. The result is hypoxia at the cellular level and, ultimately, metabolic acidosis. Additionally, carbon monoxide binds to iron-containing enzymes within the cells, leading to worsening cellular acidosis.

When assessing the patient with possible toxic inhalation, determine the nature of the inhalant or combusted material.

Content Review

TOXIC INHALATION: MANAGEMENT SEQUENCE

Assure safety of rescue personnel

Remove patient from toxic environment

Maintain an open airway

Provide humidified, high concentration oxygen.

Assessment

With carbon-monoxide poisoning, determine the source of exposure, its length, and the location.

When confronted by a patient suffering possible carbon-monoxide poisoning, determine the source of exposure, its length, and the location. Less time is required to develop a significant exposure in a closed space compared to one in an area that is fairly well ventilated.

Signs and symptoms of carbon-monoxide poisoning include headache, nausea and vomiting, confusion, agitation, loss of coordination, chest pain, loss of consciousness, and even seizures. On physical examination, the skin may be cyanotic or it may be bright cherry red (a very late finding). There may be other signs of hypoxia such as peripheral cyanosis or confusion.

Management

Content Review

CARBON MONOXIDE INHALATION: MANAGEMENT SEQUENCE

Assure safety of rescue personnel

Remove patient from exposure site

Maintain an open airway

Provide high concentration oxygen.

Upon detection of carbon monoxide poisoning, first assure the safety of rescue personnel, then remove the patient from the site of exposure. Assure and maintain the airway. Administer supplemental oxygen at the highest possible concentration. If the patient is breathing spontaneously, apply a *tight-fitting* nonrebreather mask. If respiratory depression is noted, assist respirations. If shock is present, treat. Prompt transport is essential.

Hyperbaric oxygen therapy may be used in the treatment of severe carbon monoxide poisoning. Many EMS systems have protocols established whereby patients suffering carbon monoxide poisoning are transported to hospitals with hyperbaric oxygen therapy facilities. Hyperbaric oxygen increases the PaO_2, thus promoting increased oxygen uptake and displacement of the carbon monoxide from the hemoglobin.

PULMONARY EMBOLISM

A pulmonary embolism is a blood clot (thrombus) or some other particle that lodges in a pulmonary artery, effectively blocking blood flow through that vessel. This condition is potentially life threatening because it can significantly decrease pulmonary blood flow, thus leading to hypoxemia (inadequate levels of oxygen in the blood). Pulmonary thromboembolism accounts for 50,000 deaths annually in the U.S. In fact, one in five cases of sudden death are caused by pulmonary emboli. The great majority of patients with pulmonary emboli survive; only one in ten cases of documented pulmonary emboli result in death.

The incidence of pulmonary emboli is increased in certain populations. Any condition that results in immobility of the extremities can increase the risk of thromboembolism. Such conditions include recent surgery, long-bone fractures (with immobilization in casts or splints), bedridden condition, or prolonged immobilization as with long distance travel. Venous pooling that occurs during pregnancy can also lead to pulmonary emboli. Certain disease states increase the likelihood of blood clot formation. These include cancer, infections, thrombophlebitis, atrial fibrillation, and sickle cell anemia. Also, the incidence of thromboembolic disease is increased in patients taking oral birth control pills, particularly among smokers.

Pathophysiology

Sources of pulmonary emboli include air embolism, such as can occur during the placement of a central line; fat embolism, which can occur following a fracture; amniotic fluid embolism; and blood clots. It is also possible for a foreign body (such as part of a venous catheter) to become dislodged in the venous circulation. The vast majority of cases, however, are caused by blood clots that develop in the deep venous system of the lower extremities.

As a rule, a significant amount of blood passes through the veins of the lower extremity. During normal use of our legs, muscular contractions propel the blood through the venous system with the aid of valves that are present in the lower extremity veins. This action prevents blood from flowing backward through the venous system. When there is infection, venous injury, or any other condition that leads to pooling of blood in the deep veins of the lower extremity, clot formation occurs. If a portion of the clot becomes dislodged, it will pass through the right side of the heart and become lodged in the pulmonary vasculature.

When a pulmonary embolism occurs, the blockage of blood flow through the affected artery causes the right heart to pump against increased resistance. This results in an increase in pulmonary capillary pressure. The area of the lung supplied by the occluded pulmonary vessel can no longer effectively function in gas exchange since it receives no effective blood supply. The major derangement in patients with pulmonary emboli is a perfusion disorder. The involved lung segment is still ventilated, producing a ventilation-perfusion mismatch.

Assessment

Signs and symptoms of a patient suffering a pulmonary embolism will vary, depending upon the size and location of the obstruction. The patient suffering acute pulmonary embolism may report a sudden onset of severe unexplained dyspnea, which may or may not be associated with pleuritic chest pain. The patient may also report a cough which is usually not productive but may occasionally produce blood (hemoptysis). There may be a recent history of immobilization such as hip fracture, surgery, or debilitating illness.

The patient with acute pulmonary embolism may have a sudden onset of severe unexplained dyspnea, with or without pleuritic chest pain.

The physical examination may reveal labored breathing, tachypnea, and tachycardia. In massive pulmonary emboli, there may be signs of right-heart failure such as jugular venous distention and, in some cases, falling blood pressure. In many cases, auscultation of the chest may reveal no significant lung findings, although rare crackles (rales) and wheezing may be noted. Occasionally, a pleural friction rub (leathery sound heard with inspiration) may be heard.

Always examine the extremities. In up to 50 percent of cases, findings suggestive of deep venous thrombosis will be evident. These include a warm, swollen extremity with a thick cord palpated along the medial thigh and pain upon palpation or when extending the calf.

With suspected pulmonary embolism, always examine the extremities. In up to 50 percent of cases, findings suggestive of deep venous thrombosis will be evident.

In extreme cases, the patient may present with extreme confusion as the result of hypoxia, severe cyanosis, profound hypotension, and even cardiac arrest. Physical examination may reveal petechiae (small hemorrhagic spots) on the arms and chest wall in these cases.

Management

As with all respiratory conditions, your first priorities are the airway, breathing, and circulation. Remember that a large pulmonary embolism may lead to cardiac arrest. Perform CPR if needed.

If you suspect a patient is suffering a pulmonary embolism, establish and maintain an airway. Assist ventilations as required. Administer supplemental oxygen at the highest possible concentration. Endotracheal intubation may be required.

With pulmonary embolism, as with all respiratory conditions, your first priorities are the airway, breathing, and circulation. Remember that a large pulmonary embolism may lead to cardiac arrest. Be prepared to perform CPR if needed.

Establish an IV of lactated Ringer's or normal saline at a "to keep open" rate. The diagnosis of pulmonary embolism is often difficult and requires a high index of suspicion. Remember that patients with suspected pulmonary embolism may require a significant amount of care. This disorder has a high complication rate and a significant mortality. Carefully monitor the patient's vital signs and cardiac rhythm. Quickly transport the patient to a facility with the capabilities to care for the critical needs of the patient. Treatment in the hospital setting may include the use of various medications such as thrombolytic agents and blood thinners like heparin.

SPONTANEOUS PNEUMOTHORAX

A **spontaneous pneumothorax** is defined as a pneumothorax that occurs in the absence of blunt or penetrating trauma. Spontaneous pneumothorax is a common clinical condition, with 18 cases occurring for every 100,000 population. There is also a high recurrence rate. Fifty percent of patients will have a recurrent episode within two years.

There is a 5:1 ratio of male to female patients with spontaneous pneumothorax. Other risk factors include a tall, thin stature and a history of cigarette smoking. This disorder tends to develop in patients between the ages of 20 and 40 years. Patients with COPD have a higher incidence of spontaneous pneumothorax, presumably because of the presence of thinned lung tissue (blebs) that may rupture.

Pathophysiology

The primary derangement is one of ventilation as the negative pressure that normally exists in the pleural space is lost. This prevents proper expansion of the lung in concert with the chest wall. A pneumothorax occupying 15–20 percent of the chest cavity is generally well tolerated by the patient unless there is significant underlying lung disease.

Assessment

The patient with a spontaneous pneumothorax presents with a sudden onset of sharp, pleuritic chest or shoulder pain. Often, the symptoms are precipitated by coughing or lifting. Dyspnea is commonly reported. The degree of symptoms is not strictly related to the size of the pneumothorax.

The physical examination is usually not impressive. Decreased breath sounds on the involved side may be difficult to note. They may be best heard at the lung apex. Even more subtle is hyper-resonance to percussion of the chest. Occasionally, the patient may have subcutaneous emphysema, which may be palpated as a crackling under the skin overlying the chest. Tachypnea, diaphoresis, and pallor are also seen. Cyanosis is rarely found.

Management

Use the patient's symptoms and pulse oximetry readings as guides to therapy. For most cases of spontaneous pneumothorax, supplemental oxygen is all that is required. Ventilatory support and endotracheal intubation are rarely required.

Be very careful when managing patients with a spontaneous pneumothorax who require positive pressure ventilation by mask or endotracheal tube. They are at risk for the development of a *tension pneumothorax*. You may note that the patient will become physically difficult to ventilate. Hypoxia, cyanosis, and hy-

---

Pulmonary embolism has a high complication rate and significant mortality. Carefully monitor vital signs and cardiac rhythm. Transport to a facility with the capability of caring for the critical needs of the patient.

✱ spontaneous pneumothorax a pneumothorax (collection of air in the pleural space) that occurs spontaneously, in the absence of blunt or penetrating trauma.

The patient with a spontaneous pneumothorax will have a sudden onset of pleuritic chest or shoulder pain, often precipitated by coughing or lifting.

Most cases of spontaneous pneumothorax require only supplemental oxygen.

Be careful when ventilating a patient with suspected spontaneous pneumothorax. Too much pressure may result in a tension pneumothorax.

---

potension may also develop. In addition to the usual signs of a pneumothorax, the patient will develop jugular vein distention and deviation of the trachea away from the pneumothorax. Needle decompression of a tension pneumothorax may be required.

Other management measures should include placing the patient in a position of comfort. Reserve intravenous access and electrocardiographic monitoring for patients with significant symptoms or severe underlying respiratory disease. Carefully monitor such patients during transport.

HYPERVENTILATION SYNDROME

Hyperventilation syndrome is characterized by rapid breathing, chest pains, numbness, and other symptoms usually associated with anxiety or a situational reaction. However, as shown in Table 1-4, many serious medical problems can cause hyperventilation. To avoid improper treatment, consider hyperventilation to be indicative of a serious medical problem until proven otherwise.

Consider hyperventilation indicative of a serious medical problem until proven otherwise.

Pathophysiology

Hyperventilation syndrome frequently occurs in anxious patients. The patient often senses that he cannot "catch his breath." The patient will then begin to breathe rapidly. Hyperventilation in a purely anxious patient results in the excess elimination of CO_2, causing a respiratory alkalosis. This increases the amount of bound calcium, producing a relative hypocalcemia. This results in cramping of the muscles of the feet and hands, which is called *carpopedal spasm*.

Assessment

With a hyperventilating patient, you may elicit a history of fatigue, nervousness, dizziness, dyspnea, chest pain, and numbness and tingling around the mouth, hands, and feet. The physical examination will reveal an anxious patient with tachypnea and tachycardia. As noted above, spasm of the fingers and feet may also be present. If the patient has a history of seizure disorder,

Table 1-4	CAUSES OF HYPERVENTILATION SYNDROME
Acidosis	Interstitial pneumonitis, fibrosis, edema
Beta-adrenergic agonists	Metabolic disorders
Bronchial asthma	Methyxanthine derivatives
Cardiovascular disorders	Neurologic disorders
Central nervous system infection or tumors	Pain
Congestive heart failure	Pregnancy
Drugs	Pneumonia
Fever, sepsis	Progesterone
Hepatic failure	Psychogenic or anxiety hypertension
High altitude	Pulmonary disease
Hypotension	Pulmonary emboli, vascular disease
Hypoxia	Salicylate

the hyperventilation episode may precipitate a seizure. Other symptoms are related to the underlying cause of the hyperventilation syndrome.

Management

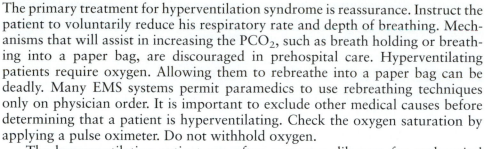
The primary treatment for hyperventilation syndrome is reassurance. Instruct the patient to voluntarily reduce his respiratory rate and depth of breathing. Mechanisms that will assist in increasing the PCO_2, such as breath holding or breathing into a paper bag, are discouraged in prehospital care. Hyperventilating patients require oxygen. Allowing them to rebreathe into a paper bag can be deadly. Many EMS systems permit paramedics to use rebreathing techniques only on physician order. It is important to exclude other medical causes before determining that a patient is hyperventilating. Check the oxygen saturation by applying a pulse oximeter. Do not withhold oxygen.

The hyperventilating patient can often present a dilemma for prehospital personnel. Although anxiety is the most common cause of hyperventilation, other more serious diseases can present in exactly the same manner. For example, pulmonary embolism or acute myocardial infarction can exhibit symptoms similar to hyperventilation syndrome.

CENTRAL NERVOUS SYSTEM DYSFUNCTION

Except in the case of drug overdose or massive stroke, central nervous system dysfunction is rarely the cause of respiratory emergencies.

Central nervous system dysfunction, with the exception of drug overdose and massive stroke, is a relatively rare cause of respiratory emergencies. However, always consider the possibility of central nervous system dysfunction in any dyspneic patient.

Pathophysiology

Central nervous system dysfunction can be a causative factor in respiratory depression and arrest. Causes include head trauma, stroke, brain tumors, and various drugs. Several medications, such as narcotics and barbiturates, make the respiratory centers in the brain less responsive to increases in $PaCO_2$. These agents also depress areas of the brain responsible for initiating respirations.

Assessment

The assessment of patients with central nervous system dysfunction should follow the same approach as for any respiratory emergency. However, you should be alert for non-respiratory system problems such as CNS trauma or drug ingestion. Be careful to note any variation in the respiratory pattern, which can be an indication of central nervous system dysfunction.

Management

With suspected central nervous system dysfunction, establish and maintain an open airway. If respiratory depression is noted or respirations are absent, initiate mechanical ventilation with supplemental oxygen and establish an IV of normal saline at a "to keep open" rate.

If central nervous system dysfunction is suspected, establish and maintain an open airway. If respiratory depression is noted or if respirations are absent, initiate mechanical ventilation. Administer supplemental oxygen, and establish an

IV of normal saline at a "to keep open" rate. Direct specific therapy at the underlying problem, if it is known.

DYSFUNCTION OF THE SPINAL CORD, NERVES, OR RESPIRATORY MUSCLES

Several disease processes can affect the spinal cord, nerves, and/or respiratory muscles. Dysfunction of these structures can lead to hypoventilation and progressive hypoxemia.

Pathophysiology

Numerous disorders can interfere with respiratory function. These include spinal cord trauma, polio, amyotrophic lateral sclerosis (ALS or Lou Gehrig's Disease), and myasthenia gravis. Viral infections, in certain cases, can cause dysfunction of the nervous system. An example of this is *Guillian-Barré Syndrome (GBS)*. In GBS, the myelin-covering of the nerve is damaged resulting in relative loss of nerve impulse conduction. This affects virtually every peripheral nerve. Approximately 30% of patients with GBS will require ventilatory assistance, as the nerves that stimulate respiration are impaired.

Certain tumors can impinge on the spinal cord, depressing respiratory function. These disorders result in an inability of the respiratory muscles to contract normally, thus causing hypoventilation. Tidal volume and minute volume are decreased. You should also be aware that patients with these disorders do not have the ability to generate an adequate cough reflex and as a result, are at risk of developing pneumonia.

Disorders that affect the spinal cord, nerves, or respiratory muscles and can interfere with respiratory function include spinal cord trauma, polio, ALS, myasthenia gravis, and tumors that impinge on the spinal cord.

Assessment

Patients with possible dysfunction of the spinal cord, nerves, or respiratory muscles may have a history of trauma that is not readily apparent. Always question the patient about injuries or falls. If there is any doubt about a possible injury, act accordingly and immobilize the cervical spine. Also, inquire about signs of symptoms that may suggest a problem with the peripheral nerves. These include such findings as numbness, pain, or sensory dysfunction. The assessment of patients with possible dysfunction of the spinal cord, nerves, or respiratory muscles should follow the same approach as for any respiratory emergency. However, be alert for subtle findings that may indicate a problem with the peripheral nervous system. Always be ready to protect the airway and support ventilation if the patient has symptoms of possible airway obstruction or respiratory failure.

Management

Management of spinal cord and respiratory muscle dysfunction is purely supportive. Establish an airway, and provide ventilatory support. If myasthenia gravis is present and if transport time is long, the physician may request the administration of one of several agents effective in treating such patients.

Management of spinal cord and respiratory muscle dysfunction is purely supportive.

SUMMARY

No matter the underlying cause of respiratory dysfunction, the primary treatment is to establish and maintain the airway, administer oxygen, and assist ventilations as required.

Respiratory emergencies are commonly encountered in prehospital care. It is important to recognize that all respiratory disorders may produce derangements in ventilation, perfusion, or diffusion. Recognition and treatment must be prompt. Understanding the underlying cause of the respiratory disorder can guide therapy. The primary treatment is to correct hypoxia. Necessary steps include establishing and maintaining the airway, assisting ventilations as required, and administering supplemental oxygen. Appropriate pharmacological agents may be subsequently ordered by medical direction.

YOU MAKE THE CALL

You and your partner respond to the scene of a 69-year-old male patient who is reported to have difficulty breathing. Once you are sure the scene is safe, you enter and find a very dyspneic patient breathing 56 times per minute. His pulse is strong and rapid at 140 beats per minute. He is using accessory muscles and has cyanosis about the lips and fingers. The patient is confused. His wife states that he has both COPD and lung cancer and reports that he has been a very heavy smoker up until the last few months. He has also had an increasing cough and fever over the past few days. The patient's initial pulse oximetry reading is 82 percent.

1. What pathophysiologic abnormality of the respiratory system do you suspect?
2. How would you initially manage this patient?
3. Why is the finding of cough and fever significant in this patient?

See Suggested Responses at the back of this book.

FURTHER READING

Dalton, A.L., D. Limmer, J.J. Mistovich, H.A. Werman. "Dyspnea" in *Advanced Medical Life Support*. Upper Saddle River, N.J.: Brady/Prentice Hall, 1999.

Marieb, E.N., ed. "The Respiratory System." In *Human Anatomy and Physiology*. 4th edition. Addison Wesley, 1999.

Seely, R.R., T.D. Stephens, and P. Tate, eds. *Respiratory System in Anatomy and Physiology*. 3rd Ed. Saint Louis: Mosby, 1995.

Thibodeau, G.A., K.T. Patton, eds. "Anatomy of the Respiratory System and Physiology of the Respiratory System." In *Anatomy and Physiology*. 3rd edition. Saint Louis: Mosby, 1996.

ON THE WEB

Visit Brady's Paramedic Website at www.bradybooks.com/paramedic.

CHAPTER 2

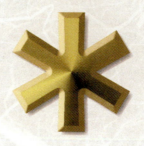

Cardiology

Objectives

Part 1: Cardiovascular Anatomy and Physiology, ECG Monitoring, and Dysrhythmia Analysis (begins on p. 69)

After reading Part 1 of this chapter, you should be able to:

1. Describe the incidence, morbidity, and mortality of cardiovascular disease. (pp. 68, 258)
2. Discuss prevention strategies that may reduce the morbidity and mortality of cardiovascular disease. (p. 68)
3. Identify the risk factors most predisposing to coronary artery disease. (p. 68)
4. Describe the anatomy of the heart, including the position in the thoracic cavity, layers of the heart, chambers of the heart, and location and function of cardiac valves. (pp. 70–75)
5. Identify the major structures of the vascular system, the factors affecting venous return, the components of cardiac output, and the phases of the cardiac cycle. (pp. 76–78)
6. Define preload, afterload, and left ventricular end-diastolic pressure and relate each to the pathophysiology of heart failure. (p. 78)

Continued

Objectives Continued

7. Identify the arterial blood supply to any given area of the myocardium. (p. 75)

8. Compare and contrast the coronary arterial distribution to the major portions of the cardiac conduction system. (pp. 75, 78–80)

9. Identify the structure and course of all divisions and subdivisions of the cardiac conduction system. (pp. 78–84)

10. Identify and describe how the heart's pacemaking control, rate, and rhythm are determined. (pp. 78–84)

11. Explain the physiological basis of conduction delay in the AV node. (pp. 83–84)

12. Define the functional properties of cardiac muscle. (pp. 77–84)

13. Define the events comprising electrical potential. (pp. 77–84)

14. List the most important ions involved in myocardial action potential and their primary function in this process. (p. 82)

15. Describe the events involved in the steps from excitation to contraction of cardiac muscle fibers. (pp. 77–84)

16. Describe the clinical significance of Starling's law. (p. 78)

17. Identify the structures of the autonomic nervous system and their effect on heart rate, rhythm, and contractility. (pp. 78–80)

18. Define and give examples of positive and negative inotropism, chronotropism, and dromotropism. (p. 80)

19. Discuss the pathophysiology of cardiac disease and injury. (pp. 97–157)

20. Explain the purpose of ECG monitoring and its limitations. (p. 84)

21. Correlate the electrophysiological and hemodynamic events occurring throughout the entire cardiac cycle with the various ECG wave forms, segments, and intervals. (pp. 88–95)

22. Identify how heart rates, durations, and amplitudes may be determined from ECG recordings. (pp. 88–95)

23. Relate the cardiac surfaces or areas represented by the ECG leads. (p. 85)

24. Differentiate among the primary mechanisms responsible for producing cardiac dysrhythmias. (pp. 94–95, 97–157)

25. Describe a systematic approach to the analysis and interpretation of cardiac dysrhythmias. (pp. 95–97)

26. Describe the dysrhythmias originating in the sinus node, the AV junction, the atria, and the ventricles. (pp. 99–157)

27. Describe the process and pitfalls of differentiating wide QRS complex tachycardias. (pp. 144–145)

28. Describe the conditions of pulseless electrical activity. (pp. 154–155)

29. Describe the phenomena of reentry, aberration, and accessory pathways. (pp. 98, 115, 157)

30. Identify the ECG changes characteristically produced by electrolyte imbalances and specify their clinical implications. (p. 157)

31. Identify patient situations where ECG rhythm analysis is indicated. (pp. 97–157)

32. Recognize the ECG changes that may reflect evidence of myocardial ischemia and injury and their limitations. (pp. 94–95)

33. Correlate abnormal ECG findings with clinical interpretation. (pp. 97–157)

34. Identify the major mechanical, pharmacological, and electrical therapeutic objectives in the treatment of the patient with any dysrhythmia. (pp. 97–157)

35. Describe artifacts that may cause confusion when evaluating the ECG of a patient with a pacemaker. (pp. 84–85, 152–153)

36. List the possible complications of pacing. (p. 153)

37. List the causes and implications of pacemaker failure. (p. 153)

Objectives Continued

38. Identify additional hazards that interfere with artificial pacemaker function. (p. 153)

39. Recognize the complications of artificial pacemakers as evidenced on an ECG. (pp. 152–153)

Part 2: Assessment and Management of the Cardiovascular Patient (begins on p. 158)

After reading Part 2 of this chapter, you should be able to:

40. Identify and describe the components of the focused history as it relates to the patient with cardiovascular compromise. (pp. 162–166)

41. Identify and describe the details of inspection, auscultation, and palpation specific to the cardiovascular system. (pp. 166–170)

42. Identify and define the heart sounds and relate them to hemodynamic events in the cardiac cycle. (pp. 168–169)

43. Describe the differences between normal and abnormal heart sounds. (pp. 168–169)

44. Define pulse deficit, pulsus paradoxus, and pulsus alternans. (pp. 164, 205)

45. Identify the normal characteristics of the point of maximal impulse (PMI). (p. 169)

46. Based on field impressions, identify the need for rapid intervention for the patient in cardiovascular compromise. (pp. 160–170)

47. Describe the incidence, morbidity, and mortality associated with myocardial conduction defects. (pp. 186, 198, 240–254)

48. Identify the clinical indications, components, and the function of transcutaneous and permanent artificial cardiac pacing. (pp. 152–153, 186, 188–189)

49. Explain what each setting and indicator on a transcutaneous pacing system represents and how the settings may be adjusted. (pp. 188–189)

50. Describe the techniques of applying a transcutaneous pacing system. (pp. 188–189)

51. Describe the characteristics of an implanted pacemaking system. (pp. 152–153)

52. Describe the epidemiology, morbidity, mortality, and pathophysiology of angina pectoris. (pp. 191, 194)

53. Describe the assessment and management of a patient with angina pectoris. (pp. 194–196)

54. Identify what is meant by the OPQRST of chest pain assessment. (pp. 162–163)

55. List other clinical conditions that may mimic signs and symptoms of coronary artery disease and angina pectoris. (pp. 191, 194)

56. Identify the ECG findings in patients with angina pectoris. (pp. 194–195)

57. Based on the pathophysiology and clinical evaluation of the patient with chest pain, list the anticipated clinical problems according to their life-threatening potential. (pp. 191, 194)

58. Describe the epidemiology, morbidity, mortality, and pathophysiology of myocardial infarction. (pp. 196–197)

59. List the mechanisms by which a myocardial infarction may be produced from traumatic and nontraumatic events. (p. 196)

60. Identify the primary hemodynamic changes produced in myocardial infarction. (pp. 196–197)

61. List and describe the assessment parameters to be evaluated in a patient with a suspected myocardial infarction. (pp. 196–197)

62. Identify the anticipated clinical presentation of a patient with a suspected acute myocardial infarction. (pp. 197–199)

63. Differentiate the characteristics of the pain/discomfort occurring in angina pectoris and acute myocardial infarction. (pp. 197–198)

64. Identify the ECG changes characteristically seen during evolution of an acute myocardial infarction. (p. 198)
65. Identify the most common complications of an acute myocardial infarction. (pp. 196–199)
66. List the characteristics of a patient eligible for thrombolytic therapy. (pp. 198–201)
67. Describe the "window of opportunity" as it pertains to reperfusion of a myocardial injury or infarction. (pp. 198–199)
68. Based on the pathophysiology and clinical evaluation of the patient with a suspected acute myocardial infarction, list the anticipated clinical problems according to their life-threatening potential. (pp. 197–201)
69. Specify the measures that may be taken to prevent or minimize complications in the patient suspected of myocardial infarction. (pp. 199–201)
70. Describe the most commonly used cardiac drugs in terms of therapeutic effect and dosages, routes of administration, side effects, and toxic effects. (pp. 175–180)
71. Describe the epidemiology, morbidity, mortality, and physiology associated with heart failure. (pp. 202–204)
72. Identify the factors that may precipitate or aggravate heart failure. (pp. 202–204)
73. Define acute pulmonary edema and describe its relationship to left ventricular failure. (p. 202)
74. Differentiate between early and late signs and symptoms of left ventricular failure and those of right ventricular failure. (pp. 203–204)
75. Define and explain the clinical significance of paroxysmal nocturnal dyspnea, pulmonary edema, and dependent edema. (pp. 204–205)
76. List the interventions prescribed for the patient in acute congestive heart failure. (pp. 205–206)
77. Describe the most commonly used pharmacological agents in the management of congestive heart failure in terms of therapeutic effect, dosages, routes of administration, side effects, and toxic effects. (pp. 175–180, 206)
78. Define and describe the incidence, mortality, morbidity, pathophysiology, assessment, and management of the following cardiac related problems (pp. 206–216):
    • Cardiac tamponade
    • Hypertensive emergency
    • Cardiogenic shock
    • Cardiac arrest
79. Identify the limiting factor of pericardial anatomy that determines intrapericardiac pressure. (p. 206)
80. Describe how to determine if pulsus paradoxus, pulsus alternans, or electrical alternans is present. (pp. 205–207)
81. Explain the essential pathophysiological defect of hypertension in terms of Starling's law of the heart. (pp. 204, 209–210)
82. Rank the clinical problems of patients in hypertensive emergencies according to their sense of urgency. (p. 208)
83. Identify the drugs of choice for hypertensive emergencies, cardiogenic shock, and cardiac arrest, including their indications, contraindications, side effects, route of administration, and dosages. (pp. 175–180, 209, 212, 213–214)
84. Describe the major systemic effects of reduced tissue perfusion caused by cardiogenic shock. (pp. 209–210)
85. Explain the primary mechanisms by which the heart may compensate for a diminished cardiac output and describe their efficiency in cardiogenic shock. (pp. 209–210)
86. Identify the clinical criteria and progressive stages of cardiogenic shock. (pp. 209–210)
87. Describe the dysrhythmias seen in cardiac arrest. (p. 213)
88. Explain how to confirm asystole using the 3-lead ECG. (p. 213)

89. Define the terms *defibrillation* and *synchronized cardioversion.* (pp. 180–181, 183)
90. Specify the methods of supporting the patient with a suspected ineffective implanted defibrillation device. (p. 182)
91. Describe resuscitation and identify circumstances and situations where resuscitation efforts would not be initiated. (pp. 213–216)
92. Identify communication and documentation protocols with medical direction and law enforcement used for termination of resuscitation efforts. (pp. 214–216)
93. Describe the incidence, morbidity, mortality, pathophysiology, assessment, and management of vascular disorders including occlusive disease, phlebitis, aortic aneurysm, and peripheral artery occlusion. (pp. 217–220)
94. Identify the clinical significance of claudication and presence of arterial bruits in a patient with peripheral vascular disorders. (pp. 217, 219, 220)
95. Describe the clinical significance of unequal arterial blood pressure readings in the arms. (p. 220)
96. Recognize and describe the signs and symptoms of dissecting thoracic or abdominal aneurysm. (pp. 218, 220)
97. Differentiate between signs and symptoms of cardiac tamponade, hypertensive emergencies, cardiogenic shock, and cardiac arrest. (pp. 206–213)
98. Utilize the results of the patient history, assessment findings, and ECG analysis to differentiate between, and provide treatment for, patients with the following conditions (pp. 160–221):
    - cardiovascular disease
    - chest pain
    - in need of a pacemaker
    - angina pectoris
    - a suspected myocardial infarction
    - heart failure
    - cardiac tamponade
    - a hypertensive emergency
    - cardiogenic shock
    - cardiac arrest
99. Based on the pathophysiology and clinical evaluation of the patient with chest pain, characterize the clinical problems according to their life-threatening potential. (pp. 191, 194)
100. Given several preprogrammed patients with cardiac complaints, provide the appropriate assessment, treatment, and transport. (pp. 160–221)

Part 3: 12 Lead ECG Monitoring and Interpretation (begins on p. 221)

After reading Part 3 of this chapter, you should be able to:

*101. Explain the placement and view of the heart provided by bipolar, unipolar (augmented), and precordial ECG leads. (pp. 224–228)
*102. Discuss QRS axis and axis deviation. (pp. 228–231)
*103. Recognize a normal 12-lead ECG. (pp. 231–232)
*104. Explain the evolution and localization of acute myocardial infarction. (pp. 232–240)
*105. Recognize 12-lead ECG tracings of a variety of conduction abnormalities. (pp. 240–254)
*106. Explain prehospital 12-lead ECG monitoring procedures. (pp. 255–258)

Note: The asterisked objectives are not included in the DOT Paramedic curriculum.

CASE STUDY

The crew of Paramedic Unit 112 is called to a local nursing home to evaluate Mr. Evan Henry, an 80-year-old male with chest pain. It is Sunday afternoon, and Mr. Henry's family has been visiting from out of town. Not used to all the attention and excitement, Mr. Henry has developed substernal chest pain that radiates to his left arm. He has a history of this type of pain, but it usually resolves after one or two sublingual nitroglycerin tablets. This time, however, the nitroglycerin tablets have failed to alleviate his pain. Because of this, the nursing home staff has activated the EMS system.

Today, Unit 112 is staffed by paramedics David Bratcher and Bart Betik. When the crew arrives at the nursing home, the nursing home staff meets them and shows them to Mr. Henry's room. Several worried family members are nearby. The paramedics place Mr. Henry on a cardiac monitor, establish an intravenous line, and administer oxygen. They perform an initial assessment and a focused history and physical exam. While Bart is listening to Mr. Henry's chest, the patient suddenly screams and collapses. A quick check finds him to be pulseless and apneic. The monitor reveals coarse ventricular fibrillation. David charges the defibrillator and delivers a 200-joule shock. The ECG remains unchanged and David delivers a second shock, this time at 300-joules. Mr. Henry remains in ventricular fibrillation. David again charges the defibrillator and delivers a third shock at 360-joules. Unfortunately, the patient and ECG remain the same.

An engine company arrives within two minutes. The crew helps to continue CPR while Bart places an endotracheal tube. The patient is ventilated with 100 percent oxygen. An end-tidal carbon dioxide detector and good, equal breath sounds confirm proper placement of the endotracheal tube. David administers 1 mg of epinephrine 1:10,000 intravenously. Following this, a fourth countershock is delivered at 360-joules. This converts the patient to a slow idioventricular rhythm. This rhythm subsequently improves to a sinus tachycardia with a weak pulse. The pulse becomes stronger and cardiac compressions are stopped. Two minutes later, the blood pressure is 110 mmHg by palpation. The ECG shows a few premature ventricular contractions developing. David administers 100 milligrams of lidocaine intravenously and begins a lidocaine drip at 2 milligrams per minute. The paramedics and crew continue mechanical ventilation and move the patient to the ambulance.

The paramedics transport the patient to the hospital. En route, the patient starts to awaken and begins to breathe on his own. In the emergency department, a 12-lead ECG confirms the presence of an anterior wall myocardial infarction. The patient is transferred to the cardiac intensive care unit. Mr. Henry rapidly improves and is weaned from the ventilator. He subsequently undergoes cardiac rehabilitation. The attending physician discharges him back to the nursing home and prescribes three different medications.

INTRODUCTION

According to current estimates, more than 60 million Americans have some form of **cardiovascular disease (CVD)**. **Coronary heart disease (CHD)**, a type of CVD, is the single largest killer of Americans. Each year, on average, 466,000 people die of CHD. Approximately 225,000 of them, a little more than half, die before ever reaching the hospital. Another way of looking at the impact of coronary heart disease is this: An American will suffer a nonfatal heart attack every 29 seconds. About once every minute, an American will die from CHD. These deaths are usually sudden and often due to lethal cardiac rhythm disturbances that result in cardiac arrest.

Sudden death from CHD is often preventable. To decrease the chances of sudden death, the patient must recognize the signs and symptoms early and seek health care. Then, the health care system must provide definitive care promptly, usually within the first hour after the onset of symptoms.

Public education about CHD has focused on two strategies. The first is to educate the public about the risk factors for the development of CHD. This program encourages patients to modify their lifestyle to minimize these risk factors. A variety of factors have been *proven* to increase the risk of cardiovascular disease. These include:

- Smoking
- Older age
- Family history of cardiac disease
- Hypertension (high blood pressure)
- Hypercholesterolemia (excessive cholesterol in the blood)
- Carbohydrate intolerance (diabetes mellitus)
- Cocaine use
- Male gender

Factors that are *thought* to increase the risk of coronary heart disease include:

- Diet
- Obesity
- Oral contraceptives (birth control pills)
- Sedentary lifestyle
- Type A personality (competitive, aggressive, hostile)
- Psychosocial tensions (stress)

The second component of public education is to teach recognition of the signs and symptoms of heart attack. Patients can only benefit from medical intervention if they recognize the signs and symptoms and promptly access the health care system. Patients are encouraged to access the EMS system early. As a paramedic, you will treat patients who already have developed the manifestations of cardiac disease. This will be an opportunity for you to further serve your patients by teaching preventive strategies, including early recognition of symptoms, education, and alteration of lifestyle.

This chapter discusses the advanced prehospital care of cardiovascular emergencies. First, we will review the pertinent anatomy and physiology, and then we will use that knowledge to discuss assessing, recognizing, and treating cardiovascular disorders.

Part 1: Cardiovascular Anatomy and Physiology, ECG Monitoring, and Dysrhythmia Analysis

Objectives

After reading Part 1 of this chapter, you should be able to:

1. Describe the incidence, morbidity, and mortality of cardiovascular disease. (pp. 68, 258)
2. Discuss prevention strategies that may reduce the morbidity and mortality of cardiovascular disease. (p. 68)
3. Identify the risk factors most predisposing to coronary artery disease. (p. 68)
4. Describe the anatomy of the heart, including the position in the thoracic cavity, layers of the heart, chambers of the heart, and location and function of cardiac valves. (pp. 70–75)
5. Identify the major structures of the vascular system, the factors affecting venous return, the components of cardiac output, and the phases of the cardiac cycle. (pp. 76–78)
6. Define preload, afterload, and left ventricular end-diastolic pressure and relate each to the pathophysiology of heart failure. (p. 78)
7. Identify the arterial blood supply to any given area of the myocardium. (p. 75)
8. Compare and contrast the coronary arterial distribution to the major portions of the cardiac conduction system. (pp. 75, 78–80)
9. Identify the structure and course of all divisions and subdivisions of the cardiac conduction system. (pp. 78–84)
10. Identify and describe how the heart's pacemaking control, rate, and rhythm are determined. (pp. 78–84)
11. Explain the physiological basis of conduction delay in the AV node. (pp. 83–84)
12. Define the functional properties of cardiac muscle. (pp. 77–84)
13. Define the events comprising electrical potential. (pp. 77–84)
14. List the most important ions involved in myocardial action potential and their primary function in this process. (p. 82)
15. Describe the events involved in the steps from excitation to contraction of cardiac muscle fibers. (pp. 77–84)
16. Describe the clinical significance of Starling's law. (p. 78)
17. Identify the structures of the autonomic nervous system and their effect on heart rate, rhythm, and contractility. (pp. 78–80)
18. Define and give examples of positive and negative inotropism, chronotropism, and dromotropism. (p. 80)
19. Discuss the pathophysiology of cardiac disease and injury. (pp. 97–157)
20. Explain the purpose of ECG monitoring and its limitations. (p. 84)
21. Correlate the electrophysiological and hemodynamic events occurring throughout the entire cardiac cycle with the various ECG wave forms, segments, and intervals. (pp. 88–95)

22. Identify how heart rates, durations, and amplitudes may be determined from ECG recordings. (pp. 88–95)
23. Relate the cardiac surfaces or areas represented by the ECG leads. (p. 85)
24. Differentiate among the primary mechanisms responsible for producing cardiac dysrhythmias. (pp. 94–95, 97–157)
25. Describe a systematic approach to the analysis and interpretation of cardiac dysrhythmias. (pp. 95–97)
26. Describe the dysrhythmias originating in the sinus node, the AV junction, the atria, and the ventricles. (pp. 99–157)
27. Describe the process and pitfalls of differentiating wide QRS complex tachycardias. (pp. 144–145)
28. Describe the conditions of pulseless electrical activity. (pp. 154–155)
29. Describe the phenomena of reentry, aberration, and accessory pathways. (pp. 98, 115, 157)
30. Identify the ECG changes characteristically produced by electrolyte imbalances and specify their clinical implications. (p. 157)
31. Identify patient situations where ECG rhythm analysis is indicated. (pp. 97–157)
32. Recognize the ECG changes that may reflect evidence of myocardial ischemia and injury and their limitations. (pp. 94–95)
33. Correlate abnormal ECG findings with clinical interpretation. (pp. 97–157)
34. Identify the major mechanical, pharmacological, and electrical therapeutic objectives in the treatment of the patient with any dysrhythmia. (pp. 97–157)
35. Describe artifacts that may cause confusion when evaluating the ECG of a patient with a pacemaker. (pp. 84–85, 152–153)
36. List the possible complications of pacing. (p. 153)
37. List the causes and implications of pacemaker failure. (p. 153)
38. Identify additional hazards that interfere with artificial pacemaker function. (p. 153)
39. Recognize the complications of artificial pacemakers as evidenced on an ECG. (pp. 152–153)

CARDIOVASCULAR ANATOMY

The *cardiovascular system*'s two major components are the heart and the peripheral blood vessels. Prehospital care of cardiovascular patients requires a sound knowledge of the anatomy and physiology of the cardiovascular system. Accurately assessing your patient, making a correct field diagnosis, and providing the best management possible will depend on your understanding of the heart and the peripheral blood vessels and how they work.

ANATOMY OF THE HEART

The *heart* is a muscular organ, approximately the size of a closed fist. It is in the center of the chest in the mediastinum, anterior to the spine and posterior to the sternum (Figure 2-1). Approximately two-thirds of the heart's mass is to the left of the midline, with the remainder to the right. The bottom of the heart, or *apex*, is just above the diaphragm, left of the midline. The top of the heart, or *base*, lies

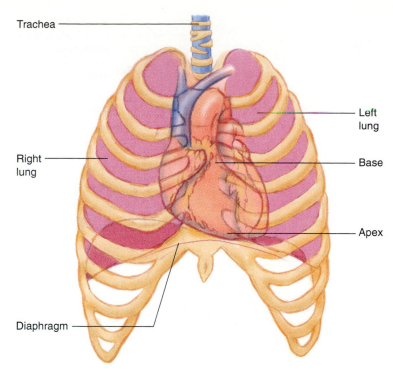

Trachea

Right lung

Diaphragm

Left lung

Base

Apex

FIGURE 2-1   Location of the heart within the chest.

at approximately the level of the second rib. The great vessels connect to the heart through the base.

Tissue Layers   The heart consists of three tissue layers: endocardium, myocardium, and pericardium (Figure 2-2). The *endocardium* is the innermost layer. It lines the heart's chambers and is bathed in blood. The *myocardium* is the thick middle layer of the heart. Its cells are unique in that they physically resemble skeletal muscle but have electrical properties similar to smooth muscle. These cells also contain specialized structures that help to rapidly conduct electrical impulses from one muscle cell to another, enabling the heart to contract. The *pericardium* is a protective sac surrounding the heart. It consists of two layers, visceral and parietal. The *visceral pericardium,* also called the *epicardium,* is the inner layer, in contact with the heart muscle itself. The *parietal pericardium* is the outer, fibrous layer. In the pericardial cavity, between these two layers, is about 25 milliliters of pericardial fluid, a straw-colored lubricant that reduces friction as the heart beats and changes position. Certain disease processes and injuries can increase the amount of fluid in this sac, compressing the heart and decreasing cardiac output.

Chambers   The heart contains four chambers (Figure 2-3). The *atria,* the two superior chambers, receive incoming blood. The *ventricles,* the two larger, inferior chambers, pump blood out of the heart. The right and left atria are separated by the *interatrial septum.* The ventricles are separated by the *interventricular septum.* Both septa contain fibrous connective tissue as well as contractile muscle. The walls of the atria are much thinner than those of the ventricles and do not contribute significantly to the heart's pumping action.

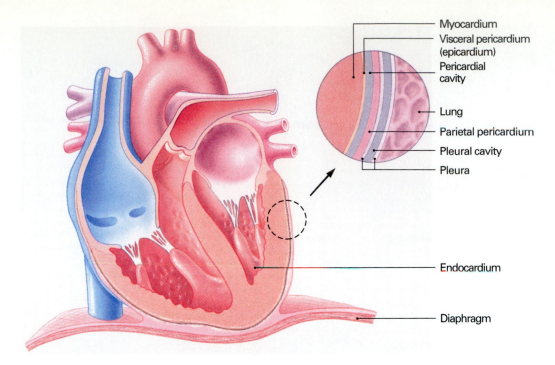

Myocardium

Visceral pericardium
(epicardium)

Pericardial
cavity

Lung

Parietal pericardium

Pleural cavity

Pleura

Endocardium

Diaphragm

FIGURE 2-2 Layers of the heart.

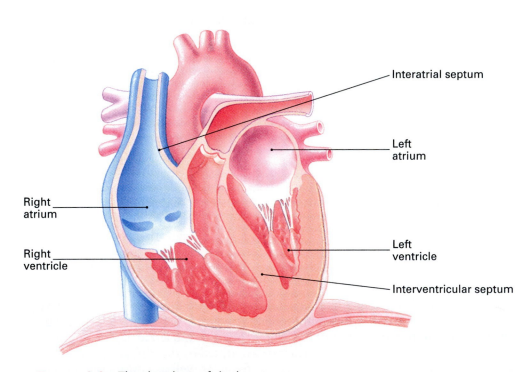

Interatrial septum

Left
atrium

Right
atrium

Left
ventricle

Right
ventricle

Interventricular septum

FIGURE 2-3 The chambers of the heart.

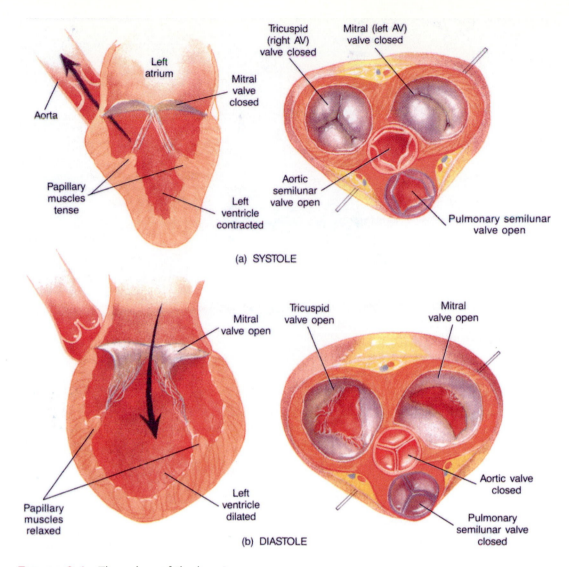

Left
atrium

Aorta

Mitral
valve
closed

Tricuspid
(right AV)
valve closed

Mitral (left AV)
valve closed

Papillary
muscles
tense

Left
ventricle
contracted

Aortic
semilunar
valve open

Pulmonary semilunar
valve open

(a) SYSTOLE

Mitral
valve open

Tricuspid
valve open

Mitral
valve open

Papillary
muscles
relaxed

Left
ventricle
dilated

Aortic valve
closed

Pulmonary
semilunar valve
closed

(b) DIASTOLE

FIGURE 2-4   The valves of the heart.

Valves The heart contains two pairs of valves, the *atrioventricular valves* and the *semilunar valves,* made of endocardial and connective tissue (Figures 2-4 and 2-5). The atrioventricular valves control blood flow between the atria and the ventricles. The right atrioventricular valve is called the *tricuspid valve* because it has three leaflets, or cusps. The left atrioventricular valve, called the *mitral valve,* has two leaflets. These valves are connected to specialized *papillary muscles* in the ventricles. When relaxed, these papillary muscles open the valves and allow blood flow between the two chambers. Specialized fibers called *chordae tendoneae* connect the valves' leaflets to the papillary muscles. They prevent the valves from prolapsing into the atria and allowing backflow during ventricular contraction.

The semilunar valves regulate blood flow between the ventricles and the arteries into which they empty. The left semilunar valve, or aortic valve, connects

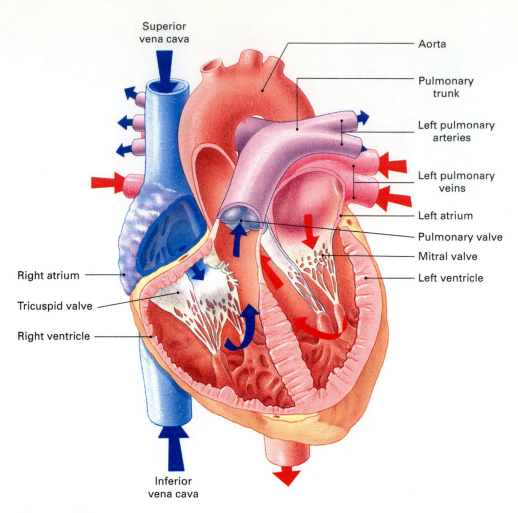

Superior
vena cava

Aorta

Pulmonary
trunk

Left pulmonary
arteries

Left pulmonary
veins

Left atrium

Pulmonary valve

Mitral valve

Left ventricle

Right atrium

Tricuspid valve

Right ventricle

Inferior
vena cava

FIGURE 2-5   Blood flow through the heart.

the left ventricle to the aorta. The right semilunar valve, or pulmonic valve, connects the right ventricle to the pulmonary artery. These valves permit one-way
movement of blood and prevent backflow.

Blood Flow   The right atrium receives deoxygenated blood from the body via
the superior and inferior venae cavae (Figure 2-5). The *superior vena cava* receives deoxygenated blood from the head and upper extremities, the *inferior vena
cava* from the areas below the heart. The right atrium pumps this blood through
the tricuspid valve and into the right ventricle. The right ventricle then pumps the
deoxygenated blood through the pulmonic valve to the *pulmonary artery* and on
to the lungs. (The pulmonary artery is the only artery in the body that carries deoxygenated blood.)

After the blood circulates through the lungs and becomes oxygenated, it returns to the left atrium via the *pulmonary veins*. (The pulmonary veins are the
only veins in the body that carry oxygenated blood.) The left atrium sends this
oxygenated blood through the mitral valve and into the left ventricle. Finally the
left ventricle pumps the blood through the aortic valve to the aorta, which feeds
the oxygenated blood to the rest of the body. Intracardiac pressures are higher
on the left than on the right because the lungs offer less resistance to blood flow
than the systemic circulation. Thus, the left myocardium is thicker than the right.

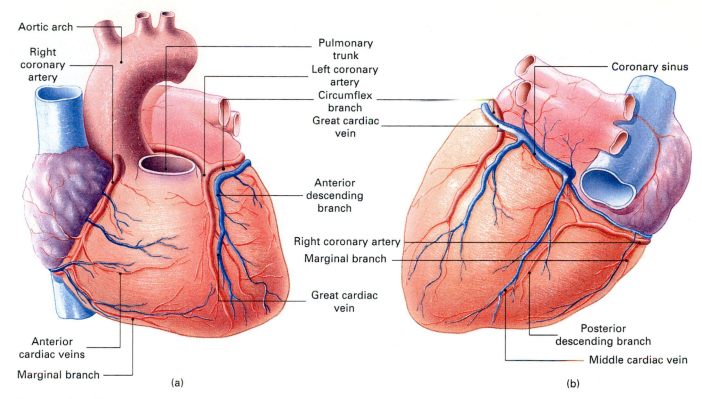

Aortic arch

Right coronary artery

Pulmonary trunk

Left coronary artery

Circumflex branch

Great cardiac vein

Anterior descending branch

Right coronary artery

Marginal branch

Great cardiac vein

Anterior cardiac veins

Marginal branch

(a)

Coronary sinus

Posterior descending branch

Middle cardiac vein

(b)

FIGURE 2-6   The coronary circulation: (a) anterior; (b) posterior.

The major vessels of the body all branch off of the aorta, which has three main parts. The *ascending aorta* comes directly from the heart. The *thoracic aorta* curves inferiorly and goes through the chest (or thorax). The *abdominal aorta* goes through the diaphragm and enters the abdomen.

Coronary Circulation   Although the endocardium is bathed in blood, the heart does not receive its nutrients from the blood within its chambers but from the *coronary arteries* (Figure 2-6). The coronary arteries originate in the aorta, just above the leaflets of the aortic valve. The main coronary arteries lie on the surface of the heart, and small penetrating arterioles supply the myocardial muscle. The *left coronary artery* supplies the left ventricle, the interventricular septum, part of the right ventricle, and the heart's conduction system. Its two major branches are the *anterior descending artery* and the *circumflex artery*. The *right coronary artery* supplies a portion of the right atrium and right ventricle and part of the conduction system. Its two major branches are the *posterior descending artery* and the *marginal artery*. (Although the blood supply to most people's hearts follows this pattern, anatomical variants do exist.) The coronary vessels receive blood during diastole, when the heart relaxes, because the aortic valve leaflets cover the coronary artery openings (*ostia*) during systole, when the heart contracts.

Blood drains from the left coronary system via the *anterior great cardiac vein* and the *lateral marginal veins*. These empty into the *coronary sinus*. The right coronary artery empties directly into the right atrium via smaller cardiac veins.

Many **anastomoses** (communications between two or more vessels) among the various branches of the coronary arteries allow *collateral circulation*. Collateral circulation is a protective mechanism that provides an alternative path for blood flow in case of a blockage somewhere in the system. This is analogous to a river's developing small tributaries to reach a larger body of water.

✱ **anastomosis** communication between two or more vessels.

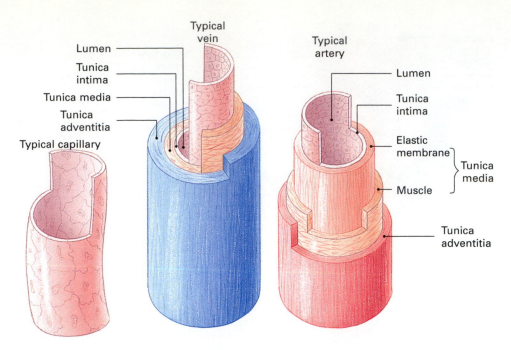

FIGURE 2-7   The layers of the peripheral arteries.

ANATOMY OF THE PERIPHERAL CIRCULATION

The peripheral circulation transports oxygenated blood from the heart to the tissues and subsequently transports deoxygenated blood back to the heart. Oxygenated blood leaves the heart via the arterial system, while deoxygenated blood returns via the venous system. (As noted earlier, the exceptions to this rule are the pulmonary artery and the pulmonary veins.)

A capillary wall consists of a single layer of cells. The walls of arteries and veins, however, comprise several layers (Figure 2-7). The arteries' and veins' innermost lining, the *tunica intima,* is a single cell layer thick. The middle layer, the *tunica media,* consists of elastic fibers and muscle. It gives blood vessels their strength and recoil, which results from the difference in pressure inside and outside the vessel. The tunica media is much thicker in arteries than in veins. The outermost lining is the *tunica adventitia,* a fibrous tissue covering. It gives the vessel strength to withstand the pressures generated by the heart's contractions. The cavity inside a vessel is the *lumen.*

The vessels' diameters vary significantly and are directly related to the amount of blood they can transport. The larger the diameter, the greater the blood flow. In fact, according to **Poiseuille's Law** the blood flow through a vessel is directly proportional to the fourth power of the vessel's radius. For example, a vessel with a relative radius of 1 would transport 1 ml per minute of blood at a pressure difference of 100 mmHg. If the vessel's radius were increased to 4, keeping the pressure difference constant, the flow would increase to 256 ml (4^4) per minute.

Arterial System   The *arterial system,* which carries oxygenated blood from the heart, functions under high pressure. The larger arterial vessels are the *arteries.* The arteries branch into smaller structures called *arterioles,* which control blood flow to various organs by their degree of resistance. The arterioles continue to divide until they become *capillaries,* which are the connection points between the arterial and venous systems. The vascular system and the tissues are able to exchange gases, fluids, and nutrients through the very thin capillary walls.

✱ **Poiseuille's Law** a law of physiology stating that blood flow through a vessel is directly proportional to the radius of the vessel to the fourth power.

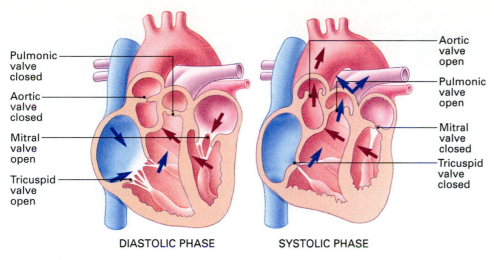

Figure labels (left diagram — DIASTOLIC PHASE):
- Pulmonic valve closed
- Aortic valve closed
- Mitral valve open
- Tricuspid valve open

Figure labels (right diagram — SYSTOLIC PHASE):
- Aortic valve open
- Pulmonic valve open
- Mitral valve closed
- Tricuspid valve closed

DIASTOLIC PHASE   SYSTOLIC PHASE

FIGURE 2-8   Relation of blood flow to cardiac contraction.

Venous System The *venous system* transports blood from the peripheral tissues back to the heart. It functions under low pressure with the aid of surrounding muscles and one-way valves within the veins. Blood enters the venous system through the capillaries, which drain into the *venules*. The venules, in turn, drain into the *veins,* the veins into the venae cavae, and the venae cavae into the atria.

CARDIAC PHYSIOLOGY

THE CARDIAC CYCLE

Although the heart's right and left sides perform different functions, they act as a unit. The right and left atria contract at the same time, filling both ventricles to their maximum capacities. Both ventricles then contract at the same time, ejecting blood into the pulmonary and systemic circulations. The pressure of the contraction closes the tricuspid and mitral valves and opens the aortic and pulmonic valves at the same time.

The **cardiac cycle** is the sequence of events that occurs between the end of one heart contraction and the end of the next. To evaluate heart sounds and read electrocardiographs, you must thoroughly understand the pumping action of the cardiac cycle (Figure 2-8). **Diastole,** the first phase of the cardiac cycle, is the *relaxation phase.* This is when ventricular filling begins. Blood enters the ventricles through the mitral and tricuspid valves. The pulmonic and aortic valves are closed. During the second phase, **systole,** the heart contracts. The atria contract first, to finish emptying their blood into the ventricles. Atrial systole is relatively quick and occurs just before ventricular contraction; in healthy hearts, this atrial "kick" boosts cardiac output. The pressure in the ventricles now increases until it exceeds the pressure in the aorta and pulmonary artery. At this point blood flows out of the ventricles through the pulmonic and aortic valves and into the arteries. The pressure also closes the mitral and tricuspid valves and, if working properly, prevents backflow of blood into the atria. When pressures in the artery exceed the pressures in the ventricles, the valves close and diastole begins again.

The normal ventricle ejects about two-thirds of the blood it contains at the end of diastole. This ratio is the **ejection fraction.** The amount of blood ejected

✳ **cardiac cycle** the period of time from the end of one cardiac contraction to the end of the next.

✳ **diastole** the period of time when the myocardium is relaxed and cardiac filling and coronary perfusion occur.

✳ **systole** the period of the cardiac cycle when the myocardium is contracting.

✳ **ejection fraction** ratio of blood pumped from the ventricle to the amount remaining at end of diastole

✱ **stroke volume** the amount of blood ejected by the heart in one cardiac contraction.

Content Review

FACTORS AFFECTING STROKE VOLUME
- Preload
- Cardiac contractility
- Afterload

✱ **preload** the pressure within the ventricles at the end of diastole; commonly called the *end-diastolic volume*.

✱ **Starling's law of the heart** law of physiology stating that the more the myocardium is stretched, up to a certain amount, the more forceful the subsequent contraction will be.

✱ **afterload** the resistance against which the heart must pump.

✱ **cardiac output** the amount of blood pumped by the heart in one minute.

is the **stroke volume.** Each time the ventricle pumps blood into the aorta, it generates a pressure wave along the major arteries, which we feel as a pulse. Stroke volume varies between 60 and 100 ml, with the average being 70 ml.

Stroke volume depends upon three factors: preload, cardiac contractility, and afterload. The heart can pump out only the blood it receives from the venous system. The pressure in the filled ventricle at the end of diastole is called **preload,** or *end-diastolic volume*. Preload influences the force and amount of the next contraction and is based on **Starling's law of the heart.** Starling's law states that the more the myocardial muscle is stretched, the greater its force of contraction will be. In other words, the greater the volume of blood filling the chamber, the more forceful the cardiac contraction. Therefore, the greater the venous return, the greater the preload and the greater the stroke volume. Myocardial muscle, however, has its limits. If stretched too far, it will not contract properly and will weaken. Think of blowing up a tire. The tension in the walls increases as you put more air in the tire. If you were to put too much air in the tire, the tire would break or bulge from the side. If either of these happened, the tension in the wall would decrease, and if you filled the tire again it would not perform as well as before. **Afterload** is the resistance against which the ventricle must contract. An increase in peripheral vascular resistance will decrease stroke volume, and conversely, a decrease in peripheral vascular resistance will allow stroke volume to increase.

Cardiac output is the volume of blood that the heart pumps in one minute. It is a function of stroke volume and heart rate, as the following formula states:

stroke volume (ml) $\times$ heart rate (bpm) = cardiac output (ml/min)

The normal heart rate is 60–100 beats per minute, and the average stroke volume is 70 ml. Thus an average cardiac output is about 5 liters/minute (5000 ml/minute), calculated as follows:

stroke volume $\times$ heart rate = cardiac output

70 ml $\times$ 70 bpm = 4900 ml/min

We have all had our blood pressure taken. Blood pressure is related to cardiac output and peripheral resistance and is calculated by the following formula:

blood pressure = cardiac output $\times$ systemic vascular resistance

Remember that cardiac output equals stroke volume times heart rate; therefore,

blood pressure = (stroke volume $\times$ heart rate) $\times$ systemic vascular resistance.

The body does its best to keep blood pressure constant by regulating the elements of this formula to compensate for changes. For instance, when stroke volume decreases, the systemic vascular resistance will increase to maintain blood pressure at a constant value. Consider, for example, a patient in shock. A shock patient has decreased cardiac output. To compensate, systemic resistance increases, reducing blood flow to the extremities, which manifests as cool, clammy skin.

NERVOUS CONTROL OF THE HEART

The sympathetic and parasympathetic components of the autonomic nervous system work in direct opposition to one another to regulate the heart. In the heart's normal state the two systems balance. In stressful situations, however, the sympathetic system becomes dominant, while during sleep the parasympathetic system dominates. The sympathetic nervous system innervates the heart through

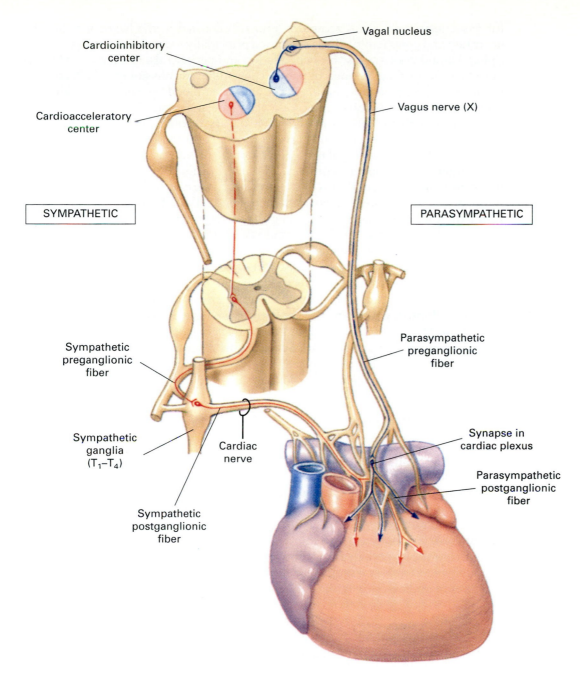

Cardioinhibitory center

Vagal nucleus

Cardioacceleratory center

Vagus nerve (X)

SYMPATHETIC

PARASYMPATHETIC

Sympathetic preganglionic fiber

Parasympathetic preganglionic fiber

Sympathetic ganglia (T_1–T_4)

Cardiac nerve

Synapse in cardiac plexus

Parasympathetic postganglionic fiber

Sympathetic postganglionic fiber

FIGURE 2-9   Nervous control of the heart.

the *cardiac plexus,* a network of nerves at the base of the heart (Figure 2-9). The sympathetic nerves arise from the thoracic and lumbar regions of the spinal cord, then leave the spinal cord and form the sympathetic chain, which runs along the spinal column. The cardiac plexus arises in turn from ganglia in the sympathetic chain and innervates both the atria and ventricles. The chemical *neurotransmitter* for the sympathetic nervous system, and thus for the cardiac plexus, is *norepinephrine.* Its release increases heart rate and cardiac contractile force, primarily through its actions on beta receptors.

The sympathetic nervous system has two principal types of receptors, alpha and beta. *Alpha receptors* are located in the peripheral blood vessels and are responsible for vasoconstriction. *Beta₁* receptors, primarily located in the heart, increase the heart rate and contractility. *Beta₂* receptors, principally located in the lungs and peripheral blood vessels, cause bronchodilation and peripheral vasodilation. Medications specific to these various receptors cause different physiological effects. For instance, beta blockers slow the heart rate and lower blood pressure by blocking the $beta_1$ receptors, whose job is to increase heart rate and contractility.

Parasympathetic control of the heart occurs through the *vagus nerve* (the tenth cranial nerve). The vagus nerve descends from the brain to innervate the heart and other organs. Vagal nerve fibers primarily innervate the atria, although some innervate the upper ventricles. The neurotransmitter for the parasympathetic nervous system, and thus the vagus nerve, is *acetylcholine*. Its release slows the heart rate and slows atrioventricular conduction. Several maneuvers can stimulate the vagus nerve, including Valsalva maneuver (forced expiration against a closed glottis, which can occur when lifting heavy objects), pressure on the carotid sinus (carotid sinus massage), and distention of the urinary bladder.

The terms *chronotropy, inotropy,* and *dromotropy* describe autonomic control of the heart. **Chronotropy** refers to heart rate. A *positive chronotropic agent* increases the heart rate. Conversely, a *negative chronotropic agent* decreases the heart rate. **Inotropy** refers to the strength of a cardiac muscular contraction. A *positive inotropic agent* strengthens the cardiac contraction, while a *negative inotropic agent* weakens it. **Dromotropy** refers to the rate of nervous impulse conduction. A positive dromotropic agent speeds impulse conduction, while a negative dromotropic agent slows conduction.

* **chronotropy** pertaining to heart rate.

* **inotropy** pertaining to cardiac contractile force.

* **dromotropy** pertaining to the speed of impulse transmission.

Role of Electrolytes

Cardiac function, both electrical and mechanical, depends heavily on electrolyte balances. Electrolytes that affect cardiac function include sodium (Na^+), calcium (Ca^{++}), potassium (K^+), chloride (Cl^-), and magnesium (Mg^{++}). Sodium plays a major role in depolarizing the myocardium. Calcium takes part in myocardial depolarization and myocardial contraction. Hypercalcemia can result in increased contractility, whereas hypocalcemia is associated with decreased myocardial contractility and increased electrical irritability. Potassium influences repolarization. Hyperkalemia decreases automaticity and conduction, whereas hypokalemia increases irritability. New research is also investigating the roles of magnesium and chloride in the cardiac cycle.

ELECTROPHYSIOLOGY

The heart comprises three types of cardiac muscle: atrial, ventricular, and specialized excitatory and conductive fibers. The atrial and ventricular muscle fibers contract in much the same way as skeletal muscle, with one major difference. Within the cardiac muscle fibers are special structures called **intercalated discs** (Figure 2-10). These discs connect cardiac muscle fibers and conduct electrical impulses quickly—400 times faster than the standard cell membrane—from one muscle fiber to the next. This speed allows cardiac muscle cells to function physiologically as a unit. That is, when one cell becomes excited, the action potential spreads rapidly across the entire group of cells, resulting in a coordinated contraction. This functional unit is a **syncytium**.

The heart has two syncytia—the *atrial syncytium* and the *ventricular syncytium*. The atrial syncytium contracts from superior to inferior, so that the atria express blood to the ventricles. The ventricular syncytium, on the other hand, contracts from inferior to superior, expelling blood from the ventricles into the aorta and pulmonary arteries. The syncytia are separated from one another by the fibrous structure that supports the valves and physically separates

* **intercalated discs** specialized bands of tissue inserted between myocardial cells that increase the rate in which the action potential is spread from cell to cell.

* **syncytium** group of cardiac muscle cells that physiologically function as a unit.

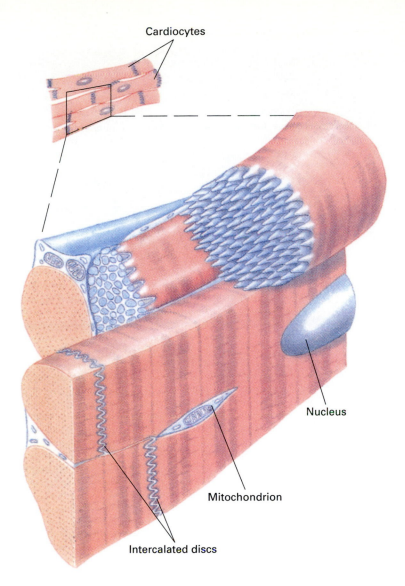

Cardiocytes

Nucleus

Mitochondrion

Intercalated discs

FIGURE 2-10   Microscopic appearance of cardiac muscle. The intercalated discs speed transmission of the electrical potential quickly from one cell to the next.

the atria from the ventricles. The only way an impulse can be conducted from the atria to the ventricles is through the *atrioventricular (AV) bundle.* Cardiac muscle functions according to an "all-or-none" principle. That is, if a single muscle fiber becomes *depolarized,* the action potential will spread through the whole syncytium. Stimulating a single atrial fiber will thus completely depolarize the atria, and stimulating a single ventricular fiber will completely depolarize the ventricles.

Cardiac Depolarization

Understanding **cardiac depolarization** is essential to interpreting electrocardiograms (ECGs). Normally, an ionic difference exists on the two sides of a cell membrane. The cell's sodium-potassium pump expels sodium (Na^+) from the cell. This leaves more negatively charged anions inside the cell than positively charged cations. Thus, the inside of the cell is more negatively charged than the outside. This difference, called the **resting potential,** can be measured experimentally by

✳ **cardiac depolarization** a reversal of charges at a cell membrane so that the inside of the cell becomes positive in relation to the outside; the opposite of the cell's resting state in which the inside of the cell is negative in relation to the outside.

✳ **resting potential** the normal electrical state of cardiac cells.

FIGURE 2-11 Schematic of ion shifts during depolarization and repolarization.

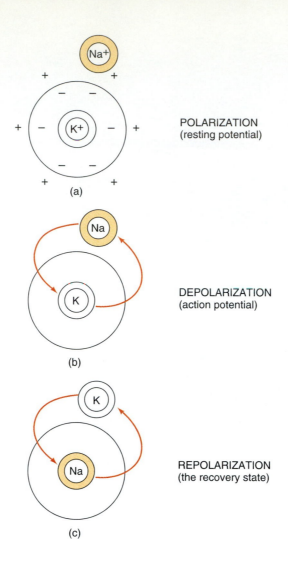

POLARIZATION
(resting potential)

(a)

DEPOLARIZATION
(action potential)

(b)

REPOLARIZATION
(the recovery state)

(c)

✳ action potential the stimulation of myocardial cells, as evidenced by a change in the membrane electrical charge, that subsequently spreads across the myocardium.

✳ repolarization return of a muscle cell to its preexcitation resting state.

placing one probe inside the cell and another outside the cell and determining the difference in millivolts. The resting potential in a myocardial cell is approximately −90 mV (Figure 2-11).

When the myocardial cell is stimulated, the membrane surrounding the cell changes instantaneously to allow sodium ions to rush into the cell, bringing with them their positive charge. This charge is so strong that it gives the inside of the cell a positive charge approximately +20 mV greater than the outside. This influx of sodium and change of membrane polarity is the **action potential**. After the influx of sodium, a slower influx of calcium ions (Ca^{++}) through the calcium channels increases the positive charge inside the cell. Once *depolarization* occurs in a muscle fiber, it is transmitted throughout the entire syncytium, via the intercalated discs, until the entire muscle mass is depolarized. Contraction of the muscle follows depolarization.

The cell membrane remains permeable to sodium for only a fraction of a second. Thereafter, sodium influx stops and potassium escapes from inside the cell. This returns the charge inside the cell to normal (negative). In addition, sodium is actively pumped outside the cell, allowing the cell to **repolarize** and return to its normal resting state.

Cardiac Conductive System

The cardiac conductive system stimulates the ventricles to depolarize in the proper direction. As mentioned earlier, the atria contract from superior to inferior, the ventricles from inferior to superior. If the depolarization impulse originated in the atria and spread passively to the ventricles, then the ventricles would depolarize from superior to inferior and would be ineffective. The cardiac conduction system, therefore, must initiate an impulse, spread it through the atria, transmit it quickly to the apex of the heart, and thence stimulate the ventricles to depolarize from inferior to superior. To do this, the conduction system relies on specialized conductive fibers comprising muscle cells that transmit the depolarization potential through the heart much faster than can regular myocardial cells.

To accomplish their task, the cells of the cardiac conductive system have the important properties of excitability, conductivity, automaticity, and contractility.

- **Excitability** The cells can respond to an electrical stimulus, like all other myocardial cells.
- **Conductivity** The cells can propagate the electrical impulse from one cell to another.
- **Automaticity** The individual cells of the conductive system can depolarize without any impulse from an outside source. This property is also called self-excitation. Generally, the cell in the cardiac conductive system with the fastest rate of discharge, or automaticity, becomes the heart's pacemaker. As a rule, the highest cell in the conductive system has the fastest rate of automaticity. Normally, this cell is in the *sinoatrial (SA) node,* high in the right atrium; however, if one pacemaker cell fails to discharge and depolarize, then the cell with the next fastest rate becomes the pacemaker.
- **Contractility** Since the cells of the cardiac conductive system are specialized cardiac muscle cells, they retain the ability to contract.

Internodal atrial pathways connect the SA node to the AV node (Figure 2-12). These internodal pathways conduct the depolarization impulse to the atrial muscle

✳ **excitability** ability of the cells to respond to an electrical stimulus.

✳ **conductivity** ability of the cells to propagate the electrical impulse from one cell to another.

✳ **automaticity** pacemaker cells' capability of self-depolarization.

✳ **contractility** ability of muscle cells to contract, or shorten.

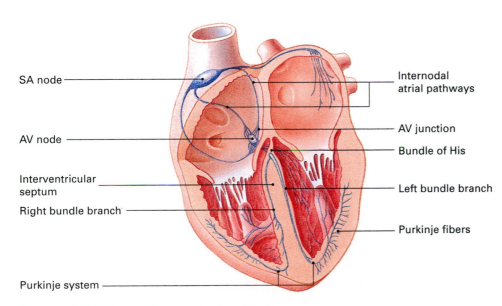

SA node

Internodal atrial pathways

AV junction

AV node

Bundle of His

Interventricular septum

Left bundle branch

Right bundle branch

Purkinje fibers

Purkinje system

FIGURE 2-12 The cardiac conductive system.

mass and through the atria to the AV junction. The AV junction (the "gatekeeper") slows the impulse and allows the ventricles time to fill. Then, the impulse passes through the AV junction into the AV node and on to the AV fibers, which conduct the impulse from the atria to the ventricles. In the ventricles the AV fibers form the *bundle of His*.

The bundle of His subsequently divides into the right and left bundle branches. The *right bundle branch* delivers the impulse to the apex of the right ventricle. From there the *Purkinje system* spreads it across the myocardium. The *left bundle branch* divides into *anterior* and *posterior fascicles* that also ultimately terminate in the Purkinje system. At the same time that the impulse is transmitted to the right ventricle, the Purkinje system spreads it across the mass of the myocardium. Repolarization predominantly occurs in the opposite direction.

Each component of the conductive system has its own intrinsic rate of self-excitation:

> SA node = 60–100 beats per minute
> AV node = 40–60 beats per minute
> Purkinje system = 15–40 beats per minute

ELECTROCARDIOGRAPHIC MONITORING

One of your most important skills as a paramedic will be obtaining and interpreting ECG rhythm strips.

* **rhythm strip** electrocardiogram printout.

One of your most important skills as a paramedic will be obtaining and interpreting electrocardiographic (ECG) **rhythm strips.** Your patient's subsequent treatment will be based upon rapid, accurate interpretation of these strips. At first, rhythm strips may seem very difficult to read, for only through classroom instruction and repeated practice can you master their interpretation. Nor will every rhythm strip you encounter be a "textbook" example; you must be comfortable with all possible variants. With practice and a systematic approach, however, you will soon be skilled in their interpretation. This section presents basic information about ECG monitoring, as well as recognizing and interpreting dysrhythmias. The additional readings recommended at the end of the chapter will help you expand this knowledge.

THE ELECTROCARDIOGRAM

* **electrocardiogram (ECG)** the graphic recording of the heart's electrical activity. It may be displayed either on paper or on an oscilloscope.

The **electrocardiogram (ECG)** is a graphic record of the heart's electrical activity. However, it tells you nothing about the heart's pumping ability, which you must evaluate by pulse and blood pressure.

The body acts as a giant conductor of electricity, and the heart is its largest generator of electrical energy. Electrodes on the skin can detect the total electrical activity within the heart at any given time. The electrical impulses on the skin surface have a very low voltage. The ECG machine amplifies these impulses and records them over time on ECG graph paper or a monitor. *Positive impulses* appear as *upward* deflections on the paper, *negative impulses* as *downward* deflections. The absence of any electrical impulse produces an *isoelectric line,* which is flat.

* **artifact** deflection on the ECG produced by factors other than the heart's electrical activity.

Artifacts are deflections on the ECG produced by factors other than the heart's electrical activity. Common causes of artifacts include:

- Muscle tremors
- Shivering
- Patient movement
- Loose electrodes
- 60 hertz interference
- Machine malfunction

It is important for ECGs to be free of artifacts. When an artifact is present, you must first try to eliminate it before recording the ECG. Loose electrodes should be replaced. Occasionally, patients may be quite diaphoretic, thus preventing the electrodes from adhering well to the skin. In these cases, you may need to wipe the skin and apply tincture of Benzoin before applying the electrode.

ECG Leads

You can obtain many views of the heart's electrical activity by monitoring the voltage change through *electrodes* placed at various places on the body surface. Each pair of electrodes is a *lead*. In the hospital, 12 leads are normally used. As a rule, most EMS systems use only 3 leads in the field. In fact, one lead alone is adequate for detecting life-threatening dysrhythmias. With the advent of thrombolytic therapy and computer interpretation, however, 12-lead ECGs are becoming more common in the field, especially in rural EMS systems. (Part 3 of this chapter presents an introductory discussion of the 12-lead ECG.)

The three types of ECG leads are bipolar, augmented, and precordial. **Bipolar leads,** the kind most frequently used, have one positive electrode and one negative electrode. Any electrical impulse moving toward the positive electrode will cause a positive (upward) deflection on the ECG paper. Any electrical impulse moving toward the negative electrode will cause a negative (downward) deflection. The absence of a positive or negative deflection means either that there is no electrical impulse or that the impulse is moving perpendicular to the lead. Leads I, II, and III, commonly called *limb leads,* are bipolar. They are the most frequently used leads in the field. Table 2-1 lists their placement sites.

These three bipolar leads form **Einthoven's triangle,** named after Dr. Willem Einthoven, who invented the ECG machine (Figure 2-13). The direction from the negative to the positive electrode is the lead's *axis.* Each lead shows a different axis of the heart. Lead I, at the top of Einthoven's triangle, has an axis of 0°. Lead II forms the right side of the triangle and has an axis of 60°. Lead III forms the left side of the triangle and has an axis of 120°.

The bipolar leads provide only three views of the heart. **Augmented,** or **unipolar, leads** provide additional views that are sometimes useful. Although these leads evaluate different axes than the bipolar leads, they utilize the same electrodes. They do this by electronically combining the negative electrodes of two of the bipolar leads to obtain an axis. These augmented leads are designated aVR, aVL, and aVF. The letter *a* indicates that the lead is augmented. The letter *V* identifies it as a unipolar lead. The *R, L,* and *F* identify the extremity on which the lead is placed (R = right arm, L = left arm, and F = left foot).

In addition, six **precordial leads** can be placed across the surface of the chest to measure electrical cardiac activity on a horizontal axis. These leads help in viewing the left ventricle and septum. They are designated V_1 through V_6, with the letter *V* identifying them as unipolar leads.

Table 2-1 BIPOLAR LEAD PLACEMENT SITES

Lead	Positive Electrode	Negative Electrode
I	Left arm	Right arm
II	Left leg	Right arm
III	Left leg	Left arm

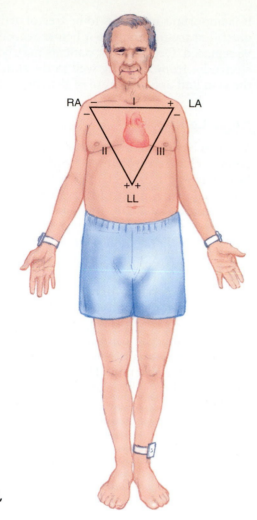

FIGURE 2-13 Einthoven's triangle as formed by Leads I, II, and III.

Routine ECG Monitoring

Whether in the ambulance, emergency department, or coronary care unit, routine ECG monitoring generally uses only one lead. The most common monitoring leads are either Lead II or the *modified chest lead 1* (MCL$_1$). Of these, Lead II is used more frequently because most of the heart's electrical current flows toward its positive axis. This gives the best view of the ECG waves and best depicts the conduction system's activity. MCL$_1$ is a special monitoring lead that some systems use selectively to help determine the origin of abnormal complexes such as premature beats. To avoid confusion, we will use Lead II as the monitor lead throughout this text.

Einthoven's triangle offers a basis for placing the leads. Usually you should place the electrodes on the chest wall instead of the extremities. This helps to reduce artifacts from arm movement. (If you use the arms, place the lead as high as possible on the extremity to decrease movement.) Make certain the skin is clean and free of hair before you place the electrodes on the chest wall. For Lead II, the positive electrode is usually placed at the apex of the heart on the chest wall (or on the left leg), the negative electrode below the right clavicle (or on the right arm). The third electrode, the ground, is placed somewhere on the left, upper chest wall (or on the left arm).

Lead II gives the best view of the ECG waves and best depicts the conduction system's activity.

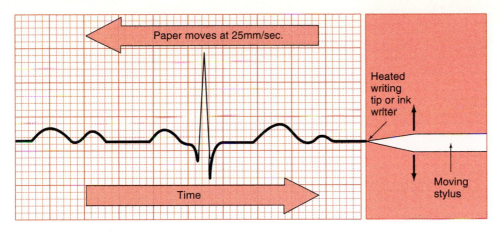

FIGURE 2-14   Recording of the ECG.

A single monitoring lead can provide considerable information, including:

- The rate of the heartbeat
- The regularity of the heartbeat
- The time it takes to conduct the impulse through the various parts of the heart

A single lead cannot provide the following information:

- The presence or location of an infarct
- Axis deviation or chamber enlargement
- Right-to-left differences in conduction or impulse formation
- The quality or presence of pumping action

ECG Graph Paper

ECG graph paper is standardized to allow comparative analysis of ECG patterns. The paper moves across the stylus at a standard speed of 25 mm/sec (Figure 2-14). The *amplitude* of the ECG *deflection* is also standardized. When properly calibrated, the ECG stylus should deflect two large boxes when one millivolt is present. Most machines have calibration buttons, and a calibration curve should be placed at the beginning of the first ECG strip. Many machines do this automatically when they are first turned on.

The ECG graph is divided into a grid of light and heavy lines. The light lines are 1 mm apart, and the heavy lines are 5 mm apart. The heavy lines thus enclose large squares, each containing twenty-five of the smaller squares formed by the lighter lines (Figure 2-15). The following relationships apply to the horizontal axis.

1 small box = 0.04 sec

1 large box = 0.20 sec (0.04 sec × 5 = 0.20 sec)

These increments measure the duration of the ECG complexes and time intervals. The vertical axis reflects the voltage amplitude in millivolts (mV). Two large boxes equal 1.0 mV.

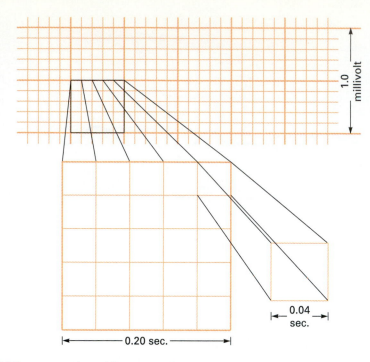

FIGURE 2-15   The ECG paper and markings.

In addition to the grid, ECG paper has time interval markings at the top. These marks are placed at three-second intervals. Each three-second interval contains 15 large boxes (0.2 sec × 15 boxes = 3.0 sec). The time markings measure heart rate.

RELATIONSHIP OF THE ECG TO ELECTRICAL EVENTS IN THE HEART

The ECG tracing's components reflect electrical changes in the heart (Figure 2-16).

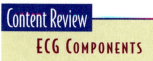

Content Review

ECG COMPONENTS
- P Wave
- QRS Complex
- T Wave
- U Wave

- *P wave.* The first component of the ECG, the P wave corresponds to atrial depolarization. On Lead II, it is a positive, rounded wave before the QRS complex (Figures 2-17–2-21).
- *QRS complex.* The QRS complex reflects ventricular depolarization. The *Q wave* is the first negative deflection after the P wave; the *R wave* is the first positive deflection after the P wave; and the *S wave* is the first negative deflection after the R wave. Not all three waves are always present, and the shape of the QRS complex can vary from individual to individual (Figure 2-22).

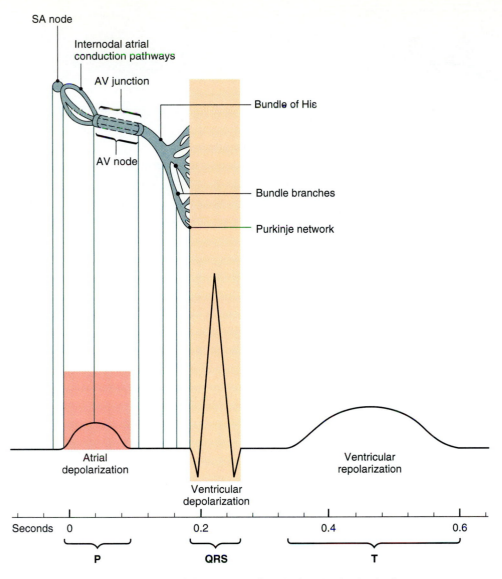

SA node

Internodal atrial conduction pathways

AV junction

Bundle of His

AV node

Bundle branches

Purkinje network

Atrial depolarization

Ventricular depolarization

Ventricular repolarization

| Seconds | 0 | 0.2 | 0.4 | 0.6 |

P   QRS   T

FIGURE 2-16   Relationship of the ECG to electrical activities in the heart.

- *T wave.* The T wave reflects repolarization of the ventricles. Normally positive in Lead II, it is rounded and usually moves in the same direction as the QRS complex (Figure 2-23).
- *U wave.* Occasionally, a U wave appears. U waves follow T waves and are usually positive. U waves may be associated with electrolyte abnormalities, or they may be a normal finding.

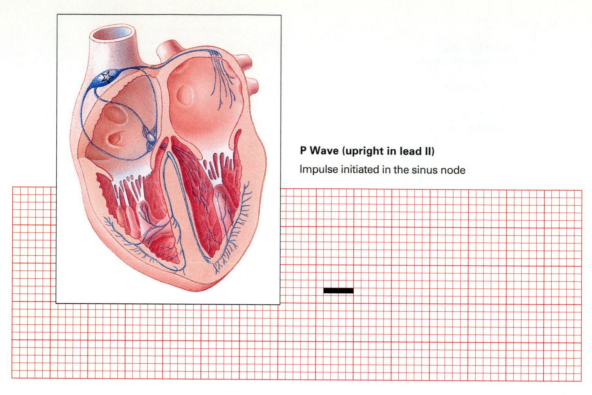

P Wave (upright in lead II)

Impulse initiated in the sinus node

FIGURE 2-17   Impulse initiation in the SA node.

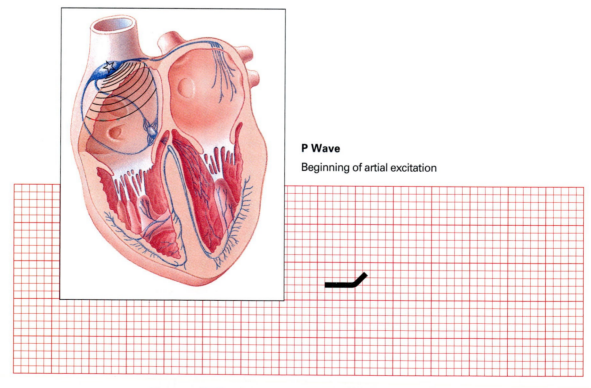

P Wave

Beginning of artial excitation

FIGURE 2-18   Beginning of atrial excitation.

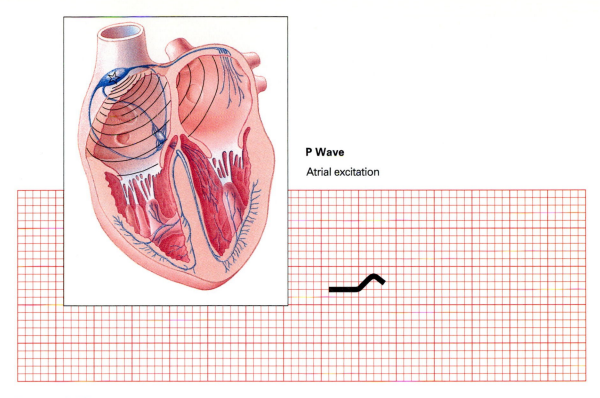

P Wave

Atrial excitation

FIGURE 2-19   Atrial excitation.

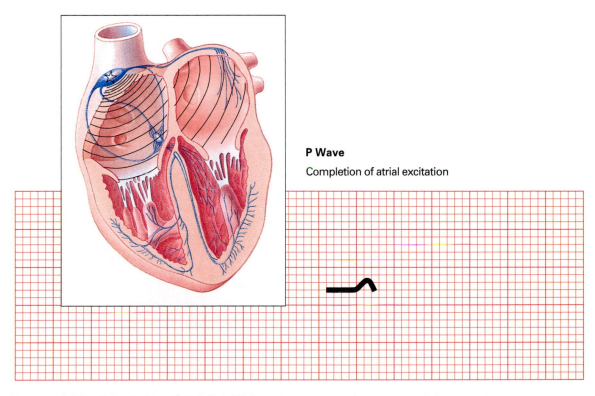

P Wave

Completion of atrial excitation

FIGURE 2-20   Completion of atrial excitation.

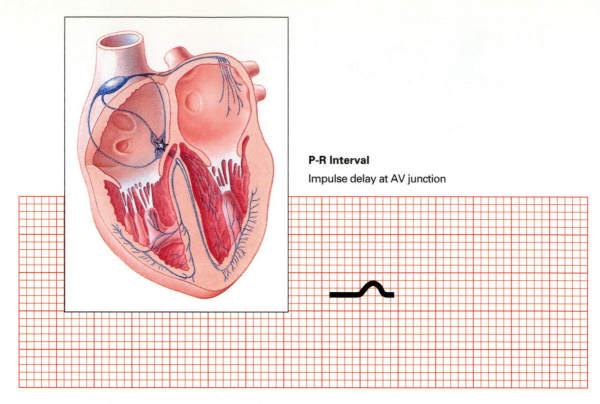

P-R Interval

Impulse delay at AV junction

FIGURE 2-21   Impulse delay at the AV junction.

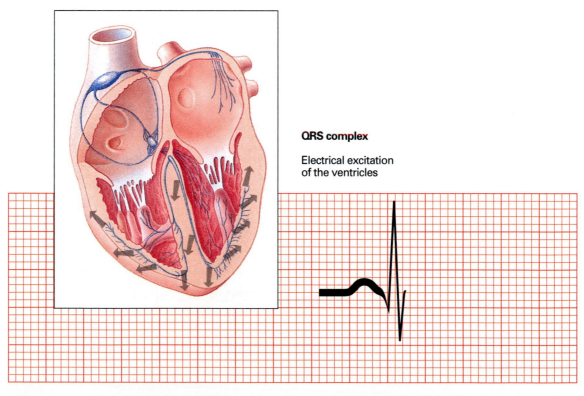

QRS complex

Electrical excitation
of the ventricles

FIGURE 2-22   Electrical excitation of the ventricles.

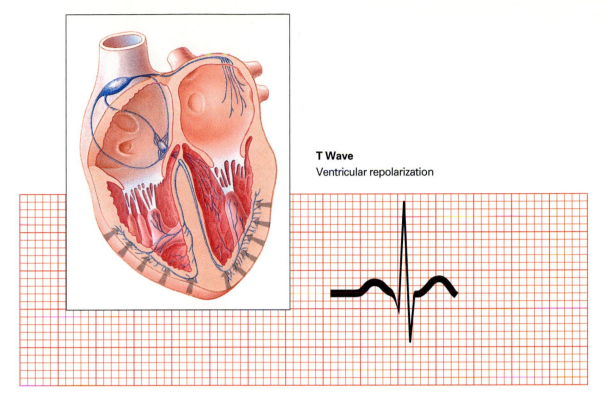

T Wave
Ventricular repolarization

FIGURE 2-23   Ventricular repolarization.

In addition to the wave forms described above, the ECG tracing reflects these important time intervals(Figure 2-24):

- *P-R interval (PRI) or P-Q interval (PQI))*. The P-R interval is the distance from the beginning of the P wave to the beginning of the QRS complex. It represents the time the impulse takes to travel from the atria to the ventricles. Occasionally, the R wave is absent, in which case this interval is called the P-Q interval. The terms P-R interval and P-Q interval may be used interchangeably.

- *QRS interval.* The QRS interval is the distance from the first deflection of the QRS complex to the last. It represents the time necessary for ventricular depolarization.

- *S-T segment.* The S-T segment is the distance from the S wave to the beginning of the T wave. Usually it is an isoelectric line; however, it may be elevated or depressed in certain disease states such as ischemia.

A normal P-R interval is 0.12-0.20 seconds. A short PRI lasts less than 0.12 seconds; a prolonged PRI lasts longer than 0.20 seconds. A prolonged PRI indicates a delay in the AV node. A normal QRS complex lasts between 0.08 and 0.12 seconds. A value of less than 0.12 seconds means that the ventricles depolarized in a normal length of time.

The **QT interval** represents the total duration of ventricular depolarization. A normal QT interval is 0.33–0.42 seconds. QT intervals and heart rate have an inverse relationship: increases in heart rate usually decrease the QT interval, while decreases in heart rate usually prolong it. A **prolonged QT interval** is thought to be related to an increased risk of certain ventricular dysrhythmias and sudden death.

Content Review

ECG TIME INTERVALS
- P-R Interval
- QRS Interval
- S-T Segment

Content Review

NORMAL INTERVAL DURATIONS
- PR   0.12–0.20 sec
- QRS   0.08–0.12 sec
- QT   0.33–0.42 sec

✱ **QT interval** period from the beginning of the QRS to the end of the T wave.

✱ **prolonged QT interval** QT interval greater than .44 seconds.

FIGURE 2-24   The ECG.

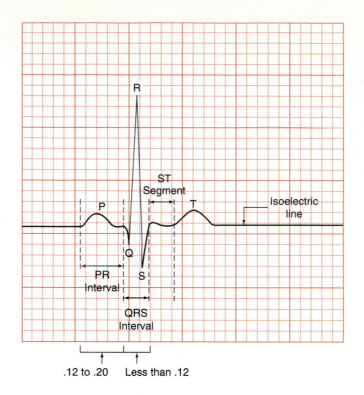

The all-or-none nature of myocardial depolarization results in an interval when the heart cannot be restimulated to depolarize. From our earlier discussion you will recall that during this time the myocardial cells have not yet repolarized and cannot be stimulated again (Figure 2-25). This **refractory period** has two parts, an **absolute refractory period** and a **relative refractory period.** During the absolute refractory period stimulation produces no depolarization whatsoever. This usually lasts from the beginning of the QRS complex to the apex of the T wave. During the relative refractory period, a sufficiently strong stimulus may produce depolarization. This usually corresponds to the T wave's down slope.

S-T Segment Changes   The S-T segment is usually an isoelectric line. Myocardial infarctions, which are caused by lack of blood flow to a part of the heart, produce changes in this line. The affected area is then electrically dead and cannot conduct electrical impulses. Myocardial infarctions usually follow this sequence:

1. Ischemia (lack of oxygen)
2. Injury
3. Necrosis (cell death, infarction)

✱ **refractory period** the period of time when myocardial cells have not yet completely repolarized and cannot be stimulated again.

✱ **absolute refractory period** the period of the cardiac cycle when stimulation will not produce any depolarization whatever.

✱ **relative refractory period** the period of the cardiac cycle when a sufficiently strong stimulus may produce depolarization.

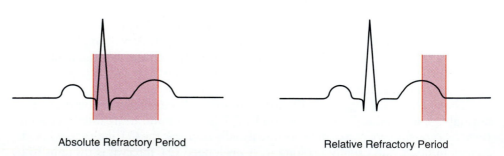

Absolute Refractory Period

Relative Refractory Period

FIGURE 2-25   Refractory periods of the cardiac cycle.

Table 2-2 OVERVIEW OF ECG LEAD GROUPINGS

Leads	Portion of the heart examined
I and aVL	The left side of the heart in a vertical plane
II, III, and aVF	The inferior (diaphragmatic) side of the heart
aVR	The right side of the heart in a vertical plane
V_1 and V_2	The right ventricle
V_3 and V_4	The intraventricular septum and the anterior wall of the left ventricle
V_5 and V_6	The anterior and lateral walls of the left ventricle

Each of these stages results in distinct S-T segment changes. Ischemia causes S-T segment depression or an inverted T wave. The inversion is usually symmetrical. Injury elevates the S-T segment, most often in the early phases of a myocardial infarction. As the tissue dies, a significant Q wave appears. As we noted earlier, small, insignificant Q waves may show up in normal ECG tracings. A significant Q wave is at least one small square wide, lasting 0.04 seconds, or is more than one-third the height of the QRS complex. Q waves may also indicate extensive transient ischemia.

Lead Systems and Heart Surfaces Using the various ECG leads is comparable to waiting for a train at a railroad crossing. You will want to know how long you have to wait (in other words, how long is the train), but you can only see the front of the train. If you had cameras at other viewpoints, you could see how long the train actually was. Similarly, by combining the different ECG leads you can view different parts of the heart.

Leads V_1–V_4 view the anterior surface of the heart. Leads I and aVL view the lateral surface of the heart. The inferior surface of the heart can be visualized in leads II, III, and aVF. These leads can show ischemia, injury, and necrotic changes and can provide information about the corresponding heart surface (Table 2-2). For example, significant S-T elevation in V_1–V_4 may indicate anterior involvement, while elevation in II, III, and aVF may indicate inferior involvement. This chapter's section on 12-lead ECG analysis discusses these leads in more detail.

Medical procedures (angioplasty) and drugs (thrombolytics) can treat acute myocardial infarction. The earlier they are initiated, the better the patient's potential outcome. Earlier identification in the field of patients with AMI will allow for earlier interventions, but the 12-lead ECG's role in out-of-hospital care remains unresolved. Its use may not be appropriate in many EMS settings. Individual EMS medical directors will determine the application and use of the 12-lead ECG in their specific EMS settings.

Earlier identification in the field of patients with AMI will allow for earlier intervention.

INTERPRETATION OF RHYTHM STRIPS

The key to interpreting rhythm strips is to approach each strip logically and systematically. Attempts to nonanalytically "eyeball" the strip often lead to incorrect interpretations. Your approach to rhythm strip interpretation should include the following basic criteria.

The key to interpreting rhythm strips is to approach each strip logically and systematically.

- Always be consistent and analytical.
- Memorize the rules for each dysrhythmia.
- Analyze a given rhythm strip according to a specific format.
- Compare your analysis to the rules for each dysrhythmia.
- Identify the dysrhythmia by its similarity to established rules.

Use ECG calipers to measure ECG tracings to assure accuracy and to avoid misinterpretation.

The health care profession uses several standard formats for ECG analysis. We will use the following five-step procedure:

1. Analyze the rate.
2. Analyze the rhythm.
3. Analyze the P-waves.
4. Analyze the P-R interval.
5. Analyze the QRS complex.

Analyzing Rate The first step in ECG strip interpretation is to analyze the heart rate. Usually this means the ventricular rate; however, if the atrial and ventricular rates differ, you must calculate both. The normal heart rate is 60–100 beats per minute. A heart rate greater than 100 beats per minute is a **tachycardia.** A heart rate less than 60 beats per minute is a **bradycardia.** You can use any of the following methods to calculate the rate.

✳ **tachycardia** a heart rate greater than 100 beats per minute.

✳ **bradycardia** a heart rate less than 60 beats per minute.

- *Six-Second Method.* Count the number of complexes in a six-second interval. Mark off a six-second interval by noting two three-second marks at the top of the ECG paper. Then multiply the number of complexes within the six-second strip by ten.
- *Heart Rate Calculator Rulers.* Commercially available heart rate calculator rulers allow you to determine heart rates rapidly. Always use them according to the accompanying directions, since variations occur among different manufacturers. Also learn a manual method so you can still calculate rates if you forget your ruler.
- *R-R Interval.* The R-R interval is related directly to heart rate. The R-R interval method is accurate only if the heart rhythm is regular. You can calculate it in the following ways:
  - Measure the duration between R waves in seconds. Divide this number into 60, giving the heart rate per minute.
    Example: $60 \div 0.65$ second = 92 (heart rate)
  - Count the number of large squares within an R-R interval, and divide the number of squares into 300.
    Example: $300 \div 3.5$ large boxes = 86 (heart rate)
  - Count the number of small squares within an R-R interval, and divide the number of squares into 1,500.
    Example: $1,500 \div 29$ small boxes = 52 (heart rate)
- *Triplicate Method.* Another method, also useful only with regular rhythms, is to locate an R wave that falls on a dark line bordering a large box on the graph paper. Then assign numbers corresponding to the heart rate to the next six dark lines to the right. The order is: 300, 150, 100, 75, 60, and 50. The number corresponding to the dark line closest to the peak of the next R wave is a rough estimate of the heart rate.

Pick one of the above methods and become comfortable with it. Use it to determine the rate on all strips that you look at.

Analyzing Rhythm The next step is to analyze the rhythm. First, measure the R-R interval across the strip. Normally, the R-R rhythm is fairly regular. Some minimal variation, associated with respirations, should be expected. If the rhythm is irregular, note whether it fits one of the following patterns.

- Occasionally irregular (only one or two R-R intervals on the strip are irregular)
- Regularly irregular (patterned irregularity or group beating)
- Irregularly irregular (no relationship among R-R intervals)

Analyzing P Waves The P waves reflect atrial depolarization. Normally, the atria depolarize away from the SA node and toward the ventricles. In Lead II, this appears as a positive, rounded P wave. When analyzing the P waves, ask yourself the following questions:

- Are P waves present?
- Are the P waves regular?
- Is there one P wave for each QRS complex?
- Are the P waves upright or inverted (compared to the QRS complex)?
- Do all the P waves look alike?

Analyzing the P-R Interval The P-R interval represents the time needed for atrial depolarization and conduction of the impulse up to the AV node. Remember, the normal P-R interval is 0.12-0.20 sec (three to five small boxes). Any deviation is an abnormal finding. The P-R interval should be consistent across the strip.

Analyzing the QRS Complex The QRS complex represents ventricular depolarization. When evaluating the QRS complex, ask yourself the following questions:

- Do all of the QRS complexes look alike?
- What is the QRS duration?

Remember, the QRS duration is usually 0.04–0.12 sec. Anything longer than 0.12 sec (three small boxes) is abnormal.

DYSRHYTHMIAS

On a normal ECG, the heart rate is between 60 and 100 beats per minute. The rhythm is regular (both P-P and R-R). The P waves are normal in shape, upright, and appear only before each QRS complex. The P-R interval lasts 0.12-0.20 sec and is constant. The QRS complex has a normal morphology, and its duration is less than 0.12 sec. All of these factors indicate a **normal sinus rhythm.** Any deviation from the heart's normal electrical rhythm is a **dysrhythmia.** The absence of cardiac electrical activity is **arrhythmia.** The causes of dysrhythmias include:

- Myocardial ischemia, necrosis, or infarction
- Autonomic nervous system imbalance
- Distention of the chambers of the heart (especially in the atria, secondary to congestive heart failure)
- Blood gas abnormalities, including hypoxia and abnormal pH
- Electrolyte imbalances (Ca^{++}, K^+, Mg^{++})

✳ normal sinus rhythm the normal heart rhythm.

✳ dysrhythmia any deviation from the normal electrical rhythm of the heart.

✳ arrhythmia the absence of cardiac electrical activity; often used interchangeably with dysrhythmia.

- Trauma to the myocardium (cardiac contusion)
- Drug effects and drug toxicity
- Electrocution
- Hypothermia
- CNS damage
- Idiopathic events
- Normal occurrences

Dysrhythmias in the healthy heart are of little significance. No matter what the etiology or type of dysrhythmia, treat the patient and his symptoms, not the dysrhythmia. You will hear this repeated over and over: Treat the patient, not the monitor.

Treat the patient, not the monitor.

MECHANISM OF IMPULSE FORMATION

Several physiologic mechanisms can cause cardiac dysrhythmias. The depolarization impulse is normally transmitted forward (*antegrade*) through the conductive system and the myocardium. In certain dysrhythmias, however, the depolarization impulse is conducted backwards (*retrograde*).

Ectopic Foci One cause of dysrhythmias is *enhanced automaticity*. This condition results when **ectopic foci** (heart cells other than the pacemaker cells) automatically depolarize, producing **ectopic** (abnormal) **beats**. Premature ventricular contractions and premature atrial contractions are examples of ectopic beats. Ectopic beats can be intermittent or sustained.

Reentry *Reentry* may cause isolated premature beats, or *tachydysrhythmias*. It occurs when ischemia or another disease process alters two branches of a conduction pathway, slowing conduction in one branch and causing a unidirectional block in the other. An antegrade depolarization wave travels slowly through the branch with ischemia and is blocked in the branch with a unidirectional block. After the depolarization wave goes through the slowed branch, it enters the branch with the unidirectional block and is conducted retrograde back to the branch's origin. By now the tissue is no longer refractory, and stimulation occurs again. This can result in rapid rhythms such as paroxysmal supraventricular tachycardia or atrial fibrillation.

CLASSIFICATION OF DYSRHYTHMIAS

Dysrhythmias can be classified in any number of ways. Some of the classification methods include:

- Nature of origin (changes in automaticity versus disturbances in conduction)
- Magnitude (major versus minor)
- Severity (life-threatening versus non-life-threatening)
- Site of origin

Classifying dysrhythmias by site of origin is closely related to basic physiology and, thus, is easy to understand. This approach divides dysrhythmias into the following categories:

- Dysrhythmias originating in the SA node
- Dysrhythmias originating in the atria

* ectopic focus nonpacemaker heart cell that automatically depolarizes; *pl.* ectopic foci.

* ectopic beat cardiac depolarization resulting from depolarization of ectopic focus.

- Dysrhythmias originating within the AV junction
- Dysrhythmias sustained in or originating in the AV junction
- Dysrhythmias originating in the ventricles
- Dysrhythmias resulting from disorders of conduction

DYSRHYTHMIAS ORIGINATING IN THE SA NODE

Dysrhythmias originating in the SA node most often result from changes in autonomic tone. However, disease can exist in the SA node itself. Dysrhythmias that originate in the SA node include:

- Sinus bradycardia
- Sinus tachycardia
- Sinus dysrhythmia
- Sinus arrest

Sinus Bradycardia

Description: Sinus bradycardia results from slowing of the SA node.

Etiology: Sinus bradycardia may result from any of the following conditions.

- Increased parasympathetic (vagal) tone
- Intrinsic disease of the SA node
- Drug effects (digitalis, propranolol, quinidine)
- Normal finding in healthy, well-conditioned persons

Rules of Interpretation/Lead II Monitoring (Figure 2-26):

Rate—less than 60
Rhythm—regular
Pacemaker site—SA node
P waves—upright and normal in morphology
P-R interval—normal (0.12–0.20 sec and constant)
QRS complex—normal (0.04–0.12 sec)

Clinical Significance: The decreased heart rate can cause decreased cardiac output, hypotension, angina, or CNS symptoms. This is especially true for rates slower than 50 beats per minute. The slow heart rate may also lead to atrial ectopic or ventricular ectopic rhythms. In a healthy athlete, sinus bradycardia may have no clinical significance.

Treatment: Treatment is generally unnecessary unless hypotension or ventricular irritability is present (Figure 2-27). Remember, treat your patient and not the monitor. If treatment is required, administer a 0.5 mg bolus of atropine sulfate. Repeat every 3–5 minutes until you have obtained a satisfactory rate or have given 0.04 mg/kg of the drug. If atropine fails, consider transcutaneous cardiac pacing (TCP), if available.

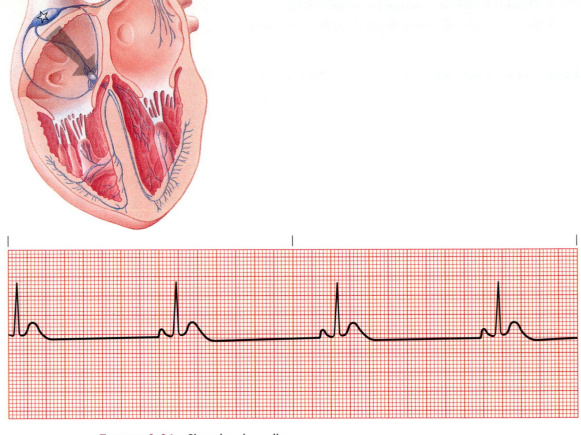

FIGURE 2-26   Sinus bradycardia.

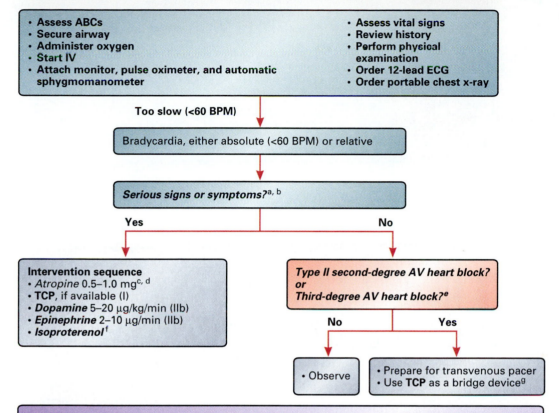

ALGORITHM: BRADYCARDIA

- Assess ABCs
- Secure airway
- Administer oxygen
- Start IV
- Attach monitor, pulse oximeter, and automatic sphygmomanometer

- Assess vital signs
- Review history
- Perform physical examination
- Order 12-lead ECG
- Order portable chest x-ray

Too slow (<60 BPM)

Bradycardia, either absolute (<60 BPM) or relative

Serious signs or symptoms?[a, b]

Yes → No →

Intervention sequence
- *Atropine* 0.5–1.0 mg[c, d]
- **TCP**, if available (I)
- **Dopamine** 5–20 μg/kg/min (IIb)
- **Epinephrine** 2–10 μg/min (IIb)
- *Isoproterenol*[f]

Type II second-degree AV heart block?
or
Third-degree AV heart block?[e]

No → Yes →

- Observe

- Prepare for transvenous pacer
- Use **TCP** as a bridge device[g]

---

a. Serious signs or symptoms must be related to the slow rate. Clinical manifestations include:
   - Symptoms (chest pain, shortness of breath, decreased level of consciousness)
   - Signs (low BP, shock, pulmonary congestion, CHF, acute MI)

b. Do not delay TCP while awaiting IV access or for *atropine* to take effect if patient is symptomatic.

c. Denervated transplanted hearts will not respond to *atropine*. Go at once to pacing, *catecholamine* infusion, or both.

d. *Atropine* should be given in repeat doses every 3–5 min up to total of 0.04 mg/kg. Consider shorter dosing intervals in severe clinical conditions. It has been suggested that *atropine* should be used with caution in atrioventricular (AV) block at the His-Purkinje level (type II AV block and new third-degree block with wide QRS complexes) (Class IIb).

e. Never treat third-degree heart block plus ventricular escape beats with *lidocaine*.

f. *Isoproterenol* should be used, if at all, with extreme caution. At low doses it is Class IIb (possibly helpful); at higher doses it is Class III (harmful).

g. Verify patient tolerance and mechanical capture. Use analgesia and sedation as needed.

FIGURE 2-27   Management of bradycardia. Adapted with permission. Journal of the American Medical Association, October 28, 1992, Volume 268, No. 16, *Guidelines for Cardiopulmonary Resuscitation and Emergency Cardiac Care*, p. 2221. © 1992 American Medical Association.

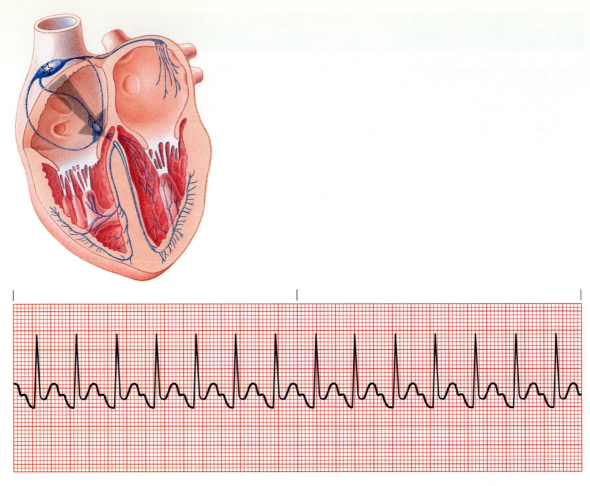

FIGURE 2-28   Sinus tachycardia.

Sinus Tachycardia

Description: Sinus tachycardia results from an increased rate of SA node discharge.

Etiology: Sinus tachycardia may result from any of the following:

- Exercise
- Fever
- Anxiety
- Hypovolemia
- Anemia
- Pump failure
- Increased sympathetic tone
- Hypoxia
- Hyperthyroidism

Rules of Interpretation/Lead II Monitoring (Figure 2-28):

Rate—greater than 100
Rhythm—regular
Pacemaker site—SA node
P waves—upright and normal in morphology
P-R interval—normal
QRS complex—normal

Clinical Significance: Sinus tachycardia is often benign. In some cases, it is a compensatory mechanism for decreased stroke volume. If the rate is greater than 140 beats per minute, cardiac output may fall because ventricular filling time is inadequate. Very rapid heart rates increase myocardial oxygen demand and can precipitate ischemia or infarct in diseased hearts. Prolonged sinus tachycardia accompanying acute myocardial infarction (AMI) is often an ominous finding suggesting cardiogenic shock.

Treatment: Treatment is directed at the underlying cause. Hypovolemia, fever, hypoxia, or other causes should be corrected.

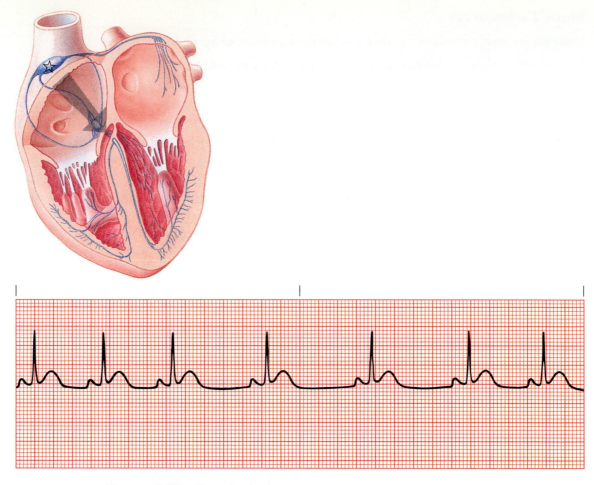

FIGURE 2-29   Sinus dysrhythmia.

Sinus Dysrhythmia

Description: *Sinus dysrhythmia* often results from a variation of the R-R interval.

Etiology: Sinus dysrhythmia is often a normal finding and is sometimes related to the respiratory cycle and changes in intrathoracic pressure. Pathologically, sinus dysrhythmia can be caused by enhanced vagal tone.

Rules of Interpretation/Lead II Monitoring (Figure 2-29):

Rate—60–100 (varies with respirations)
Rhythm—irregular
Pacemaker site—SA node
P waves—upright and normal in morphology
P-R interval—normal
QRS complex—normal

Clinical Significance: Sinus dysrhythmia is a normal variant, particularly in the young and the aged.

Treatment: Typically, none required.

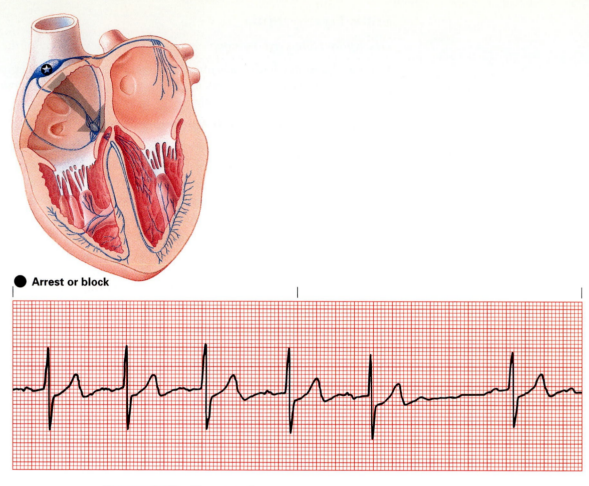

● **Arrest or block**

FIGURE 2-30   Sinus arrest.

Sinus Arrest

Description: *Sinus arrest* occurs when the sinus node fails to discharge, resulting in short periods of cardiac standstill. This standstill can persist until pacemaker cells lower in the conductive system discharge (escape beats) or until the sinus node resumes discharge.

Etiology: Sinus arrest can result from any of the following conditions.

- Ischemia of the SA node
- Digitalis toxicity
- Excessive vagal tone
- Degenerative fibrotic disease

Rules of Interpretation/Lead II Monitoring (Figure 2-30):

Rate—normal to slow, depending on the frequency and duration of the arrest

Rhythm—irregular

Pacemaker site—SA node

P waves—upright and normal in morphology

P-R interval—normal

QRS complex—normal

Clinical Significance: Frequent or prolonged episodes may compromise cardiac output, resulting in syncope (fainting) and other problems. There is always the danger of complete cessation of SA node activity. Usually, an escape rhythm develops; however, cardiac standstill occasionally can result.

Treatment: If the patient is asymptomatic, observation is all that is required. If the patient is extremely bradycardic or symptomatic, administer a 0.5 mg bolus of atropine sulfate. Repeat every 3–5 minutes until you have obtained a satisfactory rate or have administered 0.04 mg/kg of the drug. If atropine fails, consider transcutaneous cardiac pacing (TCP), if available.

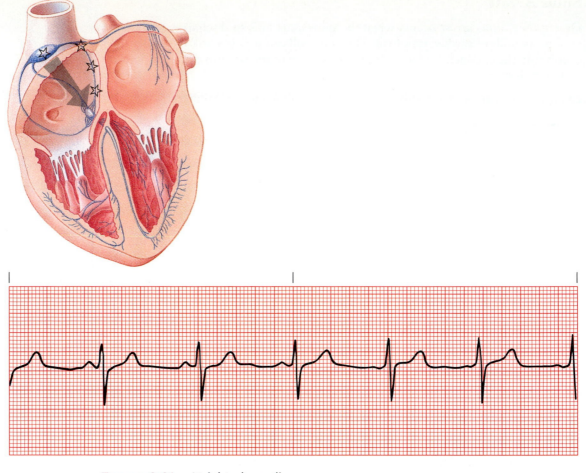

FIGURE 2-31   Atrial tachycardia.

DYSRHYTHMIAS ORIGINATING IN THE ATRIA

Dysrhythmias can originate outside the SA node in the atrial tissue or in the internodal pathways. Ischemia, hypoxia, atrial dilation, and other factors can cause atrial dysrhythmias. Dysrhythmias originating in the atria include:

- Atrial tachycardia
- Multifocal atrial tachycardia
- Premature atrial contractions
- Paroxysmal supraventricular tachycardia
- Atrial flutter
- Atrial fibrillation

Atrial Tachycardia

Description: Atrial tachycardia (also called *ectopic tachycardia* or *wandering pacemaker*) is the passive transfer of pacemaker sites from the sinus node to other latent pacemaker sites in the atria and AV junction. Often more than one pacemaker site will be present, causing variation in R-R interval and P wave morphology.

Etiology: Atrial tachycardia can result from any of the following conditions:

- A variant of sinus dysrhythmia
- A normal phenomenon in the very young or the aged
- Ischemic heart disease
- Atrial dilation

Rules of Interpretation/Lead II Monitoring (Figure 2-31):

Rate—usually normal

Rhythm—slightly irregular

Pacemaker site—varies among the SA node, atrial tissue, and the AV junction

P waves—morphology changes from beat to beat; P waves may disappear entirely

P-R interval—varies; may be less than 0.12 sec, normal, or greater than 0.20 sec

QRS Complex—normal

Clinical Significance: Atrial tachycardia usually has no detrimental effects. Occasionally, it can be a precursor of other atrial dysrhythmias such as atrial fibrillation. It sometimes indicates digitalis toxicity.

Treatment: If the patient is asymptomatic, observation is all that is required. If the patient is symptomatic, consider adenosine or verapamil.

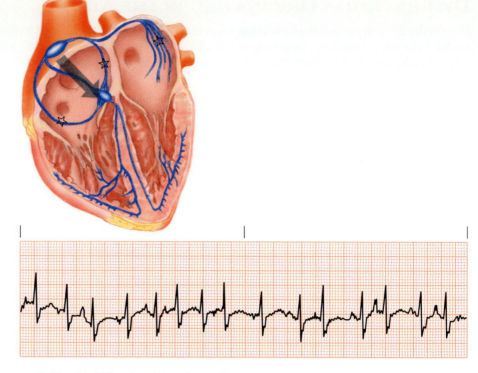

FIGURE 2-32   Multifocal atrial tachycardia.

Multifocal Atrial Tachycardia

Description: Multifocal atrial tachycardia (MAT) is usually seen in acutely ill patients. Significant pulmonary disease is seen in about 60 percent of these patients. Certain medications used to treat lung disease (such as theophylline) may worsen the dysrhythmia. Three different P waves are noted, indicating various ectopic foci.

Etiology: Multifocal atrial tachycardia can result from any of the following conditions:

- Pulmonary disease
- Metabolic disorders (hypokalemia)
- Ischemic heart disease
- Recent surgery

Rules of Interpretation/Lead II Monitoring (Figure 2-32):

Rate—more than 100

Rhythm—irregular

Pacemaker site—ectopic sites in atria

P waves—organized, discrete nonsinus P waves with at least three different forms

P-R interval—varies

QRS complex—may be less than 0.12 sec, normal, or greater than 0.20 sec, depending on the AV node's refractory status when the impulse reaches it

Clinical Significance: Frequently these patients are acutely ill; this dysrhythmia may indicate a serious underlying medical illness.

Treatment: Treatment of the underlying medical disease usually resolves the dysrhythmia. Specific antidysrhythmic therapy is frequently not needed.

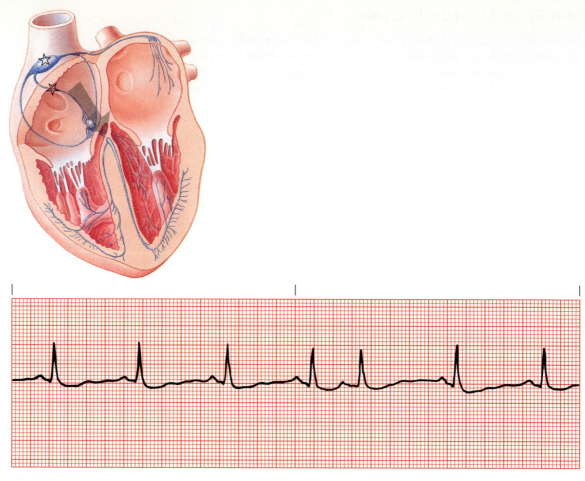

FIGURE 2-33 Premature atrial contractions.

Premature Atrial Contractions

Description: Premature atrial contractions (PACs) result from a single electrical impulse originating in the atria outside the SA node, which in turn causes a premature depolarization of the heart before the next expected sinus beat. Because it depolarizes the atrial syncytium, this impulse also depolarizes the SA node, interrupting the normal cadence. This creates a **noncompensatory pause** in the underlying rhythm.

Etiology: A premature atrial contraction can result from any of the following conditions:

- Use of caffeine, tobacco, or alcohol
- Sympathomimetic drugs
- Ischemic heart disease
- Hypoxia
- Digitalis toxicity
- No apparent cause (idiopathic)

Rules of Interpretation/Lead II Monitoring (Figure 2-33):

Rate—depends on the underlying rhythm

Rhythm—depends on the underlying rhythm; usually regular except for the PAC

Pacemaker site—ectopic focus in the atrium

P waves—the P wave of the PAC differs from the P wave of the underlying rhythm. It occurs earlier than the next expected P wave and may be hidden in the preceding T wave.

P-R interval—usually normal; can vary with the location of the ectopic focus. Ectopic foci near the SA node will have a P-R interval of 0.12 sec or greater, whereas ectopic foci near the AV node will have a P-R interval of 0.12 sec or less.

QRS complex—usually normal; may be greater than 0.12 sec if the PAC is abnormally conducted through partially refractory ventricles. In some cases, the ventricles are refractory and will not depolarize in response to the PAC. In these cases, the QRS complex is absent.

Clinical Significance: Isolated PACs are of minimal significance. Frequent PACs may indicate organic heart disease and may precede other atrial dysrhythmias.

Treatment: If the patient is asymptomatic, observation is all that is required in the field. If the patient is symptomatic, administer oxygen via a nonrebreather mask and start an IV line. Contact medical direction.

✱ **noncompensatory pause** pause following an ectopic beat where the SA node is depolarized and the underlying cadence of the heart is interrupted.

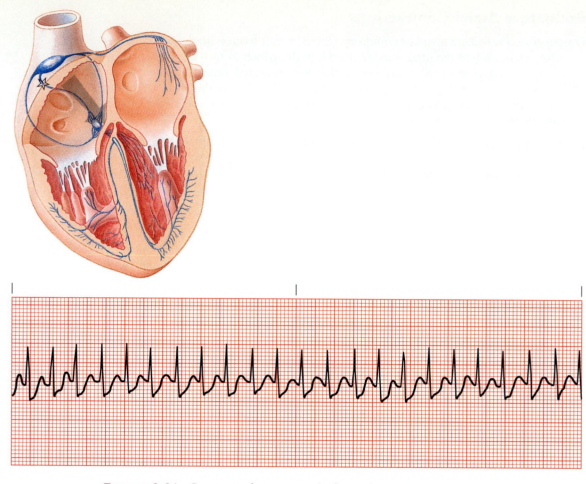

FIGURE 2-34   Paroxysmal supraventricular tachycardia.

Paroxysmal Supraventricular Tachycardia

Description: *Paroxysmal supraventricular tachycardia (PSVT)* occurs when rapid atrial depolarization overrides the SA node. It often occurs in paroxysm with sudden onset, may last minutes to hours, and terminates abruptly. It may be caused by increased automaticity of a single atrial focus or by reentry phenomenon at the AV node.

Etiology: Paroxysmal supraventricular tachycardia may occur at any age and often is not associated with underlying heart disease. It may be precipitated by stress, overexertion, smoking, or ingestion of caffeine. It is, however, frequently associated with underlying atherosclerotic cardiovascular disease and rheumatic heart disease. PSVT is rare in patients with myocardial infarction. It can occur with accessory pathway conduction such as Wolff-Parkinson-White syndrome.

Rules of Interpretation/Lead II Monitoring (Figure 2-34):

Rate—150–250 per minute

Rhythm—characteristically regular, except at onset and termination

Pacemaker site—in the atria, outside the SA node

P waves—the atrial P waves differ slightly from sinus P waves. The P wave is often buried in the preceding T wave. The P wave may be impossible to see, especially if the rate is rapid. Turning up the speed of the graph paper or oscilloscope to 50 mm/sec spreads out the complex and can help identify P waves.

P-R interval—usually normal; however, it can vary with the location of the ectopic pacemaker. Ectopic pacemakers near the SA node will have P-R intervals close to 0.12 sec, whereas ectopic pacemakers near the AV node will have P-R intervals of 0.12 sec or less.

QRS complex—normal

Clinical Significance: Young patients with good cardiac reserves may tolerate PSVT well for short periods. Patients often sense PSVT as palpitations. However, rapid rates can cause a marked reduction in cardiac output because of inadequate ventricular filling time. The reduced diastolic phase of the cardiac cycle can also compromise coronary artery perfusion. PSVT can precipitate angina, hypotension, or congestive heart failure.

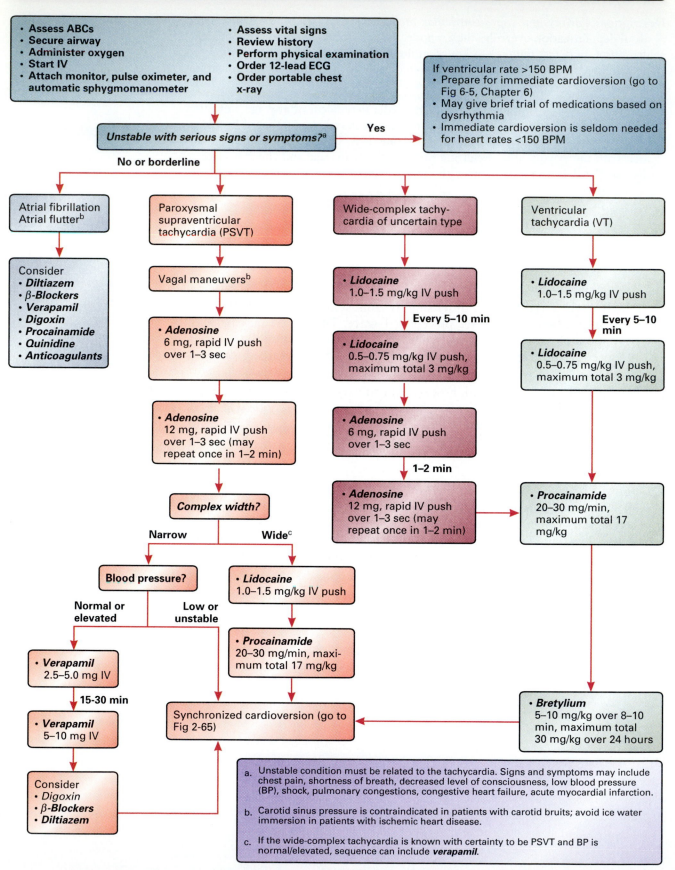

ALGORITHM: TACHYCARDIA

- Assess ABCs
- Secure airway
- Administer oxygen
- Start IV
- Attach monitor, pulse oximeter, and automatic sphygmomanometer

- Assess vital signs
- Review history
- Perform physical examination
- Order 12-lead ECG
- Order portable chest x-ray

If ventricular rate >150 BPM
- Prepare for immediate cardioversion (go to Fig 6-5, Chapter 6)
- May give brief trial of medications based on dysrhythmia
- Immediate cardioversion is seldom needed for heart rates <150 BPM

Unstable with serious signs or symptoms?[a] — **Yes**

No or borderline

Atrial fibrillation Atrial flutter[b]

Consider
- **Diltiazem**
- **β-Blockers**
- **Verapamil**
- **Digoxin**
- **Procainamide**
- **Quinidine**
- **Anticoagulants**

Paroxysmal supraventricular tachycardia (PSVT)

Vagal maneuvers[b]

- **Adenosine** 6 mg, rapid IV push over 1–3 sec

- **Adenosine** 12 mg, rapid IV push over 1–3 sec (may repeat once in 1–2 min)

Complex width?

Narrow — **Blood pressure?**

Normal or elevated
- **Verapamil** 2.5–5.0 mg IV

15-30 min

- **Verapamil** 5–10 mg IV

Consider
- **Digoxin**
- **β-Blockers**
- **Diltiazem**

Wide[c]
- **Lidocaine** 1.0–1.5 mg/kg IV push

Low or unstable

- **Procainamide** 20–30 mg/min, maximum total 17 mg/kg

Synchronized cardioversion (go to Fig 2-65)

Wide-complex tachycardia of uncertain type

- **Lidocaine** 1.0–1.5 mg/kg IV push

Every 5–10 min

- **Lidocaine** 0.5–0.75 mg/kg IV push, maximum total 3 mg/kg

- **Adenosine** 6 mg, rapid IV push over 1–3 sec

1–2 min

- **Adenosine** 12 mg, rapid IV push over 1–3 sec (may repeat once in 1–2 min)

Ventricular tachycardia (VT)

- **Lidocaine** 1.0–1.5 mg/kg IV push

Every 5–10 min

- **Lidocaine** 0.5–0.75 mg/kg IV push, maximum total 3 mg/kg

- **Procainamide** 20–30 mg/min, maximum total 17 mg/kg

- **Bretylium** 5–10 mg/kg over 8–10 min, maximum total 30 mg/kg over 24 hours

a. Unstable condition must be related to the tachycardia. Signs and symptoms may include chest pain, shortness of breath, decreased level of consciousness, low blood pressure (BP), shock, pulmonary congestions, congestive heart failure, acute myocardial infarction.

b. Carotid sinus pressure is contraindicated in patients with carotid bruits; avoid ice water immersion in patients with ischemic heart disease.

c. If the wide-complex tachycardia is known with certainty to be PSVT and BP is normal/elevated, sequence can include **verapamil**.

FIGURE 2-35   Management of paroxysmal supraventricular tachycardia. Adapted with permission. *Journal of the American Medical Association*, October 28, 1992, Volume 268, No. 16, *Guidelines for Cardiopulmonary Resuscitation and Emergency Cardiac Care*, p. 2223. ©1992 American Medical Association.

Treatment: If the patient is not tolerating the rapid heart rate, as evidenced by hemodynamic instability, attempt the following techniques in this order (Figure 2-35).

1. Vagal maneuvers. Ask the patient to perform a Valsalva maneuver. This is a forced expiration against a closed glottis, or the act of "bearing down" as if to move the bowels. This results in vagal stimulation, which may slow the heart. If this is unsuccessful, attempt carotid artery massage, if the patient is eligible. Do not attempt carotid artery massage in patients with carotid **bruits** or known cerebrovascular or carotid artery disease.

2. Pharmacological therapy. Adenosine (Adenocard) is very safe and highly effective in terminating PSVT, especially if its etiology is reentry. Administer 6 mg of adenosine by rapid IV bolus over 1–3 sec through the medication port closest to the patient's heart or central circulation. (Adenosine has a very short half-life, and you must immediately follow administration with a bolus of normal saline to allow the medication to reach its site of action while it is still effective.) If the patient does not convert after 1–2 minutes, administer a second bolus of 12 mg over 1–3 sec in the medication port closest to the patient's heart or central circulation. If this fails and the patient has a normal blood pressure, then look again at the width of the cardiac QRS. If it appears to be a narrow complex rhythm with a normal blood pressure, medical direction may request the administration of verapamil 2.5–5.0 mg. This can be repeated once in 15–30 minutes, if needed, at a dose of 5–10 milligrams. Verapamil is contraindicated in patients with a history of bradycardia, hypotension, or congestive heart failure. Do not use it with intravenous beta blockers; use it with caution in patients on chronic beta blocker therapy. Hypotension following verapamil administration can often be reversed with 0.5–1.0 gm of calcium chloride administered intravenously.

3. Electrical therapy. If the ventricular rate is greater than 150 beats per minute, or if the patient is hemodynamically unstable, use synchronized cardioversion (described later in the chapter). If time allows, sedate the patient with 5–10 mg of diazepam or 2-5 mg of midazolam (Versed) IV. Apply synchronized DC countershock of 100 joules. If this is unsuccessful, repeat the countershock at increased energy as ordered by medical direction. DC countershock is contraindicated if you suspect digitalis toxicity as the PSVT's cause.

✱ **bruit** the sound of turbulent blood flow through a vessel; usually associated with atherosclerotic disease.

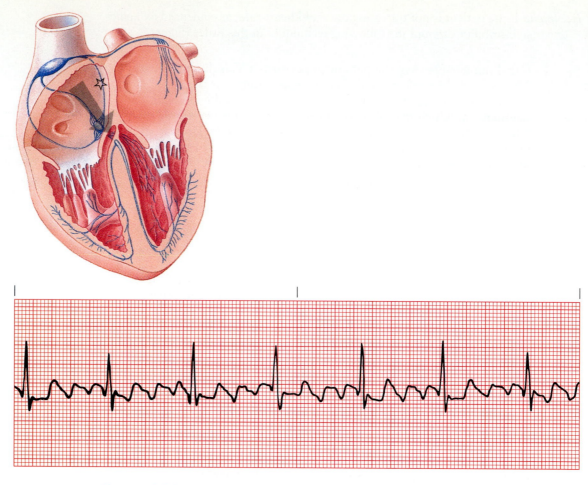

FIGURE 2-36 Atrial flutter.

Atrial Flutter

Description: Atrial flutter results from a rapid atrial reentry circuit and an AV node that physiologically cannot conduct all impulses through to the ventricles. The AV junction may allow impulses in a 1:1 (rare), 2:1, 3:1, or 4:1 ratio or greater, resulting in a discrepancy between atrial and ventricular rates. The AV block may be consistent or variable.

Etiology: Atrial flutter may occur in normal hearts, but it is usually associated with organic disease. It rarely occurs as the direct result of an MI. Atrial dilation, which occurs with congestive heart failure, is a cause of atrial flutter.

Rules of Interpretation/Lead II Monitoring (Figure 2-36):

Rate—atrial rate is 250–350 per minute. Ventricular rate varies with the ratio of AV conduction.

Rhythm—atrial rhythm is regular; ventricular rhythm is usually regular, but can be irregular if the block is variable

Pacemaker site—sites in the atria outside the SA node

P waves—flutter (F) waves are present, resembling a sawtooth or picket-fence pattern. This pattern is often difficult to identify in a 2:1 flutter. However, if the ventricular rate is approximately 150, suspect 2:1 flutter.

P-R interval—usually constant but may vary

QRS complex—normal

Clinical Significance: Atrial flutter with normal ventricular rates is generally well tolerated. Rapid ventricular rates may compromise cardiac output and result in symptoms. Atrial flutter often occurs in conjunction with atrial fibrillation and is referred to as "atrial fib-flutter."

Treatment: Treatment is indicated only for rapid ventricular rates with hemodynamic compromise (review Figure 2-35).

1. Electrical therapy. Immediate cardioversion is indicated in unstable patients—those with a heart rate greater than 150 and associated chest pain, dyspnea, a decreased level of consciousness, or hypotension. If time allows, sedate the patient with 5–10 mg of diazepam (Valium) or 2-5 mg of midazolam (Versed) IV. Then apply synchronized DC countershock of 100 joules. If this is unsuccessful, repeat the countershock at increased energy as recommended by AHA guidelines.

2. Pharmacological therapy. Occasionally you may use pharmacological therapy in stable patients with atrial flutter, especially if the rapid heart rate is causing congestive heart failure. Several medications slow the ventricular rate. The most frequently used is diltiazem (Cardizem). In addition, you may use verapamil, digoxin, beta blockers, procainamide, and quinidine. Procainamide and quinidine are often used to convert atrial flutter back to a sinus rhythm. Consult medical direction or refer to local protocols concerning pharmacological therapy for atrial flutter.

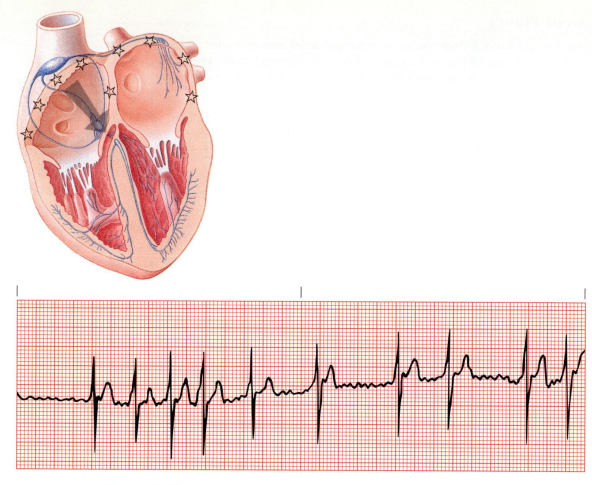

FIGURE 2-37 Atrial fibrillation.

Atrial Fibrillation

Description: Atrial fibrillation results from multiple areas of reentry within the atria or from multiple ectopic foci bombarding an AV node that physiologically cannot handle all of the incoming impulses. AV conduction is random and highly variable.

Etiology: Atrial fibrillation may be chronic and is often associated with underlying heart disease such as rheumatic heart disease, atherosclerotic heart disease, or congestive heart failure. Atrial dilation occurs with congestive heart failure and often causes atrial fibrillation.

Rules of Interpretation/Lead II Monitoring (Figure 2-37):

Rate—atrial rate is 350–750 per minute (cannot be counted); ventricular rate varies greatly depending on conduction through the AV node.

Rhythm—irregularly irregular

Pacemaker site—numerous ectopic foci in the atria

P waves—none discernible. Fibrillation (f) waves are present, indicating chaotic atrial activity.

P-R interval—none

QRS complex—normal

Clinical Significance: In atrial fibrillation, the atria fail to contract and the so-called atrial kick is lost, thus reducing cardiac output 20–25 percent. There is frequently a *pulse deficit* (a difference between the apical and peripheral pulse rates). If the rate of ventricular response is normal, as often occurs in patients on digitalis, the rhythm is usually well tolerated. If the ventricular rate is less than 60, cardiac output can fall. Suspect digitalis toxicity in patients taking digitalis with atrial fibrillation and a ventricular rate less than 60. If the ventricular response is rapid, coupled with the loss of atrial kick, cardiovascular decompensation may occur, resulting in hypotension, angina, infarct, congestive heart failure, or shock.

Treatment: Treatment is indicated only for rapid ventricular rates with hemodynamic compromise (review Figure 2-35).

1. Electrical therapy. Immediate cardioversion is indicated in unstable patients—those with heart rates greater than 150 and associated chest pain, dyspnea, a decreased level of consciousness, or hypotension. If time allows, sedate the patient with 5–10 mg of diazepam (Valium) or 2-5 mg of midazolam (Versed) IV. Then apply synchronized DC countershock of 100 joules. If this is unsuccessful, repeat the countershock at increased energy as ordered by medical direction.

2. Pharmacological therapy. Occasionally you will use pharmacological therapy in stable patients with atrial fibrillation, especially if the rapid heart rate is causing congestive heart failure. Several medications slow the ventricular rate. The most frequently used is diltiazem (Cardizem). In addition, verapamil, digoxin, beta blockers, procainamide, and quinidine can be used. Procainamide and quinidine are used to convert atrial fibrillation to a normal sinus rhythm. Atrial fibrillation is a documented risk factor for the development of stroke. As the atria fibrillate, they dilate. This allows for stagnation of blood flow within the atria and subsequent clot development. Because of this, it is sometimes prudent to administer an anticoagulant (heparin or warfarin [Coumadin]) to these patients to prevent stroke. Consult medical direction or refer to local protocols concerning pharmacological therapy of atrial fibrillation.

Patients with accessory pathways, such as in Wolff-Parkinson-White syndrome, who develop atrial flutter or atrial fibrillation, present special concerns. Usually, the electrical impulse reaches the ventricles via the accessory tract, via the AV node (normal conduction pathway), or via both. If the patient's refractory period is short in his accessory tract, more atrial impulses will be conducted down the accessory tract than through the AV node. This will result in a wide QRS complex. Rapid atrial rates occur with atrial fibrillation and flutter and can cause rapid ventricular rates. These rhythms, which have a wide complex, may resemble ventricular tachycardia. Excessive stimulation of the ventricles may actually precipitate ventricular fibrillation.

Verapamil will decrease conduction through the AV node and may shorten the refractory period of the accessory tract. Because of this, however, verapamil may accelerate the ventricular response rate and may precipitate ventricular tachycardia and ventricular fibrillation. Wolff-Parkinson-White, and the other pre-excitation syndromes, are presented in more detail later in this chapter.

DYSRHYTHMIAS ORIGINATING WITHIN THE AV JUNCTION (AV BLOCKS)

Two potential problems in the AV junction (or AV node) may result in dysrhythmias. One is an atrioventricular (AV) block, in which the electrical impulse is slowed or blocked as it passes through the AV node. The other is dysrhythmias due to a malfunction of AV junctional cells themselves.

The AV junction is an important part of the conductive system, serving two important physiological purposes (Figure 2-38). First, it effectively slows the impulse between the atria and the ventricles to allow for atrial emptying and ventricular filling. Second, it serves as a back-up pacemaker if the SA node or cells higher in the conductive system fail to fire. Part of the AV tissues function as a pacemaker node and other parts serve as the junction between the atria and the ventricles.

FIGURE 2-38 Organization of the AV node.

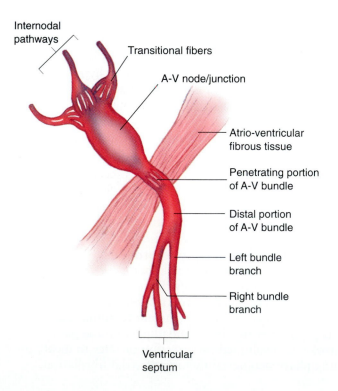

Internodal pathways

Transitional fibers

A-V node/junction

Atrio-ventricular fibrous tissue

Penetrating portion of A-V bundle

Distal portion of A-V bundle

Left bundle branch

Right bundle branch

Ventricular septum

The internodal fibers that blend to form the AV junction are called *transitional fibers*. These small fibers slow the impulse. The transitional fibers then blend into the AV junction. The lower portion of the AV node penetrates the fibrous tissue that separates the atria from the ventricles. This part of the node also slows impulse conduction. After penetrating the fibrous band, the AV node then becomes the AV bundle, which is also called the bundle of His. The bundle of His subsequently divides into the left and right bundle branches.

Atrioventricular Blocks

An *AV block* delays or interrupts impulses between the atria and the ventricles. These dysrhythmias can be caused by pathology of the AV junctional tissue or by a physiological block, such as occurs with atrial fibrillation or flutter. Their causes include AV junctional ischemia, AV junctional necrosis, degenerative disease of the conductive system, and drug toxicity (particularly from digitalis).

AV blocks can be classified according to the site or the degree of the block. Blocks may occur at the following sites:

- At the AV node
- At the bundle of His
- Below the bifurcation of the bundle of His

Our discussion classifies AV blocks by the following degrees (traditional classification):

- First-degree AV block
- Type I second-degree AV block
- Type II second-degree AV block (Mobitz II, or Infranodal)
- Third-degree AV block

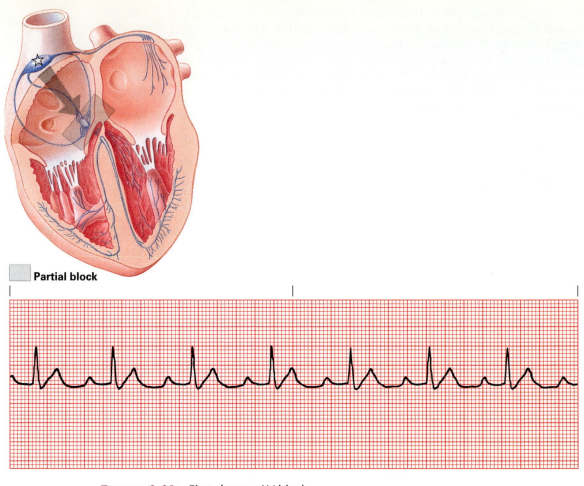

Partial block

FIGURE 2–39   First-degree AV block.

First-Degree AV Block

Description: A first-degree AV block is a delay in conduction at the level of the AV node rather than an actual block. First-degree AV block is not a rhythm in itself, but a condition superimposed upon another rhythm. The underlying rhythm must also be identified (for example, sinus bradycardia with first-degree AV block).

Etiology: AV block can occur in the healthy heart. However, ischemia at the AV junction is the most common cause.

Rules of Interpretation/Lead II Monitoring (Figure 2-39):

Rate—depends on underlying rhythm

Rhythm—usually regular; can be slightly irregular

Pacemaker site—SA node or atria

P waves—normal

P-R interval—greater than 0.20 sec (diagnostic)

QRS complex—usually less than 0.12 sec; may be bizarre in shape if conductive system disease exists in the ventricles

Clinical Significance: First-degree block is usually no danger in itself. However, a newly developed first-degree block may precede a more advanced block.

Treatment: Generally, no treatment is required except observation, unless the heart rate drops significantly. If possible, avoid drugs that slow AV conduction, such as lidocaine and procainamide.

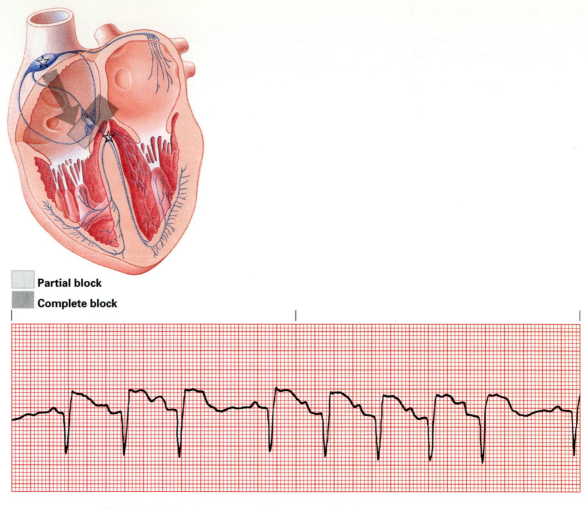

Partial block

Complete block

FIGURE 2-40   Type I second-degree AV block.

Type I Second-Degree AV Block

Description: A *type I second-degree AV block* (also called *second-degree, Mobitz I;* or *Wenckebach*), is an intermittent block at the level of the AV node. It produces a characteristic cyclic pattern in which the P-R intervals become progressively longer until an impulse is blocked (not conducted). The cycle is repetitive, and the P-P interval remains constant. The ratio of conduction (P waves to QRS complexes) is commonly 5:4, 4:3, 3:2, or 2:1. The pattern may be constant or variable.

Etiology: Low-grade AV blocks (First-degree and Second-degree Mobitz I) can occur in the healthy heart. However, ischemia at the AV junction is the most common cause. Increased parasympathetic tone and drugs are also common etiologies.

Rules of Interpretation/Lead II Monitoring (Figure 2-40):

Rate—atrial rate is unaffected; the ventricular rate may be normal or slowed

Rhythm—atrial rhythm is typically regular; ventricular rhythm is irregular because of the nonconducted beat

Pacemaker site—SA node or atria

P waves—normal; some P waves are not followed by QRS complexes

P-R interval—becomes progressively longer until the QRS complex is dropped; the cycle then repeats

QRS complex—usually less than 0.12 sec; may be bizarre in shape if conductive system disease exists in the ventricles

Clinical Significance: If beats are frequently dropped, second-degree block can compromise cardiac output by causing problems such as syncope and angina. This block is often a transient phenomenon that occurs immediately after an inferior wall myocardial infarction.

Treatment: Generally, no treatment other than observation is required. If possible, avoid drugs that slow AV conduction, such as lidocaine and procainamide. If the heart rate falls and the patient becomes symptomatic, administer 0.5 mg of atropine IV. Repeat every three to five minutes until you have obtained a satisfactory rate or have given 0.04 mg/kg of the drug. If atropine fails, consider transcutaneous cardiac pacing (TCP), if available.

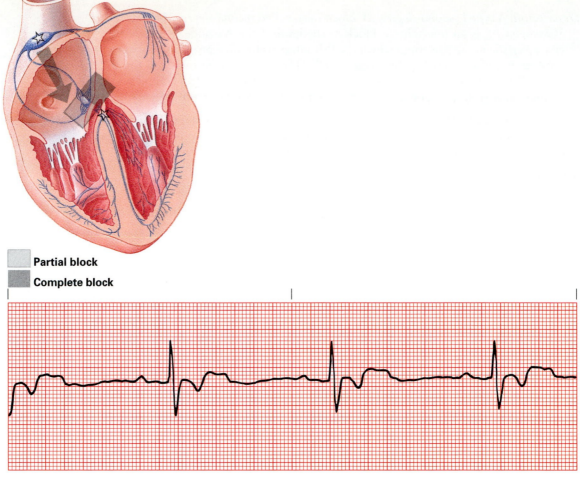

Partial block

Complete block

FIGURE 2-41   Type II second-degree AV block.

Type II Second-Degree AV Block

Description: A *type II second-degree AV block* (also called *second-degree, Mobitz II*; or *infranodal*) is an intermittent block characterized by P waves that are not conducted to the ventricles, but without associated lengthening of the P-R interval before the dropped beats. The ratio of conduction (P waves to QRS complexes) is commonly 4:1, 3:1, or 2:1. The ratio may be constant or may vary. A 2:1 Mobitz II block is often indistinguishable from a 2:1 Mobitz I block.

Etiology: Second-degree AV block, Mobitz II, is usually associated with acute myocardial infarction and septal necrosis.

Rules of Interpretation/Lead II Monitoring (Figure 2-41):

Rate—atrial rate is unaffected; ventricular rate is usually bradycardic

Rhythm—regular or irregular, depending upon whether the conduction ratio is constant or varied

Pacemaker site—SA node or atria

P waves—normal; some P waves are not followed by QRS complexes

P-R interval—constant for conducted beats; may be greater than 0.21 sec

QRS complex—may be normal; however, it is often greater than 0.12 sec because of abnormal ventricular depolarization sequence

Clinical Significance: A Mobitz II block can compromise cardiac output, causing problems such as syncope and angina if beats are frequently dropped. Since this block is often associated with cell necrosis resulting from myocardial infarction, it is considered much more serious than Mobitz I. Many Mobitz II blocks develop into full AV blocks.

Treatment: Pacemaker insertion is the definitive treatment. In the field, administer medications if stabilization is required. If the heart rate falls and the patient becomes symptomatic, administer 0.5 mg of atropine IV. Repeat every three–five minutes until you have obtained a satisfactory rate or have given 0.04 mg/kg of the drug. Use atropine with caution in patients who have high-grade blocks (second-degree Mobitz II and third-degree). The atropine may accelerate the atrial rate, but it may also worsen the AV nodal block. Consider transcutaneous cardiac pacing (TCP), if available. If the patient remains symptomatic, do not delay application of TCP while waiting for IV access or for atropine to take effect.

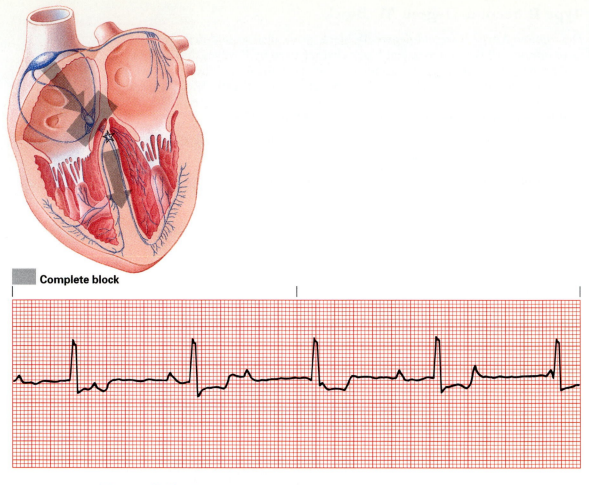

Complete block

FIGURE 2-42   Third-degree AV block.

Third-Degree AV Block

Description: A *third-degree AV block,* or *complete block,* is the absence of conduction between the atria and the ventricles resulting from complete electrical block at or below the AV node. The atria and ventricles subsequently pace the heart independently of each other. The sinus node often functions normally, depolarizing the atrial syncytium, while the escape pacemaker, located below the atria, paces the ventricular syncytium.

Etiology: Third-degree AV block can result from acute myocardial infarction, digitalis toxicity, or degeneration of the conductive system, as occurs in the elderly.

Rules of Interpretation/Lead II Monitoring (Figure 2-42):

Rate—atrial rate is unaffected. Ventricular rate is 40–60 if the escape pacemaker is junctional, less than 40 if the escape pacemaker is lower in the ventricles.

Rhythm—both atrial and ventricular rhythms are usually regular

Pacemaker site—SA node and AV junction or ventricle

P waves—normal. P waves show no relationship to the QRS complex, often falling within the T wave and QRS complex.

P-R interval—no relationship between P waves and R waves

QRS complex—greater than 0.12 sec if pacemaker is ventricular; less than 0.12 second if pacemaker is junctional

Clinical Significance: Third-degree block can severely compromise cardiac output because of decreased heart rate and loss of coordinated atrial kick.

Treatment: Pacemaker insertion is the definitive treatment. In the field, administer medications if stabilization is required. If the heart rate falls and the patient becomes symptomatic, administer 0.5 mg of atropine IV. You can repeat this every 3–5 minutes until you have obtained a satisfactory rate or have given 0.04 mg/kg of the drug. Use atropine with caution in patients with high-grade blocks (second-degree Mobitz II and third-degree). The atropine may accelerate the atrial rate, but it may also worsen the AV nodal block. Consider transcutaneous cardiac pacing (TCP), if available. If the patient remains symptomatic, do not delay application of TCP while waiting for IV access or for atropine to take effect. Never use lidocaine to treat third-degree heart block with ventricular escape beats.

Never use lidocaine to treat third-degree heart block with ventricular escape beats.

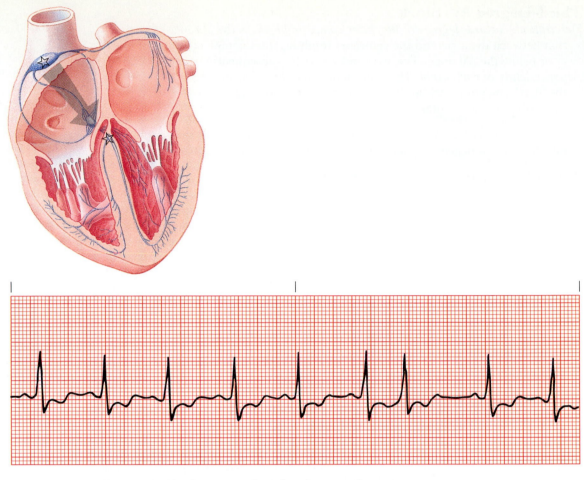

FIGURE 2-43 Premature junctional contractions.

DYSRHYTHMIAS SUSTAINED OR ORIGINATING IN THE AV JUNCTION

Dysrhythmias can originate within the AV node. The location of the pacemaker site will dictate the morphology of the P wave. Ischemia, hypoxia, and other factors have been identified as causes. Dysrhythmias originating in the AV junction include:

- Premature junctional contractions
- Junctional escape complexes and rhythm
- Accelerated junctional rhythm
- Paroxysmal junctional tachycardia

All dysrhythmias that originate in the AV junction have in common the following ECG features:

- Inverted P waves in Lead II, resulting from retrograde depolarization of the atria. The P wave's relation to QRS depolarization depends on the relative timing of atrial and ventricular depolarization. The P wave can occur before the QRS complex, if the atria depolarize first; after the QRS, if the ventricles depolarize first; or during the QRS, if the atria and ventricles depolarize simultaneously. Depolarization of the atria during ventricular depolarization masks the P wave. Some atrial complexes that originate near the AV junction can also result in inverted P waves.
- P-R interval of less than 0.12 sec
- Normal QRS complex duration

Premature Junctional Contractions

Description: Premature junctional contractions (PJCs) result from a single electrical impulse originating in the AV node that occurs before the next expected sinus beat. A PJC can result in either a **compensatory pause** or noncompensatory pause, depending on whether the SA node is depolarized. A noncompensatory pause occurs if the premature beat depolarizes the SA node and interrupts the heart's normal cadence. A compensatory pause occurs only if the SA node discharges before the premature impulse reaches it.

Etiology: A premature junctional contraction can result from any of the following conditions:

- Use of caffeine, tobacco, or alcohol
- Sympathomimetic drugs
- Ischemic heart disease
- Hypoxia
- Digitalis toxicity
- No apparent cause (idiopathic)

Rules of Interpretation/Lead II Monitoring (Figure 2-43):

Rate—depends on the underlying rhythm

Rhythm—depends on the underlying rhythm, usually regular except for the PJC

Pacemaker site—ectopic focus in the AV junction

P waves—inverted; may appear before or after the QRS complex. P waves can be masked by the QRS complex or be absent.

P-R interval—if the P wave occurs before the QRS complex, the P-R interval will be less than 0.12 sec; if the P wave occurs after the QRS complex, then technically it is an R-P interval

QRS complex—usually normal; may be greater than 0.12 sec if the PJC is abnormally conducted through partially refractory ventricles

Clinical Significance: Isolated PJCs are of minimal significance. Frequent PJCs indicate organic heart disease and may be precursors to other junctional dysrhythmias.

Treatment: If the patient is asymptomatic, only observation is required in the field.

✽ **compensatory pause** the pause following an ectopic beat where the SA node is unaffected and the cadence of the heart is uninterrupted.

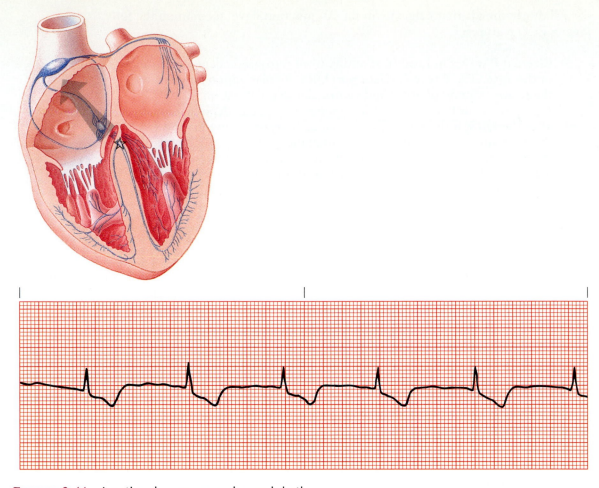

FIGURE 2-44   Junctional escape complex and rhythm.

Junctional Escape Complexes and Rhythms

Description: A *junctional escape beat,* or *junctional escape rhythm,* is a dysrhythmia that results when the rate of the primary pacemaker, usually the SA node, is slower than that of the AV node. The AV node then becomes the pacemaker. The AV node usually discharges at its intrinsic rate of 40–60 beats per minute. This is a safety mechanism that prevents cardiac standstill.

Etiology: Junctional escape rhythm has several etiologies, including increased vagal tone, which can result in SA node slowing; pathological slow SA node discharge; or heart block.

Rules of Interpretation/Lead II Monitoring (Figure 2-44):

Rate—40–60 per minute

Rhythm—irregular in single junctional escape complex; regular in junctional escape rhythm

Pacemaker site—AV junction

P waves—inverted; may appear before or after the QRS complex. The P waves can be masked by the QRS or be absent.

P-R interval—if the P wave occurs before the QRS complex, the P-R interval will be less than 0.12 sec. If the P wave occurs after the QRS complex, technically it is an R-P interval.

QRS complex—usually normal; may be greater than 0.12 sec

Clinical Significance: The slow heart rate can decrease cardiac output, possibly precipitating angina and other problems. If the rate is fairly rapid, the rhythm can be well tolerated.

Treatment: If the patient is asymptomatic, only observation is required in the field. Treatment is unnecessary unless hypotension or ventricular irritability is present. If treatment is required, administer a 0.5 mg bolus of atropine sulfate. Repeat every three–five minutes until you have obtained a satisfactory rate or have given a total of 0.04 mg/kg of the drug. If atropine fails, consider transcutaneous cardiac pacing (TCP), if available.

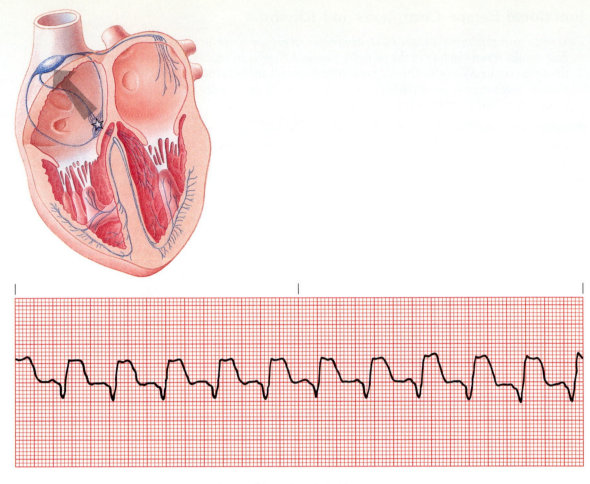

FIGURE 2-45   Accelerated junctional rhythm.

Accelerated Junctional Rhythm

Description: An *accelerated junctional rhythm* results from increased automaticity in the AV junction, causing the AV junction to discharge faster than its intrinsic rate. If the rate becomes fast enough, the AV node can override the SA node. Technically, the rate associated with an accelerated junctional rhythm is not a tachycardia. However, when compared to the intrinsic rate of the AV junctional tissue (40–60 beats per minute), it is considered accelerated.

Etiology: Accelerated junctional rhythms often result from ischemia of the AV junction.

Rules of Interpretation/Lead II Monitoring (Figure 2-45):

Rate—60–100 per minute

Rhythm—regular

Pacemaker site—AV junction

P waves—inverted; may appear before or after the QRS complex. P waves may be masked by the QRS or be absent.

P-R interval—if the P wave occurs before the QRS complex, the P-R interval will be less than 0.12 sec. If it occurs after the QRS, technically it is an R-P interval.

QRS complex—normal

Clinical Significance: An accelerated junctional rhythm is usually well tolerated. However, since ischemia is often the etiology, the patient should be monitored for other dysrhythmias.

Treatment: Prehospital treatment generally is unnecessary.

Paroxysmal Junctional Tachycardia

Description: *Paroxysmal junctional tachycardia (PJT)* develops when rapid AV junctional depolarization overrides the SA node. It often occurs in *paroxysms* (attacks with sudden onset), may last minutes or hours, and terminates abruptly. It may be caused by increased automaticity of a single AV nodal focus or by a reentry phenomenon at the AV node. Paroxysmal junctional tachycardia is often more appropriately called *paroxysmal supraventricular tachycardia (PSVT)*, since the rapid rate may make it indistinguishable from paroxysmal atrial tachycardia.

Etiology: Paroxysmal junctional tachycardia may occur at any age and may not be associated with underlying heart disease. Stress, overexertion, smoking, or ingestion of caffeine may precipitate it. However, it is frequently associated with underlying atherosclerotic heart disease (ASHD) and rheumatic heart disease. PJT rarely occurs with myocardial infarction. It can occur with accessory pathway conduction, as in Wolff-Parkinson-White syndrome.

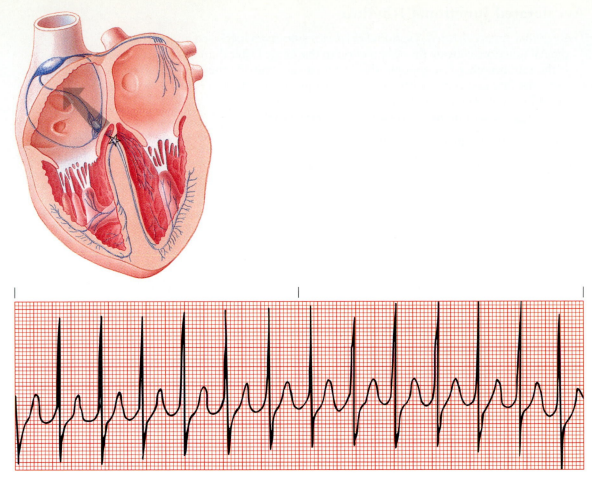

FIGURE 2-46   Paroxysmal junctional tachycardia.

Rules of Interpretation/Lead II Monitoring (Figure 2-46):

Rate—100–180 per minute

Rhythm—characteristically regular, except at onset and termination of paroxysms

Pacemaker site—AV junction

P waves—if present, P waves are inverted. They can occur before, during, or after the QRS complex. Turning up the speed of the graph paper or oscilloscope to 50 mm/sec spreads out the complex and aids in identifying P waves.

P-R interval—if the P wave occurs before the QRS complex, the P-R interval will be less than 0.12 sec. If it occurs after the QRS complex, technically it is an R-P interval.

QRS complex—normal

Clinical Significance: Young patients with good cardiac reserve may tolerate PJT well for a short time. The patient often will sense PJT as palpitations. However, rapid rates can preclude adequate ventricular filling time and markedly reduce cardiac output. The reduced diastolic phase of the cardiac cycle can also compromise coronary artery perfusion. PJT can precipitate angina, hypotension, or congestive heart failure.

Treatment: If the patient is not tolerating the rapid heart rate, as evidenced by hemodynamic instability, attempt the following techniques in this order:

1. Vagal maneuvers. Ask the patient to perform a Valsalva maneuver. This is a forced expiration against a closed glottis, or "bearing down" as if to move the bowels. This results in vagal stimulation, which may slow the heart. If this is unsuccessful, attempt carotid artery massage if the patient is eligible. (Do not attempt carotid artery massage in patients with carotid bruits or known cerebrovascular or carotid artery disease.)

2. Pharmacological therapy. Adenosine (Adenocard) is relatively safe and highly effective in terminating PJT. This is especially true if its etiology is reentry. Administer 6 mg of adenosine by rapid IV bolus over one to three seconds through the medication port closest to the patient's heart or central circulation. If the patient does not convert after one to two minutes, administer a second bolus of 12 mg over one to three seconds in the medication port closest to the patient's heart or central circulation. If this fails, and the patient has a normal blood pressure, medical direction may request the administration of verapamil. Verapamil is contraindicated in patients with a history of bradycardia, hypotension, or congestive heart failure. Do not use it with intravenous beta blockers; use it with caution in patients on chronic beta blocker therapy. Hypotension that occurs following verapamil administration can often be reversed with 0.5–1.0 gm of calcium chloride administered intravenously.

3. Electrical therapy. If the ventricular rate is greater than 150 beats per minute or the patient is hemodynamically unstable, use synchronized cardioversion. If time allows, sedate the patient with 5–10 mg of diazepam (Valium) or 2–5 milligrams of midazolam (Versed) IV. Apply synchronized DC countershock of 100 joules. If this is unsuccessful, repeat the countershock at increased energy as ordered by medical direction. DC countershock is contraindicated if you suspect digitalis toxicity as the cause of the PJT.

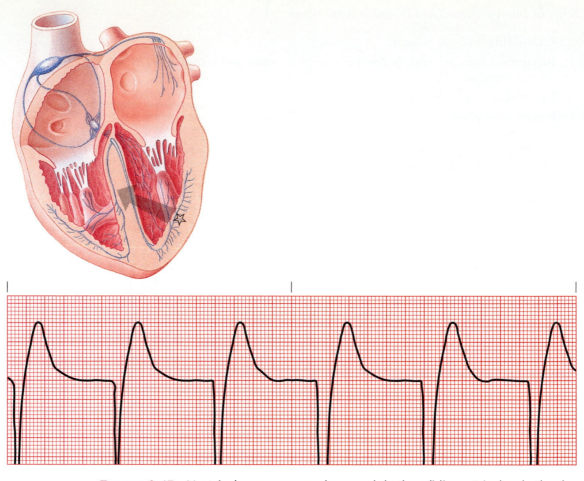

FIGURE 2-47   Ventricular escape complexes and rhythms (idioventricular rhythms).

DYSRHYTHMIAS ORIGINATING IN THE VENTRICLES

Some dysrhythmias originate within the ventricles. The pacemaker site will dictate the morphology of the QRS complex. Many factors, including ischemia, hypoxia, and medications, have been identified as causes. Dysrhythmias originating in the ventricles include:

- Ventricular escape complexes and rhythms
- Accelerated idioventricular rhythm
- Premature ventricular contraction
- Ventricular tachycardia
- Related dysrhythmia
- Ventricular fibrillation
- Asystole
- Artificial pacemaker rhythm

ECG features common to all dysrhythmias that originate in the ventricles include:

- QRS complexes of 0.12 sec or greater
- Absent P waves

Ventricular Escape Complexes and Rhythms

Description: A *ventricular escape beat* (*ventricular escape rhythm* or *idioventricular rhythm*) results either when impulses from higher pacemakers fail to reach the ventricles or when the discharge rate of higher pacemakers becomes less than that of the ventricles (normally 15–40 beats per minute). Ventricular escape rhythms serve as safety mechanisms to prevent cardiac standstill.

Etiology: Ventricular escape complexes and ventricular rhythms have several etiologies, including slowing of supraventricular pacemaker sites or high-degree AV block. They are frequently the first organized rhythms seen following successful defibrillation.

Rules of Interpretation/Lead II Monitoring (Figure 2-47):

Rate—15–40 per minute (occasionally less)

Rhythm—the rhythm is irregular in a single ventricular escape complex. Ventricular escape rhythms are usually regular unless the pacemaker site is low in the ventricular conductive system. Such placement makes regularity unreliable.

Pacemaker site—ventricle

P waves—none

P-R interval—none

QRS complex—greater than 0.12 sec and bizarre in morphology

Clinical Significance: The slow heart rate can significantly decrease cardiac output, possibly to life-threatening levels. The ventricular escape rhythm is a safety mechanism that you should not suppress. Escape rhythms can be perfusing or nonperfusing.

Treatment: Treatment depends on whether the escape rhythm is perfusing or nonperfusing. If it is perfusing, the object of treatment is to increase the heart rate. Administer a 0.5 mg bolus of atropine sulfate. Repeat every 3–5 minutes until you have obtained a satisfactory rate or have given 0.04 mg/kg of the drug. If atropine fails, consider transcutaneous cardiac pacing (TCP), if available. If the rhythm is nonperfusing, follow the pulseless electrical activity (PEA) protocol. This includes airway stabilization and CPR. Place an IV line, and administer 1 mg of epinephrine 1:10,000 IV. Direct treatment at correcting the primary problem (hypovolemia, hypoxia, cardiac tamponade, acidosis, or others). Consider a fluid challenge.

Accelerated Idioventricular Rhythm

Accelerated idioventricular rhythm is an abnormally wide ventricular dysrhythmia that usually occurs during an acute myocardial infarction. It is a sub-type of ventricular escape rhythm. Typically the rate is 60–110 beats per minute. The patient does not require treatment unless he becomes hemodynamically unstable. If this occurs, treat the ventricular focus with atropine or overdrive pacing. The principal action should be aggressive treatment of the underlying myocardial infarction as indicated, including appropriate prehospital care.

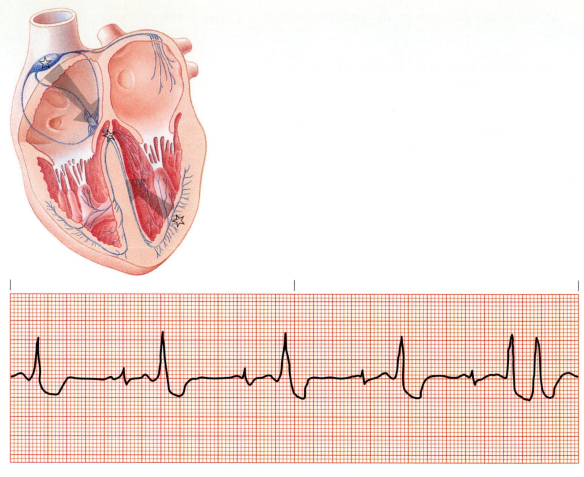

FIGURE 2-48 Premature ventricular contractions.

Premature Ventricular Contractions

Description: A *premature ventricular contraction* (*PVC,* or *ventricular ectopic*) is a single ectopic impulse arising from an irritable focus in either ventricle that occurs earlier than the next expected beat. It may result from increased automaticity in the ectopic cell or a reentry mechanism. The altered sequence of ventricular depolarization results in a wide and bizarre QRS complex and may additionally cause the T wave to occur in the direction opposite the QRS complex.

A PVC does not usually depolarize the SA node and interrupt its rhythm. That is, it does not interrupt the heart's normal cadence. The pause following the PVC is fully *compensatory.* Occasionally, an **interpolated beat** occurs when a PVC falls between two sinus beats without interrupting the rhythm.

If more than one PVC occurs, each can be classified as unifocal or multifocal. Because the PVC's morphology depends on the ectopic pacemaker's location, two PVCs of different morphologies imply two different pacemaker sites (multifocal). PVCs with the same morphology imply one pacemaker site (unifocal). If the **coupling interval** (the distance between the preceding beat and the PVC) is constant, the PVCs are most likely unifocal.

PVCs often occur in patterns of group beating. These include:

- *Bigeminy*—every other beat is a PVC
- *Trigeminy*—every third beat is a PVC
- *Quadrigeminy*—every fourth beat is a PVC

✱ **interpolated beat** a PVC that falls between two sinus beats without effectively interrupting this rhythm.

✱ **coupling interval** distance between the preceding beat and the PVC.

These terms can be applied to PACs and PJCs as well.

Repetitive PVCs are two consecutive PVCs without a normal complex in between. They can occur in groups of two (couplets) or three (triplets). More than three consecutive PVCs are often considered ventricular tachycardia.

PVCs can trigger lethal dysrhythmias such as ventricular fibrillation if they fall within the relative refractory period (the so-called R on T phenomenon). They are often classified by their relationship to the previous normal complex.

Etiologies: Etiologies for PVCs include

- Myocardial ischemia
- Increased sympathetic tone
- Hypoxia
- Idiopathic causes
- Acid-base disturbances
- Electrolyte imbalances
- Normal variant

Rules of Interpretation/Lead II Monitoring (Figure 2-48):

Rate—depends on underlying rhythm and rate of PVCs

Rhythm—interrupts regularity of underlying rhythm; occasionally irregular

Pacemaker site—ventricle

P waves—none; however, a normal sinus P wave (interpolated P wave) sometimes appears before a PVC.

P-R interval—none

QRS complex—greater than 0.12 sec and bizarre in morphology

Clinical Significance: Patients often sense PVCs as "skipped beats." In a patient without heart disease, PVCs may be insignificant. In patients with myocardial ischemia, PVCs may indicate ventricular irritability and may trigger lethal ventricular dysrhythmias. PVCs are often classified as malignant or benign. Malignant PVCs have at least one of the following traits:

- More than 6 PVCs per minute
- R on T phenomenon
- Couplets or runs of ventricular tachycardia
- Multifocal
- Associated chest pain

With most PVCs, the ventricles do not adequately fill. Because of this, you will usually not feel a pulse during the PVCs themselves. Frequent PVCs may reduce cardiac output.

PVCs can be described in terms of the Lown grading system for premature beats. The higher the grade, the more serious the ectopy:

Grade 0 = No premature beats

Grade 1 = Occasional (< 30 per hour) PVCs

Grade 2 = Frequent (> 30 per hour) PVCs

Grade 3 = Multiform (multifocal)

Grade 4 = Repetitive (couplets, salvos of 3 consecutive) PVCs

Grade 5 = R on T phenomenon

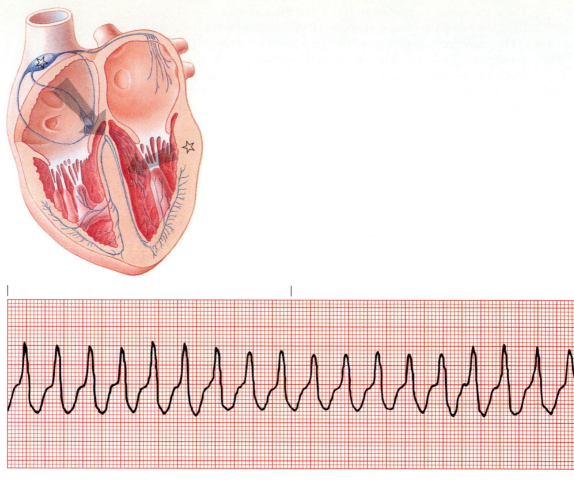

FIGURE 2-49   Ventricular tachycardia.

Treatment: If the patient has no history of cardiac disease and no symptoms, and if the PVCs are nonmalignant, no treatment is required. If the patient has a prior history of heart disease or symptoms, or if the PVCs are malignant, administer oxygen and place an IV line. If the patient is symptomatic, administer lidocaine at a dose of 1.0–1.5 mg/kg of body weight. Give an additional lidocaine bolus of 0.5–0.75 mg/kg every 5–10 minutes, if necessary, until you have given a total of 3.0 mg/kg of the drug. If the PVCs are effectively suppressed, start a lidocaine drip beginning at a rate of 2-4 mg/min. Reduce the dose in patients with decreased cardiac output (those with CHF or shock, for instance), in patients who are age 70 or greater, or in patients who have hepatic dysfunction. Give these patients a normal bolus dose first, followed by half the normal infusion. If the patient is allergic to lidocaine, or if you have given a maximum dose of lidocaine (3.0 mg/kg), consider procainamide or bretylium.

Ventricular Tachycardia

Description: Ventricular tachycardia (VT) consists of three or more ventricular complexes in succession at a rate of 100 beats per minute or more. This rhythm overrides the heart's normal pacemaker, and the atria and ventricles are asynchronous. Sinus P waves may occasionally be seen, dissociated from the QRS complexes. In *monomorphic VT* the complexes all appear the same; in *polymorphic VT* they have different sizes and shapes. One example of a polymorphic VT is *torsade de pointes.*

Etiology: As with PVCs, etiologies for ventricular tachycardia include:

- Myocardial ischemia
- Increased sympathetic tone
- Hypoxia
- Idiopathic causes
- Acid-base disturbances
- Electrolyte imbalances

Rules of Interpretation/Lead II Monitoring (Figure 2-49):

Rate—100–250 (approximately)

Rhythm—usually regular; can be slightly irregular

Pacemaker site—ventricle

P waves—if present, not associated with the QRS complexes

P-R interval—none

QRS complex—greater than 0.12 sec and bizarre in morphology

Clinical Significance: Ventricular tachycardia usually results in poor stroke volume, which, coupled with the rapid ventricular rate, may severely compromise cardiac output and coronary artery perfusion. Whether ventricular tachycardia is perfusing or nonperfusing dictates the type of treatment. Ventricular tachycardia may eventually deteriorate into ventricular fibrillation.

Treatment: If the patient is perfusing, as evidenced by the presence of a pulse, administer oxygen and place an IV line. Administer lidocaine at a dose of 1.0–1.5 mg/kg body weight intravenously. Administer additional doses of 0.5–0.75 mg/kg, until you have given a total of 3.0 mg/kg. If this treatment is unsuccessful, attempt to administer procainamide at 20–30 mg/minute to a maximum of 17 mg/kg. If procainamide fails, consider other second-line agents. Amiodarone (Cordarone) is becoming increasingly popular in the treatment of ventricular tachycardia. In the United States, it is primarily a second-line agent to lidocaine. In several of the Commonwealth countries, amiodarone is considered first-line treatment. The dose is 150–300 mg intravenously. Use synchronized cardioversion if the patient becomes unstable, as evidenced by chest pain, dyspnea, or systolic blood pressure of less than 90 mm/kg.

If the patient's condition is unstable, as evidenced by an altered level of consciousness or falling blood pressure, initiate cardioversion immediately after placing an IV line and administering oxygen. If time allows, sedate the patient first. The treatment plan is illustrated in the protocol (review Figure 2-35).

If the patient is nonperfusing, follow the protocol for ventricular fibrillation.

Torsade de Pointes *Torsade de pointes* is a polymorphic ventricular tachycardia that differs in appearance and cause from ventricular tachycardia in general. Torsade is most commonly caused by the use of certain antidysrhythmic drugs, including quinidine (Quinidex), procainamide (Pronestyl), disopyramide (Norpace), flecanide (Tambocor), sotolol (Betapace), and amiodarone (Cordarone). These agents' effects all seem to be exacerbated by the coadministration of certain nonsedating antihistamines, most notably aztemizole (Hismanol) and terfenadine (Seldane) and, in addition, the azole antifungal agents and macrolide antibiotics; erythromycin (PCE), azithromycin, (Zithromax), and clarithramycin (Biaxin). Any of these agents increase the likelihood of the patient's developing *torsade de pointes.*

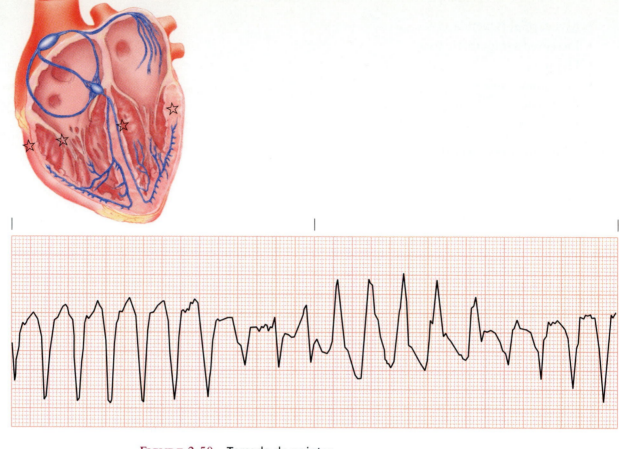

FIGURE 2-50   Torsade de pointes.

The morphology of the QRS varies from beat to beat (hence the term *torsade de pointes,* which means "twisting on a point"). In addition, the QT interval is markedly increased to 600 milliseconds or more. Torsade will usually occur in bursts that are not sustained. During the "breaks" from these bursts you should examine the rhythm strip for a prolonged Q-T interval. The QRS rate is usually between 166 and 300 beats per minute, and the R-R interval varies in an irregularly irregular pattern. The QRS complexes are wide and change in size over the span of several complexes (Figure 2-50). Attempting treatment of *torsade de pointes* with the antidysrhythmics usually used for the treatment of ventricular tachycardia can have disastrous consequences. Therefore, recognition of *torsade de pointes* as a separate dysrhythmia is essential. Treatment is 1–2 grams of magnesium sulfate placed in 100 ml of D_5W and administered over 1–2 minutes. This can be repeated every 4 hours with close monitoring of the deep tendon reflexes. Amiodarone (Cordarone) has proven effective in the treatment of torsade. Correct any underlying electrolyte problems, especially hyperkalemia.

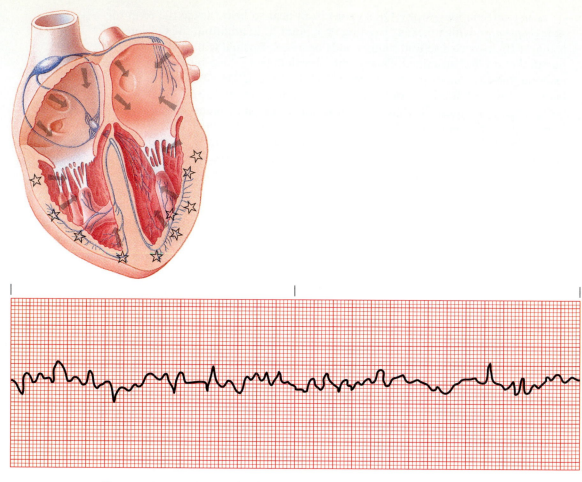

FIGURE 2-51   Ventricular fibrillation.

Ventricular Fibrillation

Description: *Ventricular fibrillation* is a chaotic ventricular rhythm usually resulting from the presence of many reentry circuits within the ventricles. There is no ventricular depolarization or contraction.

Etiology: A wide variety of causes have been associated with ventricular fibrillation. Most cases result from advanced coronary artery disease.

Rules of Interpretation/Lead II Monitoring (Figure 2-51):

Rate—no organized rhythm

Rhythm—no organized rhythm

Pacemaker site—numerous ectopic foci throughout the ventricles

P waves—usually absent

P-R interval—absent

QRS complex—absent

Clinical Significance: Ventricular fibrillation is a lethal dysrhythmia. The absence of cardiac output or an organized electrical pattern results in cardiac arrest.

Treatment: Ventricular fibrillation and nonperfusing ventricular tachycardia are treated identically. Initiate CPR. Follow this with DC countershock at 200 joules. If this is unsuccessful, repeat at 200–300 joules. If still unsuccessful, repeat at 360 joules. Subsequently, control the airway and establish an IV line. Epinephrine 1:10,000 is the drug of first choice; administer it every 3–5 minutes as required. If unsuccessful, consider second-line agents such as lidocaine, bretylium, amiodarone, procainamide, or possibly magnesium sulfate.

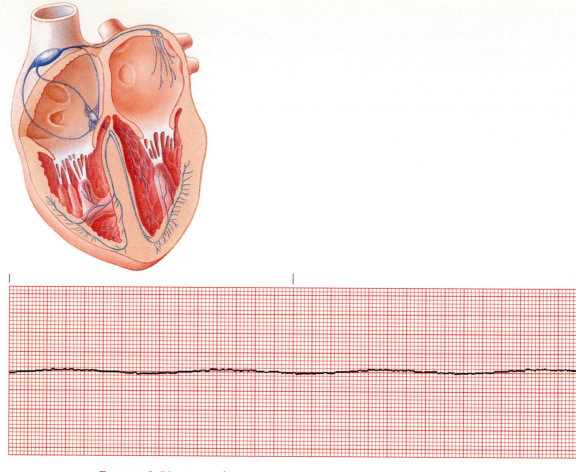

FIGURE 2-52   Asystole.

Asystole

Description: Asystole *(cardiac standstill)* is the absence of all cardiac electrical activity.

Etiology: Asystole may be the primary event in cardiac arrest. It is usually associated with massive myocardial infarction, ischemia, and necrosis. Resulting from heart blocks when no escape pacemaker takes over, asystole is often the final outcome of ventricular fibrillation.

Rules of Interpretation/Lead II Monitoring (Figure 2-52):

    Rate—no electrical activity
    Rhythm—no electrical activity
    Pacemaker site—no electrical activity
    P waves—absent
    P-R interval—absent
    QRS complex—absent

Clinical Significance: Asystole results in cardiac arrest. The prognosis for resuscitation is very poor.

Treatment: Treat asystole with CPR, airway management, oxygenation, and medications. If you have any doubt about the underlying rhythm, attempt defibrillation. Medications include epinephrine, atropine, and in certain situations, sodium bicarbonate (Figure 2-53).

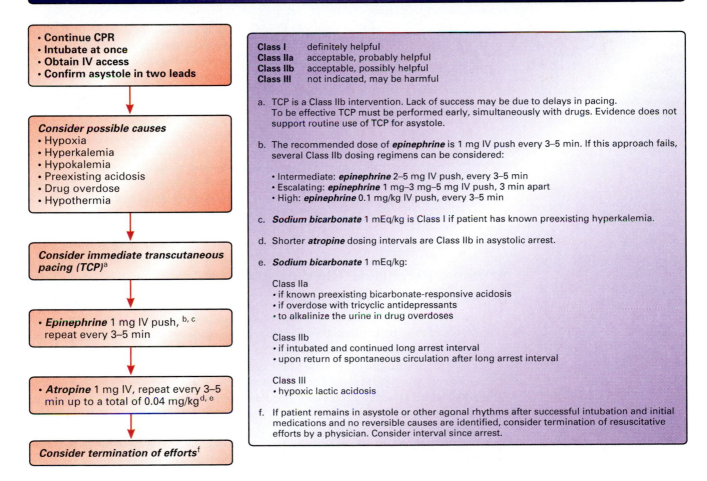

ALGORITHM: ASYSTOLE

- **Continue CPR**
- **Intubate at once**
- **Obtain IV access**
- **Confirm asystole in two leads**

Consider possible causes
- Hypoxia
- Hyperkalemia
- Hypokalemia
- Preexisting acidosis
- Drug overdose
- Hypothermia

Consider immediate transcutaneous pacing (TCP)[a]

- *Epinephrine* 1 mg IV push,[b, c] repeat every 3–5 min

- *Atropine* 1 mg IV, repeat every 3–5 min up to a total of 0.04 mg/kg[d, e]

Consider termination of efforts[f]

Class I	definitely helpful
Class IIa	acceptable, probably helpful
Class IIb	acceptable, possibly helpful
Class III	not indicated, may be harmful

a. TCP is a Class IIb intervention. Lack of success may be due to delays in pacing. To be effective TCP must be performed early, simultaneously with drugs. Evidence does not support routine use of TCP for asystole.

b. The recommended dose of *epinephrine* is 1 mg IV push every 3–5 min. If this approach fails, several Class IIb dosing regimens can be considered:

  - Intermediate: *epinephrine* 2–5 mg IV push, every 3–5 min
  - Escalating: *epinephrine* 1 mg–3 mg–5 mg IV push, 3 min apart
  - High: *epinephrine* 0.1 mg/kg IV push, every 3–5 min

c. *Sodium bicarbonate* 1 mEq/kg is Class I if patient has known preexisting hyperkalemia.

d. Shorter *atropine* dosing intervals are Class IIb in asystolic arrest.

e. *Sodium bicarbonate* 1 mEq/kg:

  Class IIa
  - if known preexisting bicarbonate-responsive acidosis
  - if overdose with tricyclic antidepressants
  - to alkalinize the urine in drug overdoses

  Class IIb
  - if intubated and continued long arrest interval
  - upon return of spontaneous circulation after long arrest interval

  Class III
  - hypoxic lactic acidosis

f. If patient remains in asystole or other agonal rhythms after successful intubation and initial medications and no reversible causes are identified, consider termination of resuscitative efforts by a physician. Consider interval since arrest.

FIGURE 2-53   Management of asystole. Adapted with permission. Journal of the American Medical Association, October 28, 1992, Volume 268, No. 16, *Guidelines for Cardiopulmonary Resuscitation and Emergency Cardiac Care,* p. 2220. ©1992 American Medical Association.

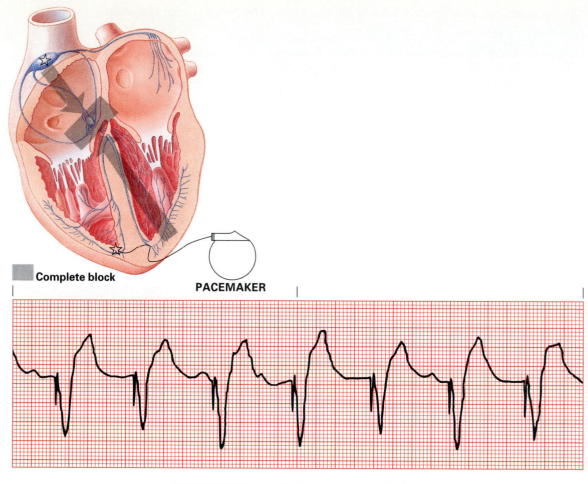

Complete block

PACEMAKER

FIGURE 2-54 Artificial pacemaker rhythm.

Artificial Pacemaker Rhythm

Description: An *artificial pacemaker rhythm* results from regular cardiac stimulation by an electrode implanted in the heart and connected to a power source. The pacemaker lead may be implanted in any of several locations in the heart, although it is most often placed in the right ventricle (ventricular pacemaker) or in both the right ventricle and the right atria (dual-chambered pacemaker.)

Fixed-rate pacemakers fire continuously at a preset rate, regardless of the heart's electrical activity. *Demand pacemakers* contain a sensing device and fire only when the natural heart rate drops below a set rate. In these cases, the pacemaker acts as an escape rhythm.

Ventricular pacemakers stimulate only the right ventricle, resulting in a rhythm that resembles an idioventricular rhythm. *Dual-chambered pacemakers,* commonly called *AV sequential pacemakers,* stimulate the atria first and then the ventricles. They are most beneficial for patients with marginal cardiac output who need the extra atrial kick to maintain cardiac output.

Pacemakers are usually inserted into patients who have chronic high-grade heart block or sick sinus syndrome or who have had episodes of severe symptomatic bradycardia.

Rules of Interpretation/Lead II Monitoring (Figure 2-54):

Rate—varies with the preset rate of the pacemaker

Rhythm—regular if pacing constantly; irregular if pacing on demand

Pacemaker site—depends on electrode placement

P waves—none produced by ventricular pacemakers. Sinus P waves may be seen but are unrelated to the paced QRS complexes. Dual-chambered pacemakers produce a P wave behind each atrial spike. A pacemaker spike is an upward or downward deflection from the baseline, which is an artifact created each time the pacemaker fires. The pacemaker spike tells you only that the pacemaker is firing. It reveals nothing about ventricular depolarization.

P-R interval—if present, varies

QRS complex—the QRS complexes associated with pacemaker rhythms are usually longer than 0.12 sec and bizarre in morphology. They often resemble ventricular escape rhythms. A QRS complex should follow each pacemaker spike. If so, the pacemaker is said to be "capturing." With demand pacemakers, some of the patient's own QRS complexes may appear. A pacemaker spike should not be associated with these complexes.

Problems with Pacemakers: Although rare, pacemakers can have problems. One cause is battery failure. Most pacemaker batteries have relatively long lives. The cardiologist can check them and usually replaces them before problems arise. If a battery fails, however, no pacing will occur and the patient's underlying rhythm, which may be bradycardic or asystolic, may return.

Occasionally, a pacemaker can *run away.* This condition, rarely seen with new pacemakers, results in a rapid discharge rate. Runaway pacemaker usually occurs when the battery runs low; newer models compensate for this by gradually increasing rate as their batteries run low.

Demand pacemakers can fail to shut down when the patient's intrinsic heart rate exceeds the rate set for the device. Thus the pacemaker competes with the patient's natural pacemaker. Occasionally, a paced beat can fall in the absolute or relative refractory period, precipitating ventricular fibrillation.

Finally, pacemakers can fail to capture if the leads become displaced or the battery fails. In such cases, pacemaker spikes are usually present without P waves or QRS complexes. Bradycardia often results.

Considerations for Management: Always examine any unconscious patient for a pacemaker. Battery packs are usually palpable under the skin, often in the shoulder or axillary region. Treat bradydysrhythmias, asystole, and ventricular fibrillation from pacemaker failure as in any other patient. You may use lidocaine to treat ventricular irritability without fear of suppressing ventricular response to the pacemaker. Defibrillate patients with pacemakers as usual, but do not discharge the paddles directly over the battery pack. If external cardiac pacing is available, you can use it until definitive care is available. Transport pacemaker failure patients promptly without prolonged field stabilization. Definitive care consists of battery replacement or temporary pacemaker insertion.

Use Of A Magnet: Applying a magnet over the pulse generator inhibits all sensing and sets the pacemaker to a predetermined rate (usually 70). The patient should carry a card with information about his particular pacemaker, since these rates are manufacturer and model dependent. Use the magnet only for short periods to avoid the unlikely development of a serious dysrhythmia (including ventricular fibrillation). The indicator for magnet use is a runaway pacemaker.

Table 2-3	SUGGESTED TREATMENT FOR UNDERLYING CAUSES OF PULSELESS ELECTRICAL ACTIVITY	
Condition	**Treatment (if allowed by local protocols)**	
Hypovolemia	Fluids	
Cardiac tamponade	Pericardiocentesis	
Tension pneumothorax	Needle thoracostomy	
Hypoxemia	Intubation/Oxygen	
Acidosis	Sodium bicarbonate	

PULSELESS ELECTRICAL ACTIVITY

Formerly termed electrical mechanical dissociation, *pulseless electrical activity (PEA)* essentially means that electrical complexes are present, but with no accompanying mechanical contractions of the heart. PEA is a perfect example of why you should treat the patient, not the monitor. Your monitor may show a textbook perfect, normal sinus rhythm, but the patient may be pulseless.

Causes of PEA include:

- Hypovolemia
- Cardiac tamponade
- Tension pneumothorax
- Hypoxemia
- Acidosis
- Massive pulmonary embolism
- Ventricular wall rupture

Administer epinephrine 1 mg every three to five minutes and treat the underlying cause(s). Table 2-3 shows suggested treatment for the different underlying causes. Early treatment can potentially reverse some of these conditions; therefore, prompt recognition and initiation of therapy are essential. Treatment for pulseless electrical activity is summarized in Figure 2-55.

DYSRHYTHMIAS RESULTING FROM DISORDERS OF CONDUCTION

Several dysrhythmias result from improper conduction through the heart. The three general categories of conductive disorders include:

- Atrioventricular blocks (discussed earlier in a separate section)
- Disturbances of ventricular conduction
- Pre-excitation syndromes

FIGURE 2-55 Management of pulseless electrical activity (PEA). Adapted with permission. Journal of the American Medical Association, October 28, 1992, Volume 268, No. 16, *Guidelines for Cardiopulmonary Resuscitation and Emergency Cardiac Care,* p. 2219. ©1992 American Medical Association.

ALGORITHM: PULSELESS ELECTRICAL ACTIVITY (PEA)

Includes
- Electromechanical Dissociation (EMD)
- Pseudo-EMD
- Idioventricular rhythms
- Ventricular escape rhythms
- Bradyasystolic rhythms
- Postdefibrillation idioventricular rhythms

• Continue CPR • Intubate at once	• Obtain IV access • Assess blood flow using Doppler ultrasound

Consider possible causes
(Parentheses = possible therapies and treatments)

- Hypovolemia (volume infusion)
- Hypoxia (ventilation)
- Cardiac tamponade (pericardiocentesis)
- Tension pneumothorax (needle decompression)
- Hypothermia (see hypothermia algorithm, Fig 10-4, Chapter 10)
- Massive pulmonary embolism (surgery, **thrombolytics**)
- Drug overdoses such as tricyclics, digitalis, β-blockers, calcium channel blockers
- Hyperkalemia[a]
- Metabolic acidosis[b]
- Massive acute myocardial infarction (Go to Fig 2-67)

- **Epinephrine** 1 mg IV push, [a, c] repeat every 3–5 min

- If absolute bradycardia (<60 BPM) or relative bradycardia, give **atropine** 1 mg IV
- Repeat every 3–5 min to a total of 0.04 mg/kg[d]

Class I definitely helpful
Class IIa acceptable, probably helpful
Class IIb acceptable, possibly helpful
Class III not indicated, may be harmful

a. **Sodium bicarbonate** 1 mEq/kg is Class I if patient has known preexisting hyperkalemia.

b. **Sodium bicarbonate** 1 mEq/kg

Class IIa
- if known preexisting bicarbonate-response acidosis
- if overdose with tricyclic antidepressants
- to alkalinize the urine in drug overdoses

Class IIb
- if intubated and continued long arrest interval
- upon return of spontaneous circulation after long arrest interval

Class III
- hypoxic lactic acidosis

c. The recommended dose of **epinephrine** is 1 mg IV push every 3–5 min. If this approach fails, several Class IIb dosing regimens can be considered:

- Intermediate: **epinephrine** 2–5 mg IV push, every 3–5 min
- Escalating: **epinephrine** 1 mg–3 mg–5 mg IV push, 3–5 min apart
- High: **epinephrine** 0.1 mg/kg IV push, every 3–5 min

d. Shorter **atropine** dosing intervals are possibly helpful in cardiac arrest (Class IIb)

Disturbances of Ventricular Conduction

Disturbances in conduction of the depolarization impulse are not limited to the AV node. Problems can arise within the ventricles as well. **Aberrant conduction** is a single supraventricular beat conducted through the ventricles in a delayed manner. **Bundle branch block** is a disorder in which all supraventricular beats are conducted through the ventricles in a delayed manner. Either the left or right bundle branch can be involved. If both branches are blocked, then a third-degree AV block exists. These complexes originate above the ventricles and should be distinguished from pure ventricular rhythms, which can have a similar QRS morphology. An *incomplete bundle branch block* has a normal QRS complex; a complete block has a wide QRS complex.

One of the two known causes of ventricular conduction disturbances is ischemia or necrosis of either the right or left bundle branch, rendering it incapable of conducting the impulse to the ventricle. The second is either a premature atrial contraction or a premature junctional contraction that reaches the ventricles or one of the bundle branches, usually the right, when it is still refractory. This often happens in atrial fibrillation because of the irregular rhythm's varying speed of repolarization.

The ECG features of ventricular conduction disturbances include a QRS complex longer than 0.12 sec because the blocked side of the heart is depolarized much more slowly than the unaffected side. The impulse passes much more slowly through the myocardium than through the rapid electrical conduction pathway. The QRS morphology is often bizarre. It can be notched or slurred, reflecting rapid depolarization through the normal conductive system and slow depolarization through the myocardium on the blocked side.

Ventricular conduction disturbances sometimes complicate ECG rhythm strip interpretation. In these cases, supraventricular beats can have abnormally wide QRS complexes. If you suspect a conduction system disturbance relating to supraventricular beats, then it is prudent to inspect some of the other leads in order to determine the problems.

Although exceptions do occur, supraventricular tachycardias caused by disturbances in conduction usually differ in several ways from wide complex tachycardias originating in the ventricles:

- A changing bundle branch block suggests supraventricular tachycardia (SVT) with aberrancy.
- A trial of carotid sinus massage may slow conduction through the AV node and may terminate a reentrant SVT or slow conduction with other supraventricular tachydysrhythmias. These maneuvers will have no effect on ventricular tachycardias.
- AV dissociation, also known as AV block, indicates a ventricular origin of the dysrhythmia.
- A full compensatory pause, usually seen after a ventricular beat, indicates ventricular tachycardia.
- Fusion beats suggest ventricular tachycardia.
- A QRS duration of longer than 0.14 sec usually indicates VT.

The patient's history may also help to differentiate the etiologies of wide complex tachycardias. In older patients with a history of myocardial infarction, congestive heart failure, or coronary artery disease, these dysrhythmias most likely have a ventricular origin.

When in doubt, treat the patient as if he has the more lethal dysrhythmia, ventricular tachycardia. In either case, use cardioversion if the patient is unstable; it is effective for both ventricular and supraventricular tachycardias.

Pre-Excitation Syndromes

Pre-excitation syndromes involve premature ventricular excitation by an impulse that bypasses the AV node. The most common of these is *Wolff-Parkinson-White (WPW) syndrome.* WPW occurs in approximately 3 of every 1,000 persons. It is characterized by a short P-R interval, generally less than 0.12 sec, and a long QRS duration, generally more than 0.12 sec. Additionally, the upstroke of the QRS often has a slur, called the *delta wave* (Figure 2-56). In WPW, conduction of the depolarization impulse from the atria to the ventricles is abnormal. The **bundle of Kent,** an extra conduction pathway between the atria and ventricles, effectively bypasses the AV node, shortening the P-R interval and prolonging the QRS complex. Most WPW patients are asymptomatic; however, the disorder is associated with a high incidence of tachydysrhythmias, usually through a reentry mechanism. WPW is also frequently associated with organic heart diseases such as atrial septal defects or mitral valve prolapse. Base treatment on the underlying rhythm.

ECG CHANGES DUE TO ELECTROLYTE ABNORMALITIES AND HYPOTHERMIA

Electrolyte imbalances can cause dysrhythmias that will appear on ECG rhythm strips. Suspect *hyperkalemia* (excessive potassium in the blood) in patients with a history of renal failure who are on dialysis. On an ECG, tall, peaked T waves in the precordial leads are an early sign of hyperkalemia. As the levels increase further, conduction decreases and the PR and QT intervals increase. At very high potassium levels, an idioventricular rhythm may develop and eventually become a classic sine wave (a wave that rises to a maximum positive level and then drops to a maximal negative level). Prominent U waves appear with *hypokalemia* (deficient potassium levels in the blood). Very low levels can widen the QRS complex.

In *hypothermia,* the Osborn wave, or J wave, is apparent. It is a slow, positive deflection at the end of the QRS complex (Figure 2-57). Other ECG changes may include:

- T wave inversion
- PR, QRS, QT prolongation.
- Sinus bradycardia
- Atrial fibrillation or flutter
- AV block
- PVCs
- Ventricular fibrillation
- Asystole

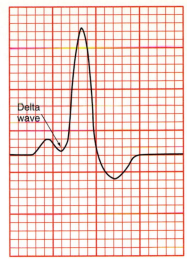

FIGURE 2-56   The delta wave of Wolf-Parkinson-White syndrome.

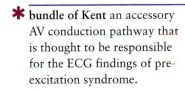

✱ bundle of Kent an accessory AV conduction pathway that is thought to be responsible for the ECG findings of pre-excitation syndrome.

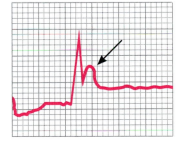

FIGURE 2-57   The Osborn ("J") wave.

Part 2: Assessment and Management of the Cardiovascular Patient

Objectives

After reading Part 2 of this chapter, you should be able to:

40. Identify and describe the components of the focused history as it relates to the patient with cardiovascular compromise. (pp. 162–166)
41. Identify and describe the details of inspection, auscultation, and palpation specific to the cardiovascular system. (pp. 166–170)
42. Identify and define the heart sounds and relate them to hemodynamic events in the cardiac cycle. (pp. 168–169)
43. Describe the differences between normal and abnormal heart sounds. (pp. 168–169)
44. Define pulse deficit, pulsus paradoxus, and pulsus alternans. (pp. 164, 205)
45. Identify the normal characteristics of the point of maximal impulse (PMI). (p. 169)
46. Based on field impressions, identify the need for rapid intervention for the patient in cardiovascular compromise. (pp. 160–170)
47. Describe the incidence, morbidity, and mortality associated with myocardial conduction defects. (pp. 186, 198, 240–254)
48. Identify the clinical indications, components, and the function of transcutaneous and permanent artificial cardiac pacing. (pp. 152–153, 186, 188–189)
49. Explain what each setting and indicator on a transcutaneous pacing system represents and how the settings may be adjusted. (pp. 188–189)
50. Describe the techniques of applying a transcutaneous pacing system. (pp. 188–189)
51. Describe the characteristics of an implanted pacemaking system. (pp. 152–153)
52. Describe the epidemiology, morbidity, mortality, and pathophysiology of angina pectoris. (pp. 191, 194)
53. Describe the assessment and management of a patient with angina pectoris. (pp. 194–196)
54. Identify what is meant by the OPQRST of chest pain assessment. (pp. 162–163)
55. List other clinical conditions that may mimic signs and symptoms of coronary artery disease and angina pectoris. (pp. 191, 194)
56. Identify the ECG findings in patients with angina pectoris. (pp. 194–195)
57. Based on the pathophysiology and clinical evaluation of the patient with chest pain, list the anticipated clinical problems according to their life-threatening potential. (pp. 191, 194)
58. Describe the epidemiology, morbidity, mortality, and pathophysiology of myocardial infarction. (pp. 196–197)
59. List the mechanisms by which a myocardial infarction may be produced from traumatic and nontraumatic events. (p. 196)
60. Identify the primary hemodynamic changes produced in myocardial infarction. (pp. 196–197)
61. List and describe the assessment parameters to be evaluated in a patient with a suspected myocardial infarction. (pp. 196–197)
62. Identify the anticipated clinical presentation of a patient with a suspected acute myocardial infarction. (pp. 197–199)

63. Differentiate the characteristics of the pain/discomfort occurring in angina pectoris and acute myocardial infarction. (pp. 197–198)
64. Identify the ECG changes characteristically seen during evolution of an acute myocardial infarction. (p. 198)
65. Identify the most common complications of an acute myocardial infarction. (pp. 196–199)
66. List the characteristics of a patient eligible for thrombolytic therapy. (pp. 198–201)
67. Describe the "window of opportunity" as it pertains to reperfusion of a myocardial injury or infarction. (pp. 198–199)
68. Based on the pathophysiology and clinical evaluation of the patient with a suspected acute myocardial infarction, list the anticipated clinical problems according to their life-threatening potential. (pp. 197–201)
69. Specify the measures that may be taken to prevent or minimize complications in the patient suspected of myocardial infarction. (pp. 199–201)
70. Describe the most commonly used cardiac drugs in terms of therapeutic effect and dosages, routes of administration, side effects, and toxic effects. (pp. 175–180)
71. Describe the epidemiology, morbidity, mortality, and physiology associated with heart failure. (pp. 202–204)
72. Identify the factors that may precipitate or aggravate heart failure. (pp. 202–204)
73. Define acute pulmonary edema and describe its relationship to left ventricular failure. (p. 202)
74. Differentiate between early and late signs and symptoms of left ventricular failure and those of right ventricular failure. (pp. 203–204)
75. Define and explain the clinical significance of paroxysmal nocturnal dyspnea, pulmonary edema, and dependent edema. (pp. 204–205)
76. List the interventions prescribed for the patient in acute congestive heart failure. (pp. 205–206)
77. Describe the most commonly used pharmacological agents in the management of congestive heart failure in terms of therapeutic effect, dosages, routes of administration, side effects, and toxic effects. (pp. 175–180, 206)
78. Define and describe the incidence, mortality, morbidity, pathophysiology, assessment, and management of the following cardiac related problems (pp. 206–216):
   • Cardiac tamponade
   • Hypertensive emergency
   • Cardiogenic shock
   • Cardiac arrest
79. Identify the limiting factor of pericardial anatomy that determines intrapericardiac pressure. (p. 206)
80. Describe how to determine if pulsus paradoxus, pulsus alternans, or electrical alternans is present. (pp. 205–207)
81. Explain the essential pathophysiological defect of hypertension in terms of Starling's law of the heart. (pp. 204, 209–210)
82. Rank the clinical problems of patients in hypertensive emergencies according to their sense of urgency. (p. 208)
83. Identify the drugs of choice for hypertensive emergencies, cardiogenic shock, and cardiac arrest, including their indications, contraindications, side effects, route of administration, and dosages. (pp. 175–180, 209, 212, 213–214)
84. Describe the major systemic effects of reduced tissue perfusion caused by cardiogenic shock. (pp. 209–210)

85. Explain the primary mechanisms by which the heart may compensate for a diminished cardiac output and describe their efficiency in cardiogenic shock. (pp. 209–210)
86. Identify the clinical criteria and progressive stages of cardiogenic shock. (pp. 209–210)
87. Describe the dysrhythmias seen in cardiac arrest. (p. 213)
88. Explain how to confirm asystole using the 3-lead ECG. (p. 213)
89. Define the terms *defibrillation* and *synchronized cardioversion*. (pp. 180–181, 183)
90. Specify the methods of supporting the patient with a suspected ineffective implanted defibrillation device. (p. 182)
91. Describe resuscitation and identify circumstances and situations where resuscitation efforts would not be initiated. (pp. 213–216)
92. Identify communication and documentation protocols with medical direction and law enforcement used for termination of resuscitation efforts. (pp. 214–216)
93. Describe the incidence, morbidity, mortality, pathophysiology, assessment, and management of vascular disorders including occlusive disease, phlebitis, aortic aneurysm, and peripheral artery occlusion. (pp. 217–220)
94. Identify the clinical significance of claudication and presence of arterial bruits in a patient with peripheral vascular disorders. (pp. 217, 219, 220)
95. Describe the clinical significance of unequal arterial blood pressure readings in the arms. (p. 220)
96. Recognize and describe the signs and symptoms of dissecting thoracic or abdominal aneurysm. (pp. 218, 220)
97. Differentiate between signs and symptoms of cardiac tamponade, hypertensive emergencies, cardiogenic shock, and cardiac arrest. (pp. 206–213)
98. Utilize the results of the patient history, assessment findings, and ECG analysis to differentiate between, and provide treatment for, patients with the following conditions (pp. 160–221):
    - cardiovascular disease
    - chest pain
    - in need of a pacemaker
    - angina pectoris
    - a suspected myocardial infarction
    - heart failure
    - cardiac tamponade
    - a hypertensive emergency
    - cardiogenic shock
    - cardiac arrest
99. Based on the pathophysiology and clinical evaluation of the patient with chest pain, characterize the clinical problems according to their life-threatening potential. (pp. 191, 194)
100. Given several preprogrammed patients with cardiac complaints, provide the appropriate assessment, treatment, and transport. (pp. 160–221)

The key to providing the best possible cardiovascular care is to take a systematic, step-by-step approach with every patient.

Airway, breathing, and circulatory problems and shock are always the most critical issues during the first minute of patient care.

ASSESSMENT OF THE CARDIOVASCULAR PATIENT

The key to providing your cardiovascular patient with the best possible medical care is to take a systematic, step-by-step approach. When you initially contact your patient, always determine the most important problems first. Airway, breathing, circulatory problems, and shock are always the most critical issues during the first minute of patient care. What may have caused any life-threatening problems does not matter at this point. In some instances such as cardiac arrest, your focus during prehospital care may never go beyond these four concerns.

After you have managed any life-threatening problems, the focused history and physical examination will help you form your field diagnosis. Cardiovascular diseases may affect the myocardium, the electrical conductive system, the pericardium, or the blood vessels. They may also involve a combination of these problems or problems associated with other systems, such as diabetes. Diseases of the myocardium include myocardial infarction, heart failure, or cardiogenic shock. In electrical conductive illnesses, the heart rate is either too fast or too slow. Although pericardial emergencies such as pericarditis or pericardial tamponade are usually diagnosed clinically by the physical examination findings, the focused history (blunt/penetrating trauma or recent infection, for example) may help you to recognize them. Vascular problems may include coronary artery occlusion, peripheral venous or arterial occlusion, or pulmonary embolism.

In the field, therapeutic treatments are generally limited to:

- Administering nitrates, aspirin, and analgesics for symptomatic chest pain
- Treating pulmonary edema
- Giving analgesics in peripheral vascular emergencies

In your on-going assessment, continually reevaluate your initial management. Based on the patient's needs, you will transport him in the appropriate mode to the appropriate facility. As with any patient, your management of the cardiac patient should include patient advocacy as well as communication and emotional support for the patient and his family. You must also effectively communicate the details of your assessment and management to the receiving staff. Additionally, your knowledge of nontransport criteria, education and prevention, proper documentation, and on-going quality assurance will all contribute to providing optimum care.

Your assessment of the patient with a cardiovascular emergency should vary according to the acuity of the situation. Patients with serious illnesses should have a limited, yet focused exam. Patients who are less seriously ill should receive a more comprehensive assessment. It is important to remember that the cardiovascular system affects virtually every other body system. Signs of cardiac disease may initially be evident only in the respiratory system as dyspnea. A comprehensive exam, however, will often reveal subtle findings that point to cardiovascular disease as the cause.

SCENE SIZE-UP AND INITIAL ASSESSMENT

After ascertaining that the scene is safe, begin an initial cardiovascular assessment. This allows you to identify life-threatening problems and set transport priorities. First, determine the patient's level of responsiveness. Is he speaking with you or unresponsive? Then move on to the ABCs. Make sure his airway is patent and free of debris and blood. Suction the airway if appropriate. Next, check the patient's rate and depth of breathing. Listen for the presence or absence of breath sounds. Certain breath sounds such as moist rales should heighten your suspicion of cardiovascular disease. Note the effort or "work" of breathing. If the patient is not breathing, initiate manual ventilation and intubate as soon as possible. Check for the rate and quality of pulses. If no pulse is present, immediately begin cardiopulmonary resuscitation. The skin can indicate the degree of perfusion present. Look for

- Color
- Temperature
- Moisture
- Turgor
- Mobility
- Edema

Finally, check the patient's blood pressure. Is he in shock? Is this a hypertensive emergency? Treat all life-threatening conditions as you find them.

FOCUSED HISTORY

After you have completed your initial cardiovascular assessment and treated life-threatening conditions, proceed with your focused history, using the SAMPLE format (*S*ymptoms, *A*llergies, *M*edications, *P*ast medical history, *L*ast oral intake, and *E*vents preceding the incident).

Common Symptoms

Cardiac disease can manifest itself in several ways. Some common chief complaints and symptoms include:

Chest pain is the most common presenting symptom in cases of cardiac disease.

- Chest pain or discomfort
- Dyspnea
- Cough
- Syncope
- Palpitation

Not all patients who have cardiac disease will have chest pain.

Chest Pain Chest pain or discomfort that may radiate to the shoulder, neck, jaw, or back is a common symptom of cardiac disease. Always remember, however, that not all patients who have cardiac disease will have chest pain. This is especially true in diabetic patients, who may have a myocardial infarction with no pain at all. Also remember that chest pain can be benign and may have no association with cardiac disease. Differentiating between benign and life-threatening chest pain is extremely difficult; do not attempt it in the field. If a cardiac etiology is even a remote possibility, treat the patient accordingly.

Follow the OPQRST acronym to obtain the patient's description of the pain.

- *Onset.* Ask about the onset of the pain. When did it begin? What was the patient doing when it started? If the patient has had chest pain in the past, ask him to compare it to previous episodes. For instance, if he had a major heart attack in the past and tells you his present pain is the same, then strongly suspect that it is also from his heart.

- *Provocation/Palliation.* What provoked the pain? Is it exertional or nonexertional? The relationship of pain to exertion is very important. During exertion, the heart muscle needs more oxygen. If it does not receive the additional oxygen, the muscle becomes ischemic and the patient has pain (angina). He may tell you that he is now walking shorter distances before the pain begins, indicating lessening blood flow to the heart. Untreated, this may lead to pain at rest and, eventually, infarction. What alleviates the pain (palliation)? Is the pain related to movement or inspiration?

- *Quality.* Ask the patient to describe the quality of the pain. Ask open-ended questions and allow the patient to characterize this symptom in his own words. Common descriptive words include sharp, tearing, pressure, and heaviness.

- *Region/Radiation.* The patient may complain of pain radiating to other regions of his body, most commonly his arms, neck, jaw, and back.

- *Severity.* Ask the patient to rate the pain on a scale of one to ten, with one being very little and ten being the worst pain he has ever felt. This can also be a useful gauge of your management's effectiveness. Some systems will use a pain scale of one to five. Regardless of the scale, it is important that the scale used is standardized in the system. It can be problematic if a paramedic asks a patient to rate his pain on a scale of one to five, but when the patient gets to the hospital, the nurse or doctor is using a scale of one to ten. Although seemingly trivial, this can significantly affect patient care.

- *Timing.* Check the timing of the pain. How long has the pain lasted? Always determine the time the pain began and record it. The onset and duration of pain directly affect decisions about the use of thrombolytic drugs. Is the pain constant or intermittent? Is it getting worse? better? Does it occur at rest or with activity?

Dyspnea Because of the heart's close relationship with the respiratory system, many cardiac patients have dyspnea (labored breathing). Dyspnea is often associated with myocardial infarction and in some patients may be the only symptom. Also, patients with congestive heart failure will experience increased dyspnea when lying down.

When confronted with a dyspneic patient, ask about the following:

- *Duration.* How long has it lasted? Is it continuous or intermittent?
- *Onset.* Was the onset sudden or rapid?
- *Provocation/palliation.* Does anything aggravate or relieve the dyspnea? Is it exertional or nonexertional?
- *Orthopnea.* Does sitting upright give relief?

Cough Frequently, patients who cough have chest pain. Is the cough dry or productive? Did the patient pull a chest muscle during coughing? Try to determine if the coughing results from congestive heart failure.

Other Related Signs and Symptoms Other related signs and symptoms to look for and ask about include:

- *Level of consciousness.* The level of consciousness indicates brain perfusion. An alteration in the level of consciousness can be due to problems within the cardiovascular system.
- *Diaphoresis (perspiration)* Cardiac problems significantly affect the autonomic nervous system. Stimulation of the sympathetic nervous system can result in marked diaphoresis.
- *Restlessness and anxiety.* Restlessness and anxiety are among the earliest symptoms when a patient is experiencing lowered brain perfusion, whether due to decreased oxygenation, decreased blood supply, or both.

- *Feeling of impending doom.* The significant and massive stimulation of the sympathetic nervous system associated with severe cardiovascular emergencies can cause a feeling of impending doom. This is a part of the "fight or flight" response. A patient with a sensation of impending doom can be experiencing a significant cardiovascular event.

- *Nausea and/or vomiting.* Nausea and vomiting are common during cardiovascular events such as myocardial ischemia. This often results from slowed peristalsis due to sympathetic stimulation.

- *Fatigue.* Fatigue is a generalized finding associated with many diseases. In patients with cardiovascular disease, it can be caused by anemia, poor oxygenation, or poor overall cardiovascular system functioning.

- *Palpitations.* Palpitations are a sensation that the heart is beating fast or skipping beats. This can result from tachycardia or simply from increased awareness of the heart's normal function.

- *Edema.* Edema is the accumulation of fluid in third (interstitial) spaces. It accompanies poor cardiac function and often indicates chronic cardiovascular disease.
  - *Extremities.* Ambulatory patients usually will develop edema in the extremities, due to the effects of gravity.
  - *Sacral.* Sacral, or presacral edema, is seen in bed-bound patients. Fluid collects in the lowest part of the patient's body, usually around the sacrum.

- *Headache.* Headache is a factor in cardiovascular disease for several reasons. First, decreased CNS perfusion can result in headaches. These are often severe. Many patients with established heart disease take nitroglycerin or other nitrate drugs. Excess administration of nitrates can cause a severe headache and may indicate worsening heart disease.

- *Syncope.* Syncope is a brief loss of consciousness due to a transient decrease in cerebral blood flow. It occurs in certain cardiac dysrhythmias and in ischemic lesions where blood flow to the heart may be impaired, reducing cardiac output and interrupting CNS perfusion. Severe pain can also cause syncope as well as other forms of psychic stress.

- *Behavioral change.* A behavioral change may very subtly indicate cardiovascular disease. More common in the elderly, it may point to either an acute or chronic decrease in cerebral blood flow.

- *Anguished facial expression.* The pain that accompanies myocardial ischemia can be quite severe. This, coupled with the effects of sympathetic nervous system stimulation, may cause the patient to exhibit anguished facial expressions.

- *Activity limitations.* Decreased cardiac performance can significantly limit a patient's physical activities. These limitations may develop slowly and be considered chronic or develop quickly and be considered acute.

- *Trauma.* Trauma, especially unexplained trauma, can be due to a temporary decrease in CNS perfusion. Unexplained facial injuries or bruises may indicate a cardiovascular problem.

Many of the signs and symptoms of cardiovascular disease can be subtle. Always assess for them and look for any sign or symptom patterns that point to cardiovascular disease.

Allergies

Ask about the patient's allergies. Is he allergic to any medications? Does he have an allergy to X-ray dye (IVP dye)? Try to differentiate between true medication allergies and undesirable side effects of a particular medication. For instance, the patient who tells you he breaks out in hives and stops breathing if he takes penicillin is having an allergic reaction. The patient who says he gets abdominal upset from aspirin is, most likely, experiencing a side effect. If in doubt, withhold the medication and contact medical direction.

If in doubt about a possible medication allergy, withhold the medication and contact medical direction.

Medications

The patient's current use of prescription medications is important. What medications is he currently taking? Has he recently changed any medications? The following drugs may be especially significant:

- Nitroglycerin (Nitrostat)
- Propranolol (Inderal) and other beta blockers
- Digitalis (Lanoxin)
- Diuretics (Lasix, Maxzide, Dyazide)
- Antihypertensives (Vasotec, Prinivil, Capoten)
- Antidysrhythmics (Mexitil, Quinaglute, Tambocor)
- Lipid lowering agents (Mevacor, Lopid)

Also question the patient in detail about his compliance with his medications. Does he take his medications? Does he take the right amount? Does he take them at the right time? With the high cost of medications and limited coverage by prescription plans, more and more patients are not taking their prescriptions. Some may even borrow a friend's medication, a dangerous practice, since it may be the wrong dosage or even the wrong drug.

The patient's use of nonprescription drugs is also important. Ask if he takes any over-the-counter medications. Numerous drugs interact, and you must be aware of all medications the patient is currently taking, prescription or otherwise. Try to bring all drug containers with you to the hospital if doing so will not adversely prolong transport time. This information is very important for the hospital staff. Recreational drug use is another major problem. For example, cocaine causes vasoconstriction of the blood vessels and can lead to myocardial infarction and severe hypertension, often in the absence of coronary artery disease. These effects can last up to two weeks. Even though this question may make you uncomfortable, you must ask it.

Try to bring all of the patient's prescription and nonprescription drug containers to the hospital with you.

Past Medical History

Avoid spending excessive time obtaining a cardiac patient's past medical history. If the patient's condition permits, however, a past medical history may help you determine if his symptoms are attributable to a cardiac condition.

- Does the patient have a history of coronary artery disease, angina, or a previous myocardial infarction? If so, chances are good that his symptoms are cardiac in origin. Comparing his prior symptoms to his present ones is helpful. If he tells you this pain is just like his previous heart attack, then he likely is experiencing another.

- Has the patient had any prior heart problems? Ask about the following:
  - Valvular disease (rheumatic heart disease)
  - Aneurysm
  - Previous cardiac surgery
  - Congenital cardiac anomalies
  - Pericarditis or other inflammatory cardiac disease
  - Congestive heart failure (CHF)
- What other medical problems does the patient have? Ask about the following:
  - Pulmonary disease/COPD
  - Diabetes mellitus
  - Renal (kidney) disease
  - Hypertension
  - Peripheral vascular disease
- Does anyone in the patient's family have cardiac disease? At what age did it first develop? Cardiac disease before the age of 50 in a close relative should heighten your concern about heart disease. If a family member had a cardiac event at a young age, especially sudden death, your patient is also at risk earlier in life. Has anyone in his family died of heart disease? At what age? Also ask if the family has a history of stroke, diabetes, or hypertension.
- Does the patient smoke? Does he know his cholesterol level? These are other modifiable risk factors for cardiac disease.

Last Oral Intake

When was the patient's last oral intake? If the patient ingested a meal high in saturated fats before the onset of symptoms, then gall bladder disease should be considered as a possible etiology. Also inquire if the patient has had an increase in caffeine intake and ask when he last drank a caffeinated beverage.

Events Preceding the Incident

What was the patient doing before the onset of symptoms? Was there emotional upset? Had he just completed a strenuous task such as mowing the yard? Has he recently started a new exercise program? Did the symptoms begin while the patient was having sex? Does the patient take Viagra? The development of chest pain during sexual intercourse is not uncommon. However, patients often will not volunteer this information. Asking about intimate events such as this may be uncomfortable, but it is necessary for optimal patient care.

PHYSICAL EXAMINATION

After addressing any life-threatening problems you find in the initial assessment, begin the physical exam. Be systematic and thorough, and remember to look (inspect), listen (auscultate), and feel (palpate) while performing your detailed examination.

Inspection

During your inspection, look for:

- *Tracheal Position.* The trachea should be midline. Movement toward a side may indicate a pneumothorax. Inspect the neck veins for evidence of jugular vein distention. The internal jugular veins are major vessels. Thus, jugular vein distention often evidences an increase in central venous pressure (Figure 2-58). Pump failure or cardiac tam-

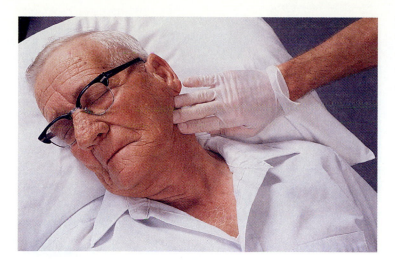

ponade can cause back pressure in the systemic circulation and jugular vein engorgement. Try to have the patient seated at a 45° angle, not lying flat, for this examination. Remember, however, that jugular vein distention is often difficult to assess in an obese patient.

- *Thorax.* Watch the patient breathe. To do this properly, expose the patient's chest wall, maintaining patient privacy if possible. Evidence of labored breathing includes retractions and accessory muscle use. Retractions are visible depressions in the soft tissues between the ribs that occur with increased respiratory effort. Accessory muscle use involves muscles of the neck, back, and abdomen. Normally these muscles play a small role in breathing, but patients with labored breathing put them to greater use. A patient with chronic obstructive pulmonary disease (COPD) may have an increased anteroposterior (AP) diameter and may appear "barrel-chested." Examination of the thorax can provide a great deal of information about the patient, including chronic problems such as COPD. The presence of a sternotomy scar, especially in an older patient, is a significant indicator of heart disease.

- *Epigastrium.* While the chest wall is exposed, inspect the epigastrium. Look for abdominal distention and visible pulsations. This may mean the patient has an aortic aneurysm with dissection or rupture.

- *Peripheral and Presacral Edema.* Chronic back pressure in the systemic venous circulation causes peripheral and presacral edema. These symptoms are most obvious in dependent parts such as the ankles (Figure 2-59). Often in bedridden patients you must inspect and palpate the sacral region for edema. Edema is generally classified as either mild or pitting. To distinguish between them, press firmly on the edematous part. If the depression remains after you remove pressure, the edema is pitting; otherwise it is mild.

- *Skin.* Several changes in the skin can be associated with cardiovascular disease. Pale and diaphoretic skin indicates peripheral vasoconstriction and sympathetic stimulation. It accompanies heart disease and other problems. A mottled appearance often indicates chronic cardiac failure.

- *Subtle Signs Of Cardiac Disease.* Look for subtle indicators of cardiac disease. Observe for signs that a patient is being treated for cardiac problems. These include midsternal scars from coronary artery bypass surgeries, pacemakers, or nitroglycerin skin patches.

FIGURE 2-59 Check for peripheral edema.

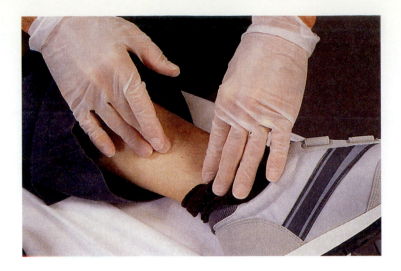

Auscultation

During your inspection listen for:

- *Breath Sounds.* Assessing breath sounds in the cardiac patient is just as important as it is in the respiratory patient. Assess the lung fields for equality. Also listen for *adventitious sounds,* those that arise or occur sporadically or in unusual locations. Such sounds as crackles (rales), wheezes, or rhonchi (whistling or snoring sounds) may indicate pulmonary congestion or edema. Patients with pulmonary edema may also have foamy, blood-tinged sputum from the mouth and nose. In severe cases, this is audible from a distance as an ominous "gurgling" sound.

- *Heart Sounds.* Avoid spending precious time auscultating heart sounds in the field. Background noise from traffic, family members, sirens, and other sources makes it very difficult to hear heart sounds, and the information you obtain generally will not affect patient management. Nonetheless, you should be familiar with normal heart sounds and be able to distinguish abnormal from normal findings (Figure 2-60). The first heart sound (S_1) is produced by closure of the AV valves (tricuspid and mitral)

FIGURE 2-60 Auscultate the chest. Listen for heart sounds.

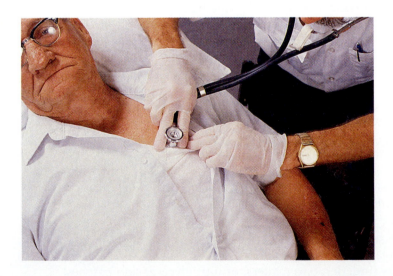

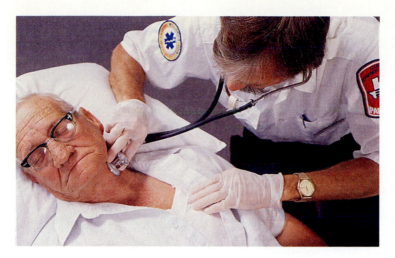

during ventricular systole. The second heart sound (S_2) is produced by closure of the aortic and pulmonary valves. S_1 and S_2 are normal. Any extra heart sounds are abnormal. The third heart sound (S_3) is associated with congestive heart failure. Occasionally, the skilled listener can hear the fourth heart sound (S_4), which occurs immediately before S_1. It is associated with increased atrial contraction. Ideally, the heart should be examined from the four classic auscultatory sites: aortic, pulmonic, mitral, and tricuspid. The point on the chest wall where the heartbeat can best be heard or felt is known as the point of maximum impulse (PMI). The PMI and examination of the heart are discussed in more detail in Volume 2, Chapter 2, Physical Examination.

An S_3 heart sound has a cadence like "Kentucky." An S_4 heart sound has a cadence like "Tennessee."

- *Carotid Artery Bruit.* Auscultation of the carotid arteries may reveal bruits (murmurs), which are a sign of turbulent blood flow through a vessel (Figure 2-61). They are audible over all major arteries, including the abdominal aorta. A bruit indicates partial blockage of the vessel, most commonly from atherosclerosis. If you detect a bruit, do not attempt carotid sinus massage. This procedure may dislodge plaque, resulting in stroke or other mishap.

Palpation

During your examination, feel for:

- *Pulse.* Determine the rate and regularity of the pulse (Figure 2-62). Also note the pulse's equality. Any pulse deficit can indicate underlying peripheral vascular disease and should be reported to medical direction.
- *Thorax.* Palpation of the thorax is extremely important as chest wall problems are quite common. These can only be elicited by palpation, which may reveal crepitus. *Crepitus* is a grating sensation that suggests the rubbing of broken bone ends or a "bubble wrap" crackling that suggests subcutaneous emphysema (air in the subcutaneous tissue). Palpapation may also reveal tenderness associated with a chest wall muscle strain, costochondritis (inflammation of the joint where the rib attaches to the sternum), or even rib fractures. It is important to remember that at least

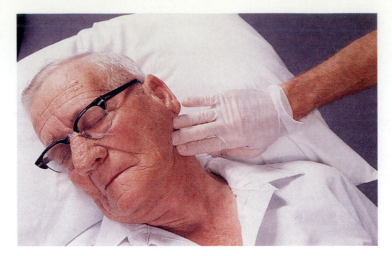

15 percent of patients with acute myocardial infarction will have associated chest wall tenderness.

- *Epigastrium.* Also feel the abdomen for pulsations and distention, which may indicate an abdominal aortic aneurysm.

Physical examination of the chest is an essential aspect of comprehensive prehospital care. Employ the standard techniques of inspection, auscultation, palpation, and occasionally, percussion. Together these skills can provide a great deal of information about chronic problems as well as the ongoing acute episode.

MANAGEMENT OF CARDIOVASCULAR EMERGENCIES

The following section discusses management techniques frequently used in cardiac emergencies. You should also become familiar with your local protocols and procedures, since they vary from system to system.

BASIC LIFE SUPPORT

Basic life support is the primary skill for managing serious cardiovascular problems.

Basic life support is the primary skill for managing serious cardiovascular problems. These include the basic airway maneuvers as well as CPR. Review basic life support techniques frequently to keep your skills at their peak.

ADVANCED LIFE SUPPORT

Most of the procedures that paramedics employ to manage cardiovascular emergencies are considered advanced life support. The number of skills will vary from system to system. Advanced prehospital skills used in managing cardiovascular emergencies include:

- ECG monitoring
- Vagal maneuvers (carotid sinus massage)
- Precordial thump
- Pharmacological management
- Defibrillation

- Synchronized cardioversion
- Transcutaneous cardiac pacing
- Diagnostic (12-lead) ECG (see Part 3 of this chapter)

Monitoring ECG in the Field

Most systems' primary tool for ECG monitoring in the field is a combination ECG monitor/defibrillator that operates on a direct current (DC) battery source (Procedure 2-1). It has the following parts:

- Paddle electrodes
- Defibrillator controls
- Synchronizer switch
- Oscilloscope
- Paper strip recorder
- Patient cable and lead wires
- Controls for monitoring
- Special features (such as data recorders)

To monitor your patient's ECG, you will place the three limb electrodes on the chest (in left arm, right arm, and left leg positions). Some manufacturers require a fourth lead on the right leg. By placing the three principal electrodes, you can monitor any of the bipolar leads (I, II, or III). On certain machines, you can also monitor the three augmented leads (aVR, aVL, or aVF) through these three electrodes. As a rule, Lead II is usually monitored, as its axis is almost the same as that of the heart. Modified chest lead 1 (MCL_1) is used occasionally and is often better for determining the site of ectopic beats.

You can also monitor your patient through the defibrillator paddles ("quick-look"). The quick-look paddles are more frequently used in cases of cardiac arrest, when there is no time to place chest electrodes. You can also use this system when the patient cable is inoperative. Among the disadvantages of quick-look paddle electrodes are that they tend to pick up more artifacts than chest electrodes and must be held in continuous contact with the chest.

To use quick-look paddles, follow these steps:

1. Turn on oscilloscope power.
2. Apply conducting gel or other medium liberally to the paddle surface.
3. Hold the paddles firmly on the chest wall with the positive electrode on the left lower chest and the negative electrode on the right upper chest. This closely simulates Lead II.
4. Observe the monitor and obtain a tracing if desired.

Chest electrodes vary from manufacturer to manufacturer. Usually to mimic Lead II, you will place the positive electrode on the patient's left lower chest and the negative electrode on his right upper chest. Placement of the ground wire varies. For MCL_1 place the positive electrode on the right lower chest wall and the negative electrode on the left upper chest wall. Again, placement of the ground wire varies. Place the electrodes to avoid large muscle masses, large quantities of chest hair, or anything that keeps the electrodes from resting flat on the skin. Also, avoid placing electrodes where you might have to place defibrillator paddles.

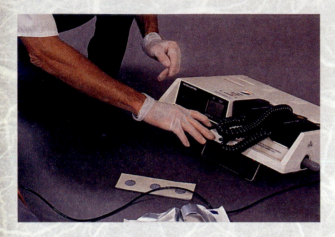

2-1a   Turn on the machine.

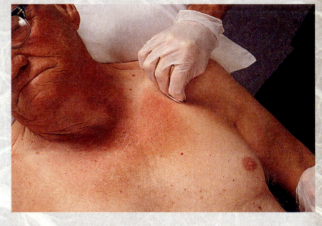

2-1b   Prepare the skin.

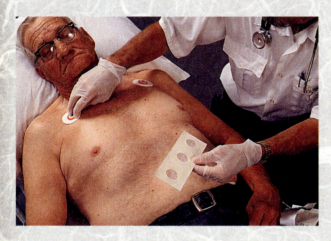

2-1c   Apply the electrodes.

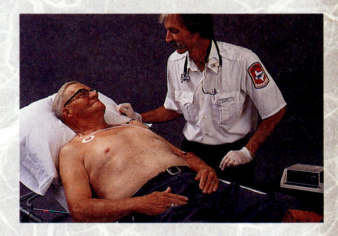

2-1d   Ask the patient to relax and remain still.

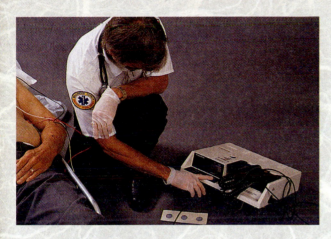

2-1e   Check the ECG.

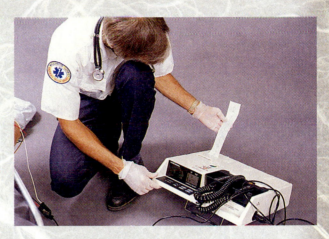

2-1f   Obtain a tracing.

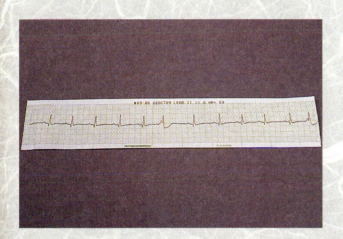

2-1g   ECG strip.

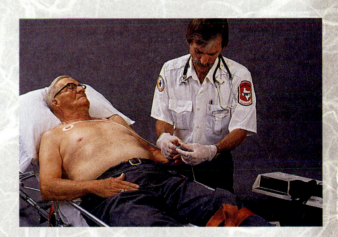

2-1h   Continue ALS care.

To place electrodes follow these steps:

1. Cleanse the skin with alcohol or abrasive pad. This removes dirt and body oil for better skin contact. If chest hair is thick, shave small amounts before placing the electrodes. If the patient is extremely diaphoretic, apply tincture of benzoin.
2. Apply electrodes to the skin surface.
3. Attach wires to the electrodes.
4. Plug the cable into the monitor.
5. Adjust gain or sensitivity to the proper level.
6. Adjust the QRS volume. (The continual beep of the ECG may disturb the patient.)
7. Obtain a baseline tracing.

Poor ECG signals are useless, and you should correct them. Their most common cause is faulty skin contact. Whenever you spot a poor signal, check for the following possible causes:

- Excessive hair
- Loose or dislodged electrode
- Dried conductive gel
- Poor placement
- Diaphoresis

An initially poor tracing may improve as the conductive gel breaks down skin resistance. Other causes of poor tracings include:

- Patient movement or muscle tremor
- Broken patient cable
- Broken lead wire
- Low battery
- Faulty grounding
- Faulty monitor

Obtain a paper printout from each patient you monitor. Be sure to adjust the stylus heat properly. Calibrate each strip when you begin monitoring so that 1 mV deflects the stylus 10 mm (two large boxes).

Again, treat the patient and not the monitor. Always compare the rhythm you see on the monitor with the patient's signs and symptoms. A patient may have a perfect rhythm on the monitor but have no pulse or blood pressure.

VAGAL MANEUVERS

For a stable patient with symptomatic tachycardia, vagal maneuvers sometimes help slow the heart rate. Ask the patient to perform a Valsalva maneuver (bearing down as if attempting to have a bowel movement) or to cough. If these are unsuccessful and the patient is eligible, attempt carotid artery massage. Do not attempt carotid artery massage on patients with carotid bruits or known cerebrovascular or carotid artery disease, as it may precipitate a stroke. Carotid sinus massage is discussed in more detail later in this chapter.

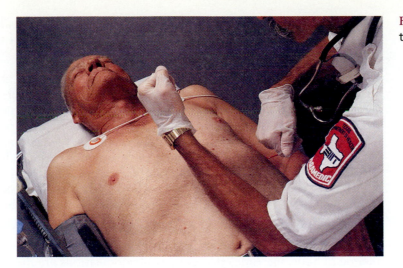

FIGURE 2–63   The precordial thump.

PRECORDIAL THUMP

The precordial thump, a blow to the midsternum with the heel of the fist, can stimulate depolarization within the heart. This is most effective when performed immediately after the onset of ventricular fibrillation or pulseless ventricular tachycardia. On occasion, the precordial thump can cause depolarization of enough ventricular cells to allow resumption of an organized rhythm. Additionally, conversions from ventricular tachycardia, complete AV block, and occasionally, ventricular fibrillation, have been reported. If no defibrillator is immediately available, you may attempt a precordial thump on a pulseless patient who has a witnessed arrest. Since the amount of energy needed to convert ventricular fibrillation increases rapidly with time, a thump is likely to succeed only if delivered early. It is not recommended in pediatric patients.

To deliver a precordial thump strike the midsternum with the heel of your fist from a distance of 10–12 inches (Figure 2-63). To avoid rib fractures and other problems, keep your arm and wrist parallel to the sternum's long axis.

PHARMACOLOGICAL MANAGEMENT

The drugs that you will use to manage cardiovascular emergencies generally fall into the categories of antidysrhythmics, sympathomimetics, and drugs used specifically for myocardial ischemia (including thrombolytics), along with other prehospital medications, some of which are used only infrequently. For more detailed information on these types of drugs, see Volume 1, Chapter 9 on pharmacology.

Antidysrhythmics

Antidysrhythmic medications control or suppress dysrhythmias. Among the more commonly used antidysrhythmics are atropine, lidocaine, procainamide, bretylium, adenosine, amiodarone, and verapamil.

Atropine Sulfate   Atropine sulfate is a parasympatholytic agent used to treat symptomatic bradycardias, especially those arising in the atria. It is an anticholinergic. It also helps in the management of asystole. Side effects include blurred vision, dilated pupils, dry mouth, tachycardia, and drowsiness. It has no contraindications in the emergency setting. It is given by IV bolus or through an endotracheal tube. Dose is

0.5 mg to 1 mg IV for bradycardia and 1.0 mg for asystole, repeated every three to five minutes for a total dose of 0.04 mg/kg. Endotracheal doses are 2.0–2.5 times the IV dose.

Lidocaine Lidocaine is a first-line antidysrhythmic used to treat and prevent life-threatening ventricular dysrhythmias. It suppresses irritable sites in the ventricle, while having little effect on unaffected myocardial tissue. Side effects include drowsiness, seizures, confusion, bradycardia, heart blocks, nausea, and vomiting. Lidocaine is contraindicated in second-degree and third-degree blocks. It is administered by IV bolus, IV drip, or through an endotracheal tube. Dose is 1.0–1.5 mg/kg slow IV push (50 mg/min) for ectopy, or normal IV push in arrest. A drip is established by mixing 1 gram into 250 cc D_5W or NaCl. The typical maintenance rate is 2–4 mg/minute. The maximum bolus dosage is 300 mg.

Procainamide Procainamide is a second-line antidysrhythmic drug to lidocaine, used for ventricular dysrhythmias refractory to lidocaine or in patients who are allergic to lidocaine. Side effects and contraindications are the same as lidocaine. It is administered by slow IV bolus and IV drip. IV bolus is 100 mg given over 5 minutes, with a maximum dose of 17 mg/kg. Discontinue it when the dysrhythmia is suppressed, hypotension ensues, the QRS is widened 50 percent, or the maximum dose is achieved. The drip rate is the same as lidocaine drip.

Bretylium Bretylium is a second-line antidysrhythmic agent used to treat life-threatening ventricular dysrhythmias, especially ventricular fibrillation. Although its antidysrhythmic effects are poorly understood, it apparently raises the ventricular fibrillation threshold. Side effects include hypotension, hypertension, dizziness, syncope, seizures, nausea, and vomiting. Bretylium is now used less frequently, due to the development of other pharmacological agents. It is administered by IV bolus and IV drip. Dose is 5 mg/kg IV push; drip rate is 1–2 mg/min. A subsequent dose of 10 mg/kg is repeated if the dysrhythmia persists. Maximum dose is 30 mg/kg.

Adenosine Adenosine is used to manage supraventricular tachydysrhythmias. It is a naturally occurring nucleoside that acts on the AV node to slow conduction and inhibit reentry pathways. Side effects include apprehension, burning sensation, heaviness in arms, hypotension, chest pressure, diaphoresis, numbness, tingling, dyspnea, tightness in the throat and/or groin pressure, headache, nausea, and vomiting. Adenosine is contraindicated in second- or third-degree blocks or in sick sinus syndrome unless a pacemaker is present. It is administered by IV rapid bolus, with the venous site as close to the heart as possible. Flush with saline rapidly, immediately after the adenosine to ensure drug delivery. The initial dose is 6 mg (rapid push), followed by a 15–30 cc saline flush. If the tachydysrhythmia is not abolished, a second dose of 12 mg may be administered. If still ineffective, a third dose of 12 mg can be administered. The maximum dose of adenosine is 30 mg.

Amiodarone Amiodarone (Cordarone) is an antidysrhythmic agent used in the management of recurring ventricular fibrillation and hemodynamically unstable ventricular tachycardia. Amiodarone is being used more frequently in the pre-hospital setting in the management of cardiac arrest. Although a second-line drug in the United States, it is considered a first-line agent in several of the Commonwealth countries. It is contraindicated in cardiogenic shock, marked sinus bradycardia, and high-degree heart blocks (2nd and 3rd degree). Hypotension is the most common side-effect. It can cause bradycardia and AV blocks. The dosage is 150–300 milligrams by slow IV infusion.

Verapamil Verapamil is a calcium channel blocker that slows the heart rate in symptomatic atrial tachycardias. It is used to terminate paroxysmal supraventricular tachycardia and to control the rapid ventricular response often seen with atrial fibrillation or flutter. It is administered by slow IV bolus. The maximum dose is 30 mg.

Sympathomimetic Agents

Sympathomimetic agents are similar to the naturally occurring hormones epinephrine and norepinephrine. They duplicate or mimic sympathetic nervous system stimulation, acting either on the alpha or beta adrenergic receptors. Alpha receptor stimulation causes peripheral vasoconstriction. Beta receptor stimulation increases heart rate, cardiac contractile force, bronchodilation, and peripheral vasodilation. Stimulating dopaminergic receptors in the renal and mesenteric blood vessels causes dilation. Commonly used sympathomimetic agents include epinephrine, norepinephrine, isoproterenol, dopamine, and dobutamine.

Epinephrine Epinephrine, which acts on both alpha and beta adrenergic receptors, is the mainstay of cardiac arrest resuscitation. It is used in ventricular fibrillation, asystole, and electromechanical dissociation. It is also sometimes used in bradycardia refractory to atropine. It is given by IV bolus, subcutaneously, and through the endotracheal tube. Dose is 1 mg of 1:10,000 solution given every three to five minutes.

Norepinephrine Norepinephrine is a sympathomimetic whose alpha agonist properties are greater than epinephrine's. It also acts on beta-receptors to a lesser degree. It is used occasionally in hemodynamically significant hypotension and cardiogenic shock, although dopamine is the first-line agent for those conditions. Norepinephrine may be effective if total peripheral resistance is low, such as in neurogenic shock. Side effects include anxiety, trembling, headache, dizziness, nausea, and vomiting. It can also cause bradycardia. Do not use norepinephrine in patients with hypotension from hypovolemia. It is administered by intravenous infusion via drip by placing 4 mg into 1000 cc of D_5W only, to yield a concentration of 4 mcg/cc. The initial loading dose is 8–12 mcg/minute to obtain a blood pressure of 80–100 mmHg systolic. The maintenance dose is 2–4 mcg/minute.

Isoproterenol Although rarely used with the advent of transcutaneous pacing, isoproterenol is a potent beta agonist that increases heart rate and cardiac contractile force. It is used in bradycardia refractory to atropine and in the management of asystole. Isoproterenol is administered by intravenous infusion. Adding 1 mg into 250 cc of D_5W or saline mixes isoproterenol, yielding 4 mcg/cc. The drip rate is 2–20 mcg/minute. Common procedure is to start with a low dose and slowly increase the dose (titrate) until a satisfactory rate is obtained. Transcutaneous pacing is preferred to isoproterenol.

Dopamine Dopamine (Intropin), a vasopressor, increases cardiac output. It stimulates both the alpha and beta receptors. As an advantage over other drugs, it often maintains renal perfusion at recommended dosages. Side effects include nervousness, headache, dysrhythmias, palpitations, chest pain, dyspnea, nausea, and vomiting. Dopamine is contraindicated for hypovolemic shock until fluid resuscitation has been completed. Dose is given via drip by mixing 800 mg into 500 cc of D_5W or saline to yield a concentration of 1600 mcg/cc (400 mg into 250 cc will also work). Dopamine's properties are dose-related: At 1–2 mcg/kg/minute, renal artery dilation occurs; at 2–10 mcg/kg/minute, it primarily affects beta receptors; at 10–15 mcg/kg/minute, it affects both alpha and beta receptors; and at 15–20 mcg/kg/minute, it primarily affects alpha receptors.

Dobutamine Like dopamine, dobutamine (Dobutrex) increases cardiac output by increasing stroke volume. It has little effect on heart rate and is occasionally used in isolated left-heart failure until other medications such as digitalis take effect. Its side effects are the same as dopamine's. Do not use dobutamine as the sole agent in hypovolemic shock unless fluid resuscitation has been completed. Dopamine is preferred over dobutamine to increase cardiac output in cardiogenic shock. Dobutamine is administered by intravenous infusion by mixing 250 mg into 250 cc of D_5W or saline, yielding a concentration of 1000 mcg/cc. Dose is 2–20 mcg/kg/minute, titrated to effect.

Drugs Used for Myocardial Ischemia

Drugs used to treat myocardial ischemia and relieve its pain include oxygen, nitrous oxide, nitroglycerin, morphine, and nalbuphine.

Oxygen Oxygen is important in emergency cardiac care. It increases the blood's oxygen content and aids oxygenation of peripheral tissues. It is indicated in any situation where hypoxia or ischemia is possible.

Nitrous Oxide Nitrous oxide (Nitronox) is purely an analgesic with no significant hemodynamic effects; however, delivery in fixed combination with 50 percent oxygen can increase myocardial oxygen supply. Nitrous oxide is self-administered by inhalation via a modified demand valve to the desired effect. Its effects subside within 2–5 minutes. Side effects include CNS depression and potential respiratory depression. Do not give nitrous oxide to patients who cannot comprehend verbal instructions or who are intoxicated with alcohol or other drugs.

Nitroglycerin Nitroglycerin is an organic nitrate that dilates peripheral arteries and veins, thus reducing preload and afterload and myocardial oxygen demand. It may cause some coronary artery dilation, increasing blood flow though the collaterals. Nitroglycerin administration often helps distinguish angina from MI. Nitroglycerin does not relieve MI symptoms, but it should be given before morphine, because it works in conjunction with morphine in an MI. Its side effects include headache, dizziness, weakness, hypotension, and tachycardia. Dosage for nitroglycerin is one tablet sublingually, repeated every 5 minutes, up to a total of three tablets. Monitor blood pressure before each dose.

NOTE: Nitroglycerin starts losing potency as soon as the bottle is opened. Always use the nitroglycerin provided on the medical intensive care unit (MICU) and check the date before administration.

Morphine Sulfate The narcotic morphine is important in managing MI. It reduces myocardial oxygen demand by reducing preload and afterload. It also acts directly on the central nervous system to relieve pain, and it reduces sympathetic nervous system discharge, which can further decrease myocardial oxygen demand. Side effects include nausea, vomiting, abdominal cramping, respiratory depression, hypotension, and potential altered mental status. Toxic effects are apnea and severe hypotension. Dosage is 1–2 mg increments slow IV push, titrated to pain relief. Monitor blood pressure before each dose.

Nalbuphine Some EMS systems use nalbuphine (Nubain) instead of morphine. It is an effective analgesic but lacks morphine's desirable hemodynamic effects. Side effects include sedation, clammy skin, dizziness, dry mouth, hypotension, hypertension, nausea, and vomiting. It is contraindicated in patients who have taken depressants or alcohol. Dose is 10–20 mg IV, intramuscularly (IM), or subcutaneously (SC).

Thrombolytic Agents

Definitive treatment of myocardial ischemia with thrombolytic agents is one of the most important recent advances in medicine. In some instances, thrombolytic therapy may be beneficial in the field. This is especially true in areas that have a long transport time to a definitive care facility. Thrombolytic agents are very expensive, and their use requires a diagnostic 12-lead ECG.

Aspirin Although not a thrombolytic, aspirin plays an important role in the treatment of cardiac ischemia. Aspirin inhibits the aggregation of platelets and is thus effective in the treatment of coronary ischemia and stroke. Its most common side effect is gastric upset, although bleeding can be a problem in selected patients. The standard dosage is one tablet (325 mg) orally. Some physicians prefer smaller doses. Baby aspirin is useful in that it can be chewed, thus more quickly reaching a therapeutic blood level.

Alteplase (Activase) (tPA) Alteplase, commonly called tPA, is a potent thrombolytic agent manufactured by recombinant DNA technology. Thus, the compound is identical to the human compound, which minimizes the chances of allergic reactions. tPA is effective if administered within 6 hours after the onset of coronary ischemia. It is given by a bolus dose followed by an infusion. The typical dose is 100 milligrams administered over $1\frac{1}{2}$ to 2 hours. Complications of tPA include hemorrhage, which can be fatal. Also, when reperfusion occurs, potentially life-threatening dysrhythmias may develop.

Relteplase (Retavase) Relteplase is another human plasminogen activator. It functions in the same fashion as tPA and has the same basic side effects and complications. Relteplase is administered as a single 10-unit bolus given by IV push over 2 minutes. A second 10-unit bolus is administered 30 minutes later. This dosing regimen makes relteplase attractive for prehospital care.

Other Prehospital Drugs

In some situations, medical direction or local protocol may recommend other drugs. These may include furosemide, diazepam, promethazine, and sodium nitroprusside.

Furosemide Furosemide (Lasix) is a potent loop diuretic that relaxes the venous system. Its effects are often seen within 5 minutes. It also has a diuretic effect that decreases intravascular fluid volume. Side effects include hypotension, ECG changes, chest pain, dry mouth, hypokalemia, hypochloremia, hyponatremia, and hyperglycemia. Furosemide should be used only in life-threatening emergencies in pregnancy, because it can cause fetal abnormalities. Dose is 40 mg slow IV push (40 mg/minute). If the patient is already taking furosemide, or another diuretic, you may need to double the dosage.

Diazepam You may administer diazepam (Valium) if the patient is extremely apprehensive or agitated. Diazepam is not an analgesic, but it will help relax the patient. Dose is 2–5 mg IV or deep IM.

Promethazine Promethazine (Phenargan) has sedative, antihistamine, antiemetic, and anticholinergic properties. It also potentiates narcotics, making it useful in an MI setting by reducing the nausea of morphine yet enhancing its effects. Its side effects are drowsiness, sedation, blurred vision, tachycardia, bradycardia, and dizziness. Promethazine is contraindicated in unresponsive patients or those taking large amounts of depressants. Extrapyramidal symptoms (dystonic symptoms) have been reported with promethazine. Dosage is 12.5–25.0 mg given slow IV push or deep IM only (25.0 mg/minute).

Sodium Nitroprusside Sodium nitroprusside (Nipride), a potent arterial and venous vasodilator, is popular for use in hypertensive crisis. It is given as an IV infusion, thus making administration more controlled and the patient's response more predictable.

Drugs Infrequently Used in the Prehospital Setting

Paramedics who work in the emergency department will encounter many medications that are not routinely used in the prehospital setting. In addition, many patients take these medications on a long-term basis.

Digitalis Digitalis (Digoxin, Lanoxin) is a cardiac glycoside. It increases the force of the cardiac contraction and cardiac output. It slows impulse conduction through the AV node and decreases the ventricular response to certain supraventricular dysrhythmias such as atrial fibrillation, atrial flutter, and paroxysmal supraventricular tachycardia. It is also used to treat heart failure. Its side effects include fatigue, muscle weakness, agitation, hallucination, headache, malaise, dizziness, vertigo, stupor, blurred vision and yellow-green halo vision, photophobia, diplopia, nausea, and vomiting. Digitalis toxicity can cause almost any dysrhythmia. In fact, digoxin frequently induces some of the same dysrhythmias it is used to treat, and these often will be refractory to traditional antidysrhythmic drugs. Digitalis is contraindicated in any digitalis-induced toxicity, ventricular fibrillation, or ventricular tachycardia not caused by CHF.

Dose is 8–12 mcg/kg IV slow IV push, over 15–20 minutes. If possible, obtain the patient's digoxin level before administering any cardiac glycoside. Most patients taking digitalis will remain therapeutic at 10–15 mcg/kg dose over a 24-hour period. Administering digitalis to patients already taking a cardiac glycoside involves complicated calculations, making it impractical for prehospital use in most settings.

Beta Blockers Beta blockers are frequently used to control dysrhythmias, high blood pressure, and angina. Many beta blockers such as propranolol (Inderal) are nonselective; others such as metoprolol are selective for B_1 or B_2 receptors. Beta blockers may precipitate congestive heart failure, heart block, and asthma in patients who are predisposed to these conditions. The beta-blocker labetolol (Trandate, Normodyne) effectively decreases blood pressure. It is given by IV bolus and infusion. The IV bolus is 20 mg over 20 minutes, and may be repeated at 40–80 mg over 10 minutes. Maximum bolus is 300 mg. Drip is established by mixing 200 mg into 160 cc D_5W; dose is 2 cc/minute.

Calcium Channel Blockers Calcium channel blockers are a relatively new class of medication. They include verapamil (Isoptin, Calan), diltiazem (Cardizem), and nifedipine (Procardia). Nifedipine is now being used, in addition to nitroglycerin, to manage angina. Like nitroglycerin, it is a vasodilator, but it works through a different mechanism. It is administered orally. Calcium channel blockers are being used increasingly for angina pectoris, dysrhythmias, hypertension, and other cardiovascular problems.

Alkalinizing Agents Alkalinizing agents such as sodium bicarbonate are used late in the management of cardiac arrest, if at all. Occasionally, metabolic acidosis from another disorder may cause PEA, asystole, ventricular tachycardia, or ventricular fibrillation. In these rare cases, sodium bicarbonate can aid in converting to a perfusing rhythm. Adequate CPR, prompt defibrillation, and appropriate drug administration should always precede the use of sodium bicarbonate. Sodium bicarbonate has few side effects and no contraindications in the emergency setting. Dose is 1 mEq/kg initially, followed by 0.5 mEq/kg every 10 minutes. When possible, dosages should be based on arterial blood gas (ABG) results.

DEFIBRILLATION

Defibrillation is the process of passing a current through a fibrillating heart to depolarize the cells and allow them to repolarize uniformly, thus restoring an organized cardiac rhythm. A critical mass of the myocardium must be depolarized

* **defibrillation** the process of passing an electrical current through a fibrillating heart to depolarize a critical mass of myocardial cells. This allows them to depolarize uniformly, resulting in an organized rhythm.

in order to suppress all of the ectopic foci. The critical mass is related to the size of the heart, but it cannot be calculated for a given individual or situation.

The *defibrillator* is an electrical capacitor that stores energy for delivery to the patient at a desired time. It consists of an adjustable high-voltage power supply, energy storage capacitor, and paddles. A current-limiting inductor connects the capacitor to the paddles. Recently, different defibrillation wave forms, most commonly biphasic wave forms, have been utilized to decrease possible tissue damage and to increase battery life. This technology evolved with the development of the compact automated external defibrillators (AEDs).

Most defibrillators use direct current (DC). Alternating current (AC) models should not be used. Direct current is more effective, more portable, and causes less muscle damage. It delivers an electrical charge of several thousand volts over a very short time, generally 4–12 milliseconds. The shock's strength is commonly expressed in energy according to the following formula:

$$\text{energy (joules)} = \text{power (watts)} \times \text{duration (seconds)}$$

The chest wall offers resistance to the electrical charge, which lowers the amount of energy actually delivered to the heart. Therefore, lowering the resistance pathway between the defibrillator paddles and the chest is important. Factors that influence chest wall resistance include:

- Paddle pressure
- Paddle-skin interface
- Paddle surface area
- Number of previous countershocks
- Inspiratory versus expiratory phase at time of countershock

The following factors influence the success of defibrillation.

- *Time until ventricular fibrillation.* In conjunction with effective CPR, defibrillation begun within four minutes after the onset of fibrillation will yield significantly improved resuscitation rates, as compared with defibrillation begun within eight minutes.
- *Condition of the myocardium.* Converting ventricular fibrillation is more difficult in the presence of acidosis, hypoxia, hypothermia, electrolyte imbalance, or drug toxicity. Secondary ventricular fibrillation (ventricular fibrillation that results from another cause) is more difficult to treat than primary ventricular fibrillation.
- *Heart size and body weight.* The effects of heart size and body weight on defibrillation are controversial. Pediatric and adult energy requirements differ, but whether size and energy level settings are related in adults is not clear.
- *Previous countershocks.* Repeated countershocks decrease transthoracic resistance, thereby allowing the defibrillator to deliver more energy to the heart at the same energy level.
- *Paddle size.* Larger defibrillator paddles are thought to be more effective and cause less myocardial damage. The ideal size for adults, however, has not been established. Generally, the paddles should be 10–13 cm in diameter. In infants, 4.5 cm paddles are adequate.
- *Paddle Placement.* For both adults and children in the emergency setting, place the paddles on the chest. Position one paddle to the right of the upper sternum, just below the clavicle. Place the other to

the left of the left nipple in an anterior axillary line immediately over the apex of the heart. Do not place paddles over the sternum. Do not place paddles over the generator of an implanted automatic defibrillator or pacemaker, which can damage or disable the device. Place the paddles approximately 5 inches from the generator. The paddles may be marked as apex (positive electrode) and sternum (negative electrode). Although reversing polarity inverts the ECG tracing, it does not affect defibrillation.

- *Paddle-skin interface.* Paddle-skin interface should have as little electrical resistance as possible. Greater resistance decreases energy delivery to the heart and increases heat production on the skin. Many available materials decrease resistance, including gels, creams, pastes, saline-soaked pads, and prepackaged gel pads. Use only creams made specifically for defibrillation, not for ECG monitoring. When using cream, make sure that it does not run and form a bridge between paddles. Never use alcohol-soaked pads; they can ignite.

- *Paddle contact pressure.* The paddle contact pressure is important. Firm, downward pressure decreases transthoracic resistance. Do not lean on the paddles, however; they may slip.

- *Properly functioning defibrillator.* The machine should deliver the amount of energy that it indicates. Therefore, frequent inspection and testing of the machine are necessary. Change and cycle the batteries as the manufacturer directs.

To perform defibrillation, use the following steps (Procedure 2-2):

1. Confirm ventricular fibrillation or pulseless ventricular tachycardia on the cardiac monitor.
2. Place the patient in a safe environment if initially in contact with some electrically conductive material such as metal or water.
3. Apply electrode gel to the paddles, or place commercial defibrillation pads on the patient's exposed thorax.
4. Turn on and charge the defibrillator to 200 joules for the first shock.
5. Ensure that the electrodes are appropriately placed on the patient's thorax with proper pressure.
6. Ensure that no one else is in contact with the patient. Verbally and visually clear everybody, including yourself, before any defibrillation attempt.
7. Deliver a defibrillatory shock by depressing both red buttons simultaneously. (Depressing only one will not deliver a shock.)
8. Reconfirm the rhythm on the monitor screen; if the patient is still in ventricular fibrillation or pulseless ventricular tachycardia, recharge the defibrillator and repeat steps 5–7 at higher energy levels.

Keep in mind the basic energy recommendations for defibrillation. After initially attempting defibrillation at 200 joules in an adult, increase dosage to a maximum of 360 joules in one or two repeat countershocks. The pediatric dosage is generally 2 joules/kg initially, repeated at 4 joules/kg if required.

EMERGENCY SYNCHRONIZED CARDIOVERSION

Synchronized cardioversion is a controlled form of defibrillation for patients who still have organized cardiac activity with a pulse. A synchronizing circuit in the defibrillator interprets the QRS cycle and delivers the electrical discharge during the R wave of the QRS complex. This reduces the likelihood of delivering the cardioversion during the vulnerable period of the QRS cycle, which can precipitate ventricular fibrillation. Synchronizing also permits the use of lower energy levels and reduces the potential for secondary dysrhythmias. Depending on the type of dysrhythmia being treated, as little as 10 joules may be adequate, especially if the origin is atrial.

Indications for emergency synchronized cardioversion in an unstable patient include:

- Perfusing ventricular tachycardia
- Paroxysmal supraventricular tachycardia
- Rapid atrial fibrillation
- 2:1 atrial flutter

The procedure for synchronized cardioversion is the same as for defibrillation. Sedate conscious patients if at all possible. Turn on the synchronizer switch, and verify that the machine is detecting the R waves (Figure 2-64). If not, you may need to reposition the electrodes. Press and hold the discharge buttons until the machine discharges on the next R wave. Some models automatically turn off the synchronizer after a cardioversion and return to defibrillation mode. To give a second synchronized shock, you must depress the synchronizer button again. If ventricular

✱ **synchronized cardioversion**
the passage of an electric current through the heart during a specific part of the cardiac cycle to terminate certain kinds of dysrhythmias.

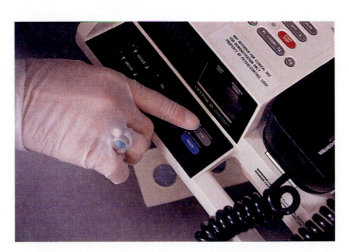

FIGURE 2–64 Activate the synchronizer.

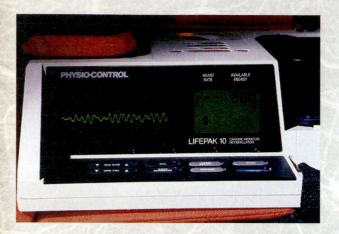

2-2a   Identify rhythm on the cardiac monitor.

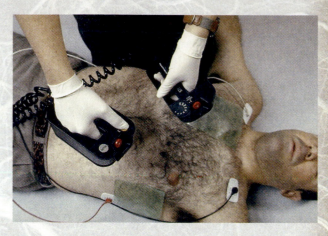

2-2b   Apply electrode gel to the paddles or place commercial defibrillation pads on the patient's exposed thorax.

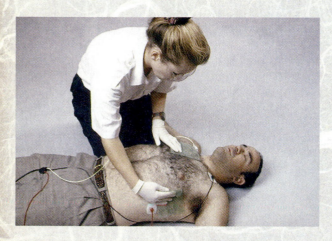

2-2c   Charge the defibrillation paddles.

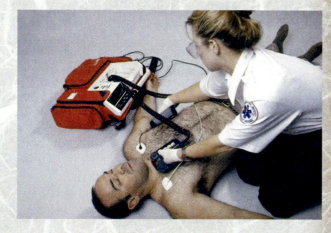

2-2d   Reconfirm the rhythm on the cardiac monitor.

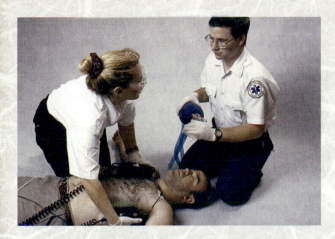

2-2e Verbally and visually clear everybody, including yourself, from the cardiac patient.

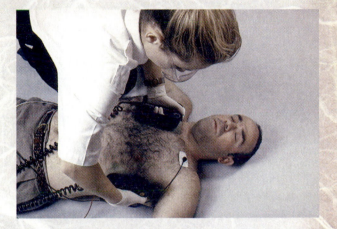

2-2f Deliver a shock by pressing both buttons simultaneously.

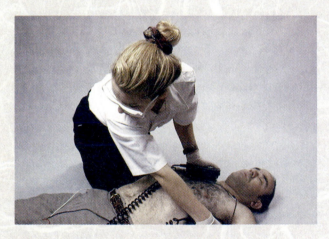

2-2g Reconfirm the rhythm on the cardiac monitor.

fibrillation occurs, you must turn off the synchronizer switch and use the machine in the defibrillation mode, because the heart produces no R wave in ventricular fibrillation and the machine will not discharge. The procedure for synchronized cardioversion is summarized in Figure 2-65.

TRANSCUTANEOUS CARDIAC PACING

Many of the newer cardiac monitor/defibrillators have a built-in cardiac pacing device that enables paramedic units to perform *transcutaneous* (external) cardiac pacing (TCP). Transcutaneous cardiac pacing allows electrical pacing of the heart through the skin via specially designed thoracic electrodes. Before the development of TCP, electrical cardiac pacing required placing an electrode through a major vein or directly into the chest. With TCP, pacing can now be provided in the prehospital setting. This is beneficial in such cases of symptomatic bradycardia as occur with high-degree AV blocks, atrial fibrillation with slow ventricular response, and other significant bradycardias (including asystole). Use transcutaneous pacing if pharmacological intervention has no effect and the patient is hypotensive or hypoperfusing.

To perform external cardiac pacing, follow these steps (Procedure 2-3):

1. Initiate IV, oxygen, and ECG monitoring.
2. Place the patient supine.
3. Confirm symptomatic bradycardia and confirm medical direction order for external cardiac pacing.
4. Apply the pacing electrodes according to the manufacturer's recommendations being sure that they interface well with the skin.
5. Connect the electrodes.
6. Set the desired heart rate on the pacemaker. This will typically range from 60 to 80 beats per minute.
7. Turn the output setting to 0.
8. Turn on the pacer.
9. Slowly increase the output until you note ventricular capture.
10. Check the pulse and blood pressure, and adjust the rate and amperage as medical direction orders.
11. Monitor the patient's response to treatment.

To manage patients in asystole, place the output on its maximum setting. Then decrease the output if capture occurs.

Occasionally, external cardiac pacing may cause patient discomfort. If this occurs, medical direction may request the administration of an analgesic.

Overdrive pacing may deter recurrent tachycardia. This involves increasing the rate above the heart's current rate in order to suppress ventricular ectopy. This is particularly useful in *torsade de pointes*. Failure of transcutaneous pacing is similar to the failure of a permanent pacemaker, as discussed earlier in the section on artificial pacemaker rhythm.

ALGORITHM: ELECTRICAL (SYNCHRONIZED) CARDIOVERSION

Tachycardia
With serious signs and symptoms related to the tachycardia

↓

If ventricular rate is >150 BPM, prepare for **immediate cardioversion**. May give brief trial of medications based on specific dysrhythmias. Immediate cardioversion is generally not needed for rates <150 BPM.

↓

Check
- Oxygen saturation
- Suction device
- IV line
- Intubation equipment

↓

Premedicate whenever possible[a]

↓

Synchronized cardioversion[b, c]

VT[d]
PSVT[e]
Atrial fibrillation   } 100 J, 200 J, 300 J, 360 J[c]
Atrial flutter[e]

a. Effective regimens have included a sedative (e.g., **diazepam, midazolam, barbiturates, etomidate, ketamine, methohexital**) with or without an analgesic agent (e.g., **fentanyl, morphine, meperidine**). Many experts recommend anesthesia if service is readily available.

b. Note possible need to resynchronize after each cardioversion.

c. If delays in synchronization occur and clinical conditions are critical, go to immediate unsynchronized shocks.

d. Treat polymorphic VT (irregular form and rate) like VF: 200 J, 200–300 J, 360 J.

e. PSVT and atrial flutter often respond to lower energy levels (start with 50 J).

FIGURE 2–65 Electrical (synchronized) cardioversion procedure. Adapted with permission. Journal of the American Medical Association, October 28, 1992, Volume 268, No. 16, *Guidelines for Cardiopulmonary Resuscitation and Emergency Cardiac Care*, p. 2224. © 1992 American Medical Association.

External pacing is of benefit in bradycardias and heart blocks that are symptomatic. The electrodes are placed on the chest as shown. The desired heart rate is selected. The current is then adjusted until "capture" of the heart's conductive system is obtained.

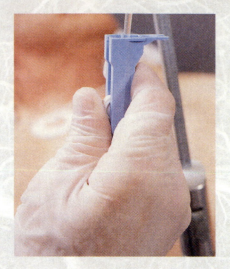

2-3a   Establish an IV line.

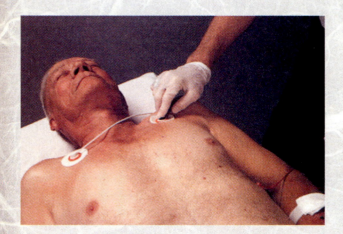

2-3b   Place ECG electrodes.

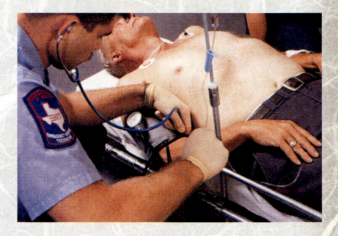

2-3c   Carefully assess vital signs and contact medical direction.

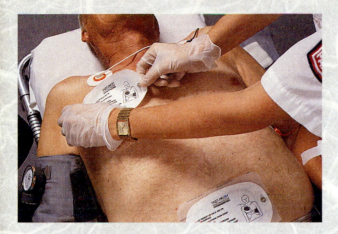

2-3d. If external pacing is ordered, apply the pacing electrodes according to the manufacturer's recommendations.

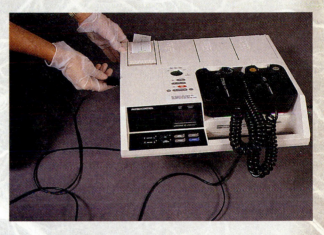

2-3e Connect the electrodes.

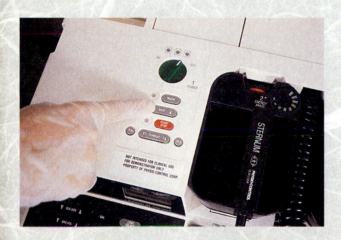

2-3f Select the desired pacing rate and current.

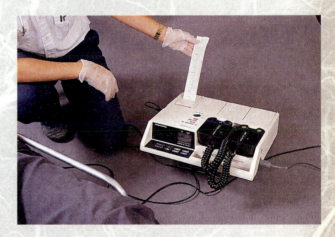

2-3g Monitor the patient's response to treatment.

CAROTID SINUS MASSAGE

Carotid sinus massage can convert paroxysmal supraventricular tachycardia into sinus rhythm by stimulating the baroreceptors in the carotid bodies. This increases vagal tone and decreases heart rate.

To perform carotid sinus massage, have atropine sulfate readily available and use the following technique (Procedure 2-4):

1. Initiate IV, oxygen, and ECG monitoring.
2. Position patient on his back, slightly hyperextending the head.
3. Gently palpate each carotid pulse separately. Auscultate each side for carotid bruits. Do not attempt carotid sinus massage if the pulse is diminished or if carotid bruits are present.
4. Tilt the patient's head to either side. Place your index and middle fingers over one artery, below the angle of the jaw and as high up on the neck as possible.
5. Firmly massage the artery by pressing it against the vertebral body and rubbing.
6. Monitor the ECG and obtain a continuous readout. Terminate massage at the first sign of slowing or heart block.
7. Maintain pressure no longer than 15–20 seconds.
8. If the massage is ineffective, you may repeat it, preferably on the other side of the patient's neck.

Complications of carotid sinus massage include dysrhythmias such as asystole, PVCs, ventricular tachycardia, or fibrillation. In addition, this procedure can interfere with cerebral circulation, causing syncope, seizure, or stroke. Increased parasympathetic tone can cause bradycardias, nausea, or vomiting.

SUPPORT AND COMMUNICATION

As with other emergencies, appropriate support and communication are an integral part of the treatment you provide for your cardiovascular patient. Time permitting, explain your treatment to the patient and his family and offer emotional support as indicated. When rapid transport is necessary, explain why. If the patient refuses transport, you will need to clearly explain the potential consequences, and use every available means to convince him of his need for appropriate treatment. As you transfer care of your patient to the receiving facility staff, you must clearly explain your findings to the receiving nurse or physician in a formal verbal briefing. This briefing should include the patient's vital information, chief complaint and history, physical exam findings, and any treatments rendered. In cardiovascular emergencies, any ECG findings will be especially important to the receiving staff.

MANAGING SPECIFIC CARDIOVASCULAR EMERGENCIES

The following section details the pathophysiology of common cardiovascular emergencies. Each section covers epidemiology, morbidity and mortality, assessment, and management.

ANGINA PECTORIS

Angina pectoris literally means "pain in the chest." This condition, however, is much more complicated than simple pain. Angina occurs when the heart's blood supply is transiently exceeded by myocardial oxygen demands. In other words, during periods of increased oxygen demand, the coronary arteries cannot deliver an adequate amount of blood to the myocardium. This can cause ischemia of the myocardium and chest pain.

As a rule, the reduced blood flow through the coronary arteries results from atherosclerosis. Atherosclerotic plaques can develop throughout the coronary circulation. Some patients may have atherosclerotic lesions that are isolated to one vessel, while others will have diffuse disease involving several vessels. Fixed blockages in the coronary arteries decrease blood flow. Remember that blood flow through a vessel is related to its diameter. Reducing the diameter of a vessel by one-half, as can occur in atherosclerosis, drastically reduces the amount of blood that the vessel can transport.

In addition to atherosclerosis, angina can result from abnormal spasm of the coronary arteries. This disorder, commonly called **Prinzmetal's angina,** *vasospastic angina,* or *atypical angina,* can also lead to inadequate blood flow, causing pain. Approximately two-thirds of the people who have vasospastic angina also have atherosclerotic coronary artery disease. Spasm of the vessel on top of atherosclerotic blockage can cause ischemia. However, one-third of patients with vasospastic angina will have little or no coronary atherosclerosis.

Angina is generally classified as stable or unstable. *Stable angina* occurs during activity, when the heart's oxygen demands are increased. Attacks of stable angina are usually precipitated by physical or emotional stress. They are relatively brief and often respond readily to treatment. *Unstable angina,* on the other hand, occurs at rest and may not respond as readily to treatment. Because unstable angina often indicates severe atherosclerotic disease, it is also called preinfarction angina. Unstable angina usually indicates that the patient's disease process is worsening.

Angina is not a self-limiting disease. It results from underlying coronary artery disease. If it is untreated and its contributing factors are unchanged, the underlying problem remains even though the pain has resolved. Because of the nature of the episodes, angina is usually progressive (that is, it accelerates in frequency and duration). Myocardial infarction may follow a single episode of angina.

It is important to remember that there are other causes of chest pain. While cardiac ischemia is one of its major causes, chest pain can arise from problems

---

* **angina pectoris** chest pain that results when blood supply's oxygen demands exceed the heart's.

* **Prinzmetal's angina** variant of angina pectoris caused by vasospasm of the coronary arteries, not blockage per se; also called *vasospastic angina* or *atypical angina.*

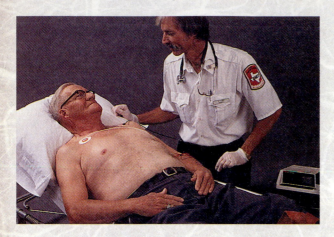

2-3a   Assess the patient.

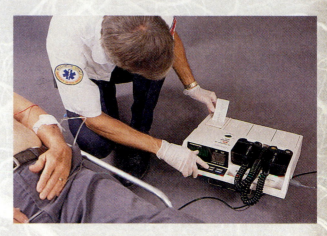

2-3b   Turn on the monitor.

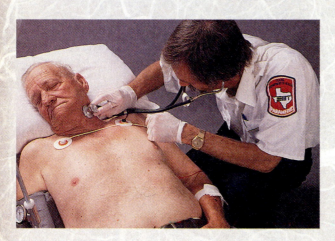

2-3c   Listen to both carotids for the presence of bruits.

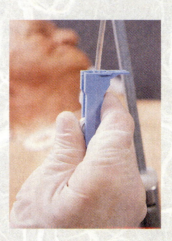

2-3d   Start an IV line.

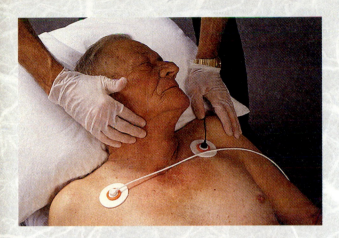

2-3e Rub either carotid. Wait.

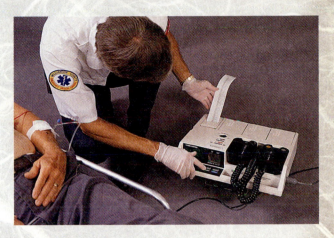

2-3f Check the rhythm.

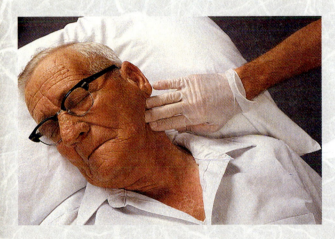

2-3g If unsuccessful, rub the other carotid.

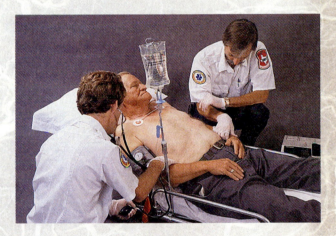

2-3h Reevalutate the patient.

in the cardiovascular system, the respiratory system, the gastrointestinal system, and the musculoskeletal system. Causes of chest pain include:

- Cardiovascular causes
  - Cardiac ischemia
  - Pericarditis (viral or autoimmune)
  - Thoracic dissection of the aorta
- Respiratory causes
  - Pulmonary embolism
  - Pneumothorax
  - Pneumonia
  - Pleural irritation (Pleurisy)
- Gastrointestinal causes
  - Cholecystitis
  - Pancreatitis
  - Hiatal hernia
  - Esophageal disease
  - Gastroesophageal reflux (GERD)
  - Peptic ulcer disease
  - Dyspepsia
- Musculoskeletal causes
  - Chest wall syndrome
  - Costochondritis
  - Acromioclavicular disease
  - Herpes zoster (shingles)
  - Chest wall trauma
  - Chest wall tumors

Diagnosing the cause of a patient's chest pain can be challenging in the hospital, let alone in the prehospital setting. As frequently occurs in emergency medicine, we look for the worst and hope for the best. Always be prepared to treat patients with chest pain as if they are suffering cardiac ischemia or another major disease process. Once you have excluded these possibilities you can consider less critical causes.

Field Assessment

When you assess an angina patient, remember that weak or absent peripheral pulses indicate potential or pending shock, which you should treat immediately. Changes in skin color such as paleness or cyanosis, or changes in temperature such as cold extremities also suggest shock.

The typical angina patient's chief complaint is a sudden onset of chest discomfort. The pain may radiate, or it may be localized to the chest. Often epigastric pain accompanies the chest pain. The patient with angina, however, often denies having chest pain, largely because he has dealt with this type of chest pain before. Although anginal episodes are common for the patient with a cardiac history, they should be considered significant when EMS is activated.

Angina usually lasts from three to five minutes, sometimes as long as fifteen minutes, and is relieved with rest and/or nitroglycerin. Atypical, or Prinzmetal, angina most often occurs at rest or without a precipitating cause. Prinzmetal angina is often accompanied by S-T segment elevation on the ECG, which can indicate myocardial tissue ischemia.

Labored breathing may or may not be present. After establishing the patency of the patient's airway, auscultate the lungs for congested breath sounds, particularly in the bases. Remember, however, the lungs may be clear. The anginal patient's heart rate and rhythm may be altered. Peripheral pulses should be equal. Typically, the blood pressure will elevate during the episode and normalize afterwards.

The contributing history may indicate that this is the patient's first recognized instance of angina, that it is a recurring event, or that the episodes are increasing in frequency or duration. A recurrence of angina or an increase in its frequency or duration is often the reason an anginal patient calls EMS. Any change in typical anginal pain is significant.

Without prolonging scene time, obtain an ECG tracing. If feasible, a 12-lead ECG is preferred for its additional diagnostic detail. After obtaining and interpreting the tracing, transmit it to the medical facility or medical direction. Typical 12-lead findings in the patient with angina are limited to patterns of ischemia: S-T depression and/or T-wave inversion. After relief of pain, the S-T depression and T-wave inversion generally will return to normal. This can take a few minutes or several hours. Occasionally the patterns may not return to normal.

Many 12-lead monitors have internal computerized pattern identification programs that will identify baseline, certain dysrhythmias, and anomalies that you might otherwise miss. These devices are most often accurate, but they do not always identify everything that may be pertinent. For example, patients experiencing Prinzmetal angina can have S-T segment elevation that dissipates after the pain has been relieved. Never trust the computer interpretation. Always overread the tracing for accuracy or telemeter it to the emergency department. The most common ECG finding in the angina patient is S-T segment depression. S-T segment changes often are not specific, however, and dysrhythmias and ectopy may not be present when the tracing is obtained.

Management

The patient experiencing angina is often apprehensive. Place him at rest in a position of physical and emotional comfort to decrease myocardial oxygen demand. Administer oxygen, generally at a high-flow rate, to increase oxygen delivery to the myocardium. Establish an IV either on scene without delaying transport or en route. If possible, and again without prolonging scene time, obtain and record a 12-lead or 3-lead ECG tracing. This is important because the ECG findings may be normal once the patient is pain free. Measure any S-T segment changes and communicate them to the receiving facility. Because a single anginal episode can be a precursor to a myocardial infarction, anticipate ECG changes such as dysrhythmias and S-T segment elevation.

Administer nitroglycerin sublingually, either as a tablet or a spray. It decreases myocardial work and, to a lesser degree, dilates coronary arteries. If the patient's symptoms persist after one or two doses of nitroglycerin, assume something more serious than angina, such as myocardial infarction. Nifedipine (Procardia), or another calcium channel blocker, is now being used, in addition to nitroglycerin, to manage angina. It is a vasodilator that works through blockade of the slow calcium channels. Consider morphine sulfate for chest pain that does not respond to nitrates or calcium channel blockers.

Patients with first episodes of angina or episodes that medication does not relieve are usually admitted to the hospital for evaluation. There is often a fine line between unstable angina and early myocardial infarction. Immediate transport is indicated if the patient does not feel relief after receiving oxygen and/or nitrates. The absence of relief indicates the patient's underlying disease process may be worsening. If the event is the beginning of a myocardial infarction, *reperfusion* (restoring blood flow to the ischemic tissue) is crucial. Hypotension can occur, especially if the patient has taken nitroglycerin. Its presence indicates transport, because it may lead to hypoperfusion of myocardial tissue. S-T segment changes, especially S-T segment elevation, indicate rapid transport. Transport should be efficient and fast but without lights and sirens unless clinically indicated. The lights and sirens could make the patient apprehensive and increase his pain.

Sometimes, the patient experiencing anginal chest pain will call EMS and then refuse transport after his chest pain is relieved. This may be due to a number of reasons, from denial to the patient's having taken older nitrates, which take longer to work. In any case, strongly encourage immediate evaluation because of the potential serious complications such as MI. Document patient refusal and be sure the patient signs the refusal and understands the potential risks. Encourage the patient to see his cardiologist or private care physician as soon as possible for follow-up.

Explain to the patient and family the reason and necessity for rapid transport, if indicated. Time permitting, also explain your treatment. Upon arrival at the emergency department, inform the physician of your findings—past history, vital signs, labored breathing, relief of pain, no relief of pain, and ECG findings, especially S-T segment findings.

MYOCARDIAL INFARCTION

✱ myocardial infarction (MI) death and subsequent necrosis of the heart muscle caused by inadequate blood supply; also *acute myocardial infarction (AMI)*.

Myocardial infarction (MI) is the death of a portion of the heart muscle from prolonged deprivation of oxygenated arterial blood. MI can also occur when the heart's oxygen demand exceeds its supply over an extended time. Myocardial infarction is most often associated with *atherosclerotic heart disease (ASHD)*. The precipitating event is commonly the formation of a *thrombus,* or blood clot, in a coronary artery already diseased from atherosclerosis. Atherosclerosis places many anginal patients at high risk for a myocardial infarction, especially those suffering from persistent or unstable angina. Myocardial infarction can also result from coronary artery spasm, microemboli (as seen with the recreational use of cocaine), acute volume overload, hypotension (from any cause), or from acute respiratory failure (acute hypoxia). Trauma can also cause myocardial infarction.

The location and size of the infarction depend on the vessel involved and the site of the obstruction (Figure 2-66.) Most infarctions involve the left ventricle. Obstruction of the left coronary artery may result in anterior, lateral, or septal infarcts. Right coronary artery occlusions usually result in infarctions of the inferior wall, posterior wall, or the right ventricle. The actual infarction is often classified as either transmural or subendocardial. In a **transmural infarction,** the entire thickness of the myocardium is destroyed. This lesion is associated with Q-wave changes on the ECG and is occasionally called a pathological Q-wave infarction. **A subendocardial infarction** involves only the subendocardial layer. Because ECG Q-wave changes usually do not accompany this type of infarction, it is often called a *non-Q wave infarction.*

✱ transmural infarction myocardial infarction that affects the full thickness of the myocardium and almost always results in a pathological Q wave in the affected leads.

✱ subendocardial infarction myocardial infarction that affects only the deeper levels of the myocardium; also called non-Q-wave infarction because it typically does not result in a significant Q wave in the affected lead.

Myocardial infarction causes varying degrees of tissue damage. First, following occlusion of the coronary artery, the affected tissue develops ischemia. If the blockage is not relieved and collateral circulation is inadequate, the tissue will infarct and die. In trauma, the usual cause of occlusion is plaque that has broken loose. The infarcted tissue becomes necrotic and eventually forms scar tissue. A ring of ischemic tissue that surrounds the area of infarcted myocardium survives primarily because of collateral circulation. This ischemic area is the site of many dysrhythmias' origins. Cardiogenic shock can develop, typically appearing first as ischemia on the 12-lead ECG (S-T depression or T-wave inversion), followed by injury (S-T elevation), and finally infarction (sometimes a pathological Q wave).

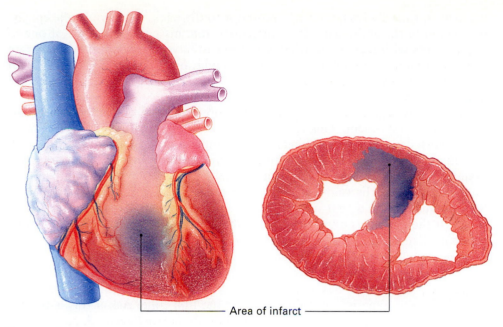

— Area of infarct —

FIGURE 2–66   Myocardial infarction.

Dysrhythmias are the most common complications of myocardial infarction. They are also the most common direct cause of death resulting from myocardial infarction. Life-threatening dysrhythmias can occur almost immediately and can result in sudden death or death within one hour after the onset of symptoms. Ventricular fibrillation or ventricular tachycardia may present early with myocardial infarction.

In addition to dysrhythmias, the destruction of a portion of the myocardial muscle mass can cause congestive heart failure. Such patients may have right heart failure, left heart failure, or both. *Heart failure* exists if the heart's pumping ability is impaired but the heart can still meet the demands of the body. That is, the heart is inefficient but adequate. If the heart cannot meet the body's oxygen demands, *inadequate tissue perfusion* results in cardiogenic shock. In cardiogenic shock, the heart is both inefficient and inadequate. Another cause of death from MI is *ventricular aneurysm* of the myocardial wall. The damaged portion of the wall weakens and in some cases bursts, resulting in sudden death. *Pump failure* resulting from extensive myocardial damage can also result in death.

The primary strategies in managing a myocardial infarction are pain relief and reperfusion. For reperfusion to be effective, rapid and safe transport is paramount. Maximum efficiency on scene and in transit is the most important care you can provide for the patient suffering an MI.

Anticipate life-threatening dysrhythmias while caring for any patient you suspect to be having a myocardial infarction.

Field Assessment

The patient's breathing may or may not be labored. Look for evidence of shock. Check for regularity of the peripheral pulses, which should be equal in the patient experiencing cardiac ischemia. Take the blood pressure; it usually elevates during the episode and normalizes afterwards.

The chief complaint in MI is chest pain. Use the OPQRST mnemonic to determine specifics about the chest pain. Typically, the onset of the chest pain is acute, severe, constant, and unrelenting. Unlike the angina patient, the MI patient's discomfort usually lasts longer than 30 minutes. The pain can radiate to the arms (primarily left), the neck, posterior to the back, or down to the epigastric region of the abdomen. Have the patient rate his pain on a scale of one to ten. Patients with true myocardial ischemia can have severe pain and may rate their chest pain with high numbers such as eight, nine, ten, or above ten. Often they will confirm an acute onset of nausea and vomiting. Neither nitroglycerin nor rest offers much pain relief.

Atypically, a patient may have mild symptoms or minimize his symptoms during your assessment. This is more common in diabetics. The patient can be vague when describing chest pain and may complain of generally not feeling well. You might easily mistake this for angina. This patient generally does not complain of vomiting and may or may not have nausea. He also will rate his pain low on a scale of ten. His vague, general descriptions may arise from many pathological causes. One is that myocardial infarctions generally evolve over 48–72 hours. If the patient is more than 24 hours into the infarction, the pain can be different than it was 12–24 hours after onset.

The patient experiencing chest pains tends to be very frightened, although this is not always the case. "A feeling of impending doom" describes the patient's fright and pain. This pain is so severe and intense that the patient fears death, especially if he is experiencing chest pain for the first time. Ask if this is the patient's first recognized episode of chest pain or a recurring event. A patient who has suffered infarction before or who has chronic angina may be less concerned with his current pain. If it is recurring, are the episodes increasing in frequency or duration? These patients often have angina-like pain with increasing frequency and/or duration. Denial is common among both the patient with a significant cardiac history and the first-time chest-pain sufferer.

After establishing the patient's airway, auscultate lung sounds. They may present clear or with congestion in the bases. The patient suffering a myocardial infarction usually presents with pallor and diaphoresis. Temperature may vary from the norm. Cold skin or extremities indicate shock. Check the heart rate and rhythm, which may be irregular, and check the peripheral pulses for equality, which MI usually does not affect. The patient's blood pressure may be elevated, normal, or lower than normal.

Apply the ECG. First examine the underlying rhythm and potential dysrhythmias. If you are using a 12-lead monitor, examine the S-T segment and Q waves. Check the S-T segment for height, depth, and overall contour. Note changes such as S-T depression, which suggests ischemia or reciprocal changes, or elevation, which suggests injury. A *pathological Q wave*—deeper than 5 mm or wider than 0.04 seconds—can indicate infarcted tissue (necrosis) or extensive transient ischemia.

Cardiac dysrhythmias are the greatest threat to the patient before he arrives at the emergency department. Of the many potential dysrhythmias, the most serious are asystole (confirmed in two leads), pulseless electrical activity (PEA), ventricular fibrillation, and ventricular tachycardia. Other dysrhythmias include narrow or wide-complex tachycardia, heart block, sinus bradycardia, and sinus tachycardia with or without ectopy. Remember, life-threatening dysrhythmias are the leading cause of death among myocardial infarction patients. Anticipate such dysrhythmias while caring for any patient you suspect to be having a myocardial infarction.

After reviewing the patient's ECG tracing, determine if he is a likely candidate for rapid transport and reperfusion. Reperfusion uses thrombolytics such as streptokinase or tPA (Activase) to stop further injury. Used properly, thrombolytics can reperfuse all ischemic tissue and much of the injured myocardial tissue, thus reducing the total damage of a myocardial infarction. They work by destroying blood clots—all clots—which, when lodged in arteries congested with plaque, are the most common cause of acute myocardial infarction. The window of time in which a thrombolytic can be given and be effective is generally considered to be six hours from the onset of symptoms. Occasionally the window will be expanded for a particularly young patient or one who is suffering serious complications. The complications associated with giving thrombolytics include hemorrhage (which can be fatal), allergic reactions, and reperfusion dysrhythmias. Unfortunately, not all myocardial infarctions are caused by blood clots. In addition, many patients have conditions that preclude them from receiving thrombolytics. These include bleeding or clotting disorders, possible blood in the stool, uncontrolled hypertension, recent trauma, recent hemorrhagic stroke, or recent surgery.

Signs of acute injury or pathological Q waves indicate rapid transport for reperfusion, if symptoms began within six hours. Ascertain as near as possible the exact time when the symptoms started, the locations of the ischemia and of the infarction if evidenced on the 12-lead, and any S-T segment changes occurring on the 12-lead. This will help the physician determine quickly if the patient is a candidate for reperfusion. If you are not certain the patient meets local criteria for thrombolytic therapy, assume he does.

After analyzing the patient's rhythm, prepare him for transport. Since reperfusion is the ultimate goal, time is of the utmost importance. Expediently treat any signs of acute ischemia, injury, or infarction. Carefully weigh treating the patient's pain while on scene against rapid transport. Whenever practical treat the patient suffering from a myocardial infarction in transit.

Many EMS systems have a checklist similar to those that emergency departments use to determine if a patient qualifies for thrombolytic therapy. While these checklists vary from area to area, their use has reduced the waiting time for patients who meet the clinical criteria for thrombolytic therapy. Standard information that should be relayed to the emergency department physician or staff includes the time of the pain's onset, S-T segment elevation, and the location of ischemia and infarction on a 12-lead.

If you are not certain the patient meets local criteria for thrombolytic therapy, assume he does.

Whenever practical treat the patient suffering from a myocardial infarction in transit.

Management

Prehospital Management of MI Treatment of the myocardial infarction patient is summarized in Figure 2-67. Keep in mind that the patient experiencing myocardial infarction is often apprehensive. Place him at rest in a position of physical and emotional comfort to decrease myocardial oxygen demand. Administer oxygen, generally at a high-flow rate, to increase oxygen delivery to the myocardium. Establish at least one IV, taking great care not to miss the vein or to have multiple misses, which could jeopardize a patient's chance of receiving thrombolytics.

Administer medications according to written protocols or upon order of medical direction. Remember, always ask the patient if he or she is allergic to any medication before giving any drug. Medications that might be indicated for the patient suspected of myocardial infarction include:

- Aspirin
- Morphine sulfate
- Promethazine (Phenergan)
- Nitroglycerin
- Nitrous oxide (Nitronox)
- Nalbuphine (Nubain)
- Atropine sulfate
- Lidocaine
- Procainamide
- Bretylium
- Adenosine

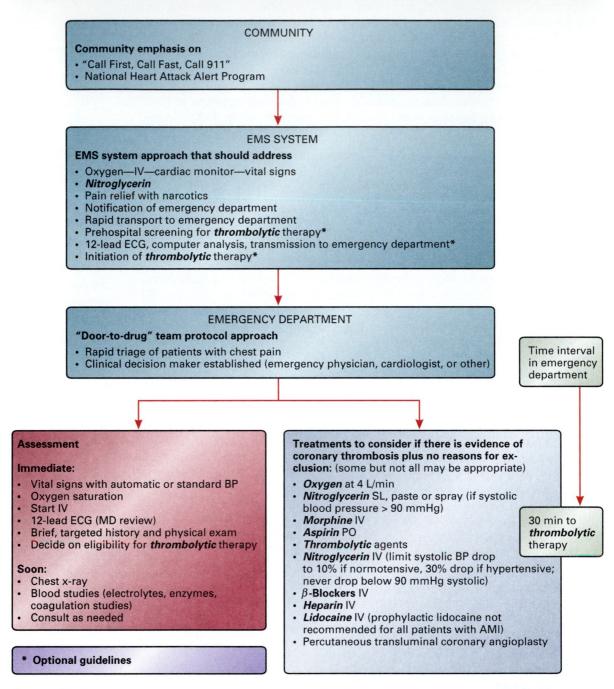

ALGORITHM: ACUTE MYOCARDIAL INFARCTION

COMMUNITY

Community emphasis on
- "Call First, Call Fast, Call 911"
- National Heart Attack Alert Program

EMS SYSTEM

EMS system approach that should address
- Oxygen—IV—cardiac monitor—vital signs
- *Nitroglycerin*
- Pain relief with narcotics
- Notification of emergency department
- Rapid transport to emergency department
- Prehospital screening for *thrombolytic* therapy*
- 12-lead ECG, computer analysis, transmission to emergency department*
- Initiation of *thrombolytic* therapy*

EMERGENCY DEPARTMENT

"Door-to-drug" team protocol approach
- Rapid triage of patients with chest pain
- Clinical decision maker established (emergency physician, cardiologist, or other)

Time interval in emergency department

Assessment

Immediate:
- Vital signs with automatic or standard BP
- Oxygen saturation
- Start IV
- 12-lead ECG (MD review)
- Brief, targeted history and physical exam
- Decide on eligibility for *thrombolytic* therapy

Soon:
- Chest x-ray
- Blood studies (electrolytes, enzymes, coagulation studies)
- Consult as needed

Treatments to consider if there is evidence of coronary thrombosis plus no reasons for exclusion: (some but not all may be appropriate)
- *Oxygen* at 4 L/min
- *Nitroglycerin* SL, paste or spray (if systolic blood pressure > 90 mmHg)
- *Morphine* IV
- *Aspirin* PO
- *Thrombolytic* agents
- *Nitroglycerin* IV (limit systolic BP drop to 10% if normotensive, 30% drop if hypertensive; never drop below 90 mmHg systolic)
- *β-Blockers* IV
- *Heparin* IV
- *Lidocaine* IV (prophylactic lidocaine not recommended for all patients with AMI)
- Percutaneous transluminal coronary angioplasty

30 min to *thrombolytic* therapy

* Optional guidelines

FIGURE 2–67   Management of myocardial infarction (MI). Adapted with permission. Journal of the American Medical Association, October 28, 1992, Volume 268, No. 16, *Guidelines for Cardiopulmonary Resuscitation and Emergency Cardiac Care,* p. 2230. ©1992 American Medical Association.

Monitor the ECG constantly. Life-threatening dysrhythmias are possible. The patient may need rapid defibrillation or synchronized cardioversion at any moment. Plan to quickly provide defibrillation, cardioconversion, or transcutaneous pacing if needed.

Transport the patient you suspect of a myocardial infarction without delay. Since most myocardial infarction patients are very apprehensive and frightened, you should transport the normotensive patient without lights and sirens. Rapid transport is indicated if the S-T segment has any changes such as depression or elevation or if pathological Q waves present on the 12-lead. If a patient exhibits S-T or Q wave anomalies, has had signs and symptoms less than three hours, or has no relief from medications, consider him a candidate for thrombolytic reperfusion. Hypotension indicates immediate transport, especially if the patient has taken nitroglycerin, because the potential hypoperfusion of myocardial tissue can compound the problem. Other factors that indicate rapid transport are any rhythm abnormalities and the presentation within six hours of the pain's onset.

If the patient is in the early stages of a myocardial infarction, the outcome of refusing transport is likely to be devastating, ranging from extensive, unnecessary myocardial damage to death. Avoid refusal at all cost, using every means at your disposal to convince the patient to be transported. If the patient still refuses, document the fact that the patient was repeatedly warned of the possible outcome and was also aware of the potential for severely decreased lifestyle or death. Have the patient sign to the fact that he understands the implications, and if at all possible, have a witness sign as well.

Explain to the patient and his family the reason and necessity for rapid transport, if indicated, and inform them of your treatment, time permitting. Upon arrival at the emergency department, inform the physician of your findings—past history, vital signs, labored breathing, relief of pain, no relief of pain, and ECG readings, especially S-T segment results.

In-Hospital Management of MI Your understanding of the management of the MI patient after you have delivered him to the emergency department is important. This is especially true if you belong to an EMS system whose paramedics also regularly staff emergency departments.

With the advent of thrombolytic therapy, many hospitals have opened specially designed chest-pain units. These facilities specialize in diagnosing and observing patients with chest pain. In addition to 12-lead ECGs, obtaining cardiac enzyme levels in chest pain patients is routine. Because dead or dying myocardial cells release cardiac enzymes, elevated levels of these enzymes indicate myocardial infarction. The enzyme levels do not increase, however, until the infarction is several hours old, so intervention ideally should occur before the enzymes have a chance to rise. Commonly assayed cardiac enzymes are lactate dehydrogenase (LDH) and creatine phosphokinase (CK). Several newer markers show promise in aiding earlier identification of myocardial injury. These include troponin (I, T, and C), myoglobin, and CK-MB (a type of CK specific for cardiac muscle).

In many chest pain patients, the diagnosis will be readily evident. In many others, however, it will remain unclear. These patients are commonly stratified according to risk. Patients with a low likelihood of cardiac ischemia may be discharged with instructions for follow-up care, which may include diagnostic tools such as stress tests. Patients with a higher likelihood of having myocardial ischemia are usually admitted to the hospital and are typically observed for 24 hours. During the patient's hospitalization, his cardiac enzyme levels are obtained several times, as is his ECG. If the tests all remain negative, the patient will usually see a cardiologist and have a stress test before going home. If the stress test is negative, the cardiologist will work up the problem as an outpatient. If the stress test is positive, additional testing is done prior to discharge. This testing includes nuclear medicine cardiac imaging (Cardiolyte) and, possibly, coronary angiography. Usually, cardiology immediately sees patients who have a high likelihood of cardiac ischemia but nondiagnostic ECGs and enzymes. These patients ordinarily are not observed but are taken directly to the cardiac lab for an angiogram.

Several treatment options are available. Patients with isolated coronary artery lesions may be candidates for percutaneous transluminal coronary angioplasty (PTCA). In these patients, lesions are identified during coronary angiography. A

The trend in emergency cardiac care is rapid cardiac catheterization and therapeutic intervention such as PTCA.

balloon catheter is then inserted into the coronary artery with the lesion. At the level of the lesion, the balloon is inflated, thus increasing the artery's diameter and reducing the relative size of the blockage. Often, the patient will have several lesions. If the arteries do not stay open following angioplasty, another alternative is to place a *stent* in the artery at the site of the lesion. The stent is a hollow tube that keeps the artery open. Patients with severe and diffuse coronary artery disease may not be candidates for angioplasty. The best option for these patients is surgical revascularization of their coronary arteries. The most common operation is the coronary artery bypass graft (CABG), in which grafts are sewn from the aorta to the coronary arteries, thus effectively bypassing the blockage. In younger patients, the surgeon may use the internal mammary artery as the source. Recently, technology has evolved to the point where some bypass grafts can be performed endoscopically. These require only small "keyhole" incisions instead of the classic sternotomy, thus markedly decreasing the pain and the recovery time. Patients whose disease is either too mild or too severe may not be candidates for surgery. These patients are managed with medication alone.

HEART FAILURE

* **heart failure** clinical syndrome in which the heart's mechanical performance is compromised so that cardiac output cannot meet the body's needs.

Heart failure is a clinical syndrome in which the heart's mechanical performance is compromised so that cardiac output cannot meet the body's needs. Heart failure is generally divided into left ventricle or right ventricle failure. Its many etiologies include valvular, coronary, or myocardial disease. Dysrhythmias can also cause or aggravate heart failure. Many other factors can contribute to heart failure, such as excess fluid or salt intake, fever (sepsis), hypertension, pulmonary embolism, or excessive alcohol or drug use. It can manifest with exertion in the patient who has an underlying disease or as a progression of the underlying disease.

Left Ventricular Failure Left ventricular failure occurs when the left ventricle fails as an effective forward pump, causing back pressure of blood into the pulmonary circulation, which often results in pulmonary edema (Figure 2-68). Its causes include various types of heart disease such as MI, valvular disease, chronic hypertension, and dysrhythmias. In left ventricular failure, the left ventricle cannot eject all of the blood that the right heart delivers to it via the lungs. Left atrial pressure rises and is subsequently transmitted to the pulmonary veins and capillaries. When pulmonary capillary pressure becomes too high, it forces the blood plasma into the alveoli, resulting in pulmonary edema. Progressive fluid accumulation in the alveoli decreases the lungs' oxygenation capacity and can cause death from hypoxia. Since MI is a common cause of left ventricular failure, you should consider that all patients with pulmonary edema may have had an MI.

Right Ventricular Failure In right ventricular failure, the right ventricle fails as an effective forward pump, resulting in back pressure of blood into the systemic venous circulation and venous congestion (Figure 2-69). The most common cause of right ventricular failure is left ventricular failure. This is because myocardial infarction is more common in the left ventricle than in the right and because chronic hypertension affects the left ventricle more adversely than the right. Right ventricular failure's other causes include systemic hypertension, which can affect both sides of the heart and can cause pure right ventricular failure. Pulmonary hypertension and *cor pulmonale* (heart failure due to pulmonary disease) result from the effects of chronic obstructive pulmonary disease (COPD). These problems are related to increased pressure in the pulmonary arteries, which results in right ventricular enlargement, right atrial enlargement, and if untreated, right heart failure.

* **pulmonary embolism (PE)** blood clot in one of the pulmonary arteries.

Pulmonary embolism (PE), a blood clot in one of the pulmonary arteries, also can cause right heart failure. If the clot is large enough to occlude a major vessel, the pressure against which the right ventricle must pump increases. This can throw the right ventricle into failure in much the same manner as pulmonary

LEFT HEART FAILURE

Signs
- Cyanosis
- Tachycardia
- Noisy Labored breathing
- Rales
- Coughing
- Blood-tinged sputum
- Gallop rhythm of the heart

Symptom
- Dyspnea

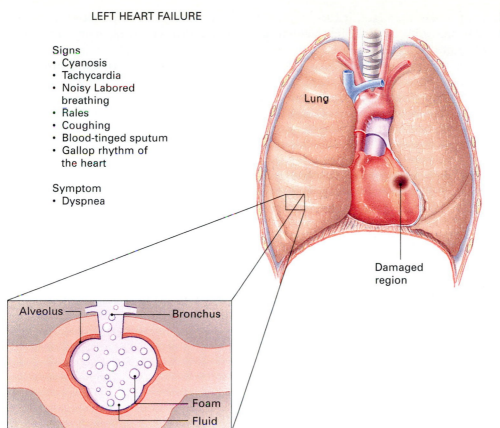

FIGURE 2–68 Left heart failure.

Lung

Damaged region

Alveolus

Bronchus

Foam

Fluid

RIGHT HEART FAILURE

Signs
- Tachycardia

- Neck veins engorging and pulsating

- Edema of body and lower extremities

- Engorged liver and spleen

- Abdominal distention (ascites)

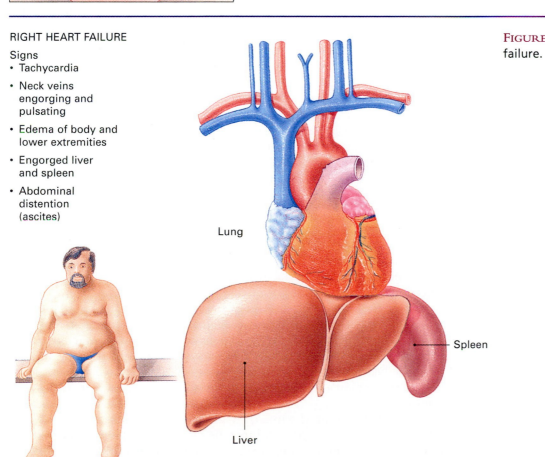

FIGURE 2–69 Right heart failure.

Lung

Spleen

Liver

hypertension. In fact, it can be considered an acute form of pulmonary hypertension. Infarct of the right atrium or ventricle, although rare, is another cause of right ventricular failure.

Starling's law of the heart enables heart failure patients to compensate, at least for a time. As you will recall from earlier in this chapter, Starling's law states that the more the myocardial muscle is stretched, the greater will be its force of contraction. Thus, the greater the preload (the volume of blood filling the chamber), the farther the myocardial muscle stretches and the more forceful the cardiac contraction. This has its limits, however. If myocardial muscle is stretched too far, it will not contract properly and the contraction will be weaker. Afterload (the resistance against which the ventricle must contract) also affects stroke volume. An increase in peripheral vascular resistance will decrease stroke volume. The reverse is also true: stroke volume will increase as peripheral vascular resistance decreases.

Congestive Heart Failure In **congestive heart failure (CHF)**, the heart's reduced stroke volume causes an overload of fluid in the body's other tissues. This presents as edema, which can be pulmonary, peripheral, sacral, or ascites (peritoneal edema). Congestive heart failure can manifest in an acute setting as pulmonary edema, pulmonary hypertension, or myocardial infarction. In the chronic setting, it can manifest as cardiomegaly (enlargement of the heart), left ventricular failure, or right ventricular failure. Heart failure can present in a first-time event, as in myocardial infarction, or in multiple events, as in left heart failure. CHF is one of the few diseases still on the rise in America. Approximately 400,000 new cases are diagnosed each year. CHF also is the most common cause of hospitalization in patients over age 65, accounting for approximately 900,000 admissions each year. Mortality is only 5 years in 50 percent of CHF patients. The end stage of this disease involves pulmonary edema and respiratory failure, followed by death. When the CHF patient calls EMS, one thing is clear; Starling's law is no longer allowing the patient to compensate.

Field Assessment

As in all cardiac emergencies, begin your assessment by checking the ABCs and managing any life threats. Often, patients with pulmonary edema will cough up large quantities of clear or pink tinged sputum. Patients with profound pulmonary edema generally have labored breathing, although this may not present until the patient begins to exert himself simply by standing or walking a few steps. Look for any changes or differences in skin color on the patient's arms, face, chest, and back. In profound CHF, mottling is often present.

Focus on the patient's chief complaint. Use the OPQRST mnemonic to elicit the patient's description of symptoms. Patients with pulmonary edema will complain of progressive or acute shortness of breath and will confirm being awakened by shortness of breath (**paroxysmal nocturnal dyspnea, or PND**). If the patient's episodes of PND are becoming more frequent, the disease process usually is worsening.

Often the heart failure patient will confirm progressive accumulation of edema or weight gain over a short time. Because many heart failure patients have an underlying cardiac or prior MI history, they may complain of mild chest pain or generalized weakness. This may be due to a weakened myocardial muscle mass, myocardial ischemia, or current MI.

Determine the patient's current medications. CHF patients are generally prescribed a loop diuretic such as Lasix or Bumex and/or hypertension medication. Many are prescribed digoxin (Lanoxin), which increases the heart's contractile force; many are oxygen dependent and may be on home oxygen. Find out if the patient has been compliant in taking medications; if not, determine how long he has been off medications. Also record and report any over-the-counter medications or herbal medications that the patient is taking, as well as any prescription medications borrowed from someone else.

Unconsciousness or an altered level of consciousness indicates pending respiratory failure. If the patient shows any sign of respiratory failure, immediately assist his breathing with 100 percent oxygen by BVM and prepare to intubate if clinically warranted.

Next assess the patient's breathing. Often, labored breathing, dyspnea, and productive cough appear. Labored breathing is the most common symptom of CHF, and it generally worsens with activity. CHF patients frequently assume the tripod position, sitting upright with both arms supporting the upper body, and confirm PND and pillow orthopnea, the inability to recline in bed without a pillow). Ask the patient how many pillows he sleeps on at night. As a rule, the more pillows, the worse the problem.

Labored breathing is the most common symptom of CHF.

Check the skin. CHF patients present with changes in the skin color, such as pallor, diaphoresis, mottling, or signs of cyanosis. Check the peripheral pulses for quality and rhythm. Also check for edema. Edema is usually found in the lower extremities, localized from the ankles to the mid-calf or the knees. Sometimes the edema will be so severe that it obliterates the distal pulses. Check the edematous area for pitting and record its severity on a scale from 0 to 4+. Edema may also be present in the sacral area of the back, especially in the bed-confined, or in the upper quadrants of abdominal cavity. Ascites (abdominal cavity edema or swelling) is very difficult to assess accurately without X-ray or ultrasound. Blood pressure may be elevated in the CHF patient, due to the body's attempt to compensate for decreased cardiac output, but this can change quickly. A decompensating patient can have a normal blood pressure that drops quickly.

The most serious complication of heart failure is pulmonary edema. Untreated pulmonary edema can quickly lead to respiratory failure. This is because the abundant serum fluid in a large portion of the alveoli inhibits oxygen exchange in the lungs and hypoxia ensues. Respiratory failure will quickly lead to death. Patients with severe pulmonary edema present with tachypnea and adventitious lung sounds. Pulmonary edema can present as crackles (rales) at both bases. Rhonchi, which indicates fluid in the larger airways of the lungs, is a sign of severe pulmonary edema. Wheezes in the CHF patient are a sign of the lungs' protective mechanisms, since bronchioles constrict in an attempt to keep additional fluid from entering the lungs. This wheezing in pulmonary edema and congestive heart failure is often called cardiac asthma. This term is confusing, however, and you should avoid using it. Consider wheezes in a geriatric patient to be pulmonary edema until proven otherwise.

Other complications of pulmonary edema are pulsus paradoxus and pulsus alternans. *Pulsus paradoxus* occurs when systolic blood pressure drops more than 10 mmHg with inspiration. This is due to compression of the great vessels or the ventricles. In *pulsus alternans,* the pulse alternates between weak and strong. Pulses may be thready or weak, and jugular vein distention (JVD) might be present. The apical pulse may be abnormal or difficult to auscultate because of abnormalities such as bulges in the heart, a displaced apex, or severe pulmonary edema. The patient may produce frothy sputum with coughing, and cyanosis may present in the late stages of CHF.

Management

In severe CHF with pulmonary edema, obtain pertinent medical history and complete the physical exam while initiating treatment. Reassess all life-threatening conditions and treat them accordingly. Do not have the patient exert himself in any way, including standing up or walking. Do not have the patient lie flat at any time. Seat him with his feet dangling. This will promote venous pooling, thus decreasing preload.

Administer high-flow oxygen. If necessary, provide positive-pressure assistance with either a demand valve if the patient can assist or a bag-valve-mask unit if he is unresponsive. When possible, establish an IV at a TKO rate. Consider placing a heparin lock or saline lock. Limiting fluids is imperative; use a minidrip set to avoid accidentally infusing excessive amounts of fluid.

Place ECG electrodes. If the patient is extremely diaphoretic, apply tincture of Benzoin first. Record a baseline ECG and keep the monitor in place throughout care.

Administer medications according to written protocols or on the order of the medical director. Some left ventricular failures result from very rapid dysrhythmias. If you suspect a dysrhythmia as a cause, treat it according to established protocols. Before giving the patient any drug, ask him or his family if he is allergic to any medication. Medications frequently used in left ventricular failure and pulmonary edema include:

- Morphine sulfate
- Nitroglycerin
- Furosemide (Lasix)
- Dopamine (Intropin)
- Dobutamine (Dobutrex)
- Promethazine (Phenergan)
- Nitrous oxide (Nitronox)

Transport the heart-failure patient as a nonemergency unless clinical conditions indicate otherwise. Conditions that indicate emergency transport include hypertension or hypotension, severe respiratory distress or pending respiratory failure, or life-threatening dysrhythmias. Remember that transporting with lights and sirens can increase the conscious patient's anxiety and worsen his condition. If nonemergency transport might compromise the patient's condition, use lights and siren. Place the patient in a position of comfort, but not lying flat.

If the patient refuses transport and is indeed in the early stages of CHF, the outcome is likely to be devastating, leading to worsening signs and symptoms, unnecessary myocardial damage, severe pulmonary edema, and even death. Avoid refusal at all costs, and use every means at your disposal to convince the patient to be transported. If he still refuses, document the fact that you repeatedly warned the patient of the possible outcome.

CARDIAC TAMPONADE

✱ **cardiac tamponade** accumulation of excess fluid inside the pericardium.

In **cardiac tamponade,** excess fluid accumulates inside the pericardium. (The normal amount of fluid between the visceral pericardium and the parietal pericardium is approximately 25 cc.) This excess fluid causes an increase in intrapericardial pressure that impairs diastolic filling and drastically decreases the amount of blood the ventricles can expel with each contraction. Chest pain or dyspnea is the chief complaint; depending on the underlying cause, the chest pain may be dull or sharp and severe.

Cardiac tamponade's onset may be gradual, as in pericarditis or as in a neoplasm such as benign or malignant cancer. Or it may be acute, as in MI or trauma. All forms of cardiac tamponade involve pericardial effusion of air, pus, serum, blood, or any combination of these four. Gradual onset usually results from an underlying condition, and overlooking or misdiagnosing the tamponade is easy. Renal disease and hypothyroidism can cause cardiac tamponade, though such instances are rare. Traumatic causes can include CPR and penetrating or nonpenetrating injuries. Whether onset is gradual or acute, cardiac tamponade can lead to death.

Field Assessment

Perform your initial assessment, including the patient's airway, breathing, and circulation. If you suspect cardiac tamponade, limit your history taking to determining the precipitating cause(s). Determine if the cause might be acute trauma such as penetrating or blunt trauma. Has the patient sustained recent trauma, including recent CPR? If you suspect a gradual onset, determine if the patient has recently had an infection or MI. Is he currently having an MI? Does he have a history of renal disease or hypothyroidism? Has he been ill? Use the OPQRST mnemonic to obtain information about the patient's symptoms.

Always consider the possibility of pericardial tamponade in a patient who received CPR, then later deteriorated.

The patient generally will present with dyspnea and orthopnea. Anterior and posterior lung sounds are usually clear. Typically, the pulse is rapid and weak. In the early stages venous pressures are often elevated, as evidenced by jugular vein distention. Blood pressure readings show a decrease in systolic pressure, pulsus paradoxus, and narrowing pulse pressures. Heart sounds are normal early on but then become muffled or faint.

Do not use the ECG, whether monitor quality or 12-lead, to diagnose cardiac tamponade; rather consider it a tool to support your clinical suspicions. The ECG is generally inconclusive, but ectopy is usually a late sign of cardiac tamponade. This is because an effusion easily irritates the heart's epicardial tissue. QRS and T-wave voltages are low, and non-specific T-wave changes occur. S-T segments may elevate. Electrical alternans (weak voltage, then normal) may appear in the P, QRS, T, and S-T segments.

Management

While obtaining any pertinent medical history and completing the physical exam, initiate treatment. Management of cardiac tamponade is primarily supportive, except when you detect shock or low perfusion. Maintain a patent airway and deliver high flow oxygen. If clinically indicated, secure the patient's airway with endotracheal intubation and maintain the patient's circulation with IV support, pharmacological agents, or CPR. Before administering any medication, ask the patient or family if he is allergic to any medications. Medications used in the treatment of cardiac tamponade include:

- Morphine sulfate
- Nitrous oxide (Nitronox)
- Furosemide (Lasix)
- Dopamine (Intropin)
- Dobutamine (Dobutrex)

Rapid transport is indicated for patients with cardiac tamponade. Remember to be supportive of the patient and family throughout your care. Upon arrival at the emergency department, inform the physician of your findings—past history, medications, vital signs, labored breathing, ECG readings, pulsus paradoxus, and shock. The therapy of choice is invasive *pericardiocentesis,* which involves aspirating fluid from the pericardium with a cardiac needle. Unless you have adequate training and local protocol permits you to do so, a physician should perform this procedure.

HYPERTENSIVE EMERGENCIES

* **hypertensive emergency** an acute elevation of blood pressure that requires the blood pressure to be lowered within one hour; characterized by end-organ changes such as hypertensive encephalopathy, renal failure, or blindness.

* **hypertensive encephalopathy** a cerebral disorder of hypertension indicated by severe headache, nausea, vomiting, and altered mental status. Neurological symptoms may include blindness, muscle twitches, inability to speak, weakness, and paralysis.

A **hypertensive emergency** is a life-threatening elevation of blood pressure. It occurs in one percent or less of patients with hypertension, usually when the hypertension is poorly controlled or untreated. A hypertensive emergency is characterized by a rapid increase in diastolic blood pressure (usually >130 mmHg) accompanied by restlessness, confusion, blurred vision, nausea, and vomiting. It often occurs with **hypertensive encephalopathy,** a condition of acute or subacute consequence of severe hypertension characterized by severe headache, vomiting, visual disturbances (including transient blindness), paralysis, seizures, stupor, and coma. On occasion, this condition may cause left ventricular failure, pulmonary edema, or stroke.

A prior history of hypertension is the precipitating cause of most hypertensive emergencies. In many cases, the patient has not complied with his hypertensive medication or other prescribed drugs. Another cause of hypertensive crisis, toxemia of pregnancy (preeclampsia), can appear at any time between the twentieth week of pregnancy and term delivery. It occurs in five percent of pregnancies and is defined as a blood pressure of at least 140/90 mmHg. Hypertension is a sign of the toxemia, not the cause. Preeclampsia poses a high risk of abruptio placentae and generally progresses to eclampsia (coma and seizures). Left untreated, it progresses to eclampsia and death for the mother and unborn fetus.

Experts estimate that more than 50 million people in the United States are hypertensive patients. Its prevalence increases with age, and it has a higher incidence among blacks, as well as a higher mortality and morbidity. With modern medications, hypertensive encephalopathy has become rare, yet it is still seen in the prehospital setting. Ischemic and hemorrhagic stroke are more common results of severe hypertension. Both hypertensive encephalopathy and stroke (ischemic or hemorrhagic) can have devastating consequences or lead to death if left untreated.

Field Assessment

After making your initial assessment, including airway, breathing, and circulation, conduct your focused history and physical examination. Generally, hypertensive patients have a chief complaint of headache, accompanied by nausea and/or vomiting, blurred vision, shortness of breath, epistaxis (nosebleed), and vertigo (dizziness). However any one of these symptoms might be the patient's only complaint. The patient may be semiconscious or unconscious or seizing. In pregnancy toxemia, the expectant mother usually has edema of the hands or face. Photosensitivity and headache are common complaints.

Determine if the patient has a history of hypertension and if he has been taking medications as prescribed. Often he has been noncompliant, taking medicines only occasionally or not at all. In some situations the patient will borrow someone else's medications or take over-the-counter medications such as herbal medications. He may be on home oxygen.

If left ventricular failure accompanies the hypertension, the lung sounds generally present with pulmonary edema; otherwise they are clear. Often the pulse is strong and at times may be bounding. By definition, hypertension is a systolic pressure greater than 160 mmHg and a diastolic pressure greater than 90 mmHg. Consider signs or symptoms of hypertensive encephalopathy associated with hypertension to be a hypertensive emergency.

The hypertensive patient's level of consciousness may be normal or altered, or he may be unconscious. His skin may be pale, flushed, or normal, cool or warm, moist or dry. Look for edema, either pitting or nonpitting. The patient may confirm PND, orthopnea, vertigo, epistaxis, tinnitus (ringing of the ears), nausea or vomiting, or visual acuities. In addition, he may have seizures or motor/sensory deficits in parts of the body or on one side. ECG findings are generally inconclusive unless the patient has an underlying cardiac condition such as angina or MI.

Management

Place the patient in a position of comfort, unless a potential exists for airway compromise, as in stroke. Provide airway and ventilatory support, if clinically indicated. Provide oxygen and base your transport considerations on the patient's clinical presentation. Attempt supportive IV therapy on-scene time or en route. Do not prolong on-scene time to establish an IV. Place pregnant patients on their left side and transport as smoothly and quietly as possible.

In recent years, calcium channel blockers such as nifedipine (Procardia) have been widely used to treat hypertensive emergencies. Now this practice is being questioned because evidence suggests that significantly reducing the patient's blood pressure may actually be harmful. Some systems still use loop diuretics such as Lasix or nitroglycerin to reduce the patient's blood pressure by manipulating preload and afterload. These treatments' effectiveness is also being scrutinized. Follow your local protocols. In severe cases, especially if hypertensive encephalopathy is present, medical direction may order one of the following medications:

Elevated blood pressures should only be treated in the prehospital setting if these are associated with end-organ changes.

- Morphine sulfate
- Furosemide (Lasix)
- Nitroglycerin
- Sodium Nitroprusside (Nipride)
- Labetalol (Trandate, Normodyne)

Explain to the patient and family the reason and necessity for rapid transport, if indicated. Advise the patient who refuses transport of the serious complications that are likely without further medical attention. Stroke, seizures, pulmonary edema, and kidney damage are but a few possible outcomes. Avoid refusal at all costs. As always, use every means at your disposal to convince the patient to be transported. Document refusals as usual.

Upon arrival at the emergency department, inform the physician of your findings—vital signs, history, labored breathing, pulmonary edema, hand or facial edema, and neurological deficits.

CARDIOGENIC SHOCK

Cardiogenic shock, the most severe form of pump failure, is shock that remains after existing dysrhythmias, hypovolemia, or altered vascular tone have been corrected. It occurs when left ventricular function is so compromised that the heart cannot meet the body's metabolic demands and the compensatory mechanisms are exhausted. This usually happens after extensive myocardial infarction, often involving more than 40 percent of the left ventricle, or with diffuse ischemia.

✱ **cardiogenic shock** the inability of the heart to meet the metabolic needs of the body, resulting in inadequate tissue perfusion.

A variety of mechanisms can cause cardiogenic shock, and its onset may be acute or progressive. Among the more common mechanical causes are tension pneumothorax and cardiac tamponade. Both affect ventricular filling, or preload, and tend to manifest acutely. Interference with ventricular emptying, or afterload, as in pulmonary embolism and prosthetic valve malfunction, can also cause cardiogenic shock. Impairments in myocardial contractility, as seen in MI, myocarditis, and recreational drug use, can manifest either progressively or acutely. Trauma, too, can cause cardiogenic shock, secondary to hypovolemia or to significant underlying disease processes such as neurologic, gastroenterologic, renal, or metabolic disorders.

Cardiogenic shock is the most severe form of pump failure.

In cardiogenic shock, the body tries to compensate either by increasing the contractile force, by improving preload, by reducing the peripheral resistance, or by all three. In the early stages, a conscious patient presents with obvious signs of shock (cold extremities, weak pulses, and low blood pressure). As Starling's law loses effect, the patient's mental status diminishes and his radial pulses are no longer palpable. Finally, when preload, afterload, and contractility fail to meet vital organ demands, unconsciousness occurs and, if left untreated, the patient will die.

Cardiogenic shock can occur at any age, but it is most often seen as an end-stage event in the geriatric patient, with significant underlying disease(s). Cardiogenic shock's mortality rate is high for geriatric patients following massive MI or septic shock. This is because end-organ damage is so severe or multiple end-organ damage reaches the point that life cannot be sustained.

Cardiogenic shock has a high mortality rate.

Field Assessment

After conducting your initial assessment, including airway, breathing, and circulation, perform your focused history and physical exam. The chief complaint may range from acute onset of chest pain to shortness of breath, altered mental status or unconsciousness, or general weakness; onset may be acute or progressive. Ask about the patient's past medical history and determine if he or she has had any recent trauma. Look for evidence of a hypovolemic cause such as a gastrointestinal bleed, septic shock, and traumatic or nontraumatic internal hemorrhage. Has the patient recently suffered a myocardial infarction? Cardiogenic shock is most often associated with large anterior infarction and/or loss of 40 percent or more of the left ventricle.

The patient's medication history may be important. Large amounts of different cardiac medications may indicate the patient has significant preexisting damage or a compromised but adequate cardiac output. Also, noncompliance with prescribed medications can further insult a preexisting weakened cardiac state, and the use of borrowed or over-the-counter medications can have unpredictable effects.

The altered mental status secondary to decreased cardiac output and unconsciousness common in cardiogenic shock may begin as restlessness and progress to confusion ending in coma. Airway findings include dyspnea, productive cough, or labored breathing. Paroxysmal nocturnal dyspnea, tripoding, adventitious lung sounds, and retractions on inspiration are also common findings. Typical ECG findings include tachycardia and atrial dysrhythmias such as atrial tachycardias. Ectopy is also common.

Myocardial infarction often precedes cardiogenic shock, and symptoms are initially the same as expected with MI; however, as cardiogenic shock develops and compensatory mechanisms fail, hypotension develops. The systolic blood pressure is often less than 80 mmHg. The usual heart rhythm is sinus tachycardia, a reflection of the cardiovascular system's attempts to compensate for the decreased stroke volume. If serious dysrhythmias are present, determining whether they are the cause of the hypotension or the result of the cardiogenic shock may be difficult; therefore, you must correct any major dysrhythmias.

The patient's skin is usually cool and clammy, reflecting peripheral vasoconstriction. Tachypnea is often present, since pulmonary edema is a common complication. Pitting or nonpitting peripheral edema may be present in the lower extremities or in the sacral area and may obliterate peripheral pulses.

Management

To manage the cardiogenic shock patient, place him in a position of comfort if he is hemodynamically stable. If any pulmonary edema is present, the patient may prefer sitting upright, with both legs hanging off the stretcher. Treatment of cardiogenic shock (Figure 2-70) consists mostly of treating the underlying problem (such as MI and CHF) or treating the patient supportively. Remember to

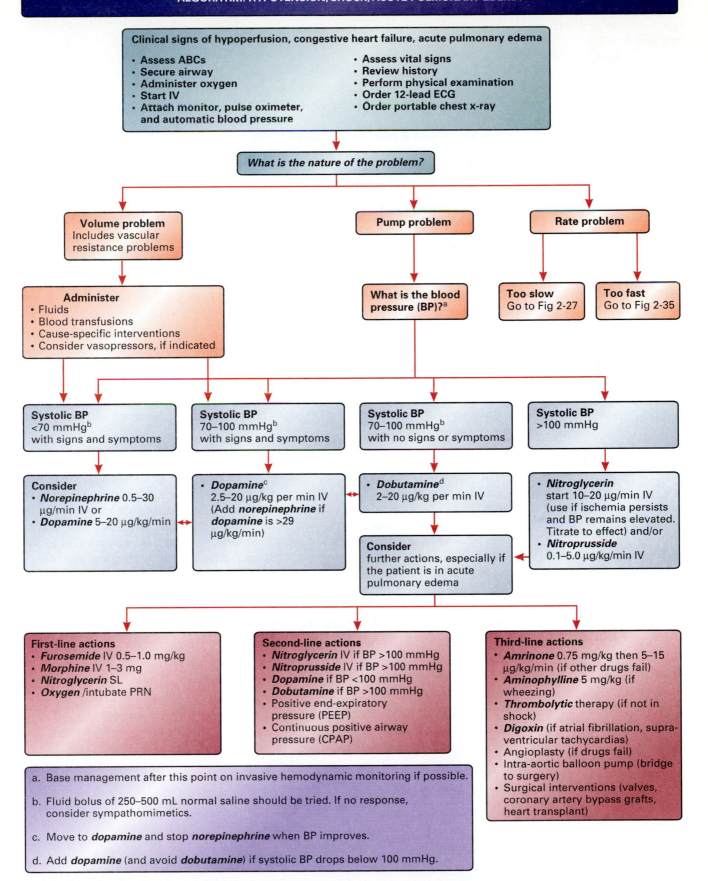

ALGORITHM: HYPOTENSION/SHOCK/ACUTE PULMONARY EDEMA

Clinical signs of hypoperfusion, congestive heart failure, acute pulmonary edema

- Assess ABCs
- Secure airway
- Administer oxygen
- Start IV
- Attach monitor, pulse oximeter, and automatic blood pressure

- Assess vital signs
- Review history
- Perform physical examination
- Order 12-lead ECG
- Order portable chest x-ray

What is the nature of the problem?

Volume problem
Includes vascular resistance problems

Pump problem

Rate problem

Administer
- Fluids
- Blood transfusions
- Cause-specific interventions
- Consider vasopressors, if indicated

What is the blood pressure (BP)?[a]

Too slow
Go to Fig 2-27

Too fast
Go to Fig 2-35

Systolic BP
<70 mmHg[b]
with signs and symptoms

Systolic BP
70–100 mmHg[b]
with signs and symptoms

Systolic BP
70–100 mmHg[b]
with no signs or symptoms

Systolic BP
>100 mmHg

Consider
- *Norepinephrine* 0.5–30 µg/min IV or
- *Dopamine* 5–20 µg/kg/min

- *Dopamine*[c] 2.5–20 µg/kg per min IV (Add *norepinephrine* if *dopamine* is >29 µg/kg/min)

- *Dobutamine*[d] 2–20 µg/kg per min IV

- *Nitroglycerin* start 10–20 µg/min IV (use if ischemia persists and BP remains elevated. Titrate to effect) and/or
- *Nitroprusside* 0.1–5.0 µg/kg/min IV

Consider
further actions, especially if the patient is in acute pulmonary edema

First-line actions
- *Furosemide* IV 0.5–1.0 mg/kg
- *Morphine* IV 1–3 mg
- *Nitroglycerin* SL
- *Oxygen* /intubate PRN

Second-line actions
- *Nitroglycerin* IV if BP >100 mmHg
- *Nitroprusside* IV if BP >100 mmHg
- *Dopamine* if BP <100 mmHg
- *Dobutamine* if BP >100 mmHg
- Positive end-expiratory pressure (PEEP)
- Continuous positive airway pressure (CPAP)

Third-line actions
- *Amrinone* 0.75 mg/kg then 5–15 µg/kg/min (if other drugs fail)
- *Aminophylline* 5 mg/kg (if wheezing)
- *Thrombolytic* therapy (if not in shock)
- *Digoxin* (if atrial fibrillation, supra-ventricular tachycardias)
- Angioplasty (if drugs fail)
- Intra-aortic balloon pump (bridge to surgery)
- Surgical interventions (valves, coronary artery bypass grafts, heart transplant)

a. Base management after this point on invasive hemodynamic monitoring if possible.

b. Fluid bolus of 250–500 mL normal saline should be tried. If no response, consider sympathomimetics.

c. Move to *dopamine* and stop *norepinephrine* when BP improves.

d. Add *dopamine* (and avoid *dobutamine*) if systolic BP drops below 100 mmHg.

FIGURE 2–70   Management of hypotension/shock/pulmonary edema. Adapted with permission. Journal of the American Medical Association, October 28, 1992, Volume 268, No. 16, *Guidelines for Cardiopulmonary Resuscitation and Emergency Cardiac Care*, p. 2227. © 1992 American Medical Association.

always treat the rate and rhythm first. Some medications that may be used to treat cardiogenic shock include:

- Vasopressors
  - Dopamine (Intropin)
  - Dobutamine (Dobutrex)
  - Norepinephrine (Levophed)

Other useful medications may include:

- Morphine sulfate
- Promethazine (Phenergan)
- Nitroglycerin
- Nitrous oxide (Nitronox)
- Furosemide (Lasix)
- Digitalis, digoxin (Lanoxin)
- Sodium bicarbonate

If the patient refuses transport, follow the general guidelines; however, remember that untreated cardiogenic shock has a grim outcome. No matter how well compensated the patient may appear, true cardiogenic shock will decompensate quickly into irreversible shock. Use every means at your disposal to convince the patient to be transported. If the patient still refuses, document accordingly.

Upon arrival at the emergency department, inform the physician of your findings—vital signs, labored breathing, pulmonary edema, dysrhythmias, or severe shock that remains despite your treatment.

Cardiac Arrest

✽ **cardiac arrest** the absence of ventricular contraction.

✽ **sudden death** death within one hour after the onset of symptoms.

Cardiac arrest and sudden death accounts for 60 percent of all deaths from coronary artery disease. **Cardiac arrest** is the absence of ventricular contraction that immediately results in systemic circulatory failure. **Sudden death** is any death that occurs within one hour of the symptoms' onset. At autopsy, actual infarction often is not present. Because severe atherosclerotic disease is common, authorities usually believe that a lethal dysrhythmia is the mechanism of death. The risk factors for sudden death are basically the same as those for atherosclerotic heart disease (ASHD) and coronary artery disease (CAD). In a large number of patients, cardiac arrest is the first manifestation of heart disease. Other causes of sudden death include:

- Drowning
- Acid-base imbalance
- Electrocution
- Drug intoxication
- Electrolyte imbalance
- Hypoxia
- Hypothermia
- Pulmonary embolism
- Stroke
- Hyperkalemia (high levels of potassium)
- Trauma
- End stage renal disease

Field Assessment

A cardiac arrest patient is unresponsive, apneic, and pulseless. Peripheral pulses are absent. After initiating CPR, place ECG leads. Dysrhythmias found in the cardiac arrest patient include ventricular fibrillation, ventricular tachycardia, asystole, or PEA. If you find asystole, you should confirm it in two or more leads.

Center questions on events prior to the arrest. Did bystanders or EMS personnel witness the arrest? Did bystanders start CPR? How much time passed from the discovery of the arrest until CPR was initiated? From discovery until EMS was activated? These questions all focus on **down time,** the duration from the beginning of the cardiac arrest until effective CPR is established. Often physicians want to know the **total down time,** which is the time from the beginning of the arrest until you deliver the patient to the emergency department. If possible, obtain the patient's past history and medications.

✳ **down time** duration from the beginning of the cardiac arrest until effective CPR is established.

✳ **total down time** duration from the beginning of the arrest until the patient's delivery to the emergency department.

Management

To manage the cardiac arrest patient properly, you must understand the terms *resuscitation, return of spontaneous circulation,* and *survival.*

- **Resuscitation** is the provision of efforts to return a spontaneous pulse and breathing to the patient in cardiac arrest.

- **Return of spontaneous circulation** (ROSC) occurs when resuscitation results in the patient's having a spontaneous pulse. ROSC patients may or may not have a return of breathing, and may or may not survive.

- **Survival** means that the patient is resuscitated and survives to be discharged from the hospital. Many resuscitated patients reach ROSC, but not all resuscitated patients survive.

✳ **resuscitation** provision of efforts to return a spontaneous pulse and breathing.

✳ **return of spontaneous circulation** resuscitation results in the patient's having a spontaneous pulse.

✳ **survival** when a patient is resuscitated and survives to be discharged from the hospital.

Basic life support is the mainstay of prehospital cardiac care.

Begin management of airway, breathing, and circulation simultaneously. When resuscitation is indicated, start CPR immediately. Remember that basic life support is the mainstay of treatment for cardiac arrest. Ventilate the patient with a bag-valve mask and 100 percent oxygen. Intubate or insert an alternative airway as quickly as possible. If changes in the ECG indicate defibrillation or synchronized cardioversion, perform it in conjunction with CPR, stopping CPR only to apply the pads or paddles and to deliver the shock(s). Make sure no one touches the patient when you deliver any shock. If the patient has an internal pacemaker or defibrillator, treat the arrest normally, taking care not to defibrillate over the device.

After establishing CPR and advanced airway management, perform IV access. The site of venipuncture should be as close to the heart as possible—for example, the antecubital area (bend of the forearm and humerus) or the external jugular vein. Follow all intravenous medications with a 30–45 second flush. After each flush, set the IV at a to-keep-open (TKO) drip rate.

Pharmacological agents that might be used in a cardiac arrest setting are:

- Atropine sulfate
- Lidocaine
- Procainamide
- Bretylium
- Epinephrine
- Norepinephrine
- Isoproterenol

- Dopamine
- Dobutamine
- Sodium bicarbonate

Postarrest stabilization requires extreme vigilance.

Management of the successful postcardiac arrest patient generally presents an unusual situation. The patient's blood pressure can return at low, normal, or high readings because of the drugs used in resuscitation. In addition, the pulse can return at bradycardic, normal, or tachycardic rates. Ventricular ectopy is the most serious concern. If the patient presented in ventricular fibrillation or ventricular tachycardia during the arrest, or if ectopy presents in the postarrest, use an antidysrhythmic agent such as lidocaine. The blood pressure may return at low readings. The ideal range of the blood pressure is 80–100 mmHg in the postarrest patient. Do not be concerned if the postarrest patient does not show any signs of response. He has endured a very harsh environment, and recovery, if any, can be slow. The postarrest setting can be unnerving, with the patient's vitals and ECG changing every minute. Approach problems one at a time, and do not be fooled by a return in pulse that fades away while the monitor still has a rhythm (PEA).

Your management of all cardiac arrest patients should follow the American Heart Association guidelines for cardiopulmonary resuscitation and emergency cardiac care. Figure 2-71 summarizes the treatment for ventricular fibrillation or ventricular tachycardia (VF/VT), the cardiac arrest rhythms with the best prognosis for successful resuscitation. Also review the algorithms for asystole (Figure 2-53) and pulseless electrical activity (PEA) (Figure 2-55).

Once you have established advanced life support, move the patient to the MICU as quickly as possible, while taking great care to avoid disrupting IVs, endotracheal intubation, CPR, or pharmacological treatment. Transport the patient to the nearest appropriate facility as safely and as smoothly as possible using lights and siren. Offer emotional support to the patient throughout your care. Upon arrival at the emergency department, inform the physician of your findings, especially down time, total down time, changes in rhythm, or return of pulses.

Withholding and Terminating Resuscitation

In some situations, the certainty that the patient will not survive indicates not initiating resuscitation efforts. Rigor mortis, fixed dependent lividity (pooling of the blood), decapitation, decomposition, and incineration are all situations in which you should withhold resuscitation.

In addition, withhold resuscitation efforts if the patient has an out-of-hospital advanced directive. A physician must sign and date the advanced directive, and it must state conditions that apply to the patient at the time of the arrest. For example, the directive may state that resuscitation should be withheld if the patient has an end-stage terminal illness. Each state and many local regions treat advanced directives differently. Review local protocol and medical direction before you might have to decide whether to honor an advanced directive.

In other instances, poor prognosis and survivability of many cardiac arrest patients makes termination of resuscitation a consideration. Some of the *inclusion* criteria for termination of resuscitation are:

- 18 years old or older
- Arrest is presumed cardiac in origin and not associated with a treatable cause such as hypothermia, overdose, or hypovolemia
- Successful and maintained endotracheal intubation
- ACLS standards have been applied throughout the arrest

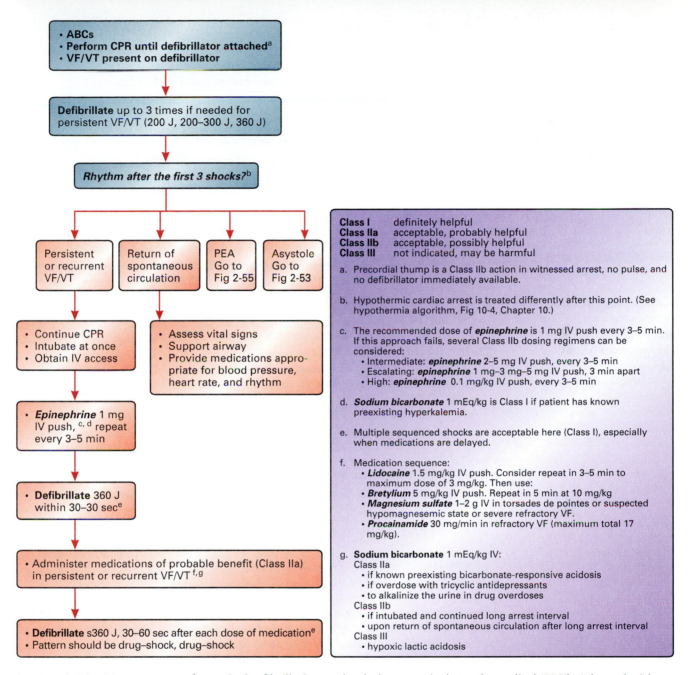

ALGORITHM: VENTRICULAR FIBRILLATION/PULSELESS VENTRICULAR TACHYCARDIA (VF/VT)

- ABCs
- Perform CPR until defibrillator attached[a]
- VF/VT present on defibrillator

Defibrillate up to 3 times if needed for persistent VF/VT (200 J, 200–300 J, 360 J)

Rhythm after the first 3 shocks?[b]

| Persistent or recurrent VF/VT | Return of spontaneous circulation | PEA Go to Fig 2-55 | Asystole Go to Fig 2-53 |

- Continue CPR
- Intubate at once
- Obtain IV access

- Assess vital signs
- Support airway
- Provide medications appropriate for blood pressure, heart rate, and rhythm

- **Epinephrine** 1 mg IV push,[c, d] repeat every 3–5 min

- **Defibrillate** 360 J within 30–30 sec[e]

- Administer medications of probable benefit (Class IIa) in persistent or recurrent VF/VT[f,g]

- **Defibrillate** ≤360 J, 30–60 sec after each dose of medication[e]
- Pattern should be drug–shock, drug–shock

Class I definitely helpful
Class IIa acceptable, probably helpful
Class IIb acceptable, possibly helpful
Class III not indicated, may be harmful

a. Precordial thump is a Class IIb action in witnessed arrest, no pulse, and no defibrillator immediately available.

b. Hypothermic cardiac arrest is treated differently after this point. (See hypothermia algorithm, Fig 10-4, Chapter 10.)

c. The recommended dose of **epinephrine** is 1 mg IV push every 3–5 min. If this approach fails, several Class IIb dosing regimens can be considered:
- Intermediate: **epinephrine** 2–5 mg IV push, every 3–5 min
- Escalating: **epinephrine** 1 mg–3 mg–5 mg IV push, 3 min apart
- High: **epinephrine** 0.1 mg/kg IV push, every 3–5 min

d. **Sodium bicarbonate** 1 mEq/kg is Class I if patient has known preexisting hyperkalemia.

e. Multiple sequenced shocks are acceptable here (Class I), especially when medications are delayed.

f. Medication sequence:
- **Lidocaine** 1.5 mg/kg IV push. Consider repeat in 3–5 min to maximum dose of 3 mg/kg. Then use:
- **Bretylium** 5 mg/kg IV push. Repeat in 5 min at 10 mg/kg
- **Magnesium sulfate** 1–2 g IV in torsades de pointes or suspected hypomagnesemic state or severe refractory VF.
- **Procainamide** 30 mg/min in refractory VF (maximum total 17 mg/kg).

g. **Sodium bicarbonate** 1 mEq/kg IV:
Class IIa
- if known preexisting bicarbonate-responsive acidosis
- if overdose with tricyclic antidepressants
- to alkalinize the urine in drug overdoses
Class IIb
- if intubated and continued long arrest interval
- upon return of spontaneous circulation after long arrest interval
Class III
- hypoxic lactic acidosis

FIGURE 2–71   Management of ventricular fibrillation and pulseless ventricular tachycardia (VF/VT). Adapted with permission. Journal of the American Medical Association, October 28, 1992, Volume 268, No. 16, *Guidelines for Cardiopulmonary Resuscitation and Emergency Cardiac Care*, p. 2217. ©1992 American Medical Association.

- On-scene ALS efforts have been sustained for 25 minutes, or the patient remains in asystole through four rounds of ALS drugs
- Patient's rhythm is asystolic or agonal when the decision to terminate is made, and this rhythm persists until the resuscitation efforts are actually terminated
- Victims of blunt trauma who present in asystole or develop asystole on scene

Depending on local protocol, the *exclusion* criteria for termination of resuscitation may include:

- Under 18 years old
- Etiology that could benefit from in-hospital treatment (such as hypothermia)
- Persistent or recurring ventricular tachycardia or fibrillation
- Transient return of a pulse
- Signs of neurological viability
- Arrest witnessed by EMS personnel
- Family or responsible party opposed to termination

Criteria that should not be considered as either inclusionary or exclusionary:

- The patient's age if 18 or over (for example, geriatric)
- Down time before EMS arrival
- Presence of a nonofficial do-not-resuscitate (DNR) order
- Quality-of-life evaluations by EMS

Review local protocol and medical direction before attempting termination of resuscitation.

Review local protocol and medical direction before attempting termination of resuscitation. Most systems use documented protocols and direct communication with an on-line medical director or physician to approve or deny termination of resuscitation. The medical director or physician may base his decision on the following information:

- Medical condition of the patient
- Known etiological factors
- Therapy rendered
- Family's presence and appraisal of the situation
- Communication of any resistance or uncertainty on the part of the family
- Maintain continuous documentation, including the ECG

The family should receive grief support. This requires EMS personnel or a community agency to be in place soon after termination of resuscitation. EMS personnel deal not only with the living or viable but also with the families of lost loved ones, especially when they have witnessed the death. Many systems employ assigned personnel to support the family after termination of resuscitation. In other systems, paramedics on the scene provide support until a predetermined person from another local agency can arrive. Although this supportive role can be uncomfortable, it will be part of your job.

Law enforcement regulations require that all local, state, or federal laws pertaining to a death be followed. These, too, may vary from region to region, but their basic principles are the same. The officer discusses the death certificate with the attending physician. He will determine if the event or patient requires assignment to a medical examiner, if the nature of the death is suspicious in any way, or if the physician is at all hesitant to sign the death certificate. The officer also may be required to assign the patient to a medical examiner if he does not have a physician. Check with local law enforcement agencies to determine their protocol.

PERIPHERAL VASCULAR AND OTHER CARDIOVASCULAR EMERGENCIES

In addition to cardiac arrest, MI, and hypertension emergencies, other common cardiovascular emergencies involve the arterial and venous systems. Such disorders are generally classified as traumatic or nontraumatic. Nontraumatic vascular emergencies typically arise from preexisting conditions or from a disease process.

Atherosclerosis

The major underlying factor in many cardiovascular emergencies is **atherosclerosis,** a progressive degenerative disease of the medium-sized and large arteries. Atherosclerosis affects the aorta and its branches, the coronary arteries, and the cerebral arteries, among others. It results from fats (lipids and cholesterol) deposited under the tunica intima (inner lining) of the involved vessels. The fat causes an injury response in the tunica intima, which subsequently damages the tunica media (middle layer) as well. Over time, calcium is deposited, causing plaques, where small hemorrhages can occur. These hemorrhages in turn lead to scarring, fibrosis, larger plaque build-up, and aneurysm. The involved arteries can become completely blocked, either by additional plaque, by a blood clot, or by an aneurysm that results from tearing in the arterial wall.

The results of atherosclerosis are evident in many disease processes. First, disruption of the vessel's intimal surface destroys the vessel's elasticity. This condition, **arteriosclerosis,** can cause hypertension and other related problems. Second, atherosclerosis can reduce blood flow through the affected vessel; common manifestations include angina pectoris and intermittent **claudication.** Frequently, thrombosis will develop, totally obstructing the vessel or the tissues it supplies. Myocardial infarction is a classic example of this process.

Aneurysm

Aneurysm is a nonspecific term meaning dilation of a vessel. The types of aneurysm include:

- Atherosclerotic
- Dissecting
- Infectious
- Congenital
- Traumatic

Most aneurysms result from atherosclerosis and involve the aorta, because the blood pressure there is the highest of any vessel in the body. An aneurysm occurs when blood surges into the aortic wall through a tear in the aortic tunica intima. Infectious aneurysms are most commonly associated with syphilis and are rare. Congenital aneurysms can occur with several disease states such as Marfan's syndrome, a hereditary disease that affects the connective tissue. Aortic aneurysm occurs in people with this disease because it involves the connective tissue within the vessel wall. Those affected may experience sudden death, usually from spontaneous rupture of the aorta, often at a fairly young age.

Abdominal Aortic Aneurysm Abdominal aortic aneurysm commonly results from atherosclerosis and occurs most frequently in the aorta, below the renal arteries and above the bifurcation of the common iliac arteries (Figure 2-72). It is ten times more common in men than in women and most prevalent between ages 60 and 70.

* **atherosclerosis** a progressive, degenerative disease of the medium-sized and large arteries.

* **arteriosclerosis** a thickening, loss of elasticity, and hardening of the walls of the arteries from calcium deposits.

* **claudication** severe pain in the calf muscle due to inadequate blood supply. It typically occurs with exertion and subsides with rest.

* **aneurysm** the ballooning of an arterial wall, resulting from a defect or weakness in the wall.

FIGURE 2–72 Rupture of an abdominal aortic aneurysm.

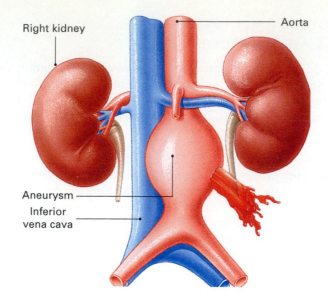

Signs and symptoms of an abdominal aneurysm include:

- Abdominal pain
- Back and flank pain
- Hypotension
- Urge to defecate, caused by the retroperitoneal leakage of blood

Dissecting Aortic Aneurysm Degenerative changes in the smooth muscle and elastic tissue of the aortic media cause most **dissecting aortic aneurysms.** This can result in hematoma and, subsequently, aneurysm. The original tear often results from **cystic medial necrosis,** a degenerative disease of connective tissue often associated with hypertension and to a certain extent, aging. Predisposing factors include hypertension, which is present in 75–85 percent of cases. It occurs more frequently in patients older than 40–50, although it can occur in younger individuals, especially pregnant women. A tendency for this disease also runs in families.

Of dissecting aortic aneurysms, 67 percent involve the ascending aorta. Once dissection has started, it can extend to all of the abdominal aorta as well as its branches, including the coronary arteries, aortic valve, subclavian arteries, and carotid arteries. The aneurysm can rupture at any time, usually into the pericardial or pleural cavity.

Acute Pulmonary Embolism

Acute pulmonary embolism occurs when a blood clot or other particle lodges in a pulmonary artery and blocks blood flow through that vessel. Pulmonary emboli may be composed of air, fat, amniotic fluid, or blood clots. Factors that predispose a patient to blood clots include prolonged immobilization, *thrombophlebitis* (inflammation and clots in a vein), use of certain medications, and atrial fibrillation.

When a pulmonary embolism blocks the blood flow through a vessel, the right heart must pump against increased resistance, which in turn increases pulmonary capillary pressure. The area of the lung supplied by the occluded vessel then stops functioning, and gas exchange decreases.

The signs and symptoms of pulmonary embolism depend upon the size of the obstruction. The patient suffering acute pulmonary embolism may report a sud-

✱ **Dissecting aortic aneurysm** aneurysm caused when blood gets between and separates the layers of the aortic wall.

✱ **cystic medial necrosis** a death or degeneration of a part of the wall of an artery.

✱ **acute pulmonary embolism** blockage that occurs when a blood clot or other particle lodges in a pulmonary artery.

den onset of severe and unexplained dyspnea that may or may not be associated with chest pain. He may have a recent history of immobilization from a hip fracture, surgery, or other debilitating illness.

Acute Arterial Occlusion

An **acute arterial occlusion** is the sudden occlusion of arterial blood flow due to trauma, thrombosis, tumor, embolus, or idiopathic means. Emboli are probably the most common cause. They can arise from within the chamber (*mural emboli*), from a thrombus in the left ventricle, from an atrial thrombus secondary to atrial fibrillation, or from a thrombus caused by abdominal aortic atherosclerosis. Arterial occlusions most commonly involve vessels in the abdomen or extremities.

✻ **acute arterial occlusion** the sudden occlusion of arterial blood flow.

Vasculitis

Vasculitis is an inflammation of blood vessels. Most vasculitis stems from a variety of rheumatic diseases and syndromes. The inflammatory process is usually segmental, and inflammation within the media of a muscular artery tends to destroy the internal elastic lamina. Necrosis and hypertrophy (enlarging) of the vessel occur, and the vessel wall has a high likelihood of breaching, leaking fibrin and red blood cells into the surrounding tissue. This potentially can lead to partial or total vascular occlusion and subsequent necrosis.

✻ **vasculitis** inflammation of blood vessels.

Noncritical Peripheral Vascular Conditions

Several peripheral vascular conditions are not immediately life threatening but often require prehospital care. They include peripheral arterial atherosclerotic disease, deep venous thrombosis, and varicose veins.

Peripheral Arterial Atherosclerotic Disease **Peripheral arterial atherosclerotic disease** is a progressive degenerative disease of the medium-sized and large arteries. It affects the aorta and its branches, the brachial and femoral peripheral arteries, and the cerebral arteries. For reasons unknown it does not affect coronary arteries. It is a gradual, progressive disease, often associated with diabetes mellitus. In extreme cases, significant arterial insufficiency may lead to ulcers and gangrene. Occlusion of the peripheral arteries causes chronic and acute ischemia.

✻ **peripheral arterial atherosclerotic disease** a progressive degenerative disease of the medium-sized and large arteries.

In the chronic setting, intermittent claudication (diminished blood flow in exercising muscle) produces pain with exertion. It occurs most commonly with the calf, but can affect any leg muscle. Rest initially relieves this pain. When the disease progresses, however, the pain presents even at rest. The extremity usually appears normal, but pulses will be reduced or absent. As the ischemia worsens, the extremity becomes painful, cold, and numb, and ulceration, gangrene, and necrosis may be present. There is no edema.

In the acute setting, arterial occlusion from an embolus, aneurysm, or thrombosis occurs. The patient experiences a sudden onset of pain, coldness, numbness, and pallor. Pulses are absent distal to the occlusion. Acute occlusion may cause severe ischemia with motor and sensory deficits. Edema is not present.

Deep Venous Thrombosis **Deep venous thrombosis** is a blood clot in a vein. It most commonly occurs in the larger veins of the thigh and calf. Predisposing factors include a recent history of trauma, inactivity, pregnancy, or varicose veins.

✻ **deep venous thrombosis** a blood clot in a vein.

The patient frequently complains of gradually increasing pain and calf tenderness. Often the leg and foot are swollen because of occluded venous drainage. Leg elevation may alleviate the signs and symptoms. In some cases, the patient may be asymptomatic. Gentle palpation of the calf and thigh may reveal tenderness and, on occasion, cord-like clotted veins. Dorsiflexion of the foot may cause

Homan's sign, discomfort behind the knee. This is associated with deep venous thrombosis. The skin may be warm and red.

Varicose Veins **Varicose veins** are dilated superficial veins, usually in the lower extremities. Predisposing factors include pregnancy, obesity, and genetics. Signs and symptoms include the visible distention of the leg veins, lower leg swelling and discomfort (especially at the end of the day), and skin color and texture changes in the legs and ankles. If the condition is chronic, venous stasis ulcers, a noncritical condition, can develop. Venous stasis ulcers can rupture, but direct pressure usually can control the bleeding, which occasionally is significant.

General Assessment and Management of Vascular Disorders

Occlusion of any vessel can result in ischemia, injury, and necrosis of the affected tissue. Depending on the tissue or organ involved, untreated occlusion can cause severe disability or death. In pulmonary occlusion, hypotension and cardiac collapse can ensue quickly, and death can occur rapidly. In cerebral occlusion, debilitating seizures, paralysis, or death can occur. Mesenteric occlusion can cause necrosis, giving rise to sepsis. Or it can affect vital organs, causing a slow and agonizing death. Pulmonary embolus, aortic aneurysm, and some acute arterial occlusions can produce a hypoperfusion state, and death can be rapid.

Assessment Begin your assessment by checking airway, breathing, and circulation. Breathing is usually not affected, except in pulmonary embolus and a decompensated state of shock. In decompensated shock resulting from aneurysm, arterial occlusion, or pulmonary embolus, breathing may be labored. Circulation may be compromised or absent distal to the affected area. Check circulation for the Five *P*s:

- Pallor
- Pain
- Pulselessness
- Paralysis
- Paresthesia

Check the skin for pallor or mottling distal to the affected area. Skin temperature may appear normal systemically but cool or cold at the affected area, or it may be systemically cool and clammy, as occurs in decompensated shock.

Determine the patient's chief complaint. Depending on the type of vascular emergency, the patient may complain of a sudden or gradual onset of discomfort, and the pain may be localized. Use the OPQRST acronym to elicit the patient's description of symptoms and pain. Is the pain in the chest, abdomen, or extremity? Does it radiate or is it localized? Was its onset gradual or sudden? If there is claudication, is it relieved with rest?

Conduct your focused history and physical exam. Determine the contributing history. This may well be the patient's first recognized event, or it may be a recurrence. Patients with a prior vascular emergency are prone to reoccurrences. They may report an increase in the frequency or duration of events. Breath sounds may be clear to auscultation. Alterations in the heart rate and rhythm may occur with pulmonary embolus and aortic aneurysm. Unequal bilateral blood pressures may indicate a high thoracic aneurysm. Peripheral pulses may be diminished or absent in the affected extremity with arterial occlusion or peripheral arterial atherosclerotic disease. Bruits may be audible over the affected carotid artery. The skin may be cool, moist, or dry, reflecting diminished circulation to the affected area or extremity. ECG findings generally do not contribute to vascular emergency treatment. If dysrhythmias or ectopy are present, treat them accordingly.

***

✳ varicose veins dilated superficial veins, usually in the lower extremity.

Content Review

THE FIVE Ps OF ACUTE ARTERIAL OCCLUSION
Pallor
Pain
Pulselessness
Paralysis
Paresthesia

Management Managing the patient with a vascular emergency is mostly supportive. Place the patient in a position of comfort. Give oxygen by nonrebreather mask if you suspect pulmonary embolus, aortic aneurysm, or arterial occlusion or if any hypotension or a hypoperfusion state presents.

Before administering any drug, ask the patient or his family if he is allergic to any medications. Pharmacological agents that might be used in a vascular emergency include:

- Nitrous oxide (Nitronox)
- Morphine sulfate

Transport the patient as soon as possible. Indications for rapid transport with lights and sirens include any situation in which medications do not relieve the patient's symptoms or in which you suspect pulmonary embolism, aortic aneurysm, or arterial occlusion. Also consider any presentation of hypotension or hypoperfusion to be an emergency and transport the patient rapidly. Report your findings to the emergency department staff.

If the patient refuses transport, advise him that serious complications are likely to occur without further medical attention. Vascular emergencies can reach a point where the patient permanently loses a limb or quickly decompensates into irreversible shock. Some patients will attempt to refuse transport because they have received relief from pain medications. Use every means at your disposal to convince them to be transported. Document refusals according to general guidelines.

Part 3: 12-Lead ECG Monitoring and Interpretation

Objectives

After reading Part 3 of this chapter, you should be able to:

*101. Explain the placement and view of the heart provided by bipolar, unipolar (augmented), and precordial ECG leads. (pp. 224–228)
*102. Discuss QRS axis and axis deviation. (pp. 228–231)
*103. Recognize a normal 12-lead ECG. (pp. 231–232)
*104. Explain the evolution and localization of acute myocardial infarction. (pp. 232–240)
*105. Recognize 12-lead ECG tracings of a variety of conduction abnormalities. (pp. 240–254)
*106. Explain prehospital 12-lead ECG monitoring procedures. (pp. 255–258)

*Note: The asterisked objectives are not included in the DOT Paramedic curriculum.

An electrocardiogram (ECG) is a graphic recording of the electrical activity of the heart. For years, routine single-lead monitoring has been an intrinsic part of prehospital care. Now, with the advent of portable 12-lead ECG monitors, multi-lead monitoring is available to prehospital providers.

Single-lead ECG monitoring was principally designed to detect cardiac dysrhythmias. It did not allow for diagnosis of acute myocardial infarction, conduction abnormalities, or other electrophysiological problems. With the advent of thrombolytic therapy, however, early detection of acute myocardial infarction has become very important. The window of time from the onset of symptoms to beginning thrombolytic therapy is limited. In many instances, early diagnosis of acute myocardial infarction can be obtained in the field and thrombolytic therapy initiated either in the field or upon arrival at the emergency department.

This part of the chapter will examine the use of 12-lead ECG monitoring in prehospital care, including relevant electrophysiology, interpretation, and techniques.

REVIEWING THE CARDIAC CONDUCTIVE SYSTEM

The cardiac conductive system was discussed in detail earlier in the chapter. It consists of conductive fibers that transmit the depolarization potential rapidly through the heart. Transmission through these specialized conductive fibers is much faster than if the impulse were transmitted through regular myocardial cells.

The purpose of the cardiac conductive system is to stimulate the atria and the ventricles to contract in the proper direction and at the proper time. The mass of atrial tissue functions together as the atrial syncytium. That is, when one cell of atrial muscle becomes excited, the action potential will spread rapidly across the entire group of cells, resulting in coordinated depolarization and subsequent contraction. Likewise, the mass of ventricular tissue functions together as the ventricular syncytium. Once stimulated, the action potential quickly spreads across the entire group of cells, resulting in coordinated depolarization and contraction.

Knowledge of the cardiac conductive system is essential to understanding and interpreting 12-lead ECG tracings (review Figure 2-12). Internodal pathways connect the SA (sinoatrial) node, located high in the right atrium, to the AV (atrioventricular) node. The internodal pathways conduct the depolarization impulse from the SA node to the atrial muscle mass and, through the atria, to the AV junction. The impulse is slowed at the AV junction, allowing time for ventricular filling. Then, as the impulse passes through the AV junction, it enters the AV node. The AV node is connected to the AV fibers, which conduct the impulse from the atria to the ventricles. The AV fibers then become the bundle of His, which transmits the impulse through the interventricular septum.

The bundle of His subsequently divides into the right and left bundle branches. The right bundle branch delivers the impulse to the apex of the right ventricle, where it is spread across the myocardium by the Purkinje system. At the same time, the impulse is carried into the left bundle branch. The left bundle branch divides into the anterior and posterior fascicles, which ultimately terminate into the Purkinje system. As the impulse is transmitted to the right ventricle, the Purkinje system simultaneously spreads it across the mass of the myocardium. Repolarization predominantly occurs in the opposite direction. This normal series of electrophysiological events results in the normal ECG tracing (review Figure 2-14).

ECG RECORDING

An ECG machine records the electrical activity of the heart as detected by the various leads attached to the body. A minimum of two electrodes are required to detect the electrical activity of the heart, so each lead is comprised of a pair of electrodes. Typically, one electrode is positive and the other negative, or one electrode is positive and the other electrode functions as a reference point. (This will be explained in more detail later.) Passage of electrical current toward the positive electrode will cause a positive deflection on the recorder. A positive deflection will cause the marker or stylus to move upward. Likewise, passage of an electrical current away from the positive electrode will cause a negative deflection on the recorder. A negative deflection will cause the marker or stylus to move downward on the recorder.

The stronger the current, the greater will be the deflection of the stylus on the ECG recorder. Electrical current that flows directly toward the positive electrode will cause a greater deflection than electrical current that flows obliquely toward the positive electrode (Figure 2-73). If current flow is exactly perpendicular to the axis of the ECG lead, there will be no deflection on the graph. This

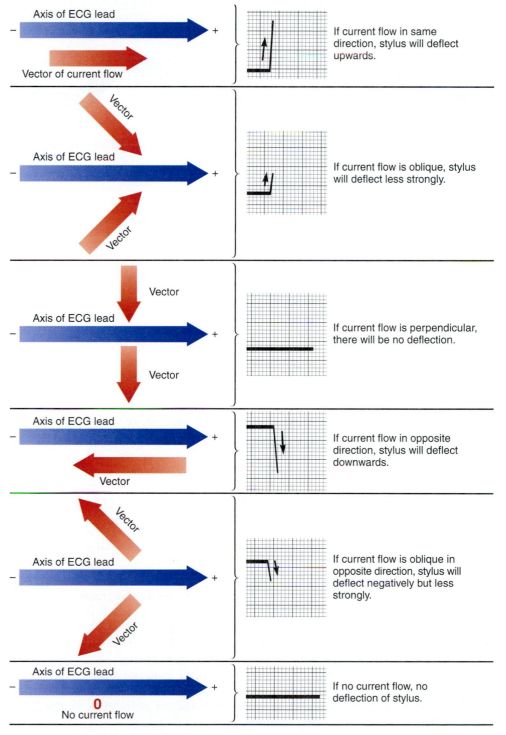

FIGURE 2–73 Results of relationships between current flow direction and ECG lead axis.

If current flow in same direction, stylus will deflect upwards.

If current flow is oblique, stylus will deflect less strongly.

If current flow is perpendicular, there will be no deflection.

If current flow in opposite direction, stylus will deflect downwards.

If current flow is oblique in opposite direction, stylus will deflect negatively but less strongly.

If no current flow, no deflection of stylus.

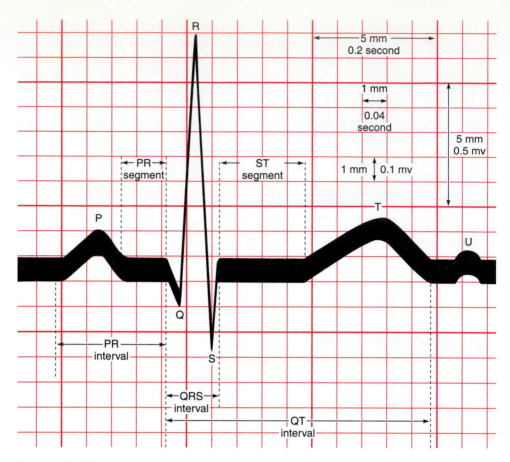

FIGURE 2–74   Electrocardiograph waves.

is because the current is flowing neither toward nor away from the electrode. In the absence of current flow, there will be no deflection on the ECG monitor.

In summary, the electrical activity of the heart is a complex combination of positive and negative current flows that can be graphically recorded on paper or an oscilloscope for monitoring (Figure 2-74).

ECG LEADS

The first ECG recording was reported by Willem Einthoven in 1903. Einthoven placed leads on the arms and legs in an effort to measure the electrical activity of the heart using a simple galvanometer. Today we still use some of the leads that Einthoven first utilized.

An ECG lead is not a single wire but a combination of two wires and their electrodes that makes a complete circuit with the electrocardiograph.

ECG leads may be bipolar, unipolar, or precordial. Leads I, II, and III are bipolar. Leads aVR, aVL, and aVF are unipolar. Together, Leads I, II, III, aVR, aVL, and aVF constitute the frontal plane leads. That is, they record the electrical activity of the heart in the frontal plane of the body utilizing electrodes on the extremities. Developed in the 1930s, the precordial leads, or "chest leads," are designed to look at the heart in the horizontal plane. They are leads V_1, V_2, V_3, V_4, V_5, and V_6 (Figure 2-75). Additional information pertaining to the ECG leads is detailed in the following sections.

Electrocardiographic Leads and Their Axes

Limb leads

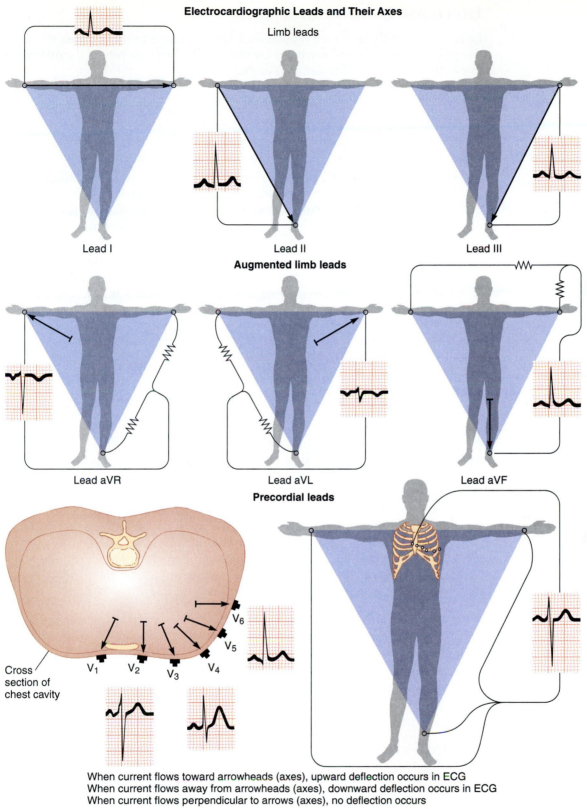

Lead I Lead II Lead III

Augmented limb leads

Lead aVR Lead aVL Lead aVF

Precordial leads

Cross section of chest cavity

V₁ V₂ V₃ V₄ V₅ V₆

When current flows toward arrowheads (axes), upward deflection occurs in ECG
When current flows away from arrowheads (axes), downward deflection occurs in ECG
When current flows perpendicular to arrows (axes), no deflection occurs

FIGURE 2–75 ECG leads and their axes.

BIPOLAR LIMB LEADS

Leads I, II, and III are called bipolar limb leads because two electrodes of opposite polarity (positive and negative) are utilized. These leads record the difference in electrical potential between two limbs.

- *Lead I.* In Lead I, the negative electrode is placed on the right arm and the positive electrode is placed on the left arm. Thus, when the electrical current moves through the heart from the right arm toward the left arm, Lead I will record a positive deflection.
- *Lead II.* In Lead II, the negative electrode is placed on the right arm and the positive electrode is placed on the left leg. Thus, when the electrical current moves through the heart from the right arm toward the left leg, Lead II will record a positive deflection.
- *Lead III.* In Lead III, the negative electrode is placed on the left arm and the positive electrode is placed on the left leg. Thus, when the electrical current moves through the heart from the left arm toward the left leg, Lead III will record a positive deflection.

These leads form "Einthoven's Triangle" around the heart (Figure 2-76). The two arms and the left leg form the corners of the triangle. It is important to point out that electrodes are typically attached to both legs. The right leg is typically used as a ground or a spare, as recordings obtained from either leg are virtually identical. (Usually, the leads are placed on the chest wall rather than the limbs.)

UNIPOLAR OR AUGMENTED LIMB LEADS

The unipolar, or augmented, limb leads utilize the same electrodes as the bipolar limb leads. These leads allow a different "look" at the heart by using two of the electrodes as a single electrode. To achieve this, two selected leads are combined in the ECG machine after each has been run through a resistor to reduce the current flow. This effectively provides a functional electrode halfway between the combined leads. The term *unipolar* refers to the resulting arrangement of one polarized (positive) electrode and the combined leads, which serve as a nonpolarized reference point. To increase the deflection's amplitude, the ground lead is disconnected, thus the term *augmented lead* (Figure 2-77).

- *Lead aVR.* In Lead aVR, the positive electrode is placed on the right arm. The negative electrode is a combination of the left arm and left leg electrode.

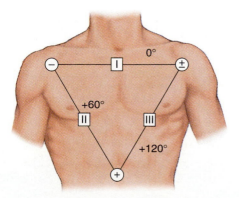

FIGURE 2–76 Einthoven's Triangle as formed by the bipolar leads.

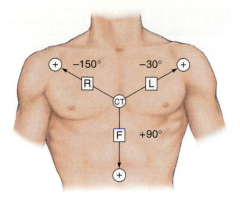

FIGURE 2-77   The pattern formed by the unipolar/augmented leads.

- *Lead aVL.* In Lead aVL, the positive electrode is placed on the left arm. The negative electrode is a combination of the right arm and left leg.
- *Lead aVF.* In Lead aVF, the positive electrode is placed on the left foot. The negative electrode is a combination of the right arm and the left arm.

All of the limb leads are in the frontal plane. If you superimpose the direction of each of these leads on a single diagram, the six leads will constitute a complete 360 degree circle (Figure 2-78). By established convention, the direction toward the left arm is considered to be 0 degrees. Some systems will use the full 360 degree circle to describe the axis of the lead in question. The radials increase clockwise in this system. Other systems will divide the circle into positive and negative halves (semi-circles). Using this system, moving clockwise, the radial coordinates are positive up to 180 degrees. Moving counterclockwise from 0 degrees, the radial coordinates are negative up to 180 degrees. Each lead can be measured on this coordinate system. Table 2-4 lists the limb leads and the direction in which they point.

This discussion will follow the semi-circle system, which is the more commonly used. Remember that both systems describe the same radials, but each uses a different frame of reference.

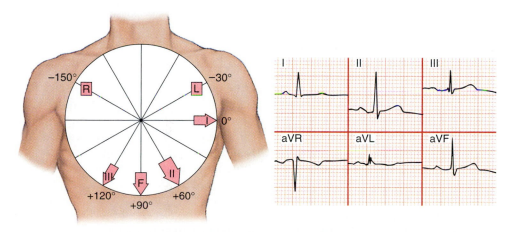

FIGURE 2-78   The hexaxial (six axes) reference system.

Table 2-4	12-LEAD ANGLES		
Lead		**Full Circle**	**Semi-Circle**
Lead I		0 degrees	0 degrees
Lead II		60 degrees	+60 degrees
Lead III		120 degrees	+120 degrees
aVR		210 degrees	−150 degrees
aVL		330 degrees	−30 degrees
aVF		90 degrees	+90 degrees

PRECORDIAL LEADS

The precordial leads provide a look at the horizontal plane of the heart. The horizontal plane is the plane that results from a section taken from front to back, from the sternum to the spine. The negative pole for the precordial leads is a common ground arranged electronically within the ECG machine by connecting all limb leads together. The positive electrode is placed on the anterior surface of the chest in positions ranging from V_1 to V_6.

- *Lead V_1.* Lead V_1 is obtained by placing the positive electrode to the right of the sternum at the fourth intercostal space.
- *Lead V_2.* Lead V_2 is obtained by placing the positive electrode to the left of the sternum at the fourth intercostal space.
- *Lead V_3.* Lead V_3 is obtained by placing the positive electrode in a line midway between Lead V_2 and Lead V_4.
- *Lead V_4.* Lead V_4 is obtained by placing the positive electrode at the mid-clavicular line at the fifth intercostal space.
- *Lead V_5.* Lead V_5 is obtained by placing the positive electrode at the anterior axillary line at the same level as V_4.
- *Lead V_6.* Lead V_6 is obtained by placing the positive electrode to the mid-axillary line at the same level as V_4.

All 12-leads record exactly the same electrical events within the heart. Each lead, however, allows us to look at these events from a different perspective.

MEAN QRS AXIS DETERMINATION

✱ **vector** a force that has both magnitude and direction.

✱ **QRS axis** reduction of all the heart's electrical forces to a single vector represented by an arrow moving in a single plane.

The heart's electrical energy is the sum of the electricity generated by each individual cardiac muscle cell. This energy exhibits both magnitude and direction. Any force that has both magnitude and direction is a **vector**. In actuality, the electrical forces of the heart move in three dimensions simultaneously during the course of each cardiac cycle. However, these forces can be averaged together at any given point in time. This averaged vector is referred to as the instantaneous vector. Ultimately, we can combine all of the instantaneous vectors occurring during the cardiac cycle into a single, averaged vector called the resultant cardiac vector or mean cardiac vector. This reduces all of the electrical forces generated by the heart's millions of cardiac cells to a single vector represented by an arrow moving in a single plane, the **QRS axis**.

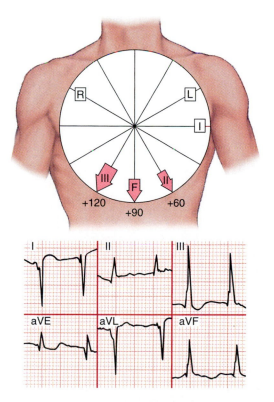

FIGURE 2–79 Axis determination.

AXIS DEVIATION

The heart's normal electrical axis is 59° degrees (−29° to +105°). In the normal tracing, Lead II should have the most positive deflection as the axis of Lead II is +60°. If the calculated axis of the heart falls outside of normal, an axis deviation exists. Any time the axis equals or exceeds +105° the patient is said to have a **right axis deviation**. Right axis deviation is abnormal and often associated with chronic obstructive pulmonary disease and pulmonary hypertension. Any time the axis of the heart is greater than or equal to −30°, a **left axis deviation** is said to exist. Left axis deviation can be associated with high blood pressure, valvular heart disease, and other disease processes.

To simplify matters, the frontal plane can be divided into quadrants (Figure 2-79). The quadrant from 0° to +90° is considered normal. The quadrant from +90° to +180° is considered right axis deviation (Figure 2-80). The quadrant

✳ **right axis deviation** a calculated axis of the heart's electrical energy that equals or exceeds +105 degrees (or in a simplified formula, from +90 to +180 degrees).

✳ **left axis deviation** a calculated axis of the heart's electrical energy that equals or exceeds −30 degrees (or in a simplified formula, from 0 to −90 degrees).

FIGURE 2–80 Right axis deviation.

FIGURE 2–81   Left axis deviation.

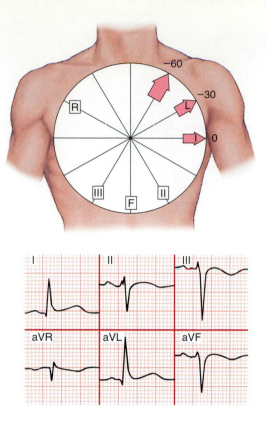

✱ indeterminate axis a calculated axis of the heart's electrical energy from −90 to −180 degrees. (Indeterminate axis is often considered to be extreme right axis deviation.)

from 0° to −90° is considered left axis deviation (Figure 2-81). Finally, the quadrant from −90° to −180° is considered **indeterminate axis.** Indeterminate axis is often considered extreme right axis deviation. While not quite as accurate, this system is effective in detecting abnormal ECG axes.

Most modern 12-lead ECG machines will electronically calculate the axis of the various waves of the ECG (P, QRS, T). These can be used to determine whether an axis deviation exists. In our discussion of cardiac axes, we have been referring to the QRS axis as it represents ventricular depolarization.

When the machine does not calculate the QRS axis, it can be calculated based on Leads I, II, and III (Figure 2-82). The heights of the QRS complexes can

FIGURE 2–82   Cardiac vector (QRS axis) calculated from Leads I, II, and III.

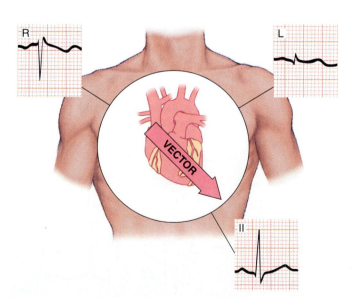

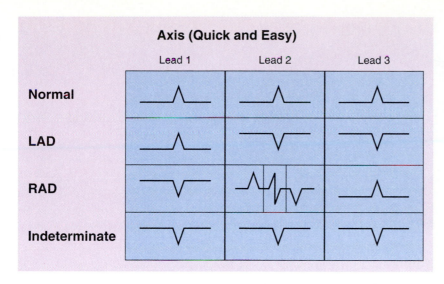

Axis (Quick and Easy)

	Lead 1	Lead 2	Lead 3
Normal			
LAD			
RAD			
Indeterminate			

FIGURE 2–83   Rapid axis determination.

be measured and plotted on a triaxial reference system. Then, the cardiac axis can be calculated. This system is of little use in the prehospital setting, as it is time consuming and requires calipers and graph paper. Alternatively, a practical system is available for rapidly estimating the electrical axis of the heart.

To rapidly determine the electrical axis of the heart, you must look at Leads I, II, and III. The system follows these steps (Figure 2-83):

1. Look at the QRS in Leads I, II, and III. If the QRS is NOT negative in any of these leads, the axis is within normal range.

2. Examine Lead I. If the QRS is negative in Lead I, look at Leads II and III. If the QRS is negative in all three leads, the axis is indeterminate. If the QRS is variable in Lead II (positive, intermediate, negative) and positive in Lead III, a right axis deviation is present.

3. Examine Lead III. If the QRS is negative in Lead III, look at Lead II. If both Lead II and III are negative, a left axis deviation is present.

Axis determination is important in interpretation of the 12-lead ECG. Bundle branch blocks, chamber enlargement, and other factors can affect the QRS axis. The role of axis determination will be discussed in greater detail later in this chapter.

THE NORMAL 12-LEAD ECG

The normal 12-lead ECG records the same series of electrical events within the heart from 12 different perspectives (Figure 2-84). This allows for examination of the heart in two planes. Many abnormalities can be detected with the 12-lead ECG. It is important to point out that the ECG records only the electrical events that occur. It does not provide any information about the heart's pumping efficiency. The ECG, like other pieces of medical information, must be used in association with a good history and physical examination, vital sign determination, and other ancillary testing and diagnostic equipment available for advanced prehospital care.

FIGURE 2–84   12-lead ECG perspectives.

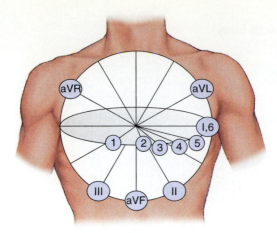

The 12-lead ECG can be presented several ways, depending on the machine being used. The most common 12-lead presentation is a 3-channel machine that provides short strips of each lead (Figure 2-85). The most common format is to place the bipolar limb leads on the left with Lead I at the top, Lead II in the middle, and Lead III at the bottom. To the right of this, in the second column, are the augmented limb leads with aVR at the top, aVL in the middle, and aVF at the bottom. To the right of the augmented limb leads are the precordial leads. Leads V_1 through V_3 are placed in the third column, and Leads V_4 through V_6 in the fourth column. This system functionally groups the leads based upon their view of the heart.

DISEASE FINDINGS

Many disease processes can affect the ECG. Among the most important of these are myocardial ischemia, injury, and infarction. A myocardial infarction is the death of a portion of the myocardium due to a loss of blood flow. Most commonly, a blood clot will form in a diseased coronary artery. This clot results in complete occlusion of the artery and stoppage of blood flow through that artery to the part of the myocardium it serves.

Initially, this will result in **myocardial ischemia.** Myocardial ischemia occurs almost immediately following loss of blood supply. The ischemic tissue is deprived of oxygen and other nutrients. Ischemic tissue can still depolarize, but ischemia tends to affect repolarization. Myocardial ischemia can cause depression of the ST segment and inversion of the T wave on the ECG. Both of these findings are due to abnormalities of repolarization. If blood supply is restored promptly to ischemic tissue, then permanent myocardial injury often can be avoided.

If myocardial ischemia is allowed to progress untreated, **myocardial injury** will occur. Myocardial injury reflects actual injury to the myocardium. The degree of injury depends upon how quickly blood supply is restored. Injured myocardium tends to be partially or completely depolarized. This tissue, often called stunned myocardium, does not contract and does not contribute to the heart's pumping ability. In addition, injured myocardium can be very irritable and can be a source of serious and potentially life-threatening dysrhythmias. With myocardial injury, current flows between the pathologically depolarized area and the normally depolarized areas. This is referred to as a **current of injury** or **injury current.** Thus, with myocardial injury, the injured tissue remains depolarized. It effectively emits a negative electrical charge into the surrounding fluids when the

---

✴ **myocardial ischemia** deprivation of oxygen and other nutrients to the myocardium (heart muscle), typically causing abnormalities in repolarization.

✴ **myocardial injury** injury to the myocardium (heart muscle), typically following myocardial ischemia that results from loss of blood and oxygen supply to the tissue. The injured myocardium tends to be partially or completely depolarized.

✴ **current of injury (injury current)** the flow of current between the pathologically depolarized area of myocardial injury and the normally depolarized areas of the myocardium.

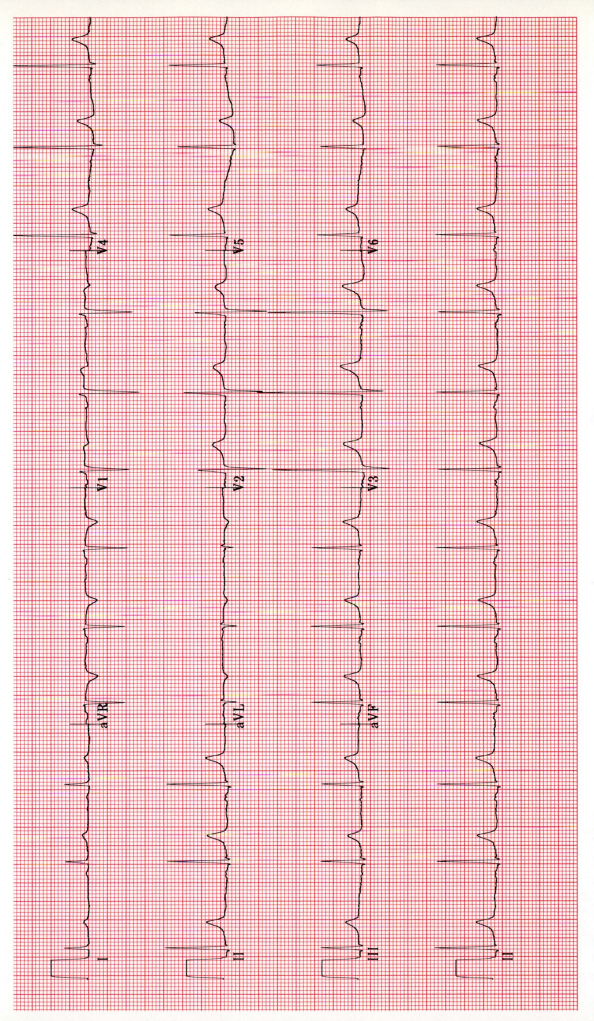

FIGURE 2–85   Normal 12-lead ECG.

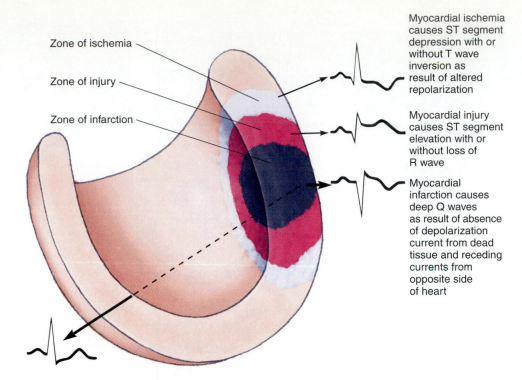

Zone of ischemia

Zone of injury

Zone of infarction

Myocardial ischemia causes ST segment depression with or without T wave inversion as result of altered repolarization

Myocardial injury causes ST segment elevation with or without loss of R wave

Myocardial infarction causes deep Q waves as result of absence of depolarization current from dead tissue and receding currents from opposite side of heart

FIGURE 2–86   The effects of myocardial ischemia, injury, and infarction.

* **myocardial infarction** death of myocardial tissue.

* **subendocardial infarction** myocardial infarction that affects only the deeper levels of the myocardium; also called non-Q-wave infarction because it typically does not result in a significant Q wave in the affected lead.

surrounding normal myocardium is positively charged. This current of injury can sometimes be seen on the ECG as elevation of the ST segment.

If the coronary occlusion persists, the myocardial tissue will subsequently die. Death of the myocardial tissue is called **myocardial infarction.** Eventually, the infarcted myocardium will be replaced by fibrous scar tissue. The scar tissue does not contract and does not depolarize in the course of cardiac depolarization. In major infarctions, the scar tissue will result in the formation of significant Q waves in the affected leads. Large areas of scar tissue can result in a ventricular aneurysm. Large aneurysms can cause chronic elevation in the ST segment, often mimicking acute myocardial injury.

All three areas (areas of ischemia, injury, and infarction) can typically be found following coronary occlusion. The outermost tissue will be ischemic (zone of ischemia). Because of collateral blood supply, oxygen and nutrients are often resupplied to this tissue before permanent injury occurs. The intermediate area will be injured (zone of injury). This area has sustained some permanent injury but still maintains some capacity for recovery. At the center of the lesion will be the most compromised tissue, or infarcted tissue (zone of infarction). This part of the myocardium will die and eventually be replaced by scar tissue. Figure 2-86 illustrates the effects of myocardial ischemia, injury, and infarction. It also illustrates the ECG changes commonly associated with each.

Myocardial infarctions may involve the whole thickness of the myocardium or only a partial thickness. The coronary arteries lie on the surface of the heart (at the epicardial level). Interruption of blood supply threatens the deeper layers (subendocardium) of the myocardium more than the superficial layers.

A myocardial infarction that affects only the deeper part of the myocardium is called a **subendocardial infarction.** The amount of tissue affected in a subendocardial infarction is typically less than in full-thickness infarctions. Subendocardial infarctions usually do not result in the development of a significant Q-wave in the affected lead. Because of this, subendocardial infarctions are often called non-Q-wave infarctions. An infarction that affects the full thickness of the myocardium is called a **transmural infarction.**

Both types of infarction can result in permanent myocardial death if appropriate intervention, such as thrombolytic therapy or percutaneous transluminal coronary angioplasty (PTCA), is not completed early in the course of the event. Transmural infarctions almost always result in the formation of a significant Q wave in the affected leads.

The goal of emergency care is to identify myocardial ischemia long before it becomes myocardial injury and infarction.

EVOLUTION OF ACUTE MYOCARDIAL INFARCTION

The precipitating event in acute myocardial infarction is occlusion of a coronary artery and interruption of blood flow to a portion of the myocardium it supplies. At this precise moment the clock starts running. In the field of emergency care, time is myocardium!

The evolution of myocardial infarction has been extensively studied. Figures 2-87 and 2-88 illustrate the events that occur in transmural and subendocardial myocardial infarctions. The following description details the evolution of a transmural myocardial infarction.

Initially, following coronary occlusion, the affected tissue will become deprived of oxygen and other nutrients and will become ischemic. Myocardial ischemia can often be demonstrated on the ECG as ST segment depression and T wave inversion in the affected leads. ST segment depression and T wave inversion may not be present at the same time. As a rule, as the quantity of ischemic tissue increases the ECG findings will become more significant.

If allowed to progress untreated, tissue at the center of the myocardial injury will transition from ischemia to injury. When a critical mass of tissue is affected, the ST segments will become elevated in the affected leads. In addition, T waves in the affected leads will become more peaked.

If blood supply has not been restored, the injured tissue will begin to die after approximately 6 hours. This infarcted tissue is lost. The ST segment will remain elevated (because of the adjoining zone of injury) and the R wave amplitude will diminish. As the infarction becomes complete over the next 48 to 72 hours, most ischemia and injury will have been replaced by infarcted tissue or will have been reperfused. This results in a decrease in ST segment elevation. Also, however, a significant Q wave will develop. A significant Q wave has a width greater than or equal to 0.04 second (one small box) or amplitude (depth) greater than or equal to one-fourth of the R wave in the same lead. T wave inversion will continue. After several months, the infarcted tissue will be replaced with a fibrous scar. By this time, the ST segment will usually return to normal and some R wave may return. T wave inversion often persists. A significant Q wave usually persists and is an indicator of an old transmural infarction.

The evolution of a subendocardial infarction is similar to that described above for a transmural infarction. However, significant Q waves typically do not occur. In addition, as the lesion heals, the ECG may return to normal, leaving no indication of a prior infarct.

LOCALIZATION OF ACUTE MYOCARDIAL INFARCTION

Each ECG lead is designed to visualize a particular part of the heart. While the bipolar and augmented limb leads evaluate the heart from the frontal plane, the precordial leads look at the heart from a horizontal plane.

✱ transmural infarction myocardial infarction that affects the full thickness of the myocardium and almost always results in a pathological Q wave in the affected leads.

Time is myocardium!

Transmural Infarction

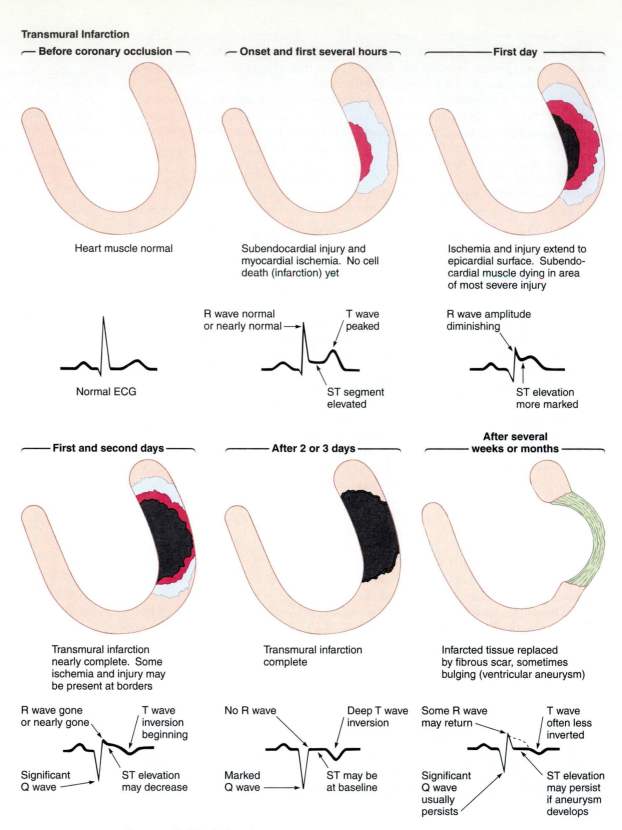

┌─ **Before coronary occlusion** ─┐

Heart muscle normal

Normal ECG

┌─ **Onset and first several hours** ─┐

Subendocardial injury and myocardial ischemia. No cell death (infarction) yet

R wave normal or nearly normal →

T wave peaked

ST segment elevated

┌─ **First day** ─┐

Ischemia and injury extend to epicardial surface. Subendocardial muscle dying in area of most severe injury

R wave amplitude diminishing

ST elevation more marked

┌─ **First and second days** ─┐

Transmural infarction nearly complete. Some ischemia and injury may be present at borders

R wave gone or nearly gone

T wave inversion beginning

Significant Q wave

ST elevation may decrease

┌─ **After 2 or 3 days** ─┐

Transmural infarction complete

No R wave

Deep T wave inversion

Marked Q wave

ST may be at baseline

After several weeks or months

Infarcted tissue replaced by fibrous scar, sometimes bulging (ventricular aneurysm)

Some R wave may return

T wave often less inverted

Significant Q wave usually persists

ST elevation may persist if aneurysm develops

FIGURE 2–87   Infarction.

236

Subendocardial Infarction

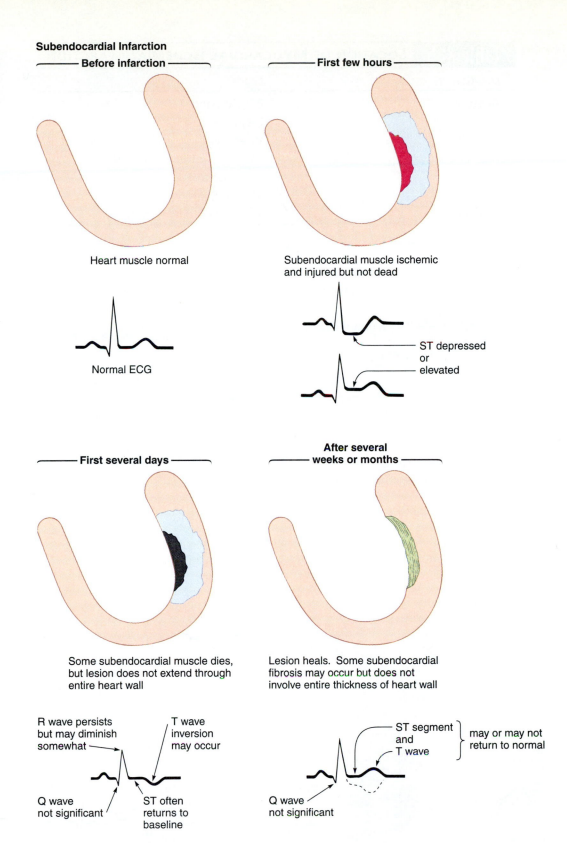

Before infarction

Heart muscle normal

Normal ECG

First few hours

Subendocardial muscle ischemic
and injured but not dead

ST depressed
or
elevated

First several days

Some subendocardial muscle dies,
but lesion does not extend through
entire heart wall

R wave persists
but may diminish
somewhat

T wave
inversion
may occur

Q wave
not significant

ST often
returns to
baseline

After several
weeks or months

Lesion heals. Some subendocardial
fibrosis may occur but does not
involve entire thickness of heart wall

ST segment
and
T wave

may or may not
return to normal

Q wave
not significant

FIGURE 2–88   Subendocardial infarction.

Table 2-5	LOCATION OF MYOCARDIAL ISCHEMIA/INFARCTION
Location	**Leads**
Anterior	I, V_2, V_3, and V_4
Anteriolateral	I, aVL, V_5, and V_6
Lateral	V_5 and V_6
High lateral	I and aVL (often with V_5, V_6)
Inferior	II, III, and aVF
Inferolateral	II, III, aVF, and V_6
True posterior	Reciprocal changes in V_1 and V_2

Various ECG leads look at a specific part of the myocardium. Abnormalities of the ECG in certain leads, with a few exceptions, indicate problems in the part of the heart those leads visualize. The following is a generalized description of the various ECG lead groupings associated with various locations of acute myocardial infarction (See Table 2-5). These descriptions are generalized and some overlapping may occur.

- *Anterior.* Leads I, V_2, V_3, and V_4 are immediately over the anterior surface of the heart. ST segment elevation, T wave inversion, and the development of significant Q waves in these leads indicate myocardial infarction involving the anterior surface of the heart (Figure 2-89). Leads V_2 and V_3 overlie the ventricular septum. Ischemic changes in these leads, and possibly in the adjoining precordial leads, are often referred to as septal infarctions.

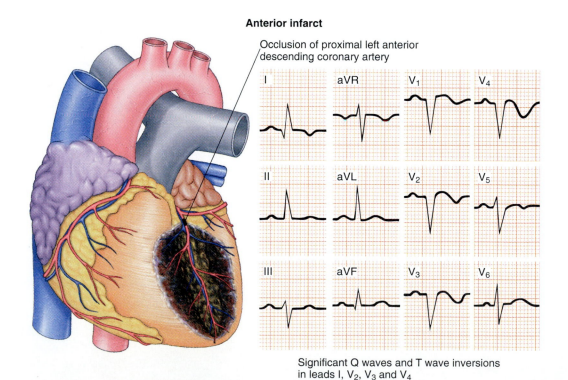

Anterior infarct

Occlusion of proximal left anterior descending coronary artery

Significant Q waves and T wave inversions in leads I, V_2, V_3 and V_4

FIGURE 2–89   Anterior infarct.

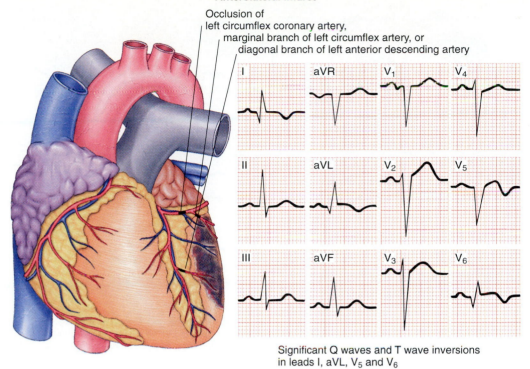

Anterolateral infarct

Occlusion of
left circumflex coronary artery,
marginal branch of left circumflex artery, or
diagonal branch of left anterior descending artery

I aVR V₁ V₄

II aVL V₂ V₅

III aVF V₃ V₆

Significant Q waves and T wave inversions
in leads I, aVL, V₅ and V₆

FIGURE 2–90   Anterolateral infarct.

- *Anterolateral.* Leads I, aVL, V_5 and V_6 examine the anterior and lateral surface of the heart. ST segment elevation, T wave inversion, and the development of significant Q waves in these leads indicate myocardial infarction involving the anterolateral surface of the heart (Figure 2-90).

- *Lateral.* Leads V_5 and V_6 visualize the lateral surface of the heart. ST segment elevation, T wave inversion, and the development of significant Q waves in these leads indicate myocardial infarction involving the lateral surface of the heart.

- *High lateral.* Leads I and aVL visualize the high lateral surface of the heart. Changes in these leads can often be seen in the other lateral leads (Leads V_5 and V_6). ST segment elevation, T wave inversion, and the development of significant Q waves in these leads indicate myocardial infarction involving the high lateral surface of the heart.

- *Inferior.* Leads II, III, and aVF visualize the inferior (diaphragmatic) surface of the heart. ST segment elevation, T wave inversion, and the development of significant Q waves in these leads indicate myocardial infarction involving the inferior surface of the heart (Figure 2-91).

- *Inferolateral.* Leads II, III, aVF, and V_6 visualize the inferolateral portion of the heart. ST segment elevation, T wave inversion, and the development of significant Q waves in these leads indicate myocardial infarction involving the inferolateral surface of the heart.

- *True posterior.* There are no ECG leads over the posterior surface of the heart. True posterior infarctions, although rare, can be diagnosed by looking for **reciprocal** changes in the anterior leads (V_1 and V_2). Normally, the R wave in Leads V_1 and V_2 is principally negative. An

✱ **reciprocal** a mirror image seen typically on the opposite wall of the injured area.

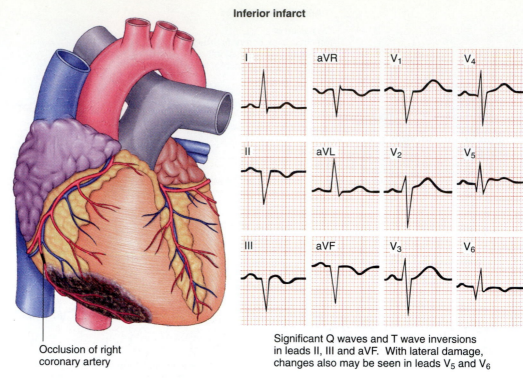

Inferior infarct

Significant Q waves and T wave inversions in leads II, III and aVF. With lateral damage, changes also may be seen in leads V_5 and V_6

Occlusion of right coronary artery

FIGURE 2–91   Inferior infarct.

unusually large R wave in Lead V_1 and V_2 can actually be a reciprocal of a posterior Q wave. Likewise, an upright T wave in these leads would be a reciprocal of posterior T wave inversion (Figure 2-92). These findings are subtle and require practice to learn. Alternatively, posterior leads (V_7 through V_{12}) can be applied to the back to confirm the presence of a true posterior myocardial infarction.

It is important to point out that the above guidelines are generalized. Individual ECG tracings will vary due to variances in body structure, underlying heart and lung disease, and other factors that can affect the ECG tracing. Thus abnormal findings may overlap somewhat in various leads. Figure 2-93 is an actual 12-lead tracing from a patient suffering an acute anterior wall myocardial infarction. Figure 2-94 is an actual 12-lead ECG from a patient with an acute anterior wall myocardial infarction with lateral extension of the infarction (anterolateral MI). Finally, Figure 2-95 is an actual 12-lead tracing taken from a patient suffering an acute inferior wall (diaphragmatic) myocardial infarction. It is important to study and periodically review actual patient ECG tracings in order to learn the various pathological changes described in this text.

CONDUCTION ABNORMALITIES

Conduction abnormalities occur when there is a delay or blockage of a part or parts of the cardiac conductive system. Conduction abnormalities can be caused by disease, drugs, and various electrolyte abnormalities.

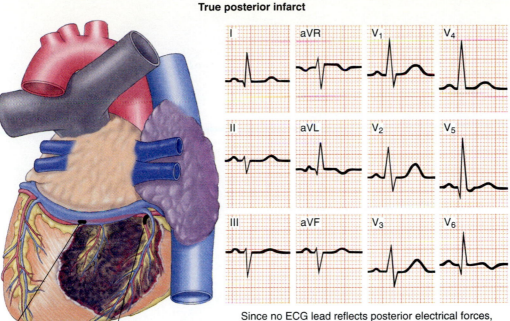

True posterior infarct

Since no ECG lead reflects posterior electrical forces, changes are reciprocal of those in anterior leads. Lead V$_1$ shows unusually large R wave (reciprocal of posterior Q wave) and upright T wave (reciprocal of posterior T wave inversion)

Occlusion of distal circumflex artery or Occlusion of posterior descending or distal right coronary arteries

FIGURE 2–92   True posterior infarct.

AV BLOCKS

AV heart blocks are some of the more common types of conduction abnormalities. AV blocks result from a delay in impulse transmission through the AV node from the atria to the ventricles.

- *First-Degree AV Block.* The simplest type of AV heart block is a first-degree AV block. In a first-degree AV block, there is a delay in transmission of the electrical impulse from the atria to the ventricles. This can be detected on the ECG by noting a PR interval of greater than 0.21 second. In a first-degree block, there is not a complete blockage of AV transmission, only a slowing of the impulse in the AV node.

- *Second-Degree AV Block (Mobitz I).* The next type of heart block is a second-degree AV block (Mobitz I). This unique type of block, also referred to as a Wenckebach phenomenon, involves a delay of impulse conduction at the AV node. Each impulse arriving at the AV junction is progressively delayed until, eventually, AV conduction is completely blocked. This results in failure of the impulse to be transmitted through to the ventricles. Typically, following the dropped beat, the cycle will repeat itself.

- *Second-Degree AV Block (Mobitz II).* A more severe form of AV heart block is a second-degree AV block (Mobitz II). In this block, certain of the impulses are conducted through the AV node while others are blocked. There is usually a recognized pattern in that one, two, or three impulses are conducted, and then one is blocked.

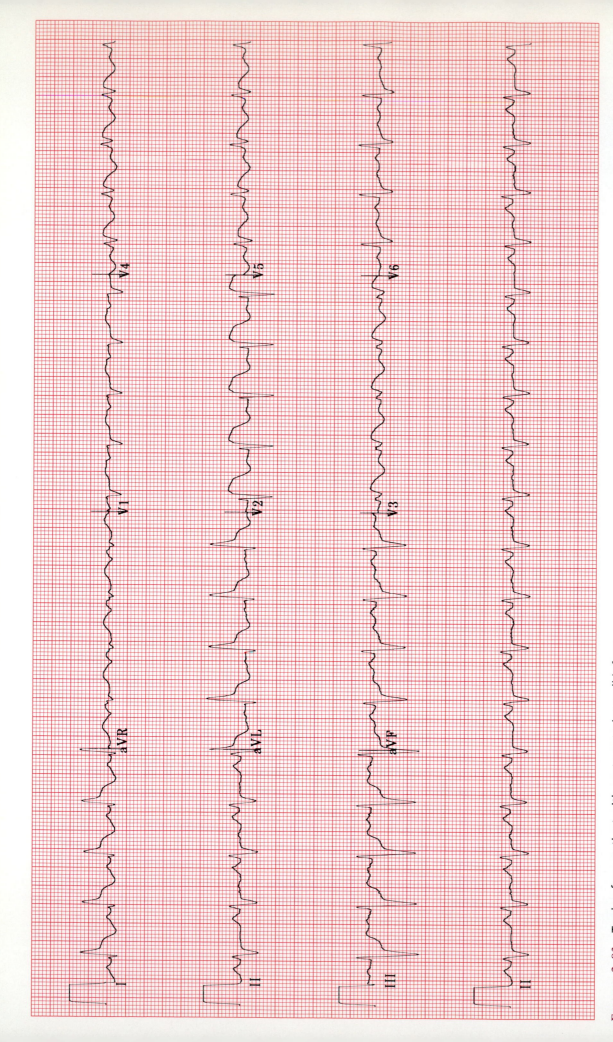

FIGURE 2–93 Tracing from patient with acute anterior wall infarct.

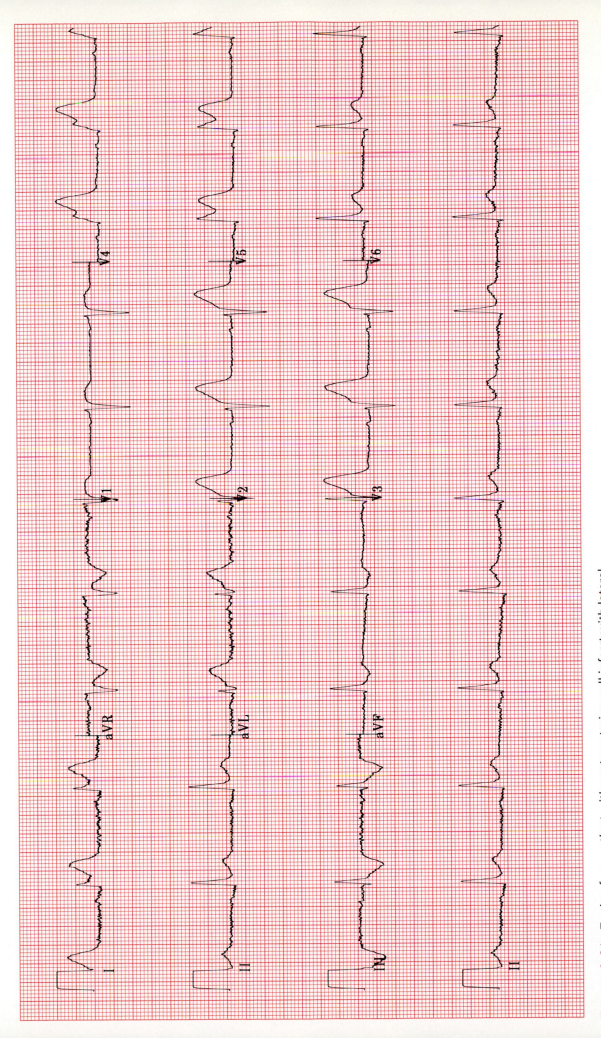

FIGURE 2–94 Tracing from patient with acute anterior wall infarct with lateral extension of the infarction (anterolateral infarct).

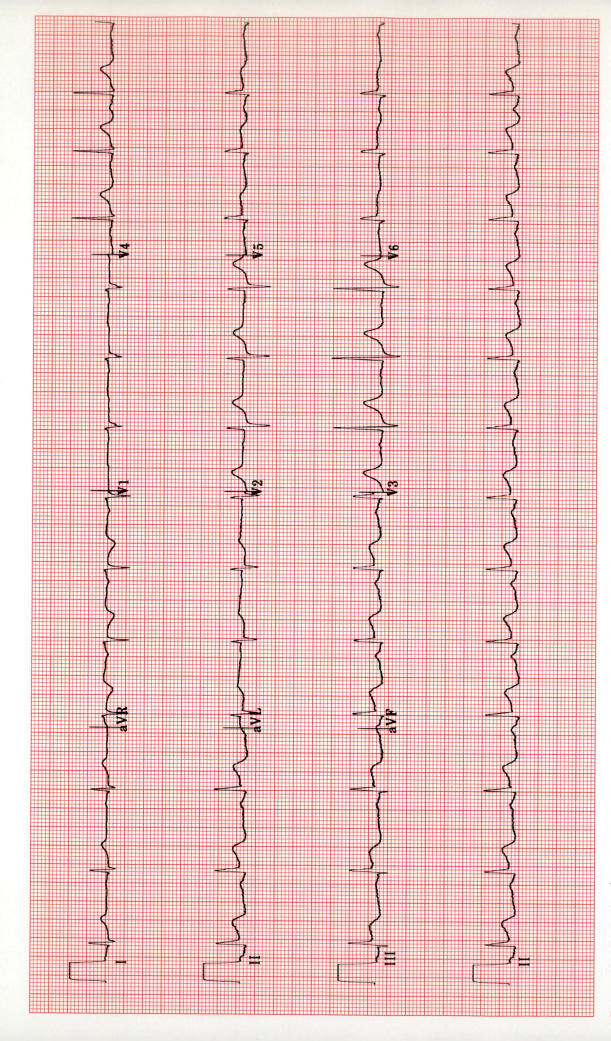

FIGURE 2–95   Tracing from a patient with acute inferior wall (diaphragmatic) infarct.

- *Third-Degree AV Block.* The most serious type of AV heart block is a third-degree AV block, also called a complete heart block. In a third-degree heart block, none of the impulses originating in the atria are conducted into the ventricles. This results in the atria and ventricles each having their own intrinsic rate. This can lead to severe bradycardia, heart failure, and in certain situations, cardiac arrest.

BUNDLE BRANCH BLOCKS

Conduction abnormalities are not limited to the AV node. Conduction defects can also occur in the right bundle branch, the left bundle branch, or even in one of the fascicles of the left bundle branch. AV blocks can be detected by single-lead monitoring. Bundle branch blocks, on the other hand, can be diagnosed only with a 12-lead tracing.

In a bundle branch block, ventricular depolarization is abnormal. The impulse will originate in the SA node, be transmitted through the internodal pathways, through the AV node, and into the bundle of His. After entering the bundle of His, the impulse is transmitted into the left and right bundle branches, and then into the Purkinje system. If the right bundle branch is blocked, the impulse will proceed down the left bundle branch. The block will prevent transmission of the impulse through the right bundle branch. The impulse must then spread from the left bundle branch, through the myocardial cells of the interventricular septum, and into the right ventricle. Likewise, blockage of the left bundle branch will cause the impulse to be spread from the right bundle branch, through the interventricular septum, and into the left ventricle.

In the case of a bundle branch block, the electrical forces traveling across the interventricular septum cannot utilize the rapid fibers of the ventricular conductive system. Because the impulse must be transmitted through the interventricular septum itself, from the functioning bundle branch to the side with the nonfunctioning bundle branch, depolarization of the affected ventricle will be delayed. This can be detected on the ECG as prolongation of the QRS complex of greater than or equal to 0.12 second. In addition, the delay in depolarization of the ventricle on the affected side can result in abnormal formation of the QRS complex.

The following discussion will address the common bundle branch blocks and hemiblocks.

- *Right Bundle Branch Block.* A right bundle branch block results from blockage of some portion of the right bundle branch. In this case, the impulse must continue down the left bundle branch and spread through the interventricular septum until the right ventricle is depolarized. This results in a delay of impulse transmission into the right ventricle causing a prolongation of the QRS complex (greater than or equal to 0.12 second). The right ventricle is a low pressure pump. Because of this, the right ventricular muscle mass is considerably smaller than the left. In the normal ECG, the electrical forces of the right ventricle are overshadowed by the more massive forces of the left ventricle. In the case of a right bundle branch block, right ventricular depolarization occurs after left ventricular depolarization. The vector of the right ventricular depolarization is rightward and anterior as compared to the left. This is because the impulse is spreading from the left ventricle to the right ventricle instead of the normal scenario where the right ventricle is stimulated by the right bundle branch.

  A complete right bundle branch block is typically characterized by a prolonged QRS complex of greater than or equal to 0.12 second. In addition, an abnormal late portion of the QRS is directed

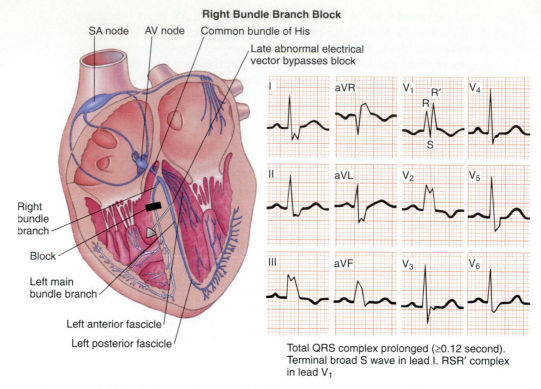

Right Bundle Branch Block

SA node AV node Common bundle of His

Late abnormal electrical vector bypasses block

Right bundle branch

Block

Left main bundle branch

Left anterior fascicle

Left posterior fascicle

I   aVR   V₁ R'   V₄
          R
          S

II   aVL   V₂   V₅

III aVF   V₃   V₆

Total QRS complex prolonged (≥0.12 second). Terminal broad S wave in lead I. RSR' complex in lead V₁

FIGURE 2–96   Right bundle branch block.

toward the right ventricle and away from the left ventricle. This typically appears as a broad S wave in Lead I. Also, a characteristic RSR′ (R-S-R prime) complex will be seen in Lead V₁ (Figure 2-96). The RSR′ (also called a "rabbit ear") reflects the abnormal septal depolarization and subsequent right ventricular depolarization. Lead V₁ lies immediately over the right ventricle and is a good lead for detecting right ventricular abnormalities.

Right bundle branch block is a rather common finding. It is a relatively thin bundle of fibers compared to the left bundle branch and is thus more susceptible to injury. Right bundle branch block can result from acute MI, drugs, electrolyte abnormalities, or general age-related deterioration of the cardiac conductive system.

- *Left Bundle Branch Block.* The left bundle branch is derived from the bundle of His. It subsequently divides into the anterior and posterior fascicles before it terminates in the Purkinje system of the left ventricle. When a left bundle branch block occurs, the left ventricle cannot be depolarized normally. Thus, the electrical impulse must be transmitted from the right ventricle, through the interventricular septum, and then into the left ventricle. As with a right bundle branch block, the depolarization impulse must spread through the interventricular septum without the aid of specialized conductive fibers. This causes a delay in impulse transmission through the interventricular septum and results in a prolongation of the QRS complex. Unlike a right bundle branch block, the direction of the forces in a left bundle branch block is from right to left, nearly the same as in the normal heart.

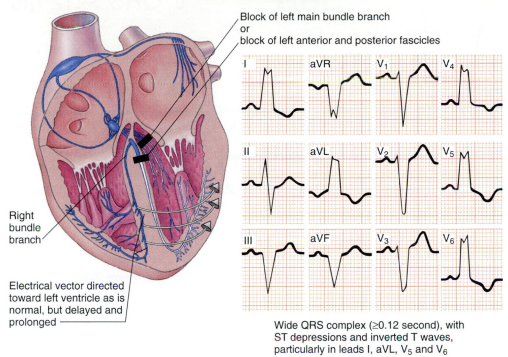

Left Bundle Branch Block

Block of left main bundle branch
or
block of left anterior and posterior fascicles

Right bundle branch

Electrical vector directed toward left ventricle as is normal, but delayed and prolonged

Wide QRS complex (≥0.12 second), with ST depressions and inverted T waves, particularly in leads I, aVL, V_5 and V_6

FIGURE 2–97   Left bundle branch block.

The QRS complexes in left bundle branch block are prolonged (greater than or equal to 0.12 second) and bizarre in appearance. Typically, wide, notched QRS complexes are seen in leads I, aVL, V_5 and V_6 (Figure 2-97). The changes are more pronounced in these leads, as they visualize the lateral aspect of the heart, which is principally the left ventricle. Deep S waves can be seen in lead V_1, V_2, or V_3 or tall R waves seen in lead I, aVL, V_5 and V_6 (as described previously).

A left bundle branch block usually indicates significant and widespread myocardial disease. Like the right bundle branch block, it too results from MI, drugs, electrolyte abnormalities, and degenerative disease of the conductive system. Most myocardial infarctions primarily affect the left ventricle. The presence of a left bundle branch block will mask ischemic changes associated with MI. Thus, a patient can suffer a significant MI, and ECG changes will not be seen because of the left bundle branch block. In fact, the presence of a left bundle branch block negates any chance of localizing an MI with a 12-lead ECG.

When a left bundle branch block is present, nothing else can be determined from the ECG in regard to ischemic changes.

An easier way to differentiate left and right bundle branch blocks is to apply the four steps of the turn-signal rule, which parallels the action of a vehicle's turn signal (Figure 2-98):

1. Determine that the QRS complex is consistently greater than .12 seconds throughout the ECG. You often can do this best by viewing the QRS duration of the precordial leads (V_1 through V_6).

2. Second, view the QRS of V_1. It lies immediately over the right ventricle and provides the best view of the superior aspect of the interventricular septum.

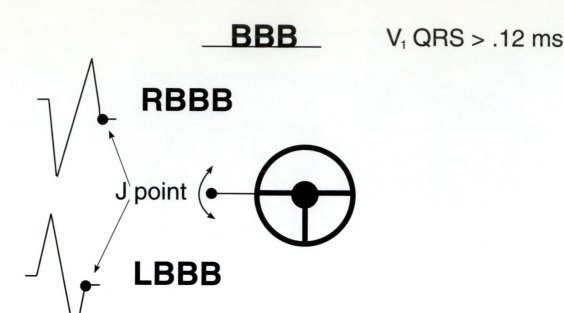

BBB V_1 QRS > .12 ms

RBBB

J point

LBBB

FIGURE 2–98   The turn-signal rule for differentiating right and left bundle branch blocks.

3. Identify the J point of the QRS, the junction between the end of the QRS and the beginning of the S-T segment.

4. Draw a horizontal line from the J point to an intersecting line of the QRS, or to the beginning of the QRS. This will produce a triangle pointing either up or down. If the triangle points up, it indicates a right bundle branch block. (If you push up a vehicle's turn signal, the signal lights indicate a right turn.) If the triangle points down, it indicates a left bundle branch block. (If you push down the turn signal lever, the lights indicate a left turn).

Detecting bundle branch blocks is important because left bundle branch blocks can mask ischemic changes associated with MI. Also some S-T elevation usually appears in the precordial leads with left bundle branch blocks, thus rendering 12-lead tracings useless in determining or localizing an MI.

- *Hemiblocks.* The left bundle branch divides into the left anterior and left posterior fascicles. Blocks can occur in either of these fascicles and are a fairly common finding.

  Left Posterior Hemiblock. A left posterior hemiblock, also called a left posterior fascicular block, results from blockage of the left posterior fascicle. Blockage of the left posterior fascicle results in a delay in depolarizing the portion of the left ventricle it innervates. A left posterior hemiblock does not typically prolong the QRS interval. In addition, the shape of the QRS complex remains relatively normal. The principal finding in a left posterior hemiblock is a rightward shift in the QRS axis. This is often difficult to diagnose, particularly if there is underlying right ventricular or pulmonary disease. Generally, the QRS axis must be greater than or equal to +120° to consider a left posterior hemiblock (Figure 2-99). Left posterior hemiblock is usually due to degenerative disease of the conductive system or ischemic heart disease.

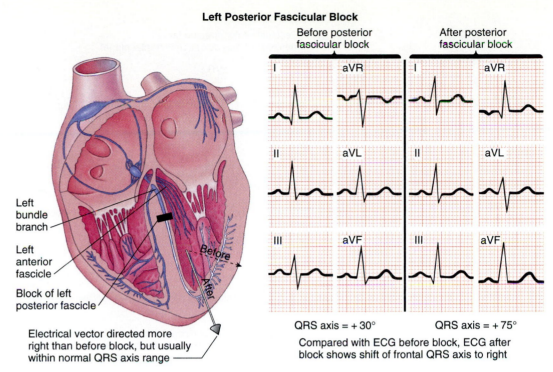

Left Posterior Fascicular Block

Before posterior fascicular block

After posterior fascicular block

I aVR I aVR

II aVL II aVL

III aVF III aVF

Left bundle branch

Left anterior fascicle

Block of left posterior fascicle

Before

After

Electrical vector directed more right than before block, but usually within normal QRS axis range

QRS axis = + 30°

QRS axis = + 75°

Compared with ECG before block, ECG after block shows shift of frontal QRS axis to right

FIGURE 2–99   Left posterior hemiblock (left posterior fascicular block).

Left Anterior Hemiblock. A left anterior hemiblock, also called a left anterior fascicular block, results from blockage of the left anterior fascicle. This block is similar to a bundle branch block, but it does *not* result in a delay in ventricular depolarization. Thus, the QRS complex is of normal duration and is generally of normal shape, without the unusual notching seen in the bundle branch blocks. The principal abnormality in a left anterior hemiblock is a shift in the QRS axis far to the left (typically more negative than −30°). This results in a negative QRS complex in Leads II, III, and aVF (Figure 2-100). A left anterior hemiblock is usually caused by degeneration of the cardiac conductive system or ischemic heart disease. It is usually a benign finding.

Figure 2-101 is an actual tracing from a patient with a left bundle branch block. Figure 2-102 is an actual tracing from a patient with a complete right bundle branch block. Both are common findings in 12-lead ECG interpretation. Remember, a left bundle branch block renders the ECG relatively useless for detecting injury or ischemia.

CHAMBER ENLARGEMENT

Although chamber enlargement rarely affects prehospital care, you should understand the condition's basic pathophysiology because it often can appear on a 12-lead ECG tracing and cause misleading patterns of ischemia.

Chamber enlargement may involve right atrial enlargement, right ventricular hypertrophy, left atrial enlargement, or left ventricular hypertrophy. **Hypertrophy** simply means enlargement without any additional cells—basically, stretching. As a rule, right atrial enlargement (RAE) is a precursor to right ventricular hypertrophy (RVH), and left atrial enlargement (LAE) is a precursor to left ventricular hypertrophy (LVH). The most common cause of chamber enlargement is disease.

✳ **hypertrophy** stretching; enlargment without any additional cells.

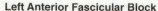

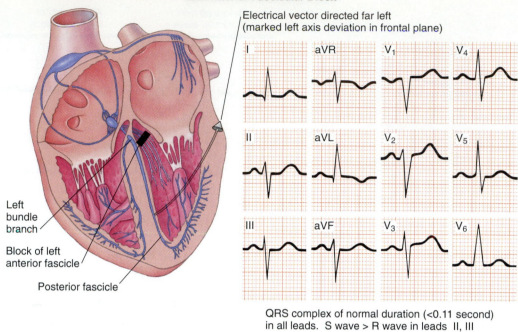

Left Anterior Fascicular Block

Electrical vector directed far left
(marked left axis deviation in frontal plane)

Left bundle branch

Block of left anterior fascicle

Posterior fascicle

QRS complex of normal duration (<0.11 second)
in all leads. S wave > R wave in leads II, III
and aVF (marked left axis deviation)

FIGURE 2–100   Left anterior hemiblock (left anterior fascicular block).

Any disease that causes long-term increased pressure in any of the heart's four chambers can cause chamber enlargement. RAE and RVH are usually caused by pulmonary disease such as COPD or emphysema. LAE and LVH are generally caused by long-term hypertension, especially if it is untreated or poorly managed.

Because the P wave represents atrial depolarization, atrial enlargement appears in the P-wave formation. The first half of the P wave, which represents right atrial depolarization, is normally rounded like a quarter-circle. The second half of the P wave, which represents left atrial depolarization, is likewise normally rounded like a quarter-circle. Right atrial enlargement appears on the 12-lead as a tall, spiked beginning of the P wave—greater than 2 mm (2 small boxes). Left atrial enlargement appears as a biphasic, widened P wave of 2.5 mm (2 1/2 small boxes). Leads II, aVL, V_1, and V_2 offer the best views of both right and left atrial enlargement (Figure 2-103).

Ventricular chamber enlargement appears in the QRS complex, which represents ventricular depolarization. Abnormally deep S waves or tall waves in the precordial leads suggest RVH or LVH. RVH generally appears as an R wave more than 7 mm tall, with a right axis deviation (RAD). To detect LVH, add the heights of the deeper S wave of V_1 or V_2 and the taller R wave of V_5 or V_6. A sum equal to or greater than 35 mm indicates LVH. Recognizing LVH is important because its S-T pattern often mimics the S-T segment elevation pattern of tissue injury (Figure 2-104).

Echocardiography is the standard method for detecting and diagnosing chamber enlargement, but 12-lead monitors programmed with internal interpretive capabilities often will detect this condition. They use complex algorithms to detect numerous, detailed and specific wave patterns in multiple leads. At best, however, the 12-lead can detect only 50 percent of chamber enlargement conditions. Nonetheless, recognizing chamber enlargement on a 12-lead tracing is important because it can give you a better insight into the extent of a patient's hypertension or COPD and because LVH can mimic the S-T segment pattern of injury.

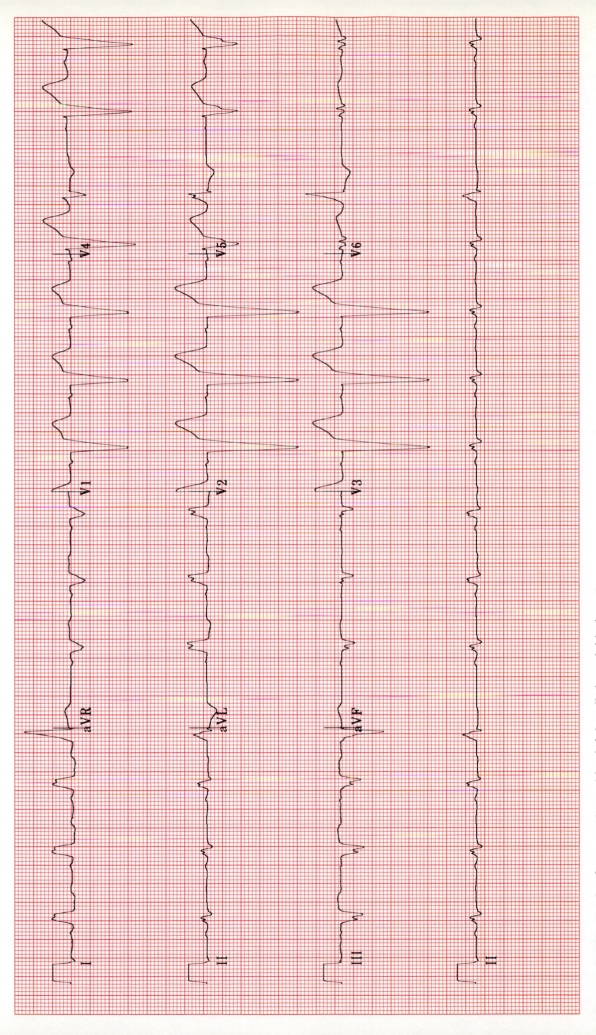

FIGURE 2–101   Tracing from a patient with a left bundle branch block.

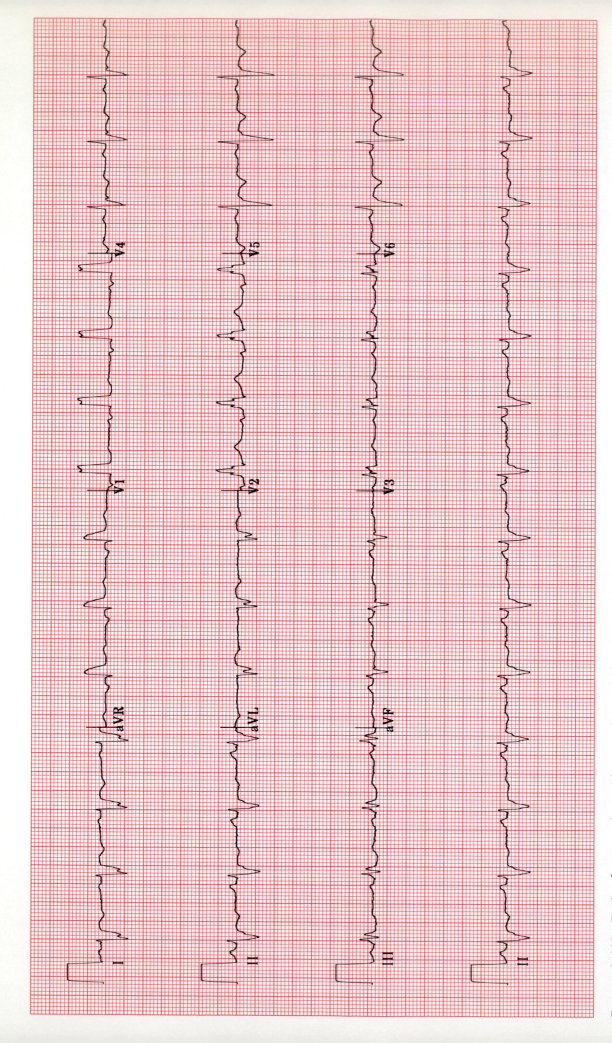

FIGURE 2–102 Tracing from a patient with a complete right bundle branch block.

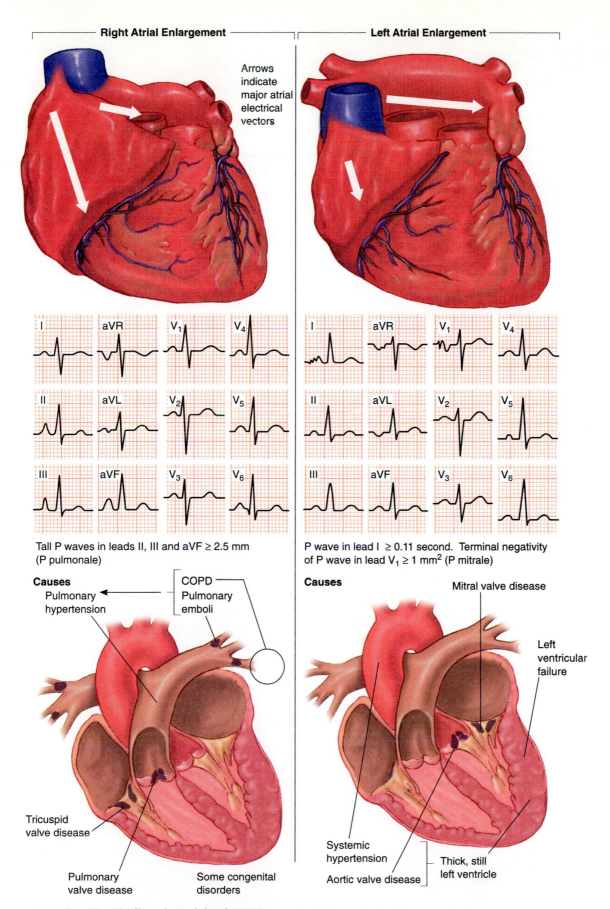

Right Atrial Enlargement

Left Atrial Enlargement

Arrows indicate major atrial electrical vectors

Tall P waves in leads II, III and aVF ≥ 2.5 mm (P pulmonale)

P wave in lead I ≥ 0.11 second. Terminal negativity of P wave in lead V_1 ≥ 1 mm^2 (P mitrale)

Causes

Pulmonary hypertension

COPD
Pulmonary emboli

Tricuspid valve disease

Pulmonary valve disease

Some congenital disorders

Causes

Mitral valve disease

Left ventricular failure

Systemic hypertension

Aortic valve disease

Thick, still left ventricle

FIGURE 2–103   Findings in atrial enlargment.

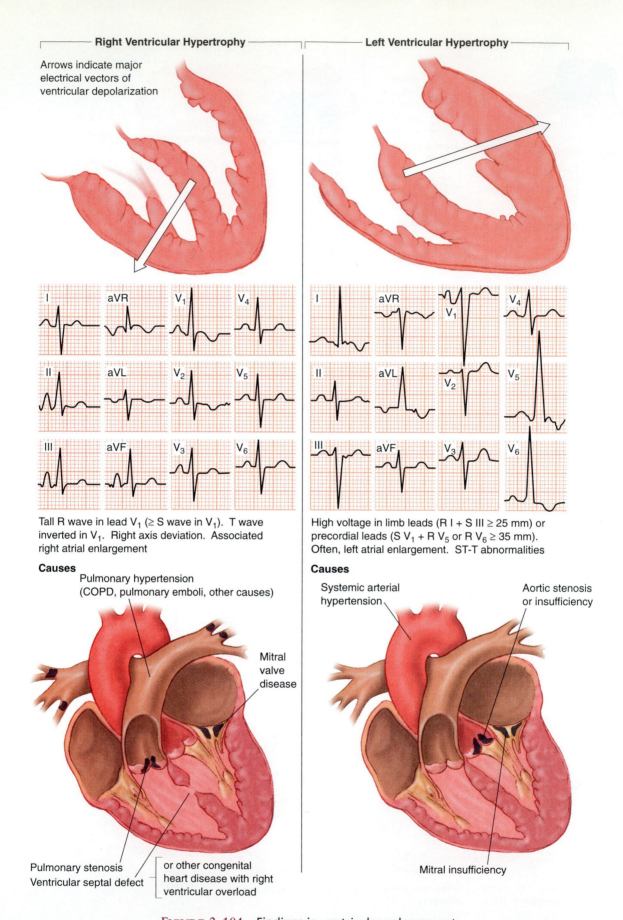

Right Ventricular Hypertrophy

Arrows indicate major electrical vectors of ventricular depolarization

I aVR V_1 V_4

II aVL V_2 V_5

III aVF V_3 V_6

Tall R wave in lead V_1 ($\geq$ S wave in V_1). T wave inverted in V_1. Right axis deviation. Associated right atrial enlargement

Causes

Pulmonary hypertension (COPD, pulmonary emboli, other causes)

Mitral valve disease

Pulmonary stenosis
Ventricular septal defect — or other congenital heart disease with right ventricular overload

Left Ventricular Hypertrophy

I aVR V_1 V_4

II aVL V_2 V_5

III aVF V_3 V_6

High voltage in limb leads (R I + S III $\geq$ 25 mm) or precordial leads (S V_1 + R V_5 or R $V_6 \geq$ 35 mm). Often, left atrial enlargement. ST-T abnormalities

Causes

Systemic arterial hypertension

Aortic stenosis or insufficiency

Mitral insufficiency

FIGURE 2–104 Findings in ventricular enlargement.

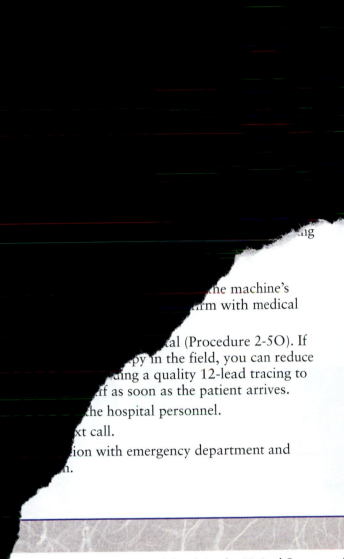

...ng

...he machine's
...rm with medical

...al (Procedure 2-5O). If
...py in the field, you can reduce
...ding a quality 12-lead tracing to
...ff as soon as the patient arrives.

...he hospital personnel.

...xt call.

...ion with emergency department and
...

...is the number one cause of death in the United States and
...s from heart attack occur within the first twenty-four
...thin the first hour. With the advent of thrombolytic ther-
...sence when managing the patient with suspected ischemic
...plays an ever-increasing role in the early recognition of pa-
...nary ischemia. In certain areas, EMS provides definitive care
...bolytic therapy in the field. This is especially important in
...ort times can be long. With cardiovascular disease, EMS can
...rence between life and death.

THE CALL

...artner on Medic 3 are dispatched to a well-kept residence
...cks from the station. The dispatch information relates the na-
...medical emergency. Upon your arrival at the residence, the
...you and shows you to a back room. The patient is a male

PREHOSPITAL ECG MONITORING

Technology has evolved to a point where portable 12-lead ECG monitoring is readily available. Many manufacturers now make 12-lead machines for prehospital care. Most machines have sophisticated electronics, many with ECG diagnostic packages. Some now have a defibrillator/pacer unit (Figure 2-105). The principles of 12-lead monitoring are similar to those for routine ECG monitoring described earlier in this chapter.

PREHOSPITAL 12-LEAD ECG MONITORING

The following skill sequence details 12-lead prehospital ECG monitoring.

1. Explain what you are going to do to the patient. Reassure him or her that the machine will not shock him.
2. Prepare all of the equipment and assure the cable is in good repair. Check to make sure there are adequate leads and materials for prepping the skin.
3. Prep the skin (Procedure 2-5A). Dirt, oil, sweat, and other materials on the skin can interfere with obtaining a quality tracing. The skin should be cleansed with an appropriate substance. If the patient is diaphoretic, dry the skin with a towel. On very hot days or in situations where the patient is very diaphoretic, tincture of Benzoin can be applied to the skin before attaching the electrode. Occasionally, it may be necessary to slightly abrade the skin to obtain a good interface. Patients with a lot of body hair may need to have the area immediately over the electrode site shaved to assure good skin/electrode interface.
4. Place the four limb leads according to the manufacturer's recommendations (Procedure 2-5B).
5. Following placement of the limb leads, prepare for placement of the precordial leads. Procedure 2-5C illustrates proper placement of the precordial leads.
6. First, place Lead V_1 by attaching the positive electrode to the right of the sternum at the fourth intercostal space (Procedure 2-5D.)

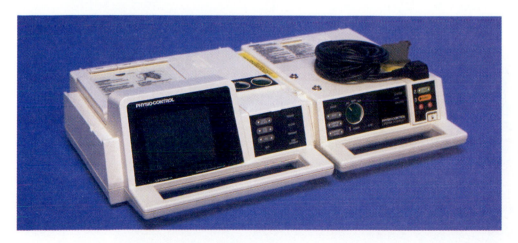

FIGURE 2–105 Prehospital 12-lead monitor.

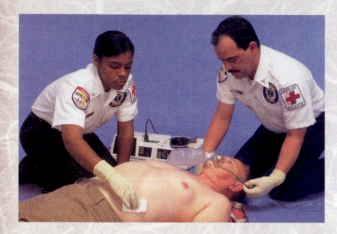

2–5a   Prep the skin.

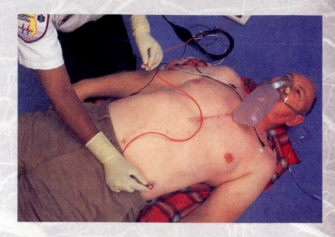

2–5b   Place the four limb leads according to the manufacturer's recommendations.

2–5g   Place lead V₃.

Lead V₁ The electrode is at the fourth intercostal space just to the right of the sternum.
Lead V₂ The electrode is at the fourth intercostal space just to the left of the sternum.
Lead V₃ The electrode is at the line midway between leads V₂ and V₄.
Lead V₄ The electrode is at the midclavicular line in the fifth interspace.
Lead V₅ The electrode is at the anterior axillary line at the same level as lead V₄.
Lead V₆ The electrode is at the midaxillary line at the same level as lead V₄.

Angle of Louis

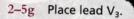

V₁ V₂ V₃ V₄ V₅ V₆

Chest Lead Placement

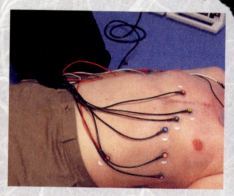

2–5j   Ensure that all leads are attached.

2–5k   Turn on the

2–5c   Proper placement of the precordial leads.

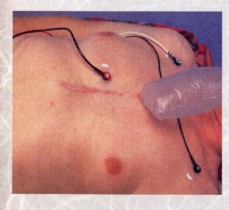

2–5d   Place lead V₁.

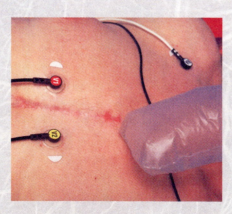

2–5e   Place lead V₂.

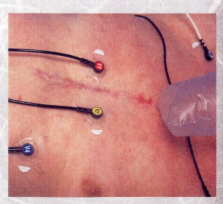

2–5f   Place lead V₄.

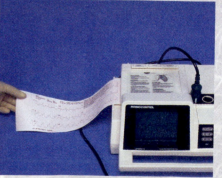

2–5m   Record the tracing.

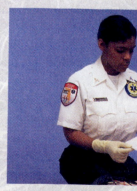

2–5n   Examine the traci

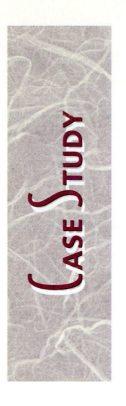
Linda applies the pulse oximeter. The patient appears well-oxygenated with an SpO₂ of 99% on the nonrebreather mask. Jack and Linda move the patient to a stretcher, being careful to protect the paralyzed extremity. They load the patient into the ambulance and transport him to the nearest emergency department with a "brain attack team."

Upon arrival at the emergency department, the patient's condition remains unchanged. His airway remains patent and his symptoms persist. A routine laboratory profile is normal. Because the patient has a hemiparesis and is unable to speak, the emergency physician orders a computed tomography (CT) scan of the brain. A neuroradiologist reads the CT scan and reports no evidence of hemorrhage in the brain. The brain attack team is consulted. They feel that thrombolytic therapy is indicated and tPA is started in the emergency department. The patient is then admitted to the neurologic intensive care unit.

Following thrombolytic therapy, the patient recovers his speech, and most of his right-sided weakness is alleviated. Several days later, the patient is discharged to the rehabilitation unit.

INTRODUCTION

Nervous system conditions and diseases affect millions of lives in the United States. Strokes attack a half million people every year, of whom 150,000 die. Epilepsy affects 2.5 million people, or approximately one percent of the U.S. population. An additional 50,000 Americans are diagnosed with Parkinson's disease each year. These are only a few examples of the impact of nervous system disorders. Millions of people are also affected by headache, multiple sclerosis, syncope, neoplasm, and other nervous system emergencies, all of which you will learn about in this chapter.

Many conditions, diseases, and injuries can cause nervous system disorders. Such disorders may be caused by internal or external factors. Modern advances and clinical studies continue to yield new medications and treatments for many conditions. Paramedics should maintain a solid knowledge of the nervous system and remain familiar with current trends and advancements in treating the neurological patient.

This chapter provides an overview of the common neurological conditions that may be encountered in the prehospital setting. It discusses the relevant anatomy and physiology of the nervous system, assessment techniques, and the recommended prehospital management.

ANATOMY AND PHYSIOLOGY

The nervous system is the body's control system.

The nervous system is the body's principal control system. This network of cells, tissues, and organs regulates nearly all bodily functions via electrical impulses transmitted through nerves, all of which are highly susceptible to hypoxia. The endocrine system is closely related to the nervous system. It exerts bodily control via hormones. You will learn more about this system in the next chapter. A third

Objectives Continued

5. Describe and differentiate the major types of seizures. (pp. 295–296)
6. Describe the phases of a generalized seizure. (pp. 295–296)
7. Define the following:
   a. Muscular dystrophy (p. 304)
   b. Multiple sclerosis (p. 304)
   c. Dystonia (p. 305)
   d. Parkinson's disease (p. 305)
   e. Trigeminal neuralgia (pp. 305–306)
   f. Bell's palsy (p. 306)
   g. Amyotrophic lateral sclerosis (p. 306)
   h. Peripheral neuropathy (pp. 276–277)
   i. Myoclonus (p. 306)
   j. Spina bifida (p. 306)
   k. Poliomyelitis (pp. 306–307)

8. Define and discuss the pathophysiology, assessment findings, and management for nontraumatic spinal injury, including:
   a. Low back pain (p. 308)
   b. Herniated intervertebral disk (p. 308)
   c. Spinal cord tumors (p. 309)
9. Differentiate between neurologic emergencies based on assessment findings. (pp. 277–286)
10. Given several preprogrammed nontraumatic neurological emergency patients, provide the appropriate assessment, management, and transport. (pp. 262–310)

CASE STUDY

A call is received by paramedic Engine Company 201 and Ambulance 68 for a "possible stroke patient." Dispatch reports that the patient is a male in his 60s with reported right-sided weakness and inability to speak. He is being assisted by bystanders in the lobby of a local bank. The response time is approximately 3 minutes. Upon arrival, the bank manager leads paramedics Jack Tory and Linda Alvarez to a corner area of the lobby where they see an elderly male sitting in a chair and being held upright by bystanders.

Jack and Linda quickly perform an initial assessment. Although unable to speak, the patient appears to be alert and cooperative. His airway is patent. His respiratory rate is 18 breaths per minute and regular. His pulse is 88 beats per minute and strong. The blood pressure is 160/90 mmHg taken in the left arm (because of the weakness in his right arm). The patient's skin is warm and dry, yet pale. The blood glucose level is 80 mg/dl. He has marked right-sided weakness but otherwise appears to be well nourished and in good overall health.

Jack quickly administers oxygen via a nonrebreather mask while Linda obtains a more detailed medical history from the patient's family. Linda places a heparin lock in the patient's left forearm while Jack places the ECG leads and turns on the monitor. The patient exhibits atrial fibrillation with a rate of 90.

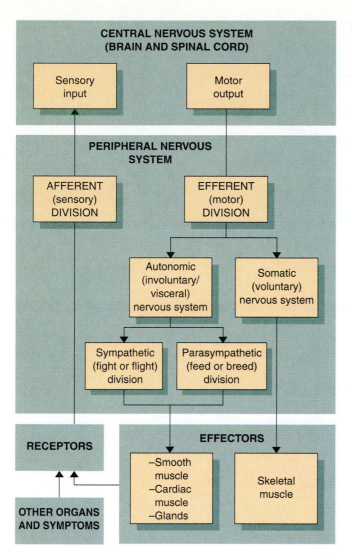

FIGURE 3-1 Overview of the nervous system.

CENTRAL NERVOUS SYSTEM (BRAIN AND SPINAL CORD)

Sensory input

Motor output

PERIPHERAL NERVOUS SYSTEM

AFFERENT (sensory) DIVISION

EFFERENT (motor) DIVISION

Autonomic (involuntary/ visceral) nervous system

Somatic (voluntary) nervous system

Sympathetic (fight or flight) division

Parasympathetic (feed or breed) division

RECEPTORS

EFFECTORS

OTHER ORGANS AND SYMPTOMS

–Smooth muscle
–Cardiac muscle
–Glands

Skeletal muscle

* **central nervous system** the brain and the spinal cord.

* **peripheral nervous system** part of the nervous system that extends throughout the body and is composed of the cranial nerves arising from the brain and the peripheral nerves arising from the spinal cord. Its subdivisions are the somatic and the autonomic nervous systems.

* **somatic nervous system** part of the nervous system controlling voluntary bodily functions.

* **autonomic nervous system** part of the nervous system controlling involuntary bodily functions. It is divided into the sympathetic and the parasympathetic systems.

* **sympathetic nervous system** division of the autonomic nervous system that prepares the body for stressful situations. Sympathetic nervous system actions include increased heart rate and dilation of the bronchioles and pupils. Its actions are mediated by the neurotransmitters epinephrine and norepinephrine.

* **parasympathetic nervous system** division of the autonomic nervous system that is responsible for controlling vegetative functions. Parasympathetic nervous system actions include decreased heart rate and constriction of the bronchioles and pupils. Its actions are mediated by the neurotransmitter acetylcholine.

system, the circulatory system, assists in regulatory functions by distributing hormones and other chemical messengers.

The nervous system consists of two main divisions—the central nervous system and the peripheral nervous system. The **central nervous system** consists of the brain and the spinal cord. The **peripheral nervous system** is somewhat more complex. As you look at Figure 3-1, note that the peripheral nervous system is divided into two major subdivisions—the **somatic nervous system**, which governs voluntary functions (those we control consciously), and the **autonomic nervous system** which has two subdivisions—the **sympathetic nervous system** and the **parasympathetic nervous system**. These two subdivisions of the autonomic nervous system work together to carry out involuntary physiological processes such as regulation of blood pressure, heart rate, and digestion.

You will learn more about these divisions of the nervous system as you continue through this chapter. As you read, it will be helpful if you think of the nervous system as a "living computer." The central nervous system is the central processing unit and the various divisions of the peripheral nervous system carry on the input and output processes.

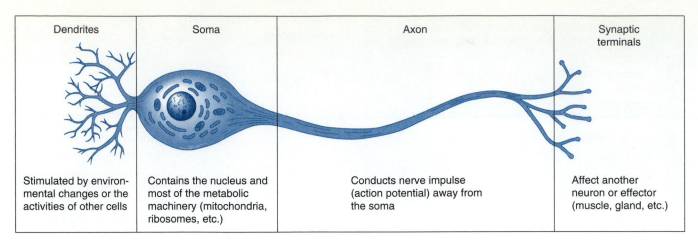

Dendrites	Soma	Axon	Synaptic terminals
Stimulated by environmental changes or the activities of other cells	Contains the nucleus and most of the metabolic machinery (mitochondria, ribosomes, etc.)	Conducts nerve impulse (action potential) away from the soma	Affect another neuron or effector (muscle, gland, etc.)

FIGURE 3-2   Anatomy of a neuron.

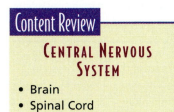

Content Review

CENTRAL NERVOUS SYSTEM

• Brain
• Spinal Cord

✱ **neuron** nerve cell; the fundamental component of the nervous system.

✱ **neurotransmitter** a substance that is released from the axon terminal of a presynaptic neuron upon excitation and that travels across the synaptic cleft to either excite or inhibit the target cell. Examples include acetylcholine, norepinephrine, and dopamine.

THE CENTRAL NERVOUS SYSTEM

Knowledge of the anatomy and physiology of the central nervous system is essential to understanding and treating nervous system emergencies.

Basic Unit—The Neuron

The fundamental unit of the nervous system is the nerve cell, or **neuron.** The neuron includes the *cell body* (soma), containing the nucleus; the *dendrites,* which transmit electrical impulses to the cell body; and the *axons,* which transmit electrical impulses away from the cell body (Figure 3-2).

The transmission of impulses in the nervous system resembles the conduction of electrical impulses through the heart. In its resting state, the neuron is positively charged on the outside and negatively charged on the inside. When electrically stimulated, sodium rapidly surges into the cell and potassium rapidly leaves it so that there is no longer a difference in electrical charge between the inside and the outside. This "depolarization," or loss of the charge difference, is subsequently transmitted down the neuron at an extremely high rate of speed.

The neuron joins with other neurons at junctions called *synapses* (Figure 3-3). The neurons never come into direct contact with each other at these synapses. Instead, upon reaching the synapse, the axon causes the release of a chemical **neurotransmitter.** This neurotransmitter, either acetylcholine or norepinephrine, then crosses the gap between the axon of the depolarized neuron and the dendrite of the adjacent neuron. The neurotransmitter stimulates the post-synaptic membrane of the connecting nerve. Acetylcholine is the neurotransmitter of the parasympathetic and voluntary (somatic) nervous systems. Norepinephrine is found in the synaptic terminals of sympathetic nerves.

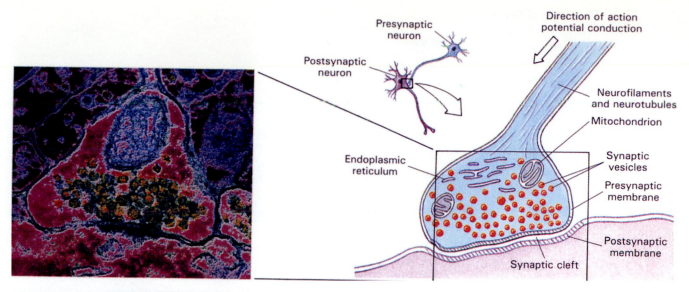

FIGURE 3-3 The synapse: (a) electron micrograph, (b) schematic.

Protective Structures

Most of the central nervous system is protected by bony structures. The brain lies within the cranial vault, protected by the skull. Covered by the scalp, the cranium consists of the bones of the head, excluding the facial bones. Bones composing the cranium include two single bones—the frontal and occipital bones—and a series of paired bones—the parietal, temporal, sphenoids, and ethmoids (Figure 3-4).

A total of 33 bones comprise the spine. They include 7 cervical vertebra, 12 thoracic vertebra, 5 lumbar vertebra, 5 sacral vertebra, and 4 coccygeal vertebra. The spinal cord is housed inside and is protected by the "spinal canal" formed by these bones (Figure 3-5).

Protective membranes called the **meninges** cover the entire central nervous system. There are three layers of meninges that pad, or cushion, the brain and spinal cord (Figure 3-6). The durable, outermost layer is referred to as the **dura mater**. The middle layer is a web-like structure known as the **arachnoid membrane**. The innermost layer, directly overlying the central nervous system, is called the **pia mater**. The space between the pia mater and the arachnoid membrane is referred to as the subarachnoid space, while the space between the dura mater and the arachnoid membrane is called the subdural space. The space outside the dura mater is called the epidural space. Both the brain and the spinal cord are bathed in **cerebrospinal fluid,** a watery, clear fluid that acts as a cushion to protect these organs from physical impact.

The Brain

The brain is the largest part of the central nervous system. The following information provides a general profile of the brain's anatomy and physiology.

✱ **meninges** membranes covering and protecting the brain and spinal cord. They consist of the pia mater, arachnoid membrane, and dura mater.

✱ **dura mater** tough outermost layer of the meninges.

✱ **arachnoid membrane** middle layer of the meninges.

✱ **pia mater** delicate innermost layer of the meninges.

✱ **cerebrospinal fluid** watery, clear fluid that acts as a cushion, protecting the brain and spinal cord from physical impact. The cerebrospinal fluid also serves as an accessory circulatory system for the central nervous system.

FIGURE 3-4 The bones of the skull.

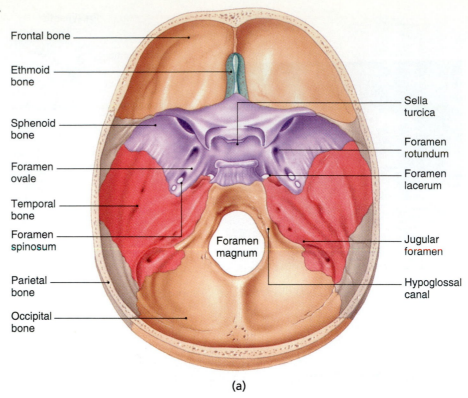

Frontal bone

Ethmoid bone

Sphenoid bone

Foramen ovale

Temporal bone

Foramen spinosum

Parietal bone

Occipital bone

Sella turcica

Foramen rotundum

Foramen lacerum

Foramen magnum

Jugular foramen

Hypoglossal canal

(a)

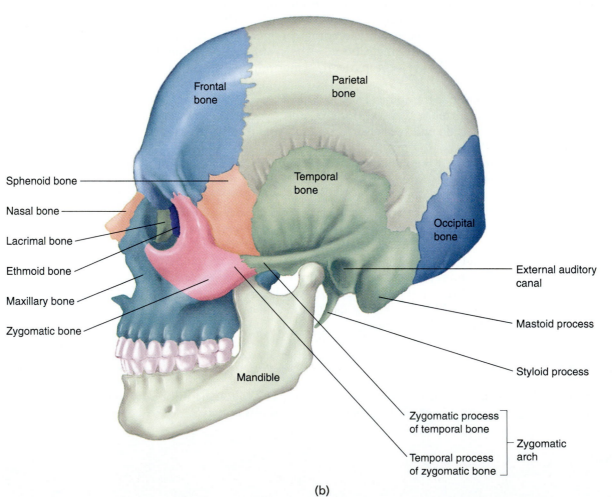

Frontal bone

Parietal bone

Sphenoid bone

Nasal bone

Lacrimal bone

Ethmoid bone

Maxillary bone

Zygomatic bone

Temporal bone

Occipital bone

External auditory canal

Mastoid process

Styloid process

Mandible

Zygomatic process of temporal bone

Temporal process of zygomatic bone

Zygomatic arch

(b)

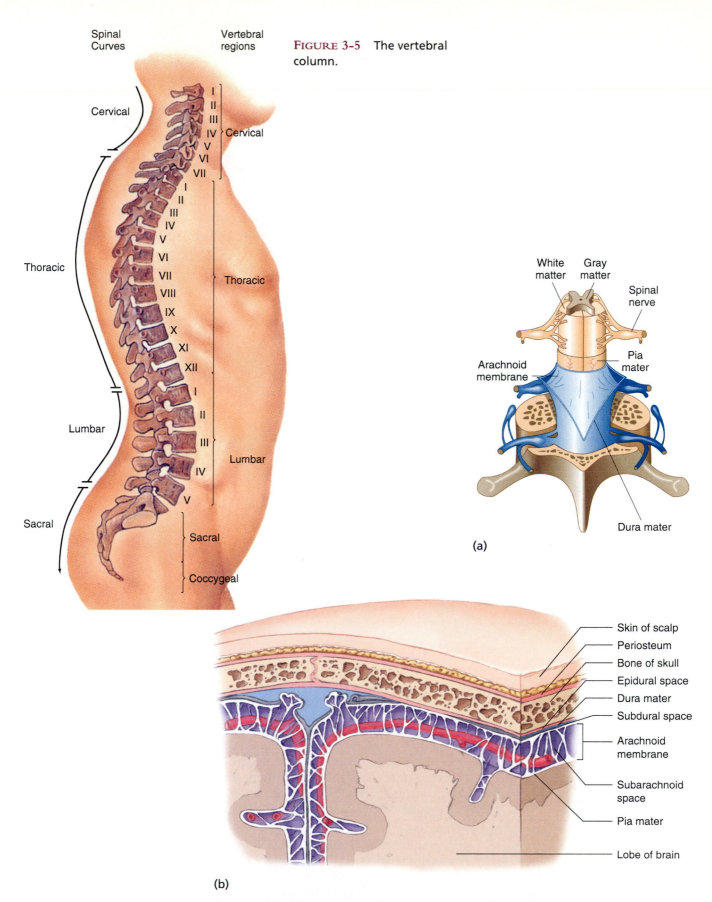

Spinal Curves

Cervical

Thoracic

Lumbar

Sacral

Vertebral regions

I
II
III
IV } Cervical
V
VI
VII

I
II
III
IV
V
VI
VII Thoracic
VIII
IX
X
XI
XII

I
II
III Lumbar
IV
V

} Sacral

} Coccygeal

FIGURE 3-5   The vertebral column.

White matter   Gray matter

Spinal nerve

Arachnoid membrane

Pia mater

Dura mater

(a)

Skin of scalp
Periosteum
Bone of skull
Epidural space
Dura mater
Subdural space
Arachnoid membrane
Subarachnoid space
Pia mater
Lobe of brain

(b)

FIGURE 3-6   The meninges: (a) posterior view of the spinal cord showing the meningeal layers; (b) the meninges of the brain.

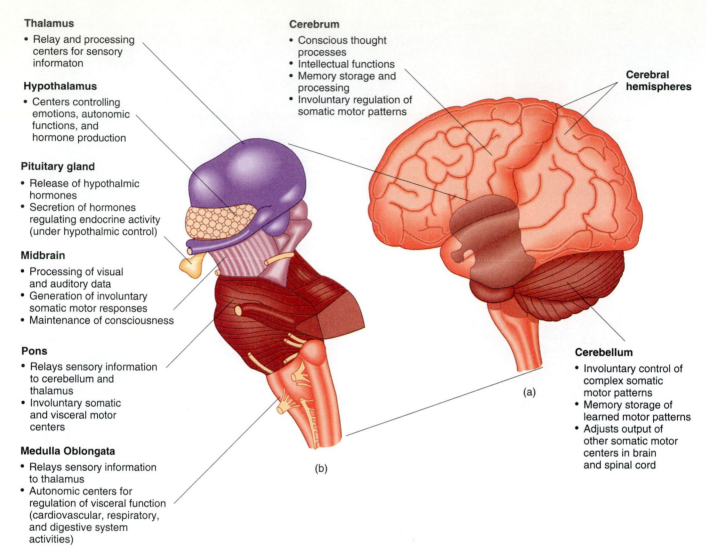

Thalamus
- Relay and processing centers for sensory informaton

Hypothalamus
- Centers controlling emotions, autonomic functions, and hormone production

Pituitary gland
- Release of hypothalmic hormones
- Secretion of hormones regulating endocrine activity (under hypothalmic control)

Midbrain
- Processing of visual and auditory data
- Generation of involuntary somatic motor responses
- Maintenance of consciousness

Pons
- Relays sensory information to cerebellum and thalamus
- Involuntary somatic and visceral motor centers

Medulla Oblongata
- Relays sensory information to thalamus
- Autonomic centers for regulation of visceral function (cardiovascular, respiratory, and digestive system activities)

Cerebrum
- Conscious thought processes
- Intellectual functions
- Memory storage and processing
- Involuntary regulation of somatic motor patterns

Cerebral hemispheres

Cerebellum
- Involuntary control of complex somatic motor patterns
- Memory storage of learned motor patterns
- Adjusts output of other somatic motor centers in brain and spinal cord

(a)

(b)

FIGURE 3-7   The human brain: (a) superficial view of the brain; (b) components of the brainstem.

✱ **cerebrum** largest part of the brain, consisting of two hemispheres. The cerebrum is the seat of consciousness and the center of the higher mental functions such as memory, learning, reasoning, judgement, intelligence, and the emotions.

✱ **diencephalon** portion of the brain lying beneath the cerebrum and above the brainstem. It contains the thalamus, hypothalamus, and the limbic system.

Divisions of the Brain Filling the cranial vault, the brain is divided into six major parts: the cerebrum, the diencephalon, the mesencephalon (midbrain), the pons, the medulla oblongata, and the cerebellum (Figure 3-7).

The cerebrum and diencephalon constitute the *forebrain*.

- *Cerebrum*. The **cerebrum** is in the anterior and middle area of the cranium. Containing two hemispheres, it is joined by a structure called the *corpus callosum*. The cerebrum governs all sensory and motor actions. It is the seat of intelligence, learning, analysis, memory, and language. The *cerebral cortex* is the outermost layer of the cerebrum.

- *Diencephalon*. Covered by the cerebrum, the **diencephalon** is sometimes called the *interbrain*. Inside it are the *thalamus, hypothalamus* (which is connected to the pituitary gland), and the *limbic system*. This area is responsible for many involuntary actions such as temperature regulation, sleep, water balance, stress response, and emotions. It plays a major role in regulating the autonomic nervous system.

The mesencephalon (midbrain), pons, and the medulla oblongata collectively form the **brainstem.** The brainstem and the cerebellum together constitute the *hindbrain.*

- *Mesencephalon, or midbrain.* The **mesencephalon,** located between the diencephalon and the pons, is responsible for certain aspects of motor coordination. The mesencephalon is the major region controlling eye movement.
- *Pons.* Between the midbrain and the medulla oblongata, the **pons** contains connections between the brain and the spinal cord.
- *Medulla Oblongata.* The **medulla oblongata** is located between the pons and the spinal cord. It marks the division between the spinal cord and the brain. Located here are major centers for controlling respiration, cardiac activity, and vasomotor activity.
- *Cerebellum.* The **cerebellum** is located in the posterior fossa of the cranial cavity. It consists of two hemispheres closely related to the brainstem and higher centers. The cerebellum coordinates fine motor movement, posture, equilibrium, and muscle tone.

Areas of Specialization Several areas of specialization are recognized within the brain and have clinical application (Figure 3-8). These include:

- *Speech.* Located in the temporal lobe of the cerebrum.
- *Vision.* Located in the occipital cortex of the cerebrum.
- *Personality.* Located in the frontal lobes of the cerebrum.
- *Balance and Coordination.* Located in the cerebellum.
- *Sensory.* Located in the parietal lobes of the cerebrum.
- *Motor.* Located in the frontal lobes of the cerebrum.
- *Reticular activating system).* The **reticular activating system (RAS)** operates in the lateral portion of the medulla, pons, and especially the midbrain. The RAS sends impulses to and receives impulses from the cerebral cortex. It is a diffuse system of interlacing nerve cells responsible for maintaining consciousness and the ability to respond to stimuli (Figure 3-9).

Vascular Supply The brain receives about 20 percent of the body's total blood flow per minute. Blood flow to the brain is provided by two systems. The *carotid system* is anterior, while the *vertebrobasilar* system is posterior. Both join at the *Circle of Willis* before entering the structures of the brain (Figure 3-10). The system is designed so that interruption of any part will not cause significant loss of blood flow to the tissues. Venous drainage of the brain is through the venous sinuses and the internal jugular veins.

Besides blood flow, cerebrospinal fluid bathes the brain and spinal cord. Several chambers within the brain, called ventricles, contain most of the intracranial volume of this fluid.

The Spinal Cord

The spinal cord is 17–18 inches long in the average adult. It leaves the brain at the medulla and proceeds, through an opening called the foramen magnum, down the spinal canal. The spinal cord, ending near the level of the first lumbar vertebra, is responsible for conducting impulses to and from the peripheral nervous system and for reflexes.

✴ brainstem part of the brain connecting the cerebral hemispheres with the spinal cord. It is comprised of the mesencephalon (midbrain), the pons, and the medulla oblongata.

✴ mesencephalon portion of the brain connecting the pons and cerebellum with the cerebral hemispheres; also called the *midbrain.* It controls motor coordination and eye movement.

✴ pons process of tissue connecting the medulla oblongata and cerebellum with upper portions of the brain.

✴ medulla oblongata lower portion of the brainstem, connecting the pons and the spinal cord. It contains major centers for control of respiratory, cardiac, and vasomotor activity.

✴ cerebellum portion of the brain located dorsally to the pons and medulla oblongata. It plays an important role in the fine motor movement, posture, equilibrium, and muscle tone.

✴ reticular activating system the system responsible for consciousness. A series of nervous tissues keeping the human system in a state of consciousness.

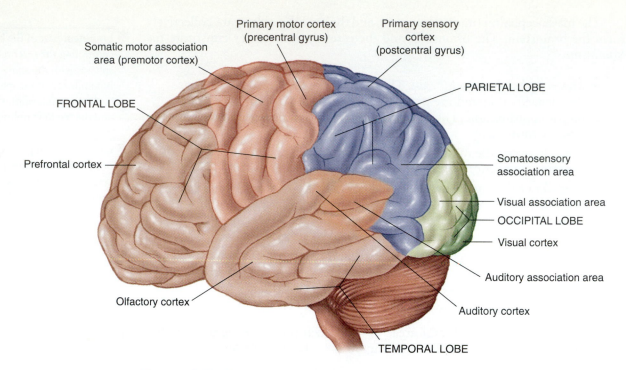

Somatic motor association
area (premotor cortex)

Primary motor cortex
(precentral gyrus)

Primary sensory
cortex
(postcentral gyrus)

FRONTAL LOBE

PARIETAL LOBE

Prefrontal cortex

Somatosensory
association area

Visual association area

OCCIPITAL LOBE

Visual cortex

Auditory association area

Olfactory cortex

Auditory cortex

TEMPORAL LOBE

FIGURE 3-8   External anatomy of the brain.

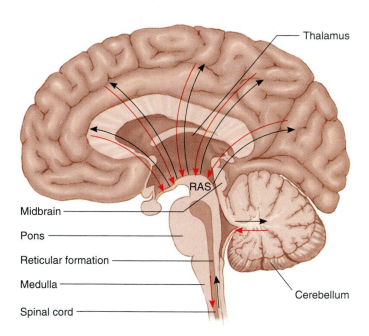

Thalamus

Midbrain

Pons

Reticular formation

Medulla

Spinal cord

RAS

Cerebellum

FIGURE 3-9   The reticular activating system (RAS) which sends and receives
messages from various parts of the brain.

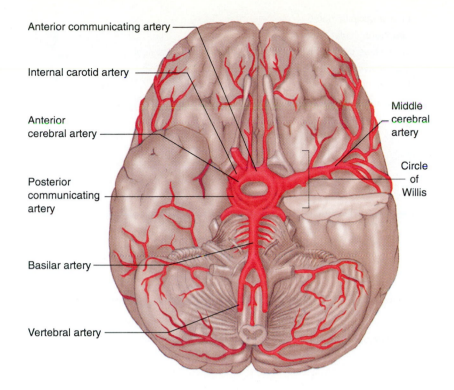

Anterior communicating artery

Internal carotid artery

Anterior cerebral artery

Posterior communicating artery

Basilar artery

Vertebral artery

Middle cerebral artery

Circle of Willis

FIGURE 3-10   An interior view of brain showing the circle of Willis, which is formed by the anterior and posterior communicating arteries.

Thirty-one pairs of nerve fibers exit the spinal cord as it descends and enters the peripheral nervous system (Figure 3-11). The dorsal roots contain afferent fibers, while the ventral roots contain efferent fibers. **Afferent** (sensory) fibers transmit impulses to the central nervous system from the body. **Efferent** (motor) fibers carry impulses from the central nervous system to the body (Figure 3-12). Each nerve root has a corresponding area of the skin, called a **dermatome,** to which it supplies sensation (Figure 3-13). Sensory deficits in a dermatomal distribution can indicate the level of a spinal cord problem. Spinal cord injury can result in damage to afferent or efferent pathways, or both. The nearer to the brainstem, the more serious the effects are likely to be.

Reflexes are protective. If a peripheral sensory nerve senses harm, such as intense heat, it sends an impulse to the spinal cord. The spinal cord then stimulates the appropriate muscles to remove the part of the body closest to the perceived threat. This process saves time as impulses do not have to go to the brain for processing. Because they are mediated in the spinal cord, reflex actions lack fine motor control.

✷ **afferent** carrying impulses toward the central nervous system. Sensory nerves are afferent nerves.

✷ **efferent** carrying impulses away from the brain or spinal cord to the periphery. Motor nerves are efferent nerves.

✷ **dermatomes** areas of the skin innervated by spinal nerves.

FIGURE 3-11 The spinal cord
and its branches.

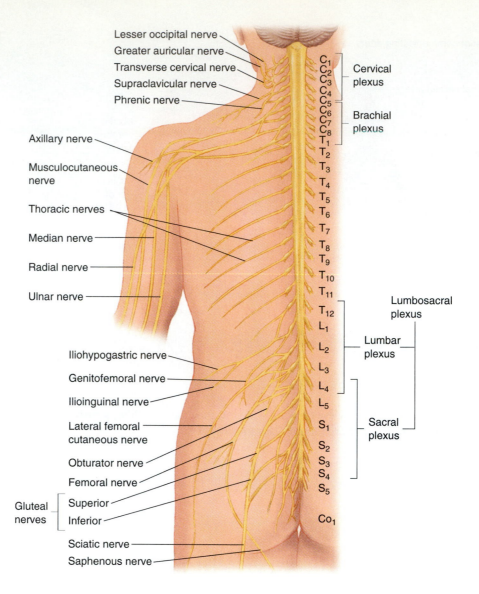

Lesser occipital nerve
Greater auricular nerve
Transverse cervical nerve
Supraclavicular nerve
Phrenic nerve

C_1
C_2
C_3
C_4 } Cervical plexus
C_5
C_6
C_7 } Brachial plexus
C_8
T_1
T_2
T_3
T_4
T_5
T_6
T_7
T_8
T_9
T_{10}
T_{11}
T_{12} } Lumbosacral plexus
L_1
L_2 } Lumbar plexus
L_3
L_4
L_5
S_1 } Sacral plexus
S_2
S_3
S_4
S_5
Co_1

Axillary nerve
Musculocutaneous nerve
Thoracic nerves
Median nerve
Radial nerve
Ulnar nerve

Iliohypogastric nerve
Genitofemoral nerve
Ilioinguinal nerve
Lateral femoral cutaneous nerve
Obturator nerve
Femoral nerve
Gluteal nerves { Superior
                  Inferior
Sciatic nerve
Saphenous nerve

FIGURE 3-12 Sectional view
of the spinal cord showing
distribution of spinal nerves.

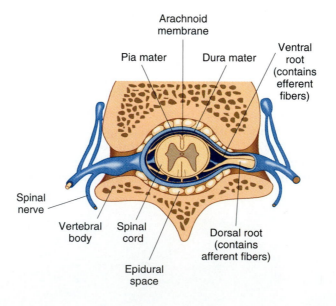

Arachnoid membrane
Pia mater
Dura mater
Ventral root (contains efferent fibers)
Spinal nerve
Vertebral body
Spinal cord
Dorsal root (contains afferent fibers)
Epidural space

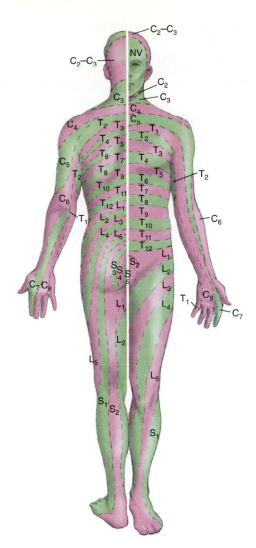

FIGURE 3-13 Dermatomes.

THE PERIPHERAL NERVOUS SYSTEM

Consisting of the cranial and the peripheral nerves, the peripheral nervous system has both voluntary and involuntary components. The twelve pairs of **cranial nerves** originate in the brain and supply nervous control to the head, neck, and certain thoracic and abdominal organs (Figure 3-14). The peripheral nerves, as described previously, originate in the spinal cord and supply nervous control to the periphery.

The four categories of peripheral nerves are:

- *Somatic Sensory.* These afferent nerves transmit sensations involved in touch, pressure, pain, temperature, and position (proprioception).
- *Somatic Motor.* These efferent fibers carry impulses to the skeletal (voluntary) muscles.
- *Visceral (Autonomic) Sensory.* These afferent tracts transmit sensations from the visceral organs. Sensations such as a full bladder or the need to defecate are mediated by visceral sensory fibers.
- *Visceral (Autonomic) Motor.* These efferent fibers exit the central nervous system and branch to supply nerves to the involuntary cardiac muscle and smooth muscle of the viscera (organs) and to the glands.

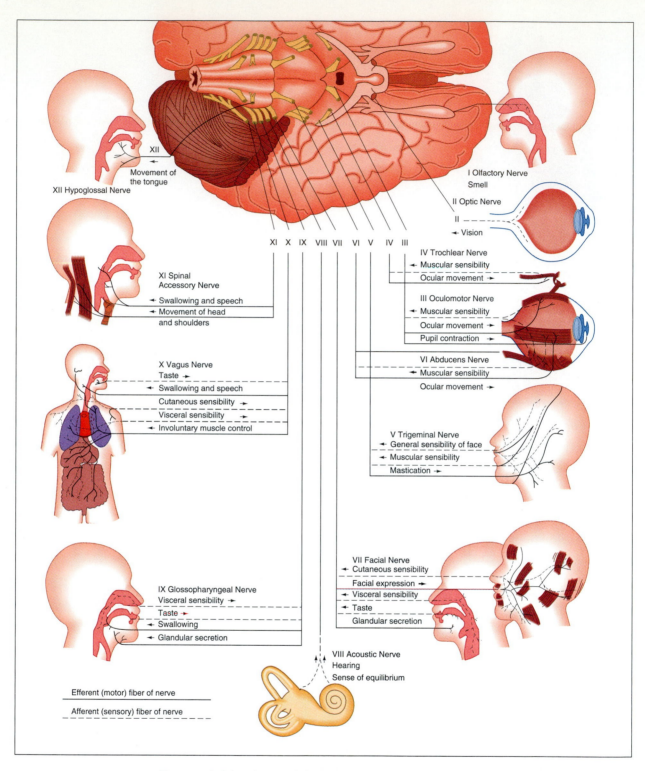

XII
Movement of
the tongue

XII Hypoglossal Nerve

**XI Spinal
Accessory Nerve**
← Swallowing and speech
← Movement of head
and shoulders

X Vagus Nerve
Taste →
← Swallowing and speech
Cutaneous sensibility →
Visceral sensibility →
← Involuntary muscle control

IX Glossopharyngeal Nerve
Visceral sensibility →
Taste →
← Swallowing
← Glandular secretion

Efferent (motor) fiber of nerve

Afferent (sensory) fiber of nerve

I Olfactory Nerve
Smell

II Optic Nerve
II
← Vision

IV Trochlear Nerve
← Muscular sensibility
Ocular movement →

III Oculomotor Nerve
← Muscular sensibility
Ocular movement →
Pupil contraction →

VI Abducens Nerve
← Muscular sensibility
Ocular movement →

V Trigeminal Nerve
← General sensibility of face
← Muscular sensibility
Mastication →

VII Facial Nerve
← Cutaneous sensibility
Facial expression →
← Visceral sensibility
← Taste
Glandular secretion

VIII Acoustic Nerve
Hearing
Sense of equilibrium

XI X IX VIII VII VI V IV III

FIGURE 3-14   The cranial nerves.

THE AUTONOMIC NERVOUS SYSTEM

The involuntary component of the peripheral nervous system, commonly called the *autonomic nervous system,* is responsible for the unconscious control of many body functions. There are two functional divisions of the autonomic nervous system—the sympathetic nervous system and the parasympathetic nervous system.

The sympathetic and parasympathetic systems are antagonistic. In their normal state, they exist in balance with each other. During stress, the sympathetic system dominates. During rest, the parasympathetic system dominates.

The Sympathetic Nervous System The sympathetic nervous system, often referred to as the "fight-or-flight" system, prepares the body for stressful situations. It is located near the thoracic and lumbar part of the spinal cord. Stimulation causes increased heart rate and blood pressure, pupillary dilation, a rise in the blood sugar, as well as bronchodilation. The neurotransmitters epinephrine and norepinephrine mediate its actions. The sympathetic nervous system is closely associated with the adrenal gland of the endocrine system.

The Parasympathetic Nervous System The parasympathetic nervous system, sometimes called the "feed-or-breed" system, is responsible for controlling vegetative functions, such as normal heart rate and blood pressure. Associated with the cranial nerves and the sacral plexus, it is mediated by the neurotransmitter acetylcholine. When stimulated, it causes a decrease in heart rate, an increase in digestive activity, pupillary constriction, and a reduction in blood glucose.

PATHOPHYSIOLOGY

A firm grasp of the pathophysiology of nontraumatic neurologic emergencies is essential in order for the paramedic to provide appropriate and timely emergency care.

ALTERATION IN COGNITIVE SYSTEMS

Consciousness is a condition in which an individual is fully responsive to stimuli and demonstrates awareness of the environment. The ability to respond to stimuli is dependent upon an intact reticular activating system (RAS). Cognition and the ability to respond to the environment rely upon an intact cerebral cortex. Therefore, altered forms of consciousness can result from dysfunction or interruption of the central nervous system.

CENTRAL NERVOUS SYSTEM DISORDERS

An alteration in mental status is the hallmark sign of central nervous system (CNS) injury or illness. Any alteration in mental status is abnormal and warrants further examination. Alterations may vary from minor thought disturbances to unconsciousness. Unconsciousness, also called **coma,** is a state in which the patient cannot be aroused, even by powerful external stimuli. There are generally two mechanisms capable of producing alterations in mental status:

- *Structural lesions.* Structural lesions (e.g., tumors, contusions) depress consciousness by destroying or encroaching upon the substance of the brain. Examples of causes of structural lesions include:
  - Brain tumor (neoplasm)
  - Degenerative disease
  - Intracranial hemorrhage
  - Parasites
  - Trauma

An alteration in mental status is the hallmark sign of central nervous system (CNS) injury or illness.

 coma a state of unconsciousness from which the patient cannot be aroused.

- *Toxic-metabolic states.* Toxic-metabolic states involve either the presence of circulating toxins or metabolites or the lack of metabolic substrates (oxygen, glucose, or thiamine). These states produce diffuse depression of both sides (hemispheres) of the cerebrum, with or without depression within the brainstem. Various causes of toxic-metabolic states include:
  - Anoxia (lack of oxygen)
  - Diabetic ketoacidosis
  - Hepatic failure
  - Hypoglycemia
  - Renal failure
  - Thiamine deficiency
  - Toxic exposure (e.g., cyanide, organophosphates)

Within the two general mechanisms (structural lesions and toxic metabolic states), there are many difficult-to-classify causes of altered mental status. Some of the more common causes are listed in the following four general categories:

- Drugs
  - Depressants (including alcohol)
  - Hallucinogens
  - Narcotics
- Cardiovascular
  - Anaphylaxis
  - Cardiac arrest
  - Stroke
  - Dysrhythmias
  - Hypertensive encephalopathy
  - Shock
- Respiratory
  - COPD
  - Inhalation of toxic gas
  - Hypoxia
- Infectious
  - AIDS
  - Encephalitis
  - Meningitis

CEREBRAL HOMEOSTASIS

The autonomic nervous system (ANS) maintains cerebral homeostasis (internal balance) and regulates and coordinates the body's vital functions, such as blood pressure, temperature regulation, respiration, and metabolism. It can be strongly affected by emotional influences, resulting in blushing, palpitations, clammy hands, and dry mouth.

PERIPHERAL NERVOUS SYSTEM DISORDERS

Peripheral neuropathy is any malfunction or damage of the peripheral nerves. It can affect muscle activity, sensation, reflexes, or internal organ function. The disorder can involve a single nerve, a *mononeuropathy,* or multiple nerves, known as *polyneuropathy.*

Mononeuropathy is usually caused by localized conditions such as trauma, compression, or infections. Fractured bones, for example, may lacerate or com-

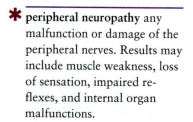

* **peripheral neuropathy** any malfunction or damage of the peripheral nerves. Results may include muscle weakness, loss of sensation, impaired reflexes, and internal organ malfunctions.

Peripheral neuropathy can affect muscle activity, sensation, reflexes, or internal organ function.

press a nerve; excessively tight tourniquets may compress and injure a nerve; and infections such as herpes zoster may affect a single segment of an afferent nerve. Another common example is carpal tunnel syndrome, a compression-type neuropathy. It is caused by compression of the median nerve that travels through the flexor tendon canal of the lower arm. Carpal tunnel syndrome can cause pain or motor dysfunction in the fingers innervated by the median nerve.

Polyneuropathy is characterized by demyelination or degeneration of peripheral nerves. It leads to sensory, motor, or mixed sensorimotor deficits. A number of conditions, such as immune disorders, toxic agents, and metabolic disorders are known causes of polyneuropathy. One example of a polyneuropathy is Guillian-Barré syndrome, which is characterized by rapidly worsening muscle weakness of the limbs that can sometimes lead to paralysis. Diabetes is one of the major causes of peripheral neuropathy. It usually affects the distal nerves of the hands and feet in the classic "stocking and glove" distribution.

Autonomic Nervous System Disorders

Disorders affecting the ANS are frequently a result of another condition. Since the control of the body's internal environment is vested in the ANS, most conditions that affect the integrity of an individual are accompanied by some changes in autonomic nervous system functioning.

GENERAL ASSESSMENT FINDINGS

Assessment of the neurological system is often difficult. Many of the signs and symptoms of nervous system dysfunction are subtle. As you conduct the scene size-up and begin the initial assessment, form a general impression of the patient and evaluate mental status before assessing the ABCs. If your initial assessment causes you to suspect nervous system dysfunction, this will prompt you to place particular emphasis on the neurological examination during the focused history and physical exam.

During the initial assessment, be alert to any signs of nervous system dysfunction. If present, these will prompt you to place particular emphasis on the neurological evaluation during the focused history and physical exam.

SCENE SIZE-UP AND INITIAL ASSESSMENT

A great deal of crucial information can be obtained while approaching the patient. Size up the scene and the surroundings as well as the patient to form a general impression. Is there evidence of toxic exposure or trauma? Look for clues that can indicate a patient's condition, such as:

General Appearance

- Is the patient conscious?
- Alert?
- Confused?
- Sitting upright?

Speech

- Can the patient speak?
- Clear and coherent?
- Full sentences?
- Slurred speech?

Skin

- Color (pink, pale, cyanotic?)
- Temperature (warm, hot, cool?)
- Moisture (diaphoretic, clammy?)

Facial drooping present?

Posture/Gait

- Upright?
- Leaning?
- Staggered?
- Steady gait?

Next, quickly check the patient's mental status through the "AVPU" method.

- **A** = The patient is alert and aware of his surroundings. A patient alert and orientated to time, place, person, and one's own person, is said to be "alert and oriented times four." Remember, no patient is "oriented" unless he has answered the questions that the paramedic has to ask.
- **V** = The patient responds to verbal stimuli. The patient responds when talked to, perhaps in a loud voice. Note if the patient delivers the answers normally or sluggishly. Also observe whether the patient has purposeful or uncoordinated movements.
- **P** = The patient responds to painful stimuli. The patient responds when tactile stimulation is used, such as a sternal rub, a squeeze of the trapezius muscle, or pinching the thenar (thumb) web space.
- **U** = The patient is unresponsive. The patient is not alert and does not respond to verbal or painful stimuli.

Assessment of cerebral functioning also includes assessing the patient's emotional status. If the patient is conscious, you can detect changes in the following:

Mood

- Is the patient's affect natural or is the patient irritable, anxious, or apathetic?
- Does the patient appear depressed? manic? happy? solemn? reserved?

Thought

- What is the patient's thought pattern? Is it logical? appropriate? scattered?

Perception

- How does the patient perceive his surroundings? Are his interactions appropriate?

Judgment

- Is the patient using reasonable and sound judgment? Is he logical?

Memory and Attention

- Is short-term memory present? long-term memory? Question family members or caregivers to obtain this information.
- Does the patient maintain conversation? pay attention? repeatedly ask or answer questions?

Any alteration from the patient's normal mental status or mood should be considered significant and warrants additional assessment.

Once a patient's level of consciousness is determined, place the greatest emphasis on maintenance of the airway. If the patient is unconscious, assume that a cervical spine injury exists and treat it appropriately. Use the modified jaw-thrust maneuver to open the airway. Once opened, insert the appropriate airway adjunct. In unresponsive patients, the tongue may be occluding the airway. In such cases, you may need only to place an oropharyngeal or nasopharyngeal airway to maintain the airway. If the patient tolerates an oropharyngeal airway, consider intubation.

Vigilantly monitor the airway in any patient with central nervous system injury. It is essential to observe for respiratory arrest that can result from increased intracranial pressure. Remain alert for an absent gag reflex and vomiting. In addition, blood from facial injuries and possible aspiration of gastric contents further threaten the patient's airway.

Observe the patient for any signs and symptoms of inadequate or impaired breathing or the presence of any abnormal respiratory patterns. Remember, the body's "breathing center" is located in the brain. Certain neurological conditions can cause these areas to malfunction and limit the patient's ability to breathe.

Complete assessment of the body's circulatory status is also a crucial part of the initial assessment. Evaluation of the heart rate, rhythm, and ECG pattern can shed light on the body's overall state of perfusion. Observe the patient's skin color, temperature, and moisture for abnormal findings such as cyanosis and moisture. A healthy adult's skin is usually warm, dry, and pink.

FOCUSED HISTORY AND PHYSICAL EXAM

Following completion of the initial assessment and correction of any immediate threats to the patient's life, turn your attention to the focused history and physical exam. This assessment should include an accurate history and a physical exam, including vital signs. Remember that any indications of nervous system dysfunction should cause you to place particular emphasis on neurological evaluation. Neurological evaluation will be detailed under "Nervous System Status" later in this chapter.

History

A thorough, accurate history of a patient is crucial in determining the current problem and subsequent treatment of a patient. One of the first steps in obtaining a thorough history involves attempting to determine whether the neurological problem is traumatic or medical. Clarification will help determine the plan for subsequent prehospital treatment. The initial history may not be easy to obtain because of the patient's altered mental status. In these cases, it is critical for you to obtain information from family, friends, or other bystanders, if available.

If the neurological emergency is due to trauma, ask the following questions:

- When did the incident occur?
- How did the incident occur, or what is the mechanism of injury?

- Was there any loss of consciousness?
- Was there evidence of incontinence? (Incontinence suggests loss of consciousness.)
- What is the patient's chief complaint?
- Has there been any change in symptoms?
- Are there any complicating factors?

If there is no evidence of a traumatic cause of the neurological emergency, ask the following questions to determine the nature of illness:

- What is the chief complaint?
- What are the details of the present illness, or the nature of the illness?
- Is there a pertinent underlying medical problem such as:
  - Cardiac disease
  - Chronic seizures
  - Diabetes
  - Hypertension
- Have these symptoms occurred before?
- Are there any environmental clues? These may include:
  - Evidence of current medications
  - Medic-Alert identification
  - Alcohol bottles or drug paraphernalia
  - Chemicals, hazardous materials

Physical Examination

The physical examination of a patient with a neurological emergency should include the standard head-to-toe examination and a more detailed neurological assessment. Pay particular attention to the pupils, respiratory status, and spinal evaluation.

Face A patient's ability to smile, frown, and wrinkle his forehead indicates an intact facial nerve (cranial nerve VII). If the patient is conscious, test these abilities. Note any drooping or facial paralysis.

Eyes The pupils are controlled by the oculomotor nerve (cranial nerve III). This nerve follows a long course through the skull and is easily compressed by brain swelling. While slight pupillary inequality is normal, abnormal pupils can be an early indicator of increasing intracranial pressure. If both pupils are dilated and do not react to light, the patient probably has a brainstem injury or has suffered serious brain anoxia. If the pupils are dilated but still react to light, the injury may be reversible. However, the patient must be transported quickly to an emergency facility capable of treating central nervous system injuries. A unilaterally dilated pupil that remains reactive to light may be the earliest sign of increasing intracranial pressure. The patient with altered mental status who presents with or develops a unilaterally dilated pupil is in the "immediate transport" category. Constricted, or pinpoint, pupils suggest a toxic etiology for the altered mental status.

A common method of assessing extraocular movement is to have the patient follow finger movements. For example, ask the patient to follow your finger to the extreme left, then up, then down. Repeat the same motions to the extreme right. These positions are referred to as the *cardinal positions of gaze*. Because extraocular movements are controlled by cranial nerves III (oculomotor), IV (trochlear), and VI (abducens), inability to look in all directions with both

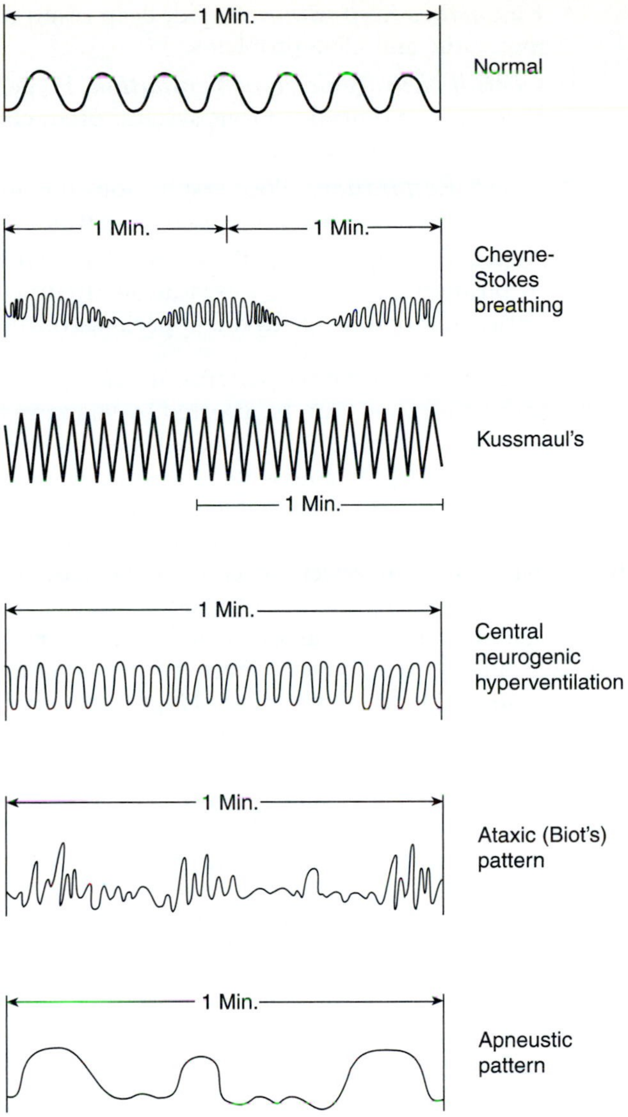

FIGURE 3-15 Respiratory patterns seen with CNS dysfunction.

eyes can be an early indication of a central nervous system problem. This is particularly important in the indication of facial trauma.

When examining a patient's pupils, it is important to check for contact lenses. Contact lenses, if present, should be removed and placed into their container or a saline solution and transported with the patient.

Nose/Mouth In the presence of facial paralysis, drooping of the patient's mouth may occur. Pay particular attention to any of these changes that may potentially compromise the patient's airway. A common way to assess for mouth droop is to ask the patient to smile. Also, ask the patient to "show your teeth." Both maneuvers will help determine whether there is any degree of facial drooping.

Respiratory Status Respiratory derangement can occur with CNS illness or injury. Any of five abnormal respiratory patterns may commonly be observed (Figure 3-15):

- *Cheyne-Stokes respiration.* A breathing pattern characterized by a period of apnea lasting 10–60 seconds, followed by gradually increasing depth and frequency of respirations.

✳ Cheyne-Stokes respiration a breathing pattern characterized by a period of apnea lasting 10-60 seconds, followed by gradually increasing depth and frequency of respirations.

General Assessment Findings **281**

✹ **Kussmaul's respiration** rapid deep respirations caused by severe metabolic and CNS problems.

✹ **central neurogenic hyperventilation** hyperventilation caused by a lesion in the central nervous system, often characterized by rapid, deep, noisy respirations.

✹ **ataxic respiration** poor respirations due to CNS damage, causing ineffective thoracic muscular coordination.

✹ **apneustic respiration** breathing characterized by a prolonged inspiration unrelieved by expiration attempts, seen in patients with damage to the upper part of the pons.

- *Kussmaul's Respiration.* Rapid, deep respirations caused by severe metabolic and CNS problems.
- *Central Neurogenic Hyperventilation.* Hyperventilation caused by a lesion in the central nervous system, often characterized by rapid, deep, noisy respirations.
- *Ataxic Respirations.* Poor respirations due to CNS damage, causing ineffective thoracic muscular coordination.
- *Apneustic Respirations.* Breathing characterized by prolonged inspiration unrelieved by expiration attempts. This is seen in patients with damage to the upper part of the pons.

Several other respiratory patterns are also possible, depending on the injury. A patient's respirations can be affected by so many factors—fear, hysteria, chest injuries, spinal cord injuries, or diabetes—that they are not as useful as other signs in monitoring the course of CNS problems. Just before death, the patient may present with central neurogenic hyperventilation.

It is important to remember that the level of carbon dioxide ($PaCO_2$) in the blood has a critical effect on cerebral vessels. The normal blood $PaCO_2$ is 40 mmHg. Increasing the $PaCO_2$ causes cerebral vasodilatation, while decreasing it results in cerebral vasoconstriction. If the patient is poorly ventilated, the $PaCO_2$ will increase, causing even further vasodilatation with a subsequent increase in intracranial pressure. Hyperventilation can decrease the $PaCO_2$ effectively causing vasoconstriction of the cerebral vessels. This will assist in minimizing brain swelling. Therefore, hyperventilate any patient who is suspected of having increased intracranial pressure at a rate of 20 breaths per minute. It is important to avoid *excessively* hyperventilating a patient so as to prevent decreasing $PaCo_2$ levels to dangerously low levels.

Cardiovascular Status Patients suffering from a neurological event are also likely to suffer changes to the cardiovascular system. Vigilant assessment of a patient's vital signs is necessary to observe these changes. Look for these changes:

- *Heart rate.* A heart rate that is too fast (tachycardia), too slow (bradycardia), or irregular (dysrhythmias).
- *ECG/rhythm.* Development of any changes to the ECG rhythm, including S-T segment changes, the onset of bradycardia, tachycardia, or potentially lethal dysrhythmias, such as ventricular fibrillation or ventricular tachycardia.
- *Bruits.* The sound of turbulent blood flow through the carotid arteries, known as a *bruit,* may be indicative of atherosclerotic disease and decreased blood flow to the brain.
- *Jugular venous distention (JVD).* Increased jugular venous pressure, known as jugular venous distention, may be present, indicating that the heart is not pumping effectively.

Nervous System Status To evaluate nervous system status, take into account sensorimotor status, motor system status, and the status of the cranial nerves.

Sensorimotor Evaluation The purpose of sensorimotor evaluation is to document loss of sensation and/or motor function. To initially assess the patient with a possible spinal injury, perform these steps:

1. If the patient is unconscious, determine the response to voice, gentle tactile stimulation, and then, if necessary, pain.
2. Evaluate the spine for pain and tenderness.

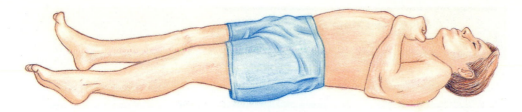

FIGURE 3-16 Patient with decorticate posturing.

3. Observe for bruises on the spine.
4. Observe for deformity of the spine.
5. Note any incontinence.
6. Check for circulation, motor function, and sensation in each extremity. Does the patient have feeling in his hands and feet? Ask the patient to wiggle his toes and push them against resistance. Compare both sides. Check bilateral grip strength. If the patient is unconscious, pain response should be observed. If the unconscious patient withdraws or localizes to the pinching of fingers and toes, there is intact sensation and motor function. This is a sign of normal or only minimally impaired cortical function.

A patient with a suspected spinal cord injury will require full spinal immobilization on a long spine board. See Volume 4, Chapter 9 for a discussion of traumatic spinal cord injury.

Both **decorticate posturing** (arms flexed, legs extended) and **decerebrate posturing** (arms and legs extended) are ominous signs of deep cerebral or upper brainstem injury (Figures 3-16 and 3-17). Flaccid paralysis usually indicates spinal cord injury.

Motor System Status   A thorough examination of the motor system of the body includes an assessment of muscle tone, strength, flexion, extension, coordination, and balance. Assess the patient for the following:

- *Muscle Tone.* Are the patient's muscles firm? Or, is atrophy present?
- *Strength.* Does the patient have adequate muscle strength? Or is weakness present? Does the patient have strong and equal grip strength?
- *Flexion/Extension.* Can the patient flex, extend, and move extremities adequately?

✳ **decorticate posture** characteristic posture associated with a lesion at or above the upper brainstem. The patient presents with the arms flexed, fists clenched, and legs extended.

✳ **decerebrate posture** sustained contraction of extensor muscles of the extremities resulting from a lesion in the brainstem. The patient presents with stiff and extended extremities and retracted head.

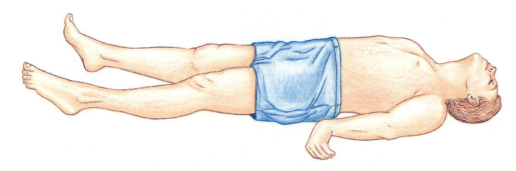

FIGURE 3-17 Patient with decerebrate posturing.

FIGURE 3-18 Glasgow Coma Scale.

Glasgow Coma Scale

Eye Opening	Spontaneous	4	
	To Voice	3	
	To Pain	2	
	None	1	
Verbal Response	Oriented	5	
	Confused	4	
	Inappropriate Words	3	
	Incomprehensible Words	2	
	None	1	
Motor Response	Obeys Commands	6	
	Localizes Pain	5	
	Withdraw (Pain)	4	
	Flexion (Pain)	3	
	Extension (Pain)	2	
	None	1	
Glasgow Coma Score Total			

TOTAL GLASGOW COMA SCALE POINTS

13 – 15 = 5

9 – 12 = 4

6 – 8 = 3

4 – 5 = 1

Conversion = Approximately One - Third Total Value

Neurologic Assessment

- *Coordination.* Are the patient's gait and movements steady and smooth? Can the patient touch finger to nose?
- *Balance.* Can the patient stand or sit upright without becoming dizzy?

Cranial Nerves Status As you learned earlier, twelve pairs of cranial nerves extend from the lower surface of the brain. Each pair is designated by a Roman numeral from I to XII. Proper and intact functioning of these nerves may be assessed during a complete neurological examination as detailed in, Volume 2, Chapter 2, "Physical Examination Techniques." Review Figure 3-14, which outlines the cranial nerves and their functions.

Further Mental Status Assessment For patients with an altered mental status or those who are unresponsive, the **Glasgow Coma Scale (GCS)** is a simple tool that can be used to evaluate and monitor the patient's condition. While it is used most commonly in trauma situations, the scale can also be a valuable tool for monitoring a medical patient's status (Figure 3-18). The scale includes three components:

- Eye opening
- Verbal response
- Motor response

✳ Glasgow Coma Scale (GCS) tool used in evaluating and quantifying the degree of coma by determining the best motor, verbal, and eye-opening response to standardized stimuli.

A number is applied to each of the components based on the patient's condition. The total score can serve as an indicator of survival. The lowest GCS score possible is 3; the highest possible score is 15. The GCS can also be used as a predictor of long-term morbidity and mortality. The following are examples of the predictive value of the GCS system:

A patient with a total score of:	Has an estimated:
8 or better	94% favorable outcome
5, 6, 7	50% favorable (adult), 90% (children)
3.4	10% favorable outcome
5, 6, 7 who drop a grade	0% favorable outcome
5, 6, 7 who improve to more than 7	80% favorable outcome

Vital Signs

Vital signs are crucial in following the course of neurological problems. Such signs can indicate changes in intracranial pressure. Increased intracranial pressure is characterized by the following changes in vital signs, sometimes collectively referred to as **Cushing's reflex:**

* Increased blood pressure
* Decreased pulse
* Decreased respirations
* Increased temperature

✱ **Cushing's reflex** a collective change in vital signs (increased blood pressure and temperature and decreased pulse and respirations) associated with increasing intracranial pressure.

A patient in the early stages of increased intracranial pressure usually exhibits a decrease in pulse rate and an increase in blood pressure and temperature. Later, if the intracranial pressure continues to rise without correction, the pulse will increase, the blood pressure will fall, and the body temperature will remain elevated. Dysrhythmias may be seen with increased intracranial pressure. Continuous ECG monitoring and pulse oximetry, if available, should be utilized to spot early signs of CNS lesions. Table 3-1 compares vital signs of a patient in shock with those of a patient with head injury and increased intracranial pressure. Remember, if you suspect that a patient has a CNS injury, take and record vital signs every five minutes.

Additional Assessment Tools

Additional technological tools may be useful in assessing and monitoring the neurological patient. Such tools should be used as adjuncts to a complete patient assessment, and they should not be relied upon as sole indicators of a patient's

Table 3-1	COMPARISON OF VITAL SIGNS IN SHOCK AND INCREASED INTRACRANIAL PRESSURE	
Vital Signs	**Shock**	**Increased ICP**
Blood pressure	Decreased	Increased
Pulse	Increased	Decreased
Respirations	Increased	Decreased
Level of Consciousness	Decreased	Decreased

condition. Paramedics should continue to base their clinical decisions on a patient's entire presentation. Use such instruments as the end-tidal CO_2 detector, pulse oximeter, and blood glucometer to gain further insight into a patient's condition.

End-Tidal CO_2 Detector The end-tidal CO_2 detector monitors the amount of carbon dioxide being exhaled by a patient while being ventilated. This device works on the premise that during exhalation CO_2 should be detected. In the apneic patient with a suspected neurological injury, the device can be used to monitor the effectiveness of the assisted ventilations. Monitoring the levels of CO_2 can assure that ventilation rate and quality are appropriate for decreasing the increased intracranial pressure.

Pulse Oximeter The pulse oximeter is an effective tool for monitoring a patient's general state of perfusion. Any patient with a pulse oximetry reading of less than 90 percent is likely to be hypoxic. In a patient who has suffered a stroke, altered mental status, or syncope, the oximeter can be a useful adjunct in monitoring a patient's condition. It can also monitor the effectiveness of airway management techniques.

Blood Glucometer A common cause of an altered mental status or focal neurological deficits is hypoglycemia. Determining the blood glucose level is often a crucial step in caring for the neurological patient. Use the glucometer to obtain an accurate blood glucose level. See Chapter 4 for a discussion of this procedure. Documented hypoglycemia should be treated with a bolus of 50% dextrose.

Geriatric Considerations in Neurological Assessment

The neurological system of the geriatric patient is susceptible to systemic illness and is often affected by other body disorders. In addition, certain neurological changes such as pupil sluggishness, loss of overall body strength, and muscle atrophy occur naturally with the aging process. Slowing of nerve conduction is another characteristic often seen in the geriatric patient. Such slowing may indicate that a little more time is necessary to obtain a complete neurological history.

The level of consciousness and overall mental status of a geriatric patient is evaluated by assessing judgment, memory, affect, mood, orientation, speech, and grooming. Interviewing family members about the patient's normal state may reveal any change in mental status. Common neurological problems of the older patient include headache, low back pain, dizziness, weakness, loss of balance, disorders like Parkinson's disease, and vascular emergencies like stroke.

ONGOING ASSESSMENT

Any patient suffering from a neurological emergency should be reassessed every five minutes during your care and during transportation. Constantly re-evaluate and monitor the patient's airway and neurological system.

MANAGEMENT OF NERVOUS SYSTEM EMERGENCIES

The primary treatment for nervous system emergencies in the field is supportive.

The primary treatment for nervous system emergencies in the field is supportive. Most conditions will not be "cured" in the prehospital setting but symptoms may be reduced or controlled. Make a strong effort to make the patient comfortable and to reduce any of the existing symptoms. Follow these steps:

- *Airway and Breathing.* Properly position any patient that you suspect has a neurological emergency and protect the airway. If there is known or possible trauma, maintain C-spine immobilization. Administer oxygen via a nonrebreather mask. If the patient is breathing inadequately or is apneic, initiate ventilatory assistance. If an airway problem is detected, first apply basic airway maneuvers such as head positioning or the modified jaw-thrust maneuver. Intubate, if indicated.

- *Circulatory Support.* Establish an IV with a crystalloid solution such as lactated Ringer's or normal saline. Alternatively, consider placing a heparin or saline lock. It is important to have an accessible route for medications. Generally, running an IV at a keep-open rate will be sufficient.

- *Pharmacological Interventions.* Medications are available to alleviate signs and symptoms in patients with neurological emergencies. Medications include dextrose, thiamine, naloxone, and diazepam.

- *Psychological Support.* Patients suffering from a nervous system emergency, acute or chronic, are likely also to suffer anxiety. Neurological deficits of any kind are frightening experiences. Provide the patient with emotional support and explain the treatment regimen. In most cases, it is appropriate to explain to the patient what is occurring and why. Careful explanation and emotional support will help allay anxiety and apprehension.

- *Transport Considerations.* Assess, provide emergency care, and package the patient as quickly and safely as possible. Rapidly transport any patient with a neurological deficit or altered mental status to an appropriate emergency department, equipped with a computerized tomography (CT) or magnetic resonance imaging (MRI) scanner and facilities capable of managing strokes with thrombolytic therapy. Modern medicine has seen the development of new advances in pharmacological and surgical interventions that are only available in the hospital setting.

The major concerns in any CNS emergency are always the airway, breathing, circulation, and, if indicated, C-spine control.

There are numerous causes of nervous system emergencies. The more common nontraumatic nervous emergencies encountered in the prehospital setting include altered mental status, seizures, stroke, transient ischemic attacks (TIA), and headache. The following discussion details the assessment and management of these frequently encountered nontraumatic nervous system emergencies.

ALTERED MENTAL STATUS

When evaluating a patient, you may find mnemonic devices useful as assessment aids. A mnemonic that may help you remember some of the common causes of altered mental status is "AEIOU-TIPS."

A = Acidosis, alcohol
E = Epilepsy
I = Infection
O = Overdose
U = Uremia (kidney failure)
T = Trauma, tumor, toxin

I = Insulin (hypoglycemia or diabetic ketoacidosis)
P = Psychosis, poison
S = Stroke, seizure

Make an effort through history-taking and patient assessment to determine the underlying cause of the altered level of consciousness. Oftentimes, however, a clear cause will not be evident and cannot be determined in the prehospital setting.

Assessment

Using the AVPU method discussed earlier, determine the patient's level of consciousness. Unresponsive patients require vigilant monitoring and protection of the airway. Use information from family, friends, or other bystanders to try to determine the underlying cause of unconsciousness. Perform a physical exam to uncover any hidden injuries, signs, or symptoms.

Management

Your initial priority is to assure that the patient's airway is open and cervical spine is immobilized (in cases of suspected head/neck injury). Simultaneously secure the patient's airway and administer supplemental oxygen. If the patient is breathing inadequately, support respirations. An unresponsive patient requires an appropriate airway adjunct. Then assess the patient's circulatory status. Evaluate the patient's heart rate, blood pressure, and monitor the cardiac rhythm.

After the above are completed, perform the following steps:

- Establish an IV of normal saline or lactated Ringer's at a keep-open rate or place a heparin or saline lock.
- Determine the blood glucose level using a reagent strip or glucometer. A serum glucose determination will assist in determining if the altered mental status is due to hypoglycemia.
- If the blood glucose level is low, administer 50 percent dextrose. This will mediate hypoglycemia, which may be the cause of the altered mental status. Even if the patient is an uncontrolled diabetic whose body is not producing enough insulin, hyperglycemia produced by administration of glucose will do limited harm in the short time before arrival at the hospital. If, however, the patient is hypoglycemic, for example from too much insulin or missing a meal, the administration of glucose can be life-saving, and the patient may respond immediately. For the alcoholic patient who is hypoglycemic, the glucose may be life-saving as well. For more information or diabetic emergencies, see Chapter 4.
- Administer naloxone if the patient is suspected of having a narcotic overdose. Naloxone, a narcotic antagonist, has proven effective in the management and reversal of overdose caused by narcotics or synthetic narcotic agents. For more information, see Chapter 8.
- If the patient is a suspected alcoholic, consider the administration of 100 mg of thiamine (vitamin B_1). It is required for the conversion of pyruvic acid to acetyl-coenzyme-A (an important step in normal metabolism). Without this conversion, a significant amount of energy available in glucose cannot be obtained. The brain is extremely sensitive to thiamine deficiency. For more information, see Chapter 8.

Chronic Alcoholism Chronic alcoholism interferes with the intake, absorption, and use of thiamine. A significant percentage of alcoholics have thiamine deficiency that can cause Wernicke's syndrome or Korsakoff's psychosis. **Wernicke's syndrome** is an acute but reversible encephalopathy (brain disease) characterized by ataxia, eye muscle weakness, and mental derangement. Of even greater concern is **Korsakoff's psychosis,** characterized by memory disorder. Once established, Korsakoff's psychosis may be irreversible. Paramedics should follow local protocols. If ordered by medical direction, administer 100 mg of thiamine IV or IM.

Increased Intracranial Pressure If an increase in intracranial pressure is likely, as occurs in a closed head injury, hyperventilate the patient at 20 breaths per minute. Decreasing the carbon dioxide level will cause cerebral vasoconstriction and will help minimize brain swelling. Use caution not to over-hyperventilate, which could decrease CO_2 levels to dangerously low levels. Medical direction may order administration of the osmotic diuretic mannitol (Osmotrol). Mannitol causes diuresis, eliminating fluid from the intravascular space through the kidneys. Many authorities feel that its oncotic effect also causes a fluid shift from the substance of the brain to the circulation, thus reducing brain edema. As with all drugs, follow local protocols.

STROKE AND INTRACRANIAL HEMORRHAGE

Stroke, also called a "brain attack," is a general term that describes injury or death of brain tissue usually due to interruption of cerebral blood flow. The term "brain attack" is used because it compares the physiology of a stroke with that of a heart attack. In both cases, oxygen deprivation causes damage to the affected tissue.

The term "brain attack" also reflects recent trends in the treatment of a stroke, which in many cases now parallels the treatment available for heart attack. Prior to 1995, prehospital care of the stroke patient was considered primarily supportive. Since then, modern medicine has discovered new therapies and has realized the importance of early intervention. Now, early recognition and rapid transport to the hospital are identified as crucial to improving the outcome for stroke patients. The National Institute of Neurological Disorders and Stroke (NINDS) suggests transport to an emergency facility with the capability to respond to a stroke patient quickly, such as a facility equipped with computed tomography (CT) and neurological services.

In addition, studies have proven that *tissue plasminogen activator (tPA,)* and other thrombolytic agents used in the treatment of heart attack, are also effective in treating certain occlusive strokes. NINDS stresses that the use of thrombolytic agents in strokes is approved by the Food and Drug Administration and is encouraged in a certain patient population. Stroke patients who may be candidates for the thrombolytic therapy must receive definitive treatment within 3 hours of onset. Because of the possibility of intervention with thrombolytics, it is crucial to determine the exact time of the onset of symptoms as accurately as possible. In addition, it is essential that the public be aware of the signs and symptoms of stroke so that EMS can be notified. Therefore, extensive public education is necessary in achieving early recognition of symptoms and appropriate intervention and treatment. Transportation to an emergency facility is crucial in achieving the best possible outcome for these patients.

Strokes are the third most common cause of death and, in middle-aged and older patients, are a frequent cause of disability. Therefore the public, particularly those with a history of atherosclerosis (hardening of the arteries), heart disease, or hypertension, should be educated on the signs and symptoms of stroke as well as the need to contact EMS at the outset of symptoms. Likewise, paramedics must understand stroke as a serious, potentially life-threatening condition that warrants rapid recognition and prompt transport.

* **Wernicke's syndrome** condition characterized by loss of memory and disorientation, associated with chronic alcohol intake and a diet deficient in thiamine.

* **Korsakoff's psychosis** psychosis characterized by disorientation, muttering delirium, insomnia, delusions, and hallucinations. Symptoms include painful extremities, bilateral wrist drop (rarely), bilateral foot drop (frequently), and pain on pressure over the long nerves.

If increased intracranial pressure is likely, hyperventilate—but do not over-hyperventilate the patient.

* **stroke** caused by either ischemic or hemorrhagic lesions to a portion of the brain, resulting in damage or destruction of brain tissue. Commonly also called a cerebrovascular accident or "brain attack."

Prompt identification and transport are critical in cases of stroke. Patients who may be candidates for thrombolytic therapy must reach definitive treatment within 3 hours of onset.

FIGURE 3-19   Etiologies of stroke.

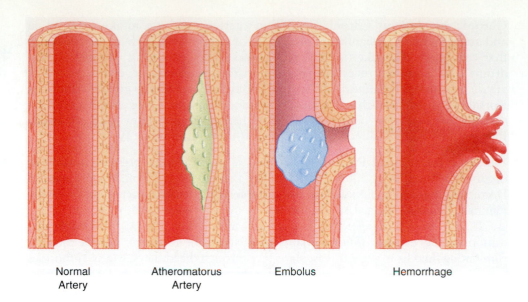

Normal Artery   Atheromatorus Artery   Embolus   Hemorrhage

Strokes can be divided into two broad categories: those caused by occlusion (blockage) of an artery and those caused by hemorrhage from a ruptured cerebral artery (Figure 3-19):

- *Occlusive Strokes.* An occlusive stroke occurs when a cerebral artery is blocked by a clot or other foreign matter. This results in *ischemia,* an inadequate blood supply to the brain tissue, and progresses to *infarction,* the death of tissues as a result of cessation of blood supply. In infarction, the tissue that has died will swell, causing further damage to nearby tissues, which only have a marginal blood supply. If swelling is severe, *herniation* (protrusion of brain tissue from the skull through the foramen magnum, the narrow opening at the base of the skull) may result. Occlusive strokes are classified as either embolic or thrombotic, depending on the cause.
  - *Embolic Strokes.* An *embolus* is a solid, liquid, or gaseous mass carried to a blood vessel from a remote site. The most common emboli are clots (thromboemboli) which usually arise from diseased blood vessels in the neck (carotid) or from abnormally contracting chambers in the heart. Atrial fibrillation often results in atrial dilation, a precursor to the formation of clots. Other types of emboli that may cause occlusion in cerebral blood vessels are air, tumor tissue, and fat. Embolic strokes occur suddenly and may be characterized by severe headaches.
  - *Thrombotic Strokes.* A *cerebral thrombus* is a blood clot that gradually develops in and obstructs a cerebral artery. As a person ages, atheromatous plaque deposits can form on the inner walls of arteries. The buildup causes a narrowing of the arteries and reduces the amount of blood that can flow through them. This process is known as atherosclerosis. Once the arteries are narrowed, platelets adhere to the roughened surface and can create a blood clot that blocks the blood flow through the cerebral artery. This ultimately results in brain tissue death. Unlike the embolic stroke, the signs and symptoms of thrombotic stroke develop gradually. This type of stroke often occurs at night and is characterized by a patient awakening with altered mental status and/or loss of speech, sensory, or motor function.

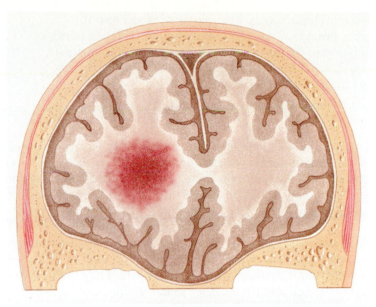

(a)

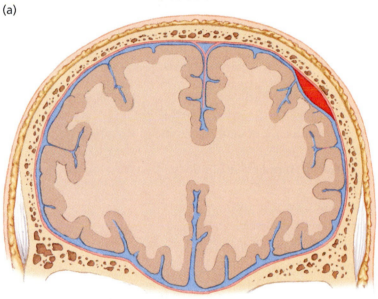

(b)

FIGURE 3-20   (a) Intracerebral hemorrhage (b) Subarachnoid hemorrhage.

- *Hemorrhagic Strokes*. Hemorrhagic strokes are usually categorized as being within the brain (intracerebral) (Figure 3-20a) or in the space around the outer surface of the brain (subarachnoid) (Figure 3-20b). Onset is often sudden and marked by a severe headache. Most intracranial hemorrhages occur in the hypertensive patient when a small vessel deep within the brain tissue ruptures. Subarachnoid hemorrhages most often result from congenital blood vessel abnormalities or from head trauma. Congenital abnormalities include aneurysms (weakened vessels) and arteriovenous malformations (collections of abnormal blood vessels). Aneurysms tend to be on the surface and may hemorrhage into the brain tissue or the subarachnoid space. Arteriovenous malformations may be within the brain, in the subarachnoid space, or both. Hemorrhage inside the brain often tears and separates normal brain tissue. The release of blood into the cavities within the brain that contain cerebrospinal fluid may paralyze vital centers. If blood in the subarachnoid space impairs drainage of cerebrospinal fluid, it may cause a rise in the intracranial pressure. Herniation of brain tissue may then occur.

Assessment

Signs and symptoms of a stroke will depend upon the type of stroke and the area of the brain damaged. Areas commonly affected are the motor, speech, and sensory centers. The onset of symptoms will be acute, and the patient may experience unconsciousness. There may be stertorous breathing (laborious breathing accompanied by snoring) due to paralysis of a portion of the soft palate. Respiratory expiration may be puffs of air out of the cheeks and mouth. The patient's pupils may be unequal, with the larger pupil on the side of the hemorrhage. Paralysis will usually involve one side of the face, one arm, and one leg. The eyes often will be turned away from the side of the body paralysis. The patient's skin may be cool and clammy. Speech disturbances, or aphasia, may also be noted.

Signs and symptom of a stroke include:

- Facial drooping
- Headache
- Confusion and agitation
- Dysphasia (difficulty in speaking)
- Aphasia (inability to speak)
- Dysarthria (impairment of the tongue and muscles essential to speech)
- Vision problems such as monocular blindness (blindness in one eye) or double vision
- Hemiparesis (weakness on one side)
- Hemiplegia (paralysis on one side)
- Paresthesia (numbness or tingling)
- Inability to recognize by touch
- Gait disturbances or uncoordinated fine motor movements
- Dizziness
- Incontinence
- Coma

Predisposing factors that may contribute to the stroke include hypertension, diabetes, abnormal blood lipid levels, oral contraceptives, sickle cell disease, and some cardiac dysrhythmias (e.g., atrial fibrillation).

Distinguishing Transient Ischemic Attacks (TIAs) Some patients may have transient stroke-like symptoms known as **TIAs,** or **transient ischemic attacks.** These indicate temporary interference with the blood supply to the brain, producing symptoms of neurological deficit. These symptoms may last for a few minutes or for several hours but usually resolve within 24 hours. After the attack, the patient will show no evidence of residual brain or neurological damage. The patient who experiences a TIA may, however, be a candidate for an eventual stroke. In fact, one third of TIA patients suffer a stroke soon thereafter.

The onset of a transient ischemic attack is usually abrupt. The specific signs and symptoms depend upon the area of the brain affected. Any one or a combi-

✱ **transient ischemic attack (TIA)** temporary interruption of blood supply to the brain.

nation of stroke symptoms may be present. In fact, it is virtually impossible to determine whether such a neurological event is due to a stroke or to a TIA in the prehospital setting.

The most common cause of a TIA is carotid artery disease. Other causes can be a small embolus, decreased cardiac output, hypotension, overmedication with antihypertensive agents, or cerebrovascular spasm.

While obtaining the history of the patient suspected of sustaining a TIA, you should try to collect information on or take note of the following factors:

- Previous neurological symptoms
- Initial symptoms and their progression
- Changes in mental status
- Precipitating factors
- Dizziness
- Palpitations
- History of hypertension, cardiac disease, sickle cell disease, or previous TIA or stroke

Management

Care for the stroke or TIA patient emphasizes early recognition, supportive measures, rapid transport, and notification of the emergency department (Figure 3-21). Aggressive airway management is a priority in caring for these patients. Field management of the stroke patient generally includes the following procedures:

- Assure scene safety, including body substance isolation.
- Establish and maintain an adequate airway. Have suction equipment readily available. Control of the patient's airway is a priority. Brain damage can affect a patient's ability to swallow and maintain an open airway.
- If patient is apneic or if breathing is inadequate, provide positive pressure ventilations at a rate of 20 per minute. Hyperventilation of the stroke patient will eliminate excessive CO_2 levels. Avoid overzealous hyperventilation that may lower CO_2 levels to detrimentally low levels causing profound cerebral vasoconstriction.
- If breathing is adequate, administer oxygen via a nonrebreather mask at 15 liters per minute.
- Complete a detailed patient history.
- Keep the patient supine or in the recovery position. If the patient has congestive heart failure, he could be maintained in a semi-upright position, if necessary.
- If an altered mental status is present or there is potential for airway compromise, place the patient in the left lateral recumbent, or recovery position.
- Determine the blood glucose level.
- Start an IV of normal saline or lactated Ringer's at a keep-open rate or place a heparin or saline lock. (Avoid dextrose solutions that may increase intracranial pressure due to increased osmotic effects.) If hypoglycemia is present, consider the administration of 50 percent dextrose by intravenous push.
- Monitor the cardiac rhythm.
- Protect the paralyzed extremities.

FIGURE 3-21 Management of suspected stroke. Adapted with permission. Journal of the American Medical Association, October 28, 1992, Volume 268, No. 16, *Guidelines for Cardiopulmonary Resuscitation and Emergency Cardiac Care*, p. 2243. © 1992 American Medical Association.

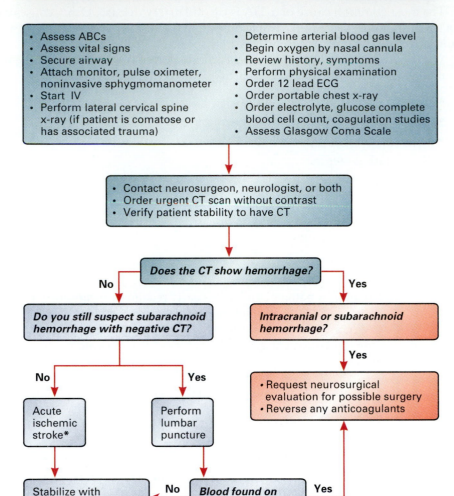

ALGORITHM: SUSPECTED STROKE

- Assess ABCs
- Assess vital signs
- Secure airway
- Attach monitor, pulse oximeter, noninvasive sphygmomanometer
- Start IV
- Perform lateral cervical spine x-ray (if patient is comatose or has associated trauma)

- Determine arterial blood gas level
- Begin oxygen by nasal cannula
- Review history, symptoms
- Perform physical examination
- Order 12 lead ECG
- Order portable chest x-ray
- Order electrolyte, glucose complete blood cell count, coagulation studies
- Assess Glasgow Coma Scale

- Contact neurosurgeon, neurologist, or both
- Order urgent CT scan without contrast
- Verify patient stability to have CT

Does the CT show hemorrhage?

No → **Do you still suspect subarachnoid hemorrhage with negative CT?**

Yes → **Intracranial or subarachnoid hemorrhage?**

Yes → • Request neurosurgical evaluation for possible surgery
• Reverse any anticoagulants

No → Acute ischemic stroke*

Yes → Perform lumbar puncture

Stabilize with appropriate therapies ← No — **Blood found on lumbar puncture?** — Yes →

* The detailed management of acute stroke is beyond the scope of the ACLS program. Management of cardiovascular emergencies in stroke victims is similar to the management in other patients. Never forget, however, that acute stroke can coexist with acute cardiovascular problems.

- Give the patient reassurance—all procedures should be explained. The patient may be unable to speak but still may be able to hear and understand.
- Rapidly transport without excessive movement or noise to an appropriate medical facility.

SEIZURES AND EPILEPSY

A **seizure** is a temporary alteration in behavior due to the massive electrical discharge of one or more groups of neurons in the brain. Seizures in any individual may be caused by stresses to the body, such as hypoxia, or a rapid lowering of

* **seizure** a temporary alteration in behavior due to the massive electrical discharge of one or more groups of neurons in the brain. Seizures can be clinically classified as generalized or partial.

blood sugar. Febrile seizures can occur in young children with sudden elevations in body temperature. Structural diseases of the brain such as tumors, head trauma, toxic eclampsia, and vascular disorders also cause seizures. The most common cause is *idiopathic epilepsy*. The term *idiopathic* means "without a known cause." The terms *epilepsy* or *epileptic* indicate nothing more than the potential to develop seizures in circumstances that would not induce them in most individuals. Seizures can provoke a great deal of anxiety in both yourself and bystanders.

To assess seizures quickly under such conditions, you need to be thoroughly familiar with their various forms.

Types of Seizures

Seizures can be clinically classified as generalized or partial. **Generalized seizures** begin as an electrical discharge in a small area of the brain but spread to involve the entire cerebral cortex, causing widespread malfunction. **Partial seizures** may remain confined to a limited portion of the brain, causing localized malfunction, or may spread and become generalized.

Generalized Seizures Generalized seizures include tonic-clonic and absence seizures. Another type, pseudoseizures, may mimic generalized seizures.

- *Tonic-Clonic.* A **tonic-clonic seizure,** also known as a *grand mal seizure,* is a generalized motor seizure, producing a loss of consciousness. It typically includes a **tonic** (increased tone) **phase,** characterized by tensed, contracted muscles, and a **clonic phase,** characterized by rhythmic jerking movements of the extremities. During the seizure episode, a patient's intercostal muscles and diaphragm become temporarily paralyzed, interrupting respirations and producing cyanosis. The patient's neck, head, face, and eye muscles may also jerk. Once respirations resume, there may be copious amounts of oral secretions (frothing) present. Incontinence is also common during a seizure. Agitation or confusion, drowsiness, or coma may also follow the seizure.

    Tonic-clonic seizures have a specific progression of events. It is descriptively convenient to refer to this progression as ranging from warning phase to period of recovery. However, not all seizure patients experience all of these events.
  - *Aura.* An aura is a subjective sensation preceding seizure activity. The aura may precede the attack by several hours or by only a few seconds. An aura may be of a psychic or a sensory nature, with olfactory, visual, auditory, or taste hallucinations. Some common types include hearing noise or music, seeing floating lights, smelling unpleasant odors, feeling an unpleasant sensation in the stomach, or experiencing tingling or twitching in a specific body area. Not all seizures are preceded by an aura.
  - *Loss of Consciousness.* The patient will become unconscious at some point after the aura sensations, if any.
  - *Tonic Phase.* This is a phase of continuous muscle tension, characterized by contraction of the patient's muscles.
  - *Hypertonic Phase.* The patient experiences extreme muscular rigidity, including hyperextension of the back.
  - *Clonic Phase.* The patient experiences muscle spasms marked by rhythmic movements. The patient's jaw usually remains clenched, making airway management difficult.
  - *Post Seizure.* The patient remains in a coma.
  - *Postictal.* The patient may awaken confused and fatigued. He may complain of a headache and may experience some neurological

Content Review

TYPES OF SEIZURES
- Generalized Seizures
  - Tonic-clonic
  - Absence
- Partial Seizures
  - Simple partial seizures
  - Complex partial seizures

✱ **generalized seizures** seizures that begin as an electrical discharge in a small area of the brain but spread to involve the entire cerebral cortex, causing widespread malfunction.

✱ **partial seizures** seizures that remain confined to a limited portion of the brain, causing localized malfunction. Partial seizures may spread and become generalized.

✱ **tonic-clonic seizure** type of generalized seizure characterized by rapid loss of consciousness and motor coordination, muscle spasms, and jerking motions.

✱ **tonic phase** phase of a seizure characterized by tension or contraction of muscles.

✱ **clonic phase** phase of a seizure characterized by alternating contraction and relaxation of muscles.

Content Review

PHASES OF A GENERALIZED SEIZURE
- Aura
- Loss of consciousness
- Tonic phase
- Hypertonic phase
- Clonic phase
- Post-seizure
- Postictal

deficit. In many cases, patients will be in this postictal state upon the arrival of paramedic crews. There may be evidence of incontinence, which supports the likelihood that seizure activity has taken place.

* **absence seizure** type of generalized seizure with sudden onset, characterized by a brief loss of awareness and rapid recovery.

- *Absence.* An **absence seizure**, also called a *petit mal seizure,* is a brief, generalized seizure that usually presents with a 10– to 30–second loss of consciousness or awareness, eye or muscle fluttering, and an occasional loss of muscle tone. Loss of consciousness may be so brief that the patient or observers may be unaware of the episode. Absence seizures are idiopathic disorders of early childhood and rarely occur after age twenty. Children who suffer frequent absence seizures are often accused of day dreaming or inattentiveness. Absence seizures may not respond to normal treatment modalities.

- *Pseudoseizures.* Pseudoseizures, also called "hysterical seizures," stem from psychological disorders. The patient presents with sharp and bizarre movements that can often be interrupted with a terse command, such as "stop it!" The seizure is usually witnessed, and there will not be a postictal period. Very rarely do patients experiencing a pseudoseizure injure themselves.

Partial Seizures Partial Seizures may be either simple or complex.

* **simple partial seizure** type of partial seizure that involves local motor, sensory, or autonomic dysfunction of one area of the body. There is no loss of consciousness.

- *Simple Partial Seizures.* **Simple partial seizures,** also sometimes called focal motor, focal sensory, or Jacksonian seizures, are characterized by chaotic movement or dysfunction of one area of the body. When there is abnormal electrical discharge from a specific portion of the brain, only those functions served by that area will have dysfunction. Simple partial seizures involve no loss of consciousness and begin as localized tonic/clonic movements. They frequently spread and can progress to generalized tonic-clonic seizures. Therefore, it is crucial that you document how such seizures begin and the course that they subsequently take.

* **complex partial seizure** type of partial seizure usually originating in the temporal lobe characterized by an aura and focal findings such as alterations in mental status or mood.

- *Complex Partial Seizures.* **Complex partial seizures,** sometimes called temporal lobe or psychomotor seizures, are characterized by distinctive auras. They include unusual smells, tastes, sounds, or the tendency of objects to look either very large and near or small and distant. Sometimes a seizure patient may visualize scenes that look very familiar (*deja vu*) or very strange. A metallic taste in the mouth is a common psychomotor seizure aura. These are focal seizures, lasting approximately 1–2 minutes. The patient experiences a loss of contact with his surroundings. Additionally, the patient may act confused, stagger, perform purposeless movement, or make unintelligible sounds. He may not understand what is said. The patient may even refuse medical aid. Some patients develop automatic behavior or show a sudden change in personality, such as abrupt explosions of rage.

Assessment

Your initial contact with the patient and bystanders will offer a unique opportunity to obtain a history that may influence your plan of management. What an untrained observer calls a seizure may be a simple fainting spell. Therefore, you need to ascertain exactly what the patient may recall or what bystanders witnessed.

Many other problems can mimic or suggest a seizure. These include migraine headaches, cardiac dysrhythmias, hypoglycemia after exercise or drug ingestion, and the tendency to faint when rising from a supine or sitting position (orthostatic hypotension). Hyperventilation, meningitis, intracranial hemorrhage, or certain tranquilizers can cause stiffness of the extremities. Decerebrate move-

A good history will be important in distinguishing a seizure from other conditions that may mimic seizure.

Table 3-2	DIFFERENTIATION BETWEEN SYNCOPE AND GENERALIZED TONIC-CLONIC SEIZURE	
Syncope	**Seizure**
Usually begins in a standing position	May begin in any position
Patient will usually remember a warning of fainting (feeling of weakness or dizziness)	May begin without warning or may be preceded by an aura
Jerking motions usually not present	Jerking motions present during unconsciousness
Patient regains consciousness almost immediately on becoming supine	Patient remains unconscious during seizure, remains drowsy during postictal period

ments, if present, may be caused by increased intracranial pressure. If you are unsure whether the patient has had a seizure, it may be more harmful than beneficial to administer an anticonvulsant medication.

It is also important to try to distinguish between syncope and true seizure (Table 3-2). Syncope patients sometimes have a short initial period of seizure-like activity (usually less than one minute), but this is not followed by a postictal state. The most common cause of fainting is vasovagal syncope associated with fatigue, emotional stress, or cardiac disease. Syncope will be discussed in greater detail later in this chapter.

When obtaining a history, remember to include the following points:

- History of seizures. This data should include length of any past seizure; whether it was generalized or focal; presence of auras, incontinence, or trauma to the tongue.
- Recent history of head trauma.
- Any alcohol and/or drug abuse.
- Recent history of fever, headache, or stiff neck.
- History of diabetes, heart disease, or stroke.
- Current medications. Most chronic seizure patients take anticonvulsant medication on a regular basis. Common anticonvulsant medications include phenytoin (Dilantin), phenobarbital, carbamazepine (Tegretol), and valproic acid (Depakote).

The physical examination of the seizure patient should include the following steps:

- Note any signs of head trauma or injury to the tongue.
- Note any evidence of alcohol and/or drug abuse.
- Document dysrhythmias.

Management

Remember that seizures tend to provoke anxiety in patients, families, and paramedics. From a medical standpoint, however, most of these situations only require managing the airway and preventing the patient from injuring himself. Because the patient may become hypo- or hyperthermic if exposed, protecting body temperature is also crucial. Field management of the seizure patient generally includes the following procedures:

- Assure scene safety.
- Maintain the airway. Do not force objects between the patient's teeth—this includes padded tongue blades. Pushing objects into the patient's mouth may cause him to vomit or to aspirate. It can also cause laryngospasm.

The prime concerns in seizure management are control of the airway and prevention of injury.

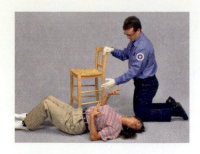

FIGURE 3-22 Protection of a seizing patient.

- Administer high-flow oxygen.
- Establish intravenous access. Initiate normal saline or lactated Ringer's solution at a keep-open rate. Do not use dextrose solutions; emergency department personnel may later administer phenytoin (Dilantin), which is incompatible with dextrose solutions.
- Determine the blood glucose level. If hypoglycemic, administer 50 percent dextrose.
- Never attempt to restrain the patient. This may injure him. However, protect the patient from hitting objects in the environment (Figure 3-22). [Note: If there is evidence of head trauma, C-spine immobilization must be considered as in any other head injury.]
- Maintain body temperature.
- Position the patient on his left side after the clonic-tonic phase (Figure 3-23).
- Suction, if required.
- Monitor cardiac rhythm.
- If seizure is prolonged (> 5 minutes), consider an anticonvulsant.
- Provide a quiet, reassuring atmosphere.
- Transport the patient in the supine or lateral recumbent position.

Status Epilepticus

✱ status epilepticus series of two or more generalized motor seizures without any intervening periods of consciousness.

Status epilepticus—two or more generalized motor seizures with no intervening return of consciousness—is a life-threatening emergency.

🗝

Status epilepticus is a series of two or more generalized motor seizures without an intervening return of consciousness. The most common cause in adults is failure to take prescribed anticonvulsant medications. Status epilepticus is a major emergency since it involves a prolonged period of apnea, which in turn can cause hypoxia of vital brain tissues. These seizures may result in respiratory arrest, severe metabolic and respiratory acidosis, extreme hypertension, increased intracranial pressure, serious elevations in body temperature, fractures of the long bones and spine, necrosis of the cardiac muscle, and severe dehydration.

The most valuable intervention is to protect the patient from airway obstruction and deliver 100 percent oxygen. Preferably this should be accomplished by bag-valve-mask assistance, since the normal ventilatory mechanisms of the patient are seriously impaired and air exchange is generally ineffective. Once the airway is maintained and ventilations are being assisted, take the following steps:

- Start an IV of normal saline at a keep-open rate.
- Monitor cardiac rhythm.

FIGURE 3-23 Place a seizing patient with no suspected spine injury on her left side.

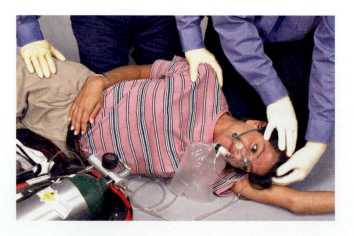

- Administer 25 gms of 50 percent dextrose IV push, if hypoglycemia is present.
- Administer 5–10 mg diazepam IV push for an adult. (Diazepam is a sedative and anticonvulsant that depresses the spread of seizure activity across the motor cortex of the brain.)
- Continue to monitor the airway. Some patients may require large doses of diazepam. Always have flumazenil (Romazicon) available in case it is needed to reverse any significant respiratory depression caused by diazepam. Remember, administration of flumazenil may result in the return of seizures. It should only be used when absolutely necessary.

SYNCOPE

As discussed earlier, **syncope** (fainting) is a neurological condition characterized by the sudden, temporary loss of consciousness caused by insufficient blood flow to the brain, with recovery of consciousness almost immediately upon becoming supine. Nearly half of all Americans will experience at least one episode of syncope during their lifetime. According to the National Institutes of Health, syncope accounts for three percent of all emergency department visits.

* **syncope** transient loss of consciousness due to inadequate flow of blood to the brain with rapid recovery of consciousness upon becoming supine; fainting.

Assessment

Focus on what caused the patient to faint, or lose consciousness. The causes of syncope can be classified into these three general categories:

- *Cardiovascular* conditions, such as dysrhythmias or mechanical problems—A heart rate that is too fast or too slow, or an abnormally functioning heart valve may trigger hypoxia in the brain and subsequent fainting.
- *Non-cardiovascular* disease, such as metabolic, neurological, or psychiatric conditions—Hypoglycemia, a transient ischemic attack, or an anxiety attack can all be causes of syncope.
- *Idiopathic,* or unknown, cause—Oftentimes, the cause of a patient's syncope remains unknown despite careful assessment and diagnostic tests.

Syncope can occur in all ages from the very young to the very old. Symptoms may include feeling faint, dizziness, lightheadedness, or a loss of consciousness without warning. Keep in mind, however, that the definition of syncope includes rapid recovery of consciousness (usually less than a minute). If a patient does not spontaneously regain consciousness within a few moments, it is NOT syncope—it is something more serious.

Syncope involves rapid recovery of consciousness. If a patient does not regain consciousness within a few moments, it is NOT syncope, but something more serious.

Management

When caring for someone who has fainted, it is important to attempt to identify the underlying cause and treat it. If no cause can be identified, anyone who loses consciousness should be transported to an appropriate emergency department and evaluated. Field management of the syncopal patient generally includes the following procedures:

- Assure scene safety.
- Establish and maintain an adequate airway.
- Administer high-flow oxygen and assist ventilations when required.
- Check circulatory status (heart rate, blood pressure, cardiac rhythm).

- Check and continuously monitor mental status.
- Start an IV of normal saline or lactated Ringer's at a keep-open rate.
- Determine the blood glucose level.
- Monitor the cardiac rhythm.
- Reassure the patient.
- Transport the patient to an emergency department.

HEADACHE

Headache can seriously disrupt a person's life. Nearly 45 million Americans suffer from chronic headaches. Of these, approximately 17 million suffer migraine headaches. An estimated 4 billion dollars is spent annually on over-the-counter pain relievers for headache.

Headache pain can be acute (sudden onset) or chronic (constant or recurring), generalized (all over) or localized (in one specific area) and can range from mild to severe. In some cases the cause is known. In others it is not. The most common types of headache can be classified into three categories:

- *Vascular.* Vascular headaches include migraines and cluster headaches. *Migraines* can last from several minutes to several days. They can be characterized by an intense or throbbing pain, photosensitivity (sensitivity to light), nausea, vomiting, and sweats. Migraines are frequently unilateral (on one side of the head) and may be preceded by an aura. *Cluster* headaches usually occur as a series of one-sided headaches that are sudden, intense, and may continue for 15 minutes to 4 hours. Symptoms may include nasal congestion, drooping eyelid, and an irritated or watery eye. Migraines occur more commonly in women, while cluster headaches generally occur in men.
- *Tension.* A significant percentage of headaches are tension headaches. Most personnel in the emergency medical field have, at one time or another, suffered from a tension headache. Sometimes such headaches occur on a daily basis. Sufferers often awake in the morning with a mild headache that gets worse during the course of the day. The tension headache produces a dull, achy pain that feels like a forceful pressure is being applied to the neck and/or head.
- *Organic.* A third, less common category includes organically caused headaches. They occur in individuals suffering from tumors, infection, or other diseases of the brain, eye, or other body system.

A continuous throbbing headache (often predominantly over the occiput) with fever, confusion, and nuchal rigidity (stiffness of the neck) are classic signs and symptoms of *meningitis*. Be alert for these features while assessing patients complaining of headache, particularly those who have also been complaining of nausea, vomiting, or rash. Chapter 11 provides further discussion on meningitis and other infectious diseases.

Assessment

When assessing a patient complaining of headache, ascertain any associated signs and symptoms, such as nausea, vomiting, blurred vision, dizziness, weakness, or watery eyes.

In addition to pain, those suffering from a headache of any type may also complain of nausea, vomiting, blurred vision, dizziness, weakness, or watery eyes. A complete and thorough history of the patient's headache is crucial to its treatment. Determine as much as you can about the pain, including:

- What was the patient doing during the onset of pain?
- Does anything provoke, or worsen, the pain (light, sound, or movement)?

- What is the quality of the pain? (Is it throbbing? crushing? tension?)
- Does the pain radiate to the neck, arm, back, or jaw?
- What is the severity of the pain (On a scale of 1–10, how does the patient rate the pain?)
- How long has the headache been present? (acute vs. chronic?)

Headache of acute onset or of a changing pattern demands immediate attention. A sudden onset of pain, description of the pain as "the worst headache in my life," or changes in the pattern of pain should all be considered characteristics of potential serious conditions, such as intracranial hemorrhage.

Management

Treatment for a victim of headache is supportive. Field management of the headache patient generally includes the following:

- Assure scene safety.
- Establish and maintain an adequate airway.
- Place the patient in a position of comfort. Patients will often place themselves in a position that best alleviates the symptoms, such as lying flat in a dark room.
- Administer high-flow oxygen and assist ventilations when required.
- Start an IV of normal saline or lactated Ringer's at a keep-open rate.
- Determine the blood glucose level.
- Monitor the cardiac rhythm.
- Reassure the patient.
- Consider antiemetics or pain control measures. Migraine headaches typically are accompanied by nausea and vomiting. Antiemetic medications, such as prochlorperazine (Compazine), have proven extremely effective in terminating migraine headaches as well as the accompanying nausea and vomiting. The current pharmacological approach to migraines first includes abortive agents such as sumatriptan (Imitrix) and prochlorperazine (Compazine). If these agents fail, then small doses of analgesics should be considered.
- Ensure a calm, quiet environment. Dimming the interior ambulance lights will help comfort the headache patient with photosensitivity.
- Transport the patient to an emergency department.

"WEAK AND DIZZY"

A frequent problem that paramedics encounter is the patient who is "weak and dizzy" or "weak all over." Generalized weakness and dizziness, although vague, can be symptoms of many diseases. Furthermore, the feeling of being weak or the feeling of being dizzy can be quire disconcerting, especially to the elderly.

Assessment

Obtain a more detailed history of the illness. Has the patient ever had symptoms like this before? Has he had vomiting and/or diarrhea? Has there been a change in his medication regimen recently or has he taken a new medication in the last 72 hours?

Patients with weakness and/or dizziness should receive a focused assessment including a neurological examination. Be alert for the presence of nystagmus (a constant, involuntary, cyclical motion of the eyeball), which can indicate a CNS or inner ear problem. Assess the various muscle groups to try and determine whether the weakness reported by the patient is localized or diffuse. Be alert for potential causes. These can be neurological, respiratory, cardiovascular, endocrine, or infectious. Many viral illnesses will cause a feeling of malaise in the early stages. Inner ear infections (labyrinthitis) often will cause dizziness, especially with sudden movements of the head. Mild volume depletion (dehydration) can cause both weakness and dizziness. Sometimes the dizzy patient will become nauseated or may actually vomit.

Management

While assessing the patient, provide supportive care. This includes:

- Assure scene safety.
- Establish and maintain an adequate airway.
- Place the patient in a position of comfort, generally with head elevated. Avoid sudden or exaggerated movement of the head as it can exacerbate symptoms.
- Administer high-flow oxygen.
- Start an IV of normal saline or lactated Ringer's at a keep-open rate. Consider a fluid bolus if the patient appears dehydrated.
- Check the blood glucose level.
- Monitor the cardiac rhythm.
- Consider the administration of an antiemetic. Often, antiemetics such as dimenhydrinate (Dramamine, Gravol) are helpful in treating dizziness and nausea. If the patient is nauseated or vomiting, consider promethezine (Phenergan) or prochlorperazine (Compazine).
- Ensure a calm, quiet environment.
- Reassure the patient.
- Transport the patient to an emergency department.

NEOPLASMS

* neoplasm literally meaning "new form"; a new or abnormal formation; a tumor.

Brain and spinal cord tumors are abnormal growths of tissue found inside the skull or the bony spinal column. The term **neoplasm** is used to describe the new growth of a tumor (as contrasted to those present at birth, known as congenital tumors). Neoplasms that affect the central nervous system occur in 40,000 Americans per year.

Neurological neoplasms can be divided into two main categories. *Benign* (non-cancerous) *tumors* are those composed of cells that grow similarly to normal cells, grow relatively slowly, and are confined to one location. *Malignant* (cancerous) *tumors* are those with growth very different from that of normal cells. They grow quickly and spread easily to other sites within the body.

Benign neoplasms in most parts of the body are not particularly harmful. Such tumors within the brain or spinal cord, however, pose a greater threat. Because the nervous system is contained within the rigid confines of the skull and spinal column, abnormal growth can place pressure on tissues and impair function. Any tumor located near any of the vital structures of the brain may seriously threaten the ability to breathe, move, or regulate other bodily functions.

Malignant tumors in most parts of the body have a tendency to spread, or *metastasize*. Most brain tumors are metastases from cancer that started somewhere else in the body. For example, breast cancers often metastasize to the brain. These metastases can grow in a single area of the brain or in several areas. However, tumors that originate in the brain or spinal cord rarely spread to other sites in the body. There are numerous types of brain tumors, which must be diagnosed in a medical facility through the use of CT or MRI scan. The cause of most tumors—and most cancers—remains imcompletely known.

Assessment

Central nervous system neoplasms present with many signs and symptoms. The clinical manifestations a patient exhibits will depend on the size, type, and the location of the tumor. As a paramedic, it is not your role to diagnose such new tumors. Instead, you will likely be called to care for someone with a previously diagnosed tumor. Or, perhaps you will be asked to assess a patient with one or more of these common signs and symptoms of a neoplasm:

- Headache (often severe and recurring frequently)
- New seizures in an adult with no history of a seizure disorder
- Nausea
- Vomiting
- Behavioral or cognitive changes
- Weakness or paralysis of one or more limbs or a side of the face
- Change in sensation of one or more limbs or a side of the face
- Lack of coordination
- Difficulty walking or unsteady gait
- Dizziness
- Double vision

Be alert for any of the classic signs and symptoms of a brain or spinal cord tumor. Obtain a thorough medical history. In addition to the SAMPLE questions, ask about the following:

- What is the state of the patient's general health?
- Has the patient had any seizure activity, headache, or nosebleed?

Ask about the type and timing of prior treatment, such as:

- Surgery for removal of a tumor
- Chemotherapy
- Radiation therapy
- Holistic therapy
- Experimental treatments

Management

Treatment of a patient with a neoplasm is primarily supportive. You should attempt to alleviate the patient's anxiety and to reduce his symptoms. Field management of the patient with a neoplasm generally includes the following:

Treatment of a patient with a neoplasm is primarily supportive.

- Assure scene safety.
- Establish and maintain an adequate airway.
- Place the patient in a position of comfort, generally with head elevated.
- Administer high-flow oxygen and assist ventilations when required.
- Start an IV of normal saline or lactated Ringer's at a keep-open rate or a saline or heparin lock.
- Monitor the cardiac rhythm.
- Consider narcotic analgesia if medical direction approves.

- Consider diazepam if seizure activity is present.
- Anti-inflammatories (dexamethasone) and diuretics may be requested by medical direction.
- Ensure a calm, quiet environment.
- Reassure the patient.
- Transport the patient to an emergency department.

BRAIN ABSCESS

A **brain abscess** is a collection of pus localized in an area of the brain. Brain abscesses are uncommon, accounting for two percent of all intracranial masses. Signs and symptoms are similar to those of a neoplasm and include headache, lethargy, hemiparesis, seizures, nuchal rigidity, nausea, and vomiting. Frequently there is also fever. Paramedic management of a patient with an abscess is supportive and similar to that for a neoplasm or meningitis.

DEGENERATIVE NEUROLOGICAL DISORDERS

A collection of diseases that selectively affect one or more functional systems of the central nervous system are known as **degenerative neurological disorders**. They generally produce symmetrical and progressive involvement of the central nervous system, affect similar areas of the brain, and produce similar clinical signs and symptoms.

Types of Degenerative Neurological Disorders

Alzheimer's Disease Alzheimer's disease is perhaps the most important of all the degenerative neurological disorders because of its frequent occurrence and devastating nature. It is the most common cause of dementia in the elderly. Alzheimer's disease results from death and disappearance of nerve cells in the cerebral cortex. This causes marked atrophy of the brain. Initially, patients will have problems with short-term memory. This will usually progress to problems with thought and intellect. The patient will develop a shuffling gait and will have stiffness of the body muscles. As the disease progresses, the patient will develop aphasia (inability to speak) and psychiatric disturbances. In the final stages the patient may become nearly decorticate, losing all ability to think, speak, and move.

Muscular Dystrophy Muscular dystrophy (MD) refers to a group of genetic diseases characterized by progressive muscle weakness and degeneration of the skeletal or voluntary muscle fibers. The heart and other involuntary muscles, are affected in some types of MD. There are several forms of MD, the most common of which is Duchenne. Some forms begin in childhood while others do not appear until middle age. The prognosis of MD varies depending on the type and progression of the disorder.

Multiple Sclerosis Multiple sclerosis (MS) refers to an unpredictable disease of the central nervous system. MS involves inflammation of certain nerve cells followed by demyelination, or the destruction of the myelin sheath, which is the fatty insulation surrounding nerve fibers of the brain and spinal cord. When the myelin sheath is damaged, the nerves are unable to properly conduct impulses. An estimated 300,000 to 400,000 Americans are presently diagnosed with MS. Most MS sufferers are women and first experience symptoms between the ages of 20 and 40.

The disease is known to involve an autoimmune attack against myelin. Signs and symptoms include weakness of one or more limbs, sensory loss, paresthesias, and changes in vision. Symptoms can wax and wane over years, and range from mild to severe. Severe cases can be debilitating, rendering a patient unable to care for himself.

Dystonias The **dystonias** are a group of disorders characterized by muscle contractions that cause twisting and repetitive movements, abnormal postures, or freezing in the middle of an action. Such movements are involuntary and sometimes painful. They may affect a single muscle, a group of muscles, or the entire body.

Early symptoms of dystonia include a deterioration in handwriting, foot cramps, or a tendency of one foot to drag after walking or running. These initial symptoms can be mild and may be noticeable only after prolonged exertion, stress, or fatigue. In many cases, they become more noticeable and widespread over time. In other individuals, there is little or no progression.

Parkinson's Disease **Parkinson's disease** belongs to a group of conditions known as motor system disorders. James Parkinson, a British physician who published a paper on what he called "the shaking palsy," first described the disease in 1817. In his paper, Dr. Parkinson described the major symptoms of the disease that would later bear his name. Since then, scientists have been searching diligently for a cause and subsequent cure.

In the 1960s, researchers identified that a naturally occurring chemical crucial to muscle activity, dopamine, is lower in victims of Parkinson's. This discovery led to the first successful treatment of the disease.

Today, more than a half million Americans are affected with Parkinson's with more than 50,000 new cases being reported every year. It affects men and women in almost equal numbers and it knows no social, economic, or geographic boundaries. The average age of onset is 60 years and it usually does not occur in patients less than 40 years old.

Parkinson's is a chronic and progressive disorder. It has four main characteristics:

- *Tremor.* Sometimes called "pill rolling," the typical tremor is a rhythmic back-and-forth motion of the thumb and forefinger. It usually begins in the hand and may progress to an arm, a foot, or the jaw.
- *Rigidity.* Most Parkinson's patients suffer rigidity, or resistance to movement. All muscles have an opposing muscle. In the healthy adult, one muscle contracts while the opposing muscle relaxes. In Parkinson's, the balance of this opposition is disturbed, leading to rigidity.
- *Bradykinesia.* Normal, spontaneous, and autonomic movement is slowed and sometimes lost. Such loss of movement is unpredictable. While one moment the patient can move easily, the next moment he cannot.
- *Postural Instability.* Impaired balance and coordination cause patients to develop a forward or backward lean, stooped posture, and the tendency to fall easily.

Victims of Parkinson's may also be plagued with depression, a slowing or "shuffling" gait, a stiff or "stone-like" face, and dementia.

Central Pain Syndrome **Central pain syndrome** is a condition that results from damage or injury to the brain, brainstem, or spinal cord. It is characterized by intense, steady pain described as burning, aching, tingling, or a "pins and needles" sensation. The syndrome may develop weeks, months, or years after an injury to the CNS. It occurs in patients who have had strokes, multiple sclerosis, limb amputations, or spinal cord injuries. Pain medications generally provide no relief for victims of central pain syndrome. Patients rely upon sedation and other methods to keep the central nervous system free from stress.

One type of chronic pain is known as trigeminal neuralgia, or *tic douloureux*. It is caused by abnormal electrical conduction along the trigeminal nerve (cranial nerve V). The condition is characterized by episodes of facial pain that are brief, yet intense. The fear of such an episode is often debilitating. Patients are treated

* **dystonias** a group of disorders characterized by muscle contractions that cause twisting and repetitive movements, abnormal postures, or freezing in the middle of an action.

* **Parkinson's disease** chronic and progressive motor system disorder characterized by tremor, rigidity, bradykinesia, and postural instability.

* **central pain syndrome** condition resulting from damage or injury to the brain, brainstem, or spinal cord characterized by intense, steady pain described as burning, aching, tingling, or a "pins and needles" sensation.

with medications such as the anti-convulsant carbamazepine (Tegretol). In select cases, surgical interventions may be used.

Bell's Palsy

Bell's palsy is the most common form of facial paralysis. It results from inflammatory reaction of the facial nerve (cranial nerve VII). The condition affects roughly 40,000 Americans every year. It is characterized by one-sided facial paralysis, the inability to close the eye, pain, tearing of the eyes, drooling, hypersensitivity to sound, and impairment of taste.

Although, the specific cause is often unknown, some causes have been identified. They are head trauma, herpes simplex virus, and Lyme disease. Treatment is usually aimed at protecting the eye. Corticosteroids may be prescribed for inflammation when pain is severe. Most patients recover within three months.

Amyotrophic Lateral Sclerosis

Amyotrophic lateral sclerosis (ALS), also known as Lou Gehrig's disease, is a progressive degeneration of specific nerve cells that control voluntary movement. Characterized by weakness, loss of motor control, difficulty speaking, and cramping, the disease eventually weakens the diaphragm, which leads to breathing problems. ALS belongs to a class of disorders known as motor neuron diseases. It affects 20,000 Americans with 5,000 new cases being reported each year.

There is currently no cure for ALS. There is also no effective therapy. However, the FDA has approved riluzole, the first drug that has been shown to prolong the lives of ALS patients. The prognosis continues to be poor. Most patients die within three to five years of being diagnosed usually as a result of pulmonary infection.

Myoclonus

Myoclonus is a term that refers to the temporary, involuntary twitching or spasm of a muscle or group of muscles. It is generally considered not a diagnosis but a symptom. It is usually one of several symptoms of a variety of nervous system disorders such as multiple sclerosis, Parkinson's, or Alzheimer's. Some simple examples of myoclonus include hiccups or muscle twitching. Pathologic myoclonus can distort normal movement and limit a person's ability to eat, walk, and talk.

Treatment of myoclonus consists of medications to reduce symptoms. Many of these drugs are also used to treat epilepsy, such as barbiturates, clonazepam, phenytoin, and sodium valproate.

Spina Bifida

Spina bifida (SB) is a neural defect that results from the failure of one or more of the fetal vertebrae to close properly during pregnancy. This leaves a portion of the spinal cord unprotected. The spinal opening can usually be repaired shortly after birth, but the nerve damage is permanent. Long term effects include physical and mobility impairments, and most individuals also have some form of learning disability. The three most common types of SB are:

- *Myelomeningocele*—the severest form and one in which the spinal cord and the meninges protrude from an opening in the spine.
- *Meningocele*—characterized by the normal development of the spinal cord, but the meninges protrude through a spinal opening.
- *Occulta*—the mildest form and one in which one or more vertebrae are malformed and covered by a layer of skin.

There is presently no cure for spina bifida. Treatment includes surgery, medications, and physiotherapy. With proper care, most children with SB live into adulthood.

Poliomyelitis

Poliomyelitis (polio) is an infectious, inflammatory viral disease of the central nervous system that sometimes results in permanent paralysis. It is characterized by fatigue, headache, fever, vomiting, stiffness of the neck, and pain to the hands and feet. New cases in the United States are rare. A vaccine developed in the 1950s caused the number of cases to decline from 50,000 to only a

---

✳ **Bell's palsy** one-sided facial paralysis with an unknown cause characterized by the inability to close the eye, pain, tearing of the eyes, drooling, hypersensitivity to sound, and impairment of taste.

✳ **amyotrophic lateral sclerosis (ALS)** progressive degeneration of specific nerve cells that control voluntary movement characterized by weakness, loss of motor control, difficulty speaking, and cramping. Also called *Lou Gehrig's disease.*

✳ **myoclonus** temporary, involuntary twitching or spasm of a muscle or group of muscles.

✳ **spina bifida (SB)** a neural defect that results from the failure of one or more of the fetal vertebrae to close properly during the first month of pregnancy.

✳ **poliomyelitis (polio)** infectious, inflammatory viral disease of the central nervous system that sometimes results in permanent paralysis.

few per year. Thousands of pre-vaccine survivors of the disease are alive today. Many of these require supportive care.

Assessment of Degenerative Neurological Disorders

When you encounter a patient with a degenerative neurological disorder, use your assessment and history-taking skills to determine the patient's chief complaint. You may be called to treat someone with an exacerbation (flare up) of one of the degenerative diseases or someone with an unrelated complaint. In either case, it is important to conduct an initial assessment, correct any life-threatening problems, and find out exactly what prompted the call to EMS.

Management of Degenerative Neurological Disorders

When caring for a patient with a degenerative neurological disease, make treating the chief complaint a priority. Do not overlook the patient's underlying condition, but don't allow it to cloud a more serious problem. After performing an initial assessment and managing any life-threatening conditions, manage the chief complaint. While providing care, consider the following about patients who suffer from a degenerative neurological disorder:

When caring for a patient with a degenerative neurological disease, make treating the chief complaint a priority. Do not allow the patient's underlying condition to cloud a more serious problem.

- *Mobility.* The ability to walk and move about freely is often taken for granted by many of us. Neurological patients often lack this ability and require assistance.
- *Communication.* Certain neurological disorders will affect a patient's ability to speak clearly and distinctly. Take the necessary time to ensure open communication. Speak with bystanders and family members to assist in gaining a thorough history.
- *Respiratory Compromise.* Exacerbations of ALS and other conditions may affect the ability to breathe. Treat any breathing problem as a priority.
- *Anxiety.* Coping with a debilitating disease is a strenuous and taxing task. Dealing with the ongoing battles with a neurological condition will cause stress—and anxiety. Approach the patient and his family with compassion and care.

The following steps may be appropriate, depending on the patient's chief complaint:

- Determine the blood glucose level. A serum glucose determination will assist in determining if an altered mental status is due to hypoglycemia.
- Establish an IV of normal saline or lactated Ringer's at a keep-open rate.
- Monitor the cardiac rhythm.
- Transport to an emergency department.

BACK PAIN AND NONTRAUMATIC SPINAL DISORDERS

Back pain is one of the most common reasons people seek health care. Millions and millions of health care dollars are spent each year on the treatment of back pain. Back pain can be classified as either traumatic or non-traumatic in origin. Many patients will develop chronic back pain. Chronic back pain is a significant cause of disability and lost time from work. EMS is occasionally called to treat persons with back pain. These calls can be due to a new injury or exacerbation of chronic back pain. In addition, some patients will develop back pain without an identifiable injury.

Low Back Pain

Back pain can be felt anywhere along the spinal column. However, low back pain (LBP) is the most common back-pain complaint. It is a common, yet debilitating condition. Low back pain is defined as back pain felt between the lower rib cage and the gluteal muscles, often radiating to the thighs.

Both chronic and new-onset low back pain are increasingly common. This complaint of low back pain is the cause of great amount of lost work time in the United States. Between 60 and 90 percent of the population experience some form of low back pain at some time in their life. Men and women are equally affected, although women over 60 years of age report low back pain symptoms more often, most likely as a result of post-menopausal osteoporosis. Occupations that involve exposure to vibrations from vehicles or machinery and those that require repetitious lifting are often implicated in low back pain. As a paramedic, you yourself are particularly at risk for back problems.

About one percent of acute low back pain results from sciatica, which causes severe pain along the path of the sciatic nerve, down the back of the thigh and inner leg. This is sometimes accompanied by motor and sensory deficits such as muscle weakness. Sciatica may be caused by compression or trauma to the sciatic nerve or its roots, often resulting from a herniated intervertebral disk or osteoarthrosis of the lumbosacral vertebrae. It may also be caused by inflammation of the sciatic nerve from metabolic, toxic, or infectious causes.

Pain occurring at the level of L-3, L-4, L-5, and S-1 may be due to inflammation of the interspinous bursae. Low back pain may also result from inflammation or sprains or strains of the muscles and ligaments that attach to the spine or from vertebral fractures. Additional causes of back pain include tumors, inflammation of the synovial sacs, rising venous pressure, degenerative joint disease, abnormal bone pressure, problems with spinal mobility, and inflammation caused by infection (osteomyelitis).

In fact, however, most low back pain is idiopathic. That is, the cause may be difficult or impossible to diagnose, even by a physician or in a hospital setting. This makes treatment of many cases of low back pain frustrating and sometimes unsuccessful.

Causes of Nontraumatic Spinal Disorders and Back Pain

Spinal problems may be caused by trauma, but many spinal disorders have nontraumatic causes. Nontraumatic spinal injuries most often result from three causes:

- Degeneration or rupture of the disks that separate the vertebrae
- Degeneration or fracture of the vertebrae
- Cyst or tumor that impinges on the spine

The type and degree of pain that results from these conditions differs from person to person.

Disk Injury The cartilaginous disks that separate the vertebrae may rupture as a result of injury or may rupture or degenerate as part of the process of aging. Degeneration may cause a narrowing of the disk that compromises spinal stability. Degenerative disk disease is more common in patients over 50 years of age.

A herniated disk occurs when the gelatinous center of the disk (the *nucleus pulposa*) extrudes through a tear in the tough outer capsule (the *anulus fibrosa*). The pain that results from these conditions usually results from pressure on the spinal cord or muscle spasm at the site. The intervetebral disks themselves have no innervation. Herniation may be caused by degenerative disk disease, by trauma, or by improper lifting. Improper lifting is the most common cause. Men aged 30 to 50 years are more prone to disk herniation than women. Herniation most commonly affects the disks at L-4, L-5, and S-1 but may also occur in C-5, C-6, and C-7.

Vertebral Injury The vertebrae themselves may break down (vertebral spondylolysis), especially the lamina or vertebral arch between the articulating facets (the areas where adjoining vertebrae contact one another). Heredity is thought to be a significant factor in the development of spondylolysis. Rotational fractures are common at these sites. Spinal fractures are frequently associated with osteoporosis (brittle bones), which tends to develop in many elderly persons.

Cysts and Tumors A cyst or tumor along the spine or intruding into the spinal canal may cause pain by pressing on the spinal cord, by causing degenerative changes in the bone, or by interrupting blood supply. The specific manifestations depend on the location and the type of the cyst or tumor.

Other Medical Causes Back pain can also be caused by medical conditions associated with neither traumatic nor nontraumatic spinal injury. For example, back pain may manifest as referred pain from disorders such as diabetic neuropathy, renal calculus, abdominal aortic aneurysm, and many other conditions such as those discussed in this chapter. It would be a mistake to assume that all back complaints are related to the spinal cord, the vertebrae, the intervetebral disks, or the muscles and ligaments surrounding the vertebrae.

Assessment

Assessment of back pain is based on the patient's chief complaint, the history, and the physical exam. When the complaint is low back pain, a precise diagnosis is likely to be difficult. Preliminary diagnosis may be based on a history of risk factors, such as an occupation requiring repetitive lifting, exposure to vibrations from vehicles or industrial machinery, or a known history of osteoporosis.

The complaint of low back pain often involves radiation of the pain from the gluteus to the thigh, leg, and foot. Usually there is history of slow onset over several weeks to months and the patient has called for your help secondary to an increase in pain and the lack of relief from warm compresses or over-the-counter analgesics. The patient may or may not recall a particular incident that has caused this "low back pain;" direct trauma is very rarely a contributing factor in this type of pain.

Just because low back pain is a common complaint that can be hard to diagnose, do not dismiss this type of complaint as "not real pain." A complete history and physical exam by a physician are necessary to determine the cause of any back pain. Diagnosis will often depend on the results of a CT or MRI scan, electromyelography, or other in-hospital testing.

In the prehospital setting, the important task is to determine if the patient's pain is caused by a life-threatening or a non-life-threatening condition. A good patient history will help in this determination. A history of work or play involving lifting or twisting and a sudden onset of pain, often associated with straining, coughing, or sneezing, may point to a mechanical type of muscle or ligament injury. A gradual onset of pain may point instead to a chronic condition such as degenerative disk disease or tumor development. The presence of associated neurological deficit may also point to a more serious underlying cause. When the complaint is back pain, be sure to inquire about prior back surgery, physical therapy, and time lost from work.

Location of the injury may be revealed by a limited range of motion in the lumbar spine, tenderness on palpation at the location of the injury, alterations in sensation, pain, and temperature at the site, pain or paresthesia below the injury (in the upper extremities with cervical injury, symptoms increasing with neck motion, with possible slight motor weakness in the biceps and triceps; similar symptoms in the lower extremities with injury to the thoracic or lumbar spine).

Keep in mind that you are very unlikely to be able to determine the cause of your patient's back pain in the field. Primarily, you need to gather information from the history and physical exam that you will report to the receiving physician and that will help you determine what degree of immobilization, if any, will be necessary during transport.

Management

Prehospital management of back pain is primarily aimed at decreasing any pain or discomfort caused by moving the patient and keeping a watchful eye for signs and symptoms of any serious underlying disorder.

Should C-spine precautions be taken with the patient complaining of back pain? Should this patient be immobilized to a long back board or a vacuum-type stretcher? These questions are best answered, "It depends." First you must consider trauma as a possible cause of the patient's pain. If there is no recent mechanism of injury, consider whether the patient has a possible history of osteoporosis or another disease that might lead to spinal fracture. In these cases, consider immobilizing the patient.

If trauma and possible fracture are ruled out, you may still undertake C-spine precautions and immobilization, because the less movement a patient is put through the more comfortable he will feel. Long-board or vacuum-stretcher immobilization may be the best mode of transportation. If in doubt, immobilize, remembering the injunction to "do no harm."

Some patients with back pain and back spasms may require parenteral analgesics and parenteral diazepam before they can even lie on the stretcher. Contact medical direction regarding analgesic and muscle relaxant therapy.

Conduct ongoing assessment en route with special attention to the airway, breathing, vital signs, and the possible presence or development of motor and sensory deficits that may indicate a critical condition and that can adversely affect the patient's breathing effort.

SUMMARY

Nervous system emergencies include a complex variety of illnesses and injuries. A thorough patient assessment and medical history will help guide your care and will prove invaluable for subsequent hospital management.

Initial field management is directed at ensuring an adequate airway and ventilation. The brain requires a constant supply of oxygen, glucose, and vitamins. After 10–20 seconds without blood flow, the patient becomes unconscious. Significant loss of oxygen (anoxia) or low blood sugar (hypoglycemia) can cause coma or seizures. Supply high-flow oxygen to patients with neurological disorders. Administer dextrose to any neurological patient with hypoglycemia.

Neurological injuries and illnesses often require treatment as soon as possible to prevent progressive damage. Patients suffering from an altered level of consciousness, stroke (brain attack), transient ischemic attack, seizures, and syncope require early intervention and transportation to the closest appropriate facility.

You will also be called to care for patients suffering from a headache, neoplasm, a degenerative neurological disorder, or a complaint of back pain. These conditions may be relatively minor, or indicative of a much more serious underlying condition. They too require a complete patient assessment, medical history, and supportive care.

Care for the neurological patient may simply be supportive. In other cases, you should provide drug therapy or other interventions to limit or reduce the presenting symptoms. Airway management remains a priority in caring for any patient with an alteration in neurological function.

YOU MAKE THE CALL

You and your partner are called to 222 East 19th Street on an unknown medical problem. Dispatch reports that the call came from a neighbor and further information is not available.

Upon arrival at the scene, you find a 64-year-old female sitting upright in a chair complaining of a "terrible headache." As you begin to interview the patient, you discover that she is having difficulty breathing and has slurred speech. You place the patient on high-flow oxygen while your partner interviews the neighbor and the patient's niece who has just arrived.

While you are taking the patient's pulse, the niece reports that her aunt is usually alert and able to speak complete sentences. Her blood pressure is 190/110, pulse 90, and her respiratory rate is 18 breaths per minute. Blood glucose level is 92 mg/dl.

En route to the hospital, the patient sits up slightly and says, "I am feeling much better now." She reports that her headache has dissipated, and you notice that her speech is no longer slurred.

1. Based on the clinical symptoms present, what might be wrong with this patient?
2. What would account for the quickly dissipating symptoms?
3. What is the priority in managing this patient's care?
4. What are the appropriate steps in caring for this patient?

See Suggested Responses at the back of this book.

FURTHER READING

Brunner, Lillian, et al. *Brunner and Suddarth's Textbook of Medical-Surgical Nursing.* 9th ed. Philadelphia: Lippincott, Williams, and Wilkins, 1999.

Dickinson, Edward. *Fire Service Emergency Care.* Upper Saddle River, N.J.: Brady, 1999.

Fauci, A.S., et al. *Harrison's Principles of Internal Medicine.* 14th ed. New York: McGraw-Hill, 1998.

Guyton, Arthur C. and John E. Hall. *Textbook of Medical Physiology.* 9th ed. Philadelphia: W.B. Saunders, 1996.

National Institute of Neurological Disorders and Stroke. *Rapid Identification and Treatment of Acute Stroke.* Bethesda, M.D.: National Institutes of Health, 1997.

Saunders, Charles E. and Mary T. Ho. *Current Emergency Diagnosis and Treatment.* 5th ed. Norwalk, CT: Appleton and Lange, 2000.

Tintanelli, J.E. et al. *Emergency Medicine: A Comprehensive Study Guide.* 5th ed. New York: McGraw-Hill, 1999.

ON THE WEB

Visit Brady's Paramedic Website at www.bradybooks.com/paramedic.

CHAPTER 4

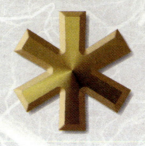

Endocrinology

Objectives

After reading this chapter, you should be able to:

1. Describe the incidence, morbidity, and mortality of endocrinologic emergencies. (pp. 326–327, 329-330, 336-337)
2. Identify the risk factors that predispose a person to endocrinologic disease. (pp. 329, 336–337, 340, 341)
3. Discuss the anatomy and physiology of organs and structures associated with endocrinologic diseases. (pp. 316–326)
4. Discuss the pathophysiology, assessment findings, need for rapid intervention and transport, and management of endocrinologic emergencies. (pp. 326–341)

5. Describe osmotic diuresis and its relationship to diabetes mellitus. (p. 329)
6. Describe the pathophysiology of adult and juvenile onset diabetes mellitus. (pp. 329–330)
7. Differentiate between the pathophysiology of normal glucose metabolism and diabetic glucose metabolism. (pp. 327–329)
8. Describe the mechanism of ketone body formation and its relationship to ketoacidosis. (pp. 328, 330–332)

Continued

9. Discuss the physiology of the excretion of potassium and ketone bodies by the kidneys. (pp. 328–329)
10. Describe the relationship of insulin to serum glucose levels. (pp. 315, 323–324)
11. Describe the effects of decreased levels of insulin on the body. (pp. 329–333)
12. Describe the effects of increased serum glucose levels on the body. (pp. 333, 336)
13. Discuss the pathophysiology, assessment findings, and management of the following endocrine emergencies:
    a. nonketotic hyperosmolar coma (pp. 332–333)
    b. diabetic ketoacidosis (pp. 330–332)
    c. hypoglycemia (pp. 333, 336)
    d. hyperglycemia (pp. 329, 330-332)
    e. thyrotoxicosis (pp. 336–338)

    f. myxedema (pp. 338–339)
    g. Cushing's syndrome (pp. 340–341)
    h. adrenal insufficiency, or Addison's disease (p. 341)
14. Describe the actions of epinephrine as it relates to the pathophysiology of hypoglycemia. (p. 333)
15. Describe the compensatory mechanisms utilized by the body to promote homeostasis when hypoglycemia is present. (pp. 315, 323–324)
16. Differentiate among different endocrine emergencies based on assessment and history. (pp. 326–341)
17. Given several scenarios involving endocrine emergency patients, provide the appropriate assessment, management, and transportation. (pp. 315–341)

CASE STUDY

Shauna White and Steve Curran leave the hospital after the Quarterly Trauma Case Conference and notify dispatch that they are in service and en route to quarters. Within minutes, they receive a dispatch call for an unknown medical emergency in a nearby residential neighborhood. The response time is less than 3 minutes. They park the unit in front of the house and don personal protective equipment. As Steve removes the stretcher and jump kit from the back of the unit, a police cruiser pulls up to the curb. The officers intercept Steve and Shauna, explaining that they were dispatched after someone called 911 to report the sounds of a possible altercation in the home.

At that moment, a woman walks up and identifies herself as Mrs. Spencer, the 911 caller. She says that she was in her garden when she heard loud sounds suddenly coming from the McKenzies' house next door. She says she was alarmed because the noise lasted for only a short time, but it sounded like items were being thrown or broken. Moreover, she knows that Mr. McKenzie is traveling out of town. Mrs. McKenzie left the house about an hour before the noise occurred. At the moment, however, all is quiet.

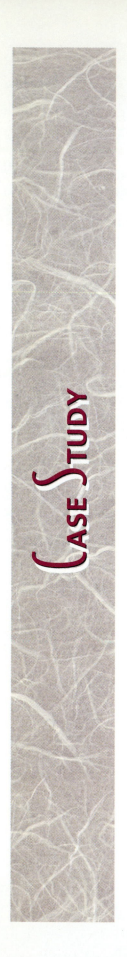

The officers caution Steve, Shauna, and Mrs. Spencer to stand clear until they secure the scene. They approach the front door, identify themselves as police, and enter the house. In less than a minute, they call out 'All clear,' and summon the paramedics. Shauna and Steve quickly enter. In the living room, they see that the furniture in one corner has been overturned, and books and magazines are strewn about the floor. An officer crouches near an adolescent male who appears to be in his mid-teens. The boy is pale and diaphoretic. He looks confused as the officer speaks to him. His clothing is out of place. Mrs. Spencer looks in from the open doorway and identifies the young man as Mark McKenzie.

Shauna's initial assessment reveals a 16-year-old male without airway compromise. He is breathing rapidly, but with good depth and volume. His carotid pulse is rapid and strong. Although the patient is conscious, he responds to Shauna with incoherent muttering. Steve quickly places a nonrebreather oxygen mask over the patient's face, then he and Shauna move him onto the stretcher. One of the police officers says he'll look around the scene for evidence of medications or illicit drugs.

Mark pulls the oxygen mask off and tries to get up and walk. Shauna replaces the mask and tries to reassure him. Finally, after he makes several more attempts to get up, Mark is gently restrained on the stretcher. Shauna begins a more detailed assessment while Steve looks for a vein to draw blood and start an intravenous line. He notes that Mark's skin is pale, cool, and clammy. Shauna observes no obvious injuries except a small bruise forming on the right cheek. In addition, she does not smell any unusual odors such as alcohol or paint fumes. Mark is not wearing a Medic Alert tag. Shauna finds that Mark's blood pressure is 130/88 mmHg, his pulse is 120 beats per minute, and his respiratory rate is 28 breaths per minute. The oxygen saturation is 99 percent on the nonrebreather mask.

Prior to starting the IV line, Steve follows protocol, filling a red-top tube with blood and obtaining a sample for immediate determination of the blood glucose level. The portable glucose detection device reports the glucose level as "LOW." As Steve gives Shauna the information, the officer returns and tells them that he found a bottle of insulin in the refrigerator with Mark's name on the label.

Hypoglycemia is potentially life threatening, and Steve immediately administers 50 milliliters of 50 percent dextrose (25 grams) intravenously per standing orders. Within minutes, Mark's skin becomes warm and dry, and he begins to speak more clearly. As Shauna prepares to contact medical direction prior to transporting Mark to the hospital for evaluation, his mother returns home. She says that Mark was diagnosed with diabetes at age 8 and is usually well controlled, but his insulin dosage was recently changed. She thanks the team but says she would prefer to contact Mark's physician, Dr. McGraw, directly rather than having Mark transported to the hospital. Shauna contacts medical direction and notifies them of the refusal of transport.

Steve aseptically discontinues Mark's IV while Shauna prepares the patient care report and transport refusal form for Mrs. McKenzie's signature. Prior to leaving the scene, Shauna reminds Mark and Mrs. McKenzie that they should not hesitate to call 911 again if they need help. She thanks the police officers for their assistance.

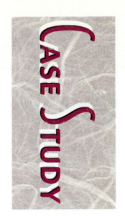

INTRODUCTION

The *endocrine system* is an important body system. Closely linked to the nervous system, it controls numerous physiological processes. Unlike the nervous system, which exerts its control through nervous impulses, the endocrine system controls the body through specialized chemical messengers called **hormones.** The fundamental structural units of the endocrine system are the **endocrine glands.** Each endocrine gland produces one or more hormones. (An example of an endocrine gland is the pancreas. Specific endocrine glands will be described later. The endocrine glands are the chief focus of this chapter.)

Endocrine glands differ from other glands in that they are ductless. Instead of releasing hormones through ducts to a local site, they secrete their hormones directly into capillaries to circulate in the blood throughout the body. In contrast, the majority of glands are **exocrine glands,** which release their chemical products through ducts and tend to have a local effect. For example, the salivary glands are a type of exocrine gland. The salivary glands are located near the pharynx and secrete digestive enzymes, such as amylase, into the pharynx.

Keep in mind these important points about endocrine glands:

* In contrast to the exocrine glands, whose effects tend to be localized, endocrine glands tend to have widespread effects.
* The hormones released by endocrine glands typically act on distant tissues. They exert a very specific effect on their target tissues.
* Some hormones, such as insulin, have many target organs. Other hormones have only a few target organs.
* Through the release of hormones, the endocrine system plays an important role in regulating body function.

As noted above, the principal product of an endocrine gland is a hormone. The term *hormone* comes from the Greek for "to set in motion," and hormones keep in motion, or regulate, numerous vital cell processes. For example, the hormones insulin and glucagon enable the body to maintain a stable blood glucose level, both after and between meals. This is an example of **homeostasis,** the natural tendency of the body to maintain an appropriate internal environment in the face of changing external conditions. Hormones such as growth hormone and thyroid hormone regulate **metabolism.** Metabolism encompasses all the cellular processes that produce the energy and molecules needed for growth or repair. In

* **hormone** chemical substance released by a gland that controls or affects processes in other glands or body systems.

* **endocrine gland** gland that secretes chemical substances directly into the blood; also called a *ductless gland.*

* **exocrine gland** gland that secretes chemical substances to nearby tissues through a duct; also called a *ducted gland.*

The effects of exocrine glands tend to be localized, while the effects of endocrine glands tend to be widespread.

* **homeostasis** the natural tendency of the body to keep the internal environment and metabolism steady and normal.

* **metabolism** the sum of cellular processes that produce the energy and molecules needed for growth and repair.

addition, hormones such as estrogen and testosterone regulate the sexual development of puberty and the subsequent reproductive function of adulthood.

Many people have endocrine disorders involving excessive or deficient hormone function. Some common conditions, such as hypothyroidism, are readily controlled by hormone replacement medication. Other hormonal disorders may have a more difficult course. You will find that the hormonal disorder diabetes mellitus is commonly involved in medical emergencies encountered in the prehospital setting.

ANATOMY AND PHYSIOLOGY

There are eight major glands in the endocrine system: the hypothalamus, pituitary gland, thyroid gland, parathyroid glands, thymus, pancreas, adrenal glands, and gonads. The pineal gland is also an endocrine gland, but much of its function remains unclear. In addition to the endocrine glands, many body tissues have been found to have endocrine function. These include the kidneys, heart, placenta, and parts of the digestive tract.

The endocrine glands are located throughout the body (Figure 4-1). Although Figure 4-1 shows an adult, remember that the thymus is primarily active

Content Review

ENDOCRINE GLANDS
Hypothalamus
Pituitary
Thyroid
Parathyroid
Thymus
Pancreas
Adrenals
Gonads
Pineal

FIGURE 4-1 The major glands of the endocrine system.

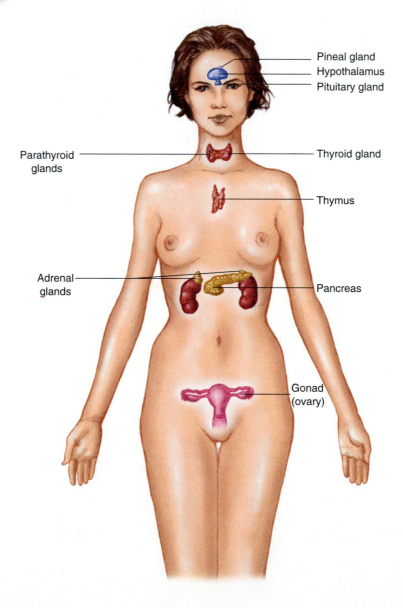

Pineal gland
Hypothalamus
Pituitary gland

Parathyroid glands

Thyroid gland

Thymus

Adrenal glands

Pancreas

Gonad (ovary)

during childhood, when it plays a role in maturation of the immune system. By adulthood, the thymus is so small that it is not visualized on chest X-rays. The hormones secreted by endocrine glands, their target tissues, and their effects are listed in Table 4-1.

HYPOTHALAMUS

The *hypothalamus* is located deep within the cerebrum of the brain. Hypothalamic cells act both as nerve cells, or neurons, and as gland cells. The hypothalamus is the junction, or connection, between the central nervous system and the endocrine system. As neurons, many hypothalamic cells receive messages from the **autonomic nervous system**—peripheral nerves that, among other functions, detect internal conditions such as blood pressure or blood glucose level and convey that information to the central nervous system through nerve impulses. Some hypothalamic cells respond by producing nerve impulses that travel to cells in the posterior pituitary gland. Other hypothalamic cells respond as gland cells by producing and releasing hormones into the stalk of tissue that connects the hypothalamus and the anterior pituitary gland.

In response to impulses from the autonomic nervous system, the hypothalamus—and other organs of the endocrine system—can release the hormones that promote homeostasis:

* *Growth hormone releasing hormone (GHRH)*
* *Growth hormone inhibiting hormone (GHIH)*
* *Corticotropin releasing hormone (CRH)*
* *Thyrotropin releasing hormone (TRH)*
* *Gonadotropin releasing hormone (GnRH)*
* *Prolactin releasing hormone (PRH)*
* *Prolactin inhibiting hormone (PIH)*

As you can see in Table 4-1, most hypothalamic hormones, including thyrotropin releasing hormone (TRH) and growth hormone releasing hormone (GHRH), stimulate secretion of pituitary hormones that rouse yet another endocrine gland or body tissue to increased activity. For example, in response to TRH the anterior pituitary releases thyroid stimulating hormone, and thyroid stimulating hormone then acts upon the thyroid gland to increase thyroid activity.

The pair of hypothalamic hormones—growth hormone releasing hormone (GHRH) and growth hormone inhibitory hormone (GHIH)—demonstrate a major trait of endocrine function: Many hormonal activities are driven not by one hormone, but rather by two hormones with opposing effects. GHRH stimulates secretion of growth hormone, and GHIH suppresses secretion of growth hormone. The actual amount of growth hormone secreted by the anterior pituitary depends on the net amount of stimulation (Figure 4-2).

PITUITARY GLAND

The *pituitary gland* is only about the size of a pea. It is divided into posterior and anterior pituitary lobes. These tissues have different embryonic origins and different functional relationships with the hypothalamus. The *posterior pituitary gland* responds to nerve impulses from the hypothalamus, whereas the *anterior pituitary gland* responds to hypothalamic hormones that travel down the stalk that connects the anterior pituitary and hypothalamus. As you look at the target

* autonomic nervous system part of the nervous system controlling involuntary bodily functions. It is divided into the sympathetic and the parasympathetic systems.

Gland and Major Hormone(s)	Target Tissues	Major Hormone Effect(s)
Hypothalamus		
Growth hormone releasing hormone, GHRH	Anterior pituitary	Stimulates release of growth hormone
Growth hormone inhibiting hormone, GHIH (or somatostatin)	Anterior pituitary	Suppresses release of growth hormone
Corticotropin releasing hormone, CRH	Anterior pituitary	Stimulates release of adrenocorticotropin
Thyrotropin releasing hormone, TRH	Anterior pituitary	Stimulates release of thyroid-stimulating hormone
Gonadotropin releasing hormone, GnRH	Anterior pituitary	Stimulates release of luteinizing hormone and follicle-stimulating hormone
Prolactin releasing hormone, PRH	Anterior pituitary	Stimulates release of prolactin
Prolactin inhibiting hormone, PIH	Anterior pituitary	Suppresses release of prolactin
Posterior pituitary gland		
Antidiuretic hormone, ADH	Kidneys	Stimulates increased reabsorption of water into blood volume
Oxytocin	Uterus and breasts of females, kidneys	Stimulates uterine contractions and milk release
Anterior pituitary gland		
Growth hormone, GH	All cells, especially growing cells	Stimulates body growth in childhood; causes switch to fats as energy source
Adrenocorticotropic hormone, ACTH	Adrenal cortexes	Stimulates release of corticosteroidal hormones cortisol and aldosterone
Thyroid-stimulating hormone, TSH	Thyroid	Stimulates release of thyroid hormones thyroxine and triiodothyronine
Follicle-stimulating hormone, FSH	Ovaries or Testes	FSH stimulates development of sex cells (ovum or sperm)
Luteinizing hormone, LH	Ovaries or Testes	LH stimulates release of hormones (estrogen, progesterone or testosterone)
Prolactin, PRL	Mammary glands	Stimulates production and release of milk
Thyroid gland		
Thyroxine, T_4	All cells	Stimulates cell metabolism
Triiodothyronine, T_3	All cells	Stimulates cell metabolism
Calcitonin	Bone	Stimulates calcium uptake by bones, decreasing blood calcium level
Parathyroid glands		
Parathyroid hormone, PTH	Bone, intestine, kidneys	Stimulates calcium release from bone, calcium uptake from GI tract, calcium reabsorption in kidney, all increasing blood calcium level
Thymus		
Thymosin	White blood cells, primarily T lymphocytes	Stimulates reproduction and functional development of T lymphocytes

Gland and Major Hormone(s)	Target Tissues	Major Hormone Effect(s)
Pancreas		
Glucagon	All cells, particularly in liver, muscle, and fat	Stimulates hepatic glycogenolysis and gluconeogenesis, increasing blood glucose level
Insulin	All cells, particularly in liver, muscle, and fat	Stimulates cellular uptake of glucose, Increased rate of synthesis of glycogen, proteins, and fats, decreasing blood glucose level
Somatostatin	Alpha and Beta cells in the pancreas	Suppresses secretion of glucagon and insulin within islets of Langerhans
Adrenal medulla		
Epinephrine (or adrenaline)	Muscle, liver, cardiovascular system	Stimulates features of "Fight-or-Flight" response to stress
Norepinephrine	Muscle, liver, cardiovascular system	Stimulates vasoconstriction
Adrenal cortex		
Glucocorticoids		
Cortisol	Most cells, particularly white blood cells (cells responsible for inflammatory and immune responses)	Stimulates glucagon-like effects, acts as anti-inflammatory and immunosuppressive agent
Mineralocorticoids		
Aldosterone	Kidneys, blood	Contributes to salt and fluid balance by stimulating kidneys to increase potassium excretion and decrease sodium excretion, increasing blood volume
Androgenic hormones		
Estrogen	Most cells	See effects under Gonads
Progesterone	Uterus	
Testosterone	Most cells	
Ovaries		
Estrogen	Most cells particularly those of female reproductive tract	Stimulates development of secondary sexual characteristics, plays role in maturation of egg prior to ovulation
Progesterone	Uterus	Stimulates uterine changes necessary for successful pregnancy
Testes		
Testosterone	Most cells, particularly those of male reproductive tract	Stimulates development of secondary sexual characteristics, plays role in development of sperm cells
Pineal gland		
Melatonin	Exact action unknown	Releases melatonin in response to light, may help determine daily, lunar, and reproductive cycles, may affect mood

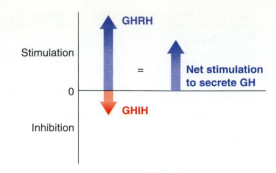

FIGURE 4-2 Regulation by hormone pairs. The net level of stimulation created by the opposing actions of growth-hormone releasing hormone (GHRH) and growth-hormone inhibitory hormone (GHIH) determines the amount of growth hormone (GH) secreted by the anterior pituitary.

tissues of the anterior pituitary in Table 4-1, you will understand why physiologists once thought of the pituitary gland as the "master gland." Its hormones have a direct impact on endocrine glands throughout the body. The term isn't used much anymore, because the dependence of the pituitary on the hypothalamus has been made clear.

As noted above, the pituitary gland has two lobes, the posterior and the anterior.

Posterior Pituitary

The posterior pituitary produces two hormones:

- *Antidiuretic hormone (ADH)*—causes retention of body water
- *Oxytocin*—causes uterine contraction and lactation

Antidiuretic hormone (ADH), also known as vasopressin, causes the kidneys to increase water reabsorption. This retention of water, or antidiuretic effect, results in increased circulating blood volume and decreased urine volume. Increased secretion of ADH is part of the homeostatic mechanism that can counteract losses of blood volume up to about 25 percent. Clinically, you will see increased ADH secretion in early shock states associated with dehydration or hemorrhage. Note that the opposite effect, decreased secretion of ADH, occurs after ingestion of alcohol and when there is a significant rise in circulating blood volume.

Although it is unlikely that a disorder in ADH secretion will present as a medical emergency, you should understand such endocrine dysfunction when patients discuss their medical histories. **Diabetes insipidus,** a disorder marked by large volumes of urine, is caused by inadequate ADH secretion relative to blood volume. The resultant reduction of blood volume, or diuretic effect, appears as excessive urine production. In a 24-hour period, the kidneys normally produce 1 to 1.5 liters of urine. In diabetes insipidus, it is not uncommon for urine output to increase to almost 20 liters per day. You can remember the characteristic urine presentation of diabetes insipidus by remembering that dilute urine has an insipid, or neutral, odor (and taste).

Oxytocin, the natural form of the drug Pitocin, stimulates uterine contraction and lactation in women who have just delivered a baby. Oxytocin actually causes the "letdown" of milk by stimulating contractile cells within the mammary glands. An infant suckling at the breast stimulates receptors in the nipples that causes the release of oxytocin from the posterior pituitary. This, in turn, causes discharge of milk so that the infant can feed. Following delivery, it is recommended that the infant be placed on the breast to suckle, thus stimulating the release of oxytocin. In addition to stimulating milk letdown, the oxytocin stimulates uterine contraction, which can help minimize post-partum bleeding.

* **diabetes insipidus** excessive urine production caused by inadequate production of antidiuretic hormone.

In both sexes, oxytocin has a mild antidiuretic effect, which is similar to that of ADH due to their chemical similarity. The relationship between oxytocin and ADH has direct application to emergency medicine. Women in preterm labor are often given an IV fluid bolus in an attempt to suppress uterine contractions without the use of drugs. This works in the following way: The administration of IV fluid bolus causes an increase in circulating blood volume, which is detected by autonomic nerves in the kidneys. An impulse is sent through the hypothalamus to the posterior pituitary, where it causes decreased secretion of ADH. This inhibition of ADH secretion in turn triggers decreased secretion of oxytocin, which contributes to the observed increase in urine production and, one hopes, the goal of suppression of preterm labor.

Anterior Pituitary

Because almost all of the anterior pituitary hormones regulate other endocrine glands, disorders directly involving the anterior pituitary are rarely a factor in endocrine emergencies. Table 4-1 lists the six hormones secreted by the anterior pituitary, as well as target tissues and hormone effects. As you can see, five of the six hormones regulate the activity of target glands, while the sixth affects almost all cells:

Five anterior pituitary hormones affect target glands.

- *Adrenocorticotropic hormone (ACTH)*—targets the adrenal cortexes
- *Thyroid-stimulating hormone (TSH)*—targets the thyroid
- *Follicle-stimulating hormone (FSH)*—targets the gonads, or sex organs
- *Luteinizing hormone (LH)*—also targets the gonads
- *Prolactin (PRL)*—targets the mammary glands of women

The sixth anterior pituitary hormone has a broader effect.

- *Growth hormone (GH)*—targets almost *all* body cells.

GH has its most significant effects in children because it is the primary stimulant of skeletal growth. In adults, GH has several physiologic effects, but the most significant is metabolic. GH causes adipose cells to release their stored fats into the blood and causes body cells to switch from glucose to fats as the primary energy source. The net effect is that the body uses up fat stores and conserves its sugar stores.

THYROID GLAND

The two lobes of the *thyroid gland* are located in the neck anterior to and just below the cartilage of the larynx, with one lobe on either side of the midline. The two lobes are connected by a small isthmus, or band of tissue, that crosses the trachea at the level of the cricoid cartilage. The thyroid produces three hormones:

- *Thyroxine (T_4)*—stimulates cell metabolism
- *Triiodothyronine (T_3)*—stimulates cell metabolism
- *Calcitonin*—lowers blood calcium levels

The thyroid is composed of tiny hollow sacs called follicles, which are filled with a thick fluid called *colloid*. The hormones *thyroxine (T_4)* and *triiodothyronine*

(T_3) are produced within the colloid. When stimulated by the pituitary hormone TSH or by environmental conditions such as cold, the thyroid gland releases these hormones to increase the general rate of cell metabolism.

The thyroid gland also contains perifollicular cells called C cells which produce a different hormone, *calcitonin.* Calcitonin lowers blood calcium levels by increasing uptake of calcium by bones and inhibiting breakdown of bone tissue. Parathyroid hormone has the opposite, or antagonistic, effect on the blood calcium level, which is covered in the following discussion of the parathyroid glands.

Disorders of excessive or deficient production of thyroid hormones T_4 and T_3, called hyperthyroidism and hypothyroidism respectively, will be discussed later in this chapter.

PARATHYROID GLANDS

Each *parathyroid gland* is very small, with a maximum diameter of 5 mm and weight of only 35–40 mg. Normally, four parathyroid glands are located on the posterior lateral surfaces of the thyroid, one pair above the other. Sometimes there are more than four parathyroid glands, but only rarely are there fewer. The parathyroid glands secrete:

- *Parathyroid hormone (PTH)*—increases blood calcium levels

PTH increases blood calcium levels through actions on three different target tissues. In bone, the primary target, PTH causes release of calcium into the blood. In the intestines, PTH converts Vitamin D into its active form, causing increased absorption of calcium. In the kidneys, PTH causes increased reabsorption of calcium. PTH is the antagonist of calcitonin, and the balance of PTH and calcitonin determines the level of blood calcium. The parathyroid glands rarely cause clinical problems. However, they can be accidentally damaged or removed during surgery or they may be damaged if the thyroid gland is irradiated. In either case, the loss of parathyroid function may result in hypocalcemia, low blood calcium levels.

THYMUS GLAND

The *thymus* is in the mediastinum just behind the sternum. It is fairly large in children but shrinks into a small remnant of fat and fibrous tissue in adults. Although the thymus is usually considered a lymphatic organ on the basis of its anatomy, its most important function is as an endocrine gland: During childhood, it secretes

- *Thymosin*—promotes maturation of T lymphocytes

Thymosin is critical to maturation of T lymphocytes, the cells responsible for cell-mediated immunity. The T of T lymphocyte stands for thymus.

PANCREAS

The pancreas, located in the upper retroperitoneum behind the stomach and between the duodenum and spleen, is composed of both endocrine and exocrine tissues. The exocrine tissues, known as *acini,* secrete digestive enzymes essential to digestion of fats and proteins into a duct that empties into the small intestine.

The microscopic clusters of endocrine tissue found within the pancreas are known as *islets of Langerhans.* Although there are one to two million islets interspersed throughout the pancreas, they comprise only about two percent of its

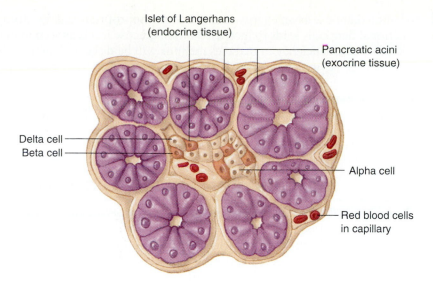

Islet of Langerhans
(endocrine tissue)

Pancreatic acini
(exocrine tissue)

Delta cell
Beta cell

Alpha cell

Red blood cells
in capillary

FIGURE 4-3   The internal
anatomy of the pancreas.

total mass. The three most important types of endocrine cells in the islets of Langerhans are termed *alpha (α), beta (β),* and *delta (δ)* (Figure 4-3). Each type produces and secretes a different hormone. In addition, the islets contain a much smaller number of cells called polypeptide cells. These cells produce pancreatic polypeptide (PP), the function of which is still unclear.

The alpha and beta cells produce two hormones essential for homeostasis of blood glucose:

- *Glucagon*—increases blood glucose
- *Insulin*—decreases blood glucose

Approximately 25 percent of islet tissue is made up of alpha cells. Alpha cells produce the hormone *glucagon.* When blood glucose level falls, alpha cells increase secretion of glucagon. Glucagon stimulates breakdown of glycogen, the complex carbohydrate that is the storage form of glucose, into individual glucose molecules that are released into the blood. This process, called **glycogenolysis,** takes place in more than one tissue, but activity in the liver is by far the most important in raising blood glucose level.

✳ **glycogenolysis** the break-down of glycogen to glucose, primarily by liver cells.

The liver is the largest and heaviest of the internal organs and so it has many cells that can contain glycogen. In addition, liver cells have the greatest capacity to store glycogen—liver cells can store 5 to 8 percent of their weight as glycogen. Compare this with the capacity of skeletal muscle (1 to 3 percent), another important storage tissue in the body. In addition to stimulating glycogenolysis, the hormone glucagon also stimulates liver breakdown of body proteins and fats with subsequent chemical conversion to glucose. This second process, which produces glucose from non-sugar sources, is called **gluconeogenesis.** Both processes contribute to homeostasis by raising the blood glucose level.

✳ **gluconeogenesis** conversion of protein and fat to form glucose.

Beta cells make up about 60 percent of islet tissue, and they produce the hormone *insulin.* Insulin is the antagonist of glucagon: Insulin lowers the blood glucose level by increasing the uptake of glucose by body cells. In addition, insulin promotes energy storage in the body by increasing the synthesis of glycogen, protein, and fat. Because the liver removes circulating insulin within 10 to 15 minutes from time of secretion, it must be secreted constantly to sustain an appropriate balance of glucagon and insulin—a balance that results in a steady supply of glucose for immediate use as an energy source and for appropriate energy storage. Loss of functional beta cells leads to increased blood glucose levels as seen in diabetes. The role of insulin deficiency in diabetes mellitus will be discussed later in this chapter.

Delta cells, which comprise about 10 percent of islet tissue, produce *somatostatin*. This hormone acts within islets to inhibit secretion of glucagon and insulin. Somatostatin also retards nutrient absorption from the intestines, although its mechanisms of action in the gut are poorly understood. As you look at Table 4-1, note that somatostatin is the same substance as growth-hormone inhibiting hormone (GHIH).

TERMINOLOGY RELATED TO GLUCOSE

You can remember terms related to glucose by performing some breakdown of your own. Look at the terms as they are listed below, where each word part is given along with its meaning and a sample sentence. Then you may want to reread the preceding discussion of glucagon and insulin, keeping the meanings of the word parts in mind as the terms appear. Keep these meanings in mind, also, when you read the discussion of diabetes mellitus later in the chapter.

Glucagon   gluco = glucose, agon = to drive
   The hormone glucagon drives an increase in blood glucose.

Glycogen   glyco = sugar, gen = origin
   The complex carbohydrate glycogen is the source for much of the blood glucose produced between meals.

Glycogenolysis   *glycogen*, lysis = to loosen or unbind
   Glycogenolysis breaks glycogen down into its component glucose molecules.

Gluconeogenesis   gluco = glucose, neo = new, genesis = origin
   New glucose molecules are synthesized from non-sugar sources through the process of gluconeogenesis.

ADRENAL GLANDS

The paired *adrenal glands* are located on the superior surface of the kidneys. Each gland has two distinct anatomical divisions with different functions. The inner portion of the adrenal gland is called the *adrenal medulla,* and its cells behave both as nerve cells and as gland cells. The adrenal medulla is intimately related to the sympathetic component of the autonomic nervous system. When sympathetic nerves carry an impulse into the adrenal medulla, its cells respond by secreting the catecholamine hormones *epinephrine* (or adrenalin) and *norepinephrine* into the bloodstream. The outer portion of the adrenal gland is called the *adrenal cortex,* and it consists of endocrine tissue. The adrenal cortex secretes three classes of steroidal hormones that differ only slightly in chemical structure but have very distinct effects in the body:

- *Glucocorticoids,* of which *cortisol* is by far the most important, account for 95 percent of adrenocortical hormone production. Like glucagon, they increase the blood glucose level by promoting gluconeogenesis and decreasing glucose utilization as an energy source. If you recall that cortisone is a commonly used medical glucocorticoid, you will realize that this class of hormones also inhibits inflammatory reactions and immune-system responses, as well as potentiates the effects of catecholamines. The anterior pituitary hormone that promotes release, ACTH, is secreted in response to stress, trauma, or serious infection.

- *Mineralocorticoids,* of which *aldosterone* is the most important, contribute to salt and fluid balance in the body by regulating sodium and potassium excretion through the kidneys.
- *Androgenic hormones* have the same effects as those secreted by gonads, and they will be covered in that discussion.

You may see disorders related to deficient or excessive secretion of adrenal hormones present as medical emergencies. They will be discussed later in this chapter.

GONADS

Some differences in the gonads are obvious: Ovaries produce eggs, whereas testes produce sperm cells. However, the gonads of both sexes share one vital function: They are the endocrine glands chiefly responsible for the sexual maturation of puberty and any subsequent reproduction.

Ovaries

The ovaries, or female gonads, are paired organs about the size of an almond that are located in the pelvis on either side of the uterus. Under the regulation of the anterior pituitary hormones FSH and LH, the ovaries produce:

- *Estrogen*
- *Progesterone*

The hormone *estrogen* promotes the development and maintenance of secondary female sexual characteristics. Estrogen also plays a role in the egg development that precedes ovulation during each menstrual cycle. *Progesterone* is familiarly known as the "hormone of pregnancy" because it is necessary for implantation of the fertilized egg and maintenance of the uterine lining throughout pregnancy. Estrogen also serves to protect the female against heart disease. When estrogen levels fall at menopause, the female's risk of developing heart disease quickly increases to the level of the male's. In addition, the ovaries produce small amounts of *testosterone,* which influences some body changes associated with puberty.

Testes

The male gonads, or *testes,* are located outside of the abdominal cavity in the scrotum. Under the regulation of the anterior pituitary hormones FSH and LH, the testes produce:

- *Testosterone*

The hormone *testosterone* promotes the development and maintenance of secondary male sexual characteristics and plays a role in development of sperm.

PINEAL GLAND

The pineal gland is located in the roof of the thalamus in the brain. Its function has remained somewhat elusive. However, it has been shown that the pineal gland releases the hormone *melatonin* in response to changes in light. For example, melatonin production is lowest during daylight hours and highest in the dark of the night. Because of this, the pineal is felt to help determine day-length and lunar cycles and plays a role in controlling the reproductive "biological clock." Melatonin may affect a person's mood. The pineal gland has been implicated in "seasonal affective disorder (SAD)," which is characterized by severe depression during the winter months. Further research will help clarify the role of melatonin.

OTHER ORGANS WITH ENDOCRINE ACTIVITY

We have discussed the principal glands of the endocrine system. Many tissues not considered part of the endocrine system have important endocrine functions. There are organs in other systems that secrete hormones directly into the blood. The placenta can be considered an endocrine gland because of its secretion of *human chorionic gonadotropin (hCG)* throughout gestation. It is the early secretion of hCG that is detected by at-home pregnancy tests. In the digestive tract, gastric and intestinal mucosa produce the hormones *gastrin* and *secretin,* both of which regulate digestive function.

Additionally, there are hormone-producing cells in the atrial walls of the heart. *Atrial natriuretic hormone (ANH)* is secreted by certain atrial cells in response to increased stretching of the atrial walls due to abnormally high blood volume or blood pressure. The hormone ANH is an antagonist to ADH and inhibits secretion of aldosterone, thus contributing to a homeostatic reduction in blood volume by increasing urine production.

The kidneys also have some endocrine function. Certain kidney cells will react to a decrease in blood volume or blood pressure by releasing the enzyme *renin.* Renin acts on *angiotensinogen,* converting it to *angiotensin I.* In the lungs, angiotensin I is converted to *angiotensin II* by *angiotensin-converting enzyme (ACE).* Angiotensin II stimulates the adrenal production of aldosterone, which causes water retention by the kidneys. This leads to increased blood volume and blood pressure. In addition to renin, the kidneys secrete the hormone *erythropoietin* that stimulates the production of red blood cells by the bone marrow. The role of erythropoietin is discussed in greater detail in Chapter 9.

ENDOCRINE DISORDERS AND EMERGENCIES

The most common endocrine emergencies you should expect to treat will involve complications of diabetes mellitus. This section explains the pathophysiology of diabetes and its complications, including ketoacidosis and hypoglycemia, as a basis for discussion of field management. In addition, the section covers endocrine emergencies involving disorders of the thyroid and adrenal glands.

DISORDERS OF THE PANCREAS

Diabetes Mellitus

✱ diabetes mellitus disorder of inadequate insulin activity, due either to inadequate production of insulin or to decreased responsiveness of body cells to insulin.

The disease **diabetes mellitus** is marked by inadequate insulin activity in the body. As noted earlier, insulin is critical to maintaining normal blood glucose levels. Glucose is important for all cells, but it is especially important for brain cells. In fact, glucose is the *only* substance that brain cells can readily and efficiently use as an energy source. In addition, insulin enables the body to store energy as glycogen, protein, and fat.

Diabetes mellitus, or sugar diabetes, is not only a serious disease but also a common and ancient one. Over 8 million Americans have been diagnosed with diabetes, and U.S. health experts believe nearly the same number of Americans may be living with undiagnosed diabetes. The disease was named in ancient times by Greek physicians who noted that affected persons produced large volumes of urine that attracted bees and other insects, hence diabetes (meaning "to syphon," or "to pass through") for excessive urine production and mellitus (meaning "honey sweet") for the presence of sugar in the urine. If you remember that mellitus means sweet and insipidus means neutral, you will remember the common trait and the major distinctions in the presentations of untreated diabetes insipidus and diabetes mellitus.

Before presenting pathophysiology, we will examine in detail the normal body handling of glucose. The discussion of glucose metabolism will focus on events at the molecular and cellular level, whereas the discussion on regulation of blood glucose will focus on events in the blood and in major target tissues such as liver, fat cells, and kidneys.

Glucose Metabolism You learned in the chapter introduction that metabolism is the sum of the processes that produce the energy and molecules needed for cell growth or repair. The word *metabolism* comes from the Greek for "to change." Two kinds of change take place within a cell. One kind builds complex molecules from simpler ones. The synthesis of glycogen from glucose is an example. The other kind breaks down complex molecules into simpler ones. The breakdown of glucose into carbon dioxide, water, and energy (in the form of adenosine triphosphate, or ATP) is an example.

The building processes within a cell are collectively called **anabolism.** The prefix *ana-* comes from the Greek for "up," and anabolic pathways build molecules of higher complexity. Breakdown processes are collectively called **catabolism.** The prefix *cata-* comes from the Greek for "down," and catabolic pathways produce molecules of lower complexity. Anabolic pathways usually require energy to drive them, and catabolic pathways often release energy as part of the process. In other words, anabolic activity uses energy while catabolic activity produces energy.

Look at the summary of effects of insulin and glucagon in Table 4-2. When materials are abundant after meals and blood glucose is high, insulin enables cells to use glucose directly and to store energy as glycogen, protein, and fat. Insulin stimulates anabolic pathways. In contrast, glucagon is the dominant hormone during periods of low blood glucose. It stimulates catabolic pathways to produce usable energy from the body's stores.

In order for anabolic pathways to proceed, insulin must first exert its stimulatory effects. Insulin acts by binding to receptors in the outer cell membrane. These receptors are proteins whose structure reacts specifically with insulin. When insulin is bound to a receptor, it changes the permeability of the membrane

* **anabolism** the constructive or "building up" phase of metabolism.

* **catabolism** the destructive or "breaking down" phase of metabolism.

Table 4-2　SUMMARY OF GLUCOSE METABOLISM

Hormonal Effects of Insulin and Glucagon

Insulin	Glucagon
Dominant hormone when blood glucose level is high	Dominant hormone when blood glucose level is low
Major Effects on Target Tissues	*Major Effects on Target Tissues*
all cells: ↑ uptake glucose	
liver: ↑ production of glycogen, protein, fat	liver: ↑ glycogenolysis → glucose
liver, fat: ↑ production of fats	liver: ↑ gluconeogenesis (protein, fat → glucose)

such that glucose enters the cell far more readily. The rate at which glucose can be transported into cells can be increased tenfold or more by the action of insulin. Without insulin activity, the amount of glucose that can enter cells is far too small to meet average body energy demands. Note the two requirements for insulin effectiveness:

1. There must be sufficient insulin circulating in the bloodstream to satisfy cellular needs.
2. Insulin must be able to bind to body cells in such a way that adequate levels of stimulation occur.

The importance of these two requirements will become clear when you learn about the two types of diabetes mellitus.

Sometimes the body cannot use glucose as a primary energy source. In diabetes, this occurs when insufficient insulin activity exists for blood glucose to be taken in and used by cells. Other conditions, such as a high-fat, low-carbohydrate diet or starvation (which can occur in conjunction with some eating disorders) cause depletion of body stores of carbohydrate. Under any of these conditions, the body slowly switches from glucose to fat as the primary energy source. Adipose cells break down fats into their component free fatty acids, and the blood concentration of fatty acids rises considerably.

Most of the fatty acid is used directly by body cells as an energy source. Some is taken in by liver cells. In the liver, catabolism of fatty acids produces acetoacetic acid. When more acetoacetic acid is released from the liver than can be used by body cells, it accumulates in the blood along with two closely related substances, acetone and β-hydroxybutyric acid. These three substances are collectively called **ketone bodies,** and their presence in biologically significant quantity in the blood is called **ketosis.** This catabolic state is significant in the context of the emergency condition called diabetic ketoacidosis, or diabetic coma.

Regulation of Blood Glucose Homeostasis of blood glucose is remarkably effective. If you draw venous blood samples from a group of healthy persons, you'll find that fasting blood glucose (generally done after an overnight fast) is usually between 80 to 90 mg glucose/dL blood. In the first hour or so after a meal, blood glucose may increase to about 120 to 140 mg/dL before falling toward the fasting, or baseline, level. The principal tissues involved in homeostasis are the alpha and beta tissues of the islets of Langerhans (producing glucagon and insulin, respectively) and the liver—as shown in Table 4-2. Liver disease, even in the presence of normal pancreatic function, can cause significant disturbances in glucose homeostasis.

A blood glucose level lower than baseline (often defined as less than 80 mg/dL) reflects **hypoglycemia,** or low blood sugar. Similarly, a blood glucose level higher than that expected shortly after a meal (often defined as greater than 140 mg/dL when drawn in a setting other than directly following a meal) reflects **hyperglycemia,** or high blood sugar. Both terms indicate the blood glucose level only, not the cause of the abnormality.

The last factor to consider in discussing regulation of blood glucose is the role of the kidneys. When blood is filtered through the glomeruli of the kidneys, glucose, along with water and many other small molecules, passes from the blood into the proximal tubule. Water, glucose, and other useful materials are then reabsorbed, while waste products that are not reabsorbed become part of the urine, which will be excreted from the body. The amount of glucose that is reabsorbed depends on the blood level of glucose that already exists. Reabsorption of glucose is essentially complete at blood glucose levels up to about 180 mg/dL. Above that level, glucose begins to be lost in urine.

✳ **ketone bodies** compounds produced during the catabolism of fatty acids, including acetoacetic acid, β-hydroxybutyric acid, and acetone.

✳ **ketosis** the presence of significant quantities of ketone bodies in the blood.

✳ **hypoglycemia** deficiency of blood glucose. Sometimes called *insulin shock.* Hypoglycemia is a medical emergency.

✳ **hyperglycemia** excessive blood glucose.

Glucose loss in urine can lead to dehydration, which has its physiologic basis in osmosis. Osmosis is the tendency of water molecules to migrate across a semipermeable membrane such that the concentrations of particles approach equivalence on both sides. Our example is the cell membranes that form the boundaries between the tubules of the kidney and the capillaries that surround them.

When glucose spills into urine, the osmotic pressure, or concentration of particulates, rises inside the kidney tubule to a level higher than that of the blood. Water follows glucose into urine to cause a marked water loss termed **osmotic diuresis**, which is the basis of the excessive urination characteristic of untreated diabetes. The term **diuresis** alone refers to increased formation and secretion of urine. The presence of glucose in urine, **glycosuria**, creates the sweet urine that added *mellitus* to *diabetes*.

Last, you should note that whenever the flow rate of fluid inside the kidney tubules rises, as in osmotic diuresis, an increase in excretion of potassium occurs. This leads to the potential for significant hypokalemia and its effects, including cardiac dysrhythmias.

Type I Diabetes Mellitus When we discussed the elements essential to normal insulin activity, the first was the presence of adequate amounts of insulin in the body. *Type I diabetes mellitus* is characterized by very low production of insulin by the pancreas. In many cases, no insulin is produced at all. Type I diabetes is commonly called juvenile-onset diabetes because of the average age at diagnosis. The term *insulin-dependent diabetes mellitus (IDDM)* is also used because patients require regular insulin injections to maintain glucose homeostasis. This type of diabetes is less common than is Type II diabetes, but it is more serious. Diabetes is regularly among the ten leading causes of death in the United States, and Type I diabetes accounts for most diabetes-related deaths.

Heredity is an important factor in determining which persons will be predisposed to development of Type I diabetes. The cause of Type I diabetes is often unclear. However, viral infection, production of autoantibodies directed against beta cells, and genetically determined early deterioration of beta cells are all possible. The immediate cause of the disease is destruction of beta cells.

In untreated Type I diabetes, blood glucose levels rise because, without adequate insulin, cells cannot take up the circulating sugar. Hyperglycemia in the range of 300 to 500 mg/dL is not uncommon. As glucose spills into urine, large amounts of water are lost, too, through osmotic diuresis. Catabolism of fat becomes significant as the body switches to fatty acids as the primary energy source. Overall, this pathophysiology accounts for the constant thirst (polydipsia), excessive urination (polyuria), ravenous appetite (polyphagia), weakness, and weight loss associated with untreated Type I diabetes. Ketosis can occur as the result of fat catabolism, and it may proceed to frank diabetic ketoacidosis, a medical emergency that you will encounter in the field and that will be discussed later in this chapter.

Type II Diabetes Mellitus The second requirement for proper insulin activity is insulin binding such that adequate stimulation of cells occurs. Type II diabetes mellitus is associated with a moderate decline in insulin production accompanied by a markedly deficient response to the insulin that is present in the body. Type II diabetes is also called adult-onset diabetes or *non-insulin-dependent diabetes mellitus (NIDDM)*.

Heredity may play a role in predisposition. In addition, obese persons are more likely to develop Type II diabetes, and obesity probably plays a role in development of the disease. Increased weight (and increased size of fat cells) causes a relative deficiency in the number of insulin receptors per cell, which makes fat cells less responsive to insulin. This type of diabetes is far more common than is

* **osmotic diuresis** greatly increased urination and dehydration that results when high levels of glucose cannot be reabsorbed into the blood from the kidney tubules and the osmotic pressure of the glucose in the tubules also prevents water reabsorption.

* **diuresis** formation and secretion of large amounts of urine.

* **glycosuria** glucose in urine, which occurs when blood glucose levels exceed the kidney's ability to reabsorb glucose.

Content Review

SYMPTOMS OF UNTREATED DIABETES MELLITUS
Polydipsia
Polyuria
Polyphagia
Weakness
Weight loss

Type I diabetes, accounting for about 90 percent of cases of diabetes mellitus. It is also less serious.

Untreated Type II diabetes typically presents with a lower level of hyperglycemia and fewer major signs of metabolic disruption. For instance, glucose use is usually sufficient to keep the body from switching to fats as the primary energy source. Thus, diabetic ketoacidosis is uncommon in these patients. However, a complication called hyperglycemic hyperosmolar nonketotic coma can occur, and you may see it as a medical emergency. It is discussed later in this chapter.

Medical treatment of Type II diabetes is less intensive than that required for Type I diabetes. Initial therapy often consists of dietary change and increased exercise in an attempt to improve body weight. If nonpharmacological therapy is insufficient to bring blood glucose levels down to the normal range, oral hypoglycemic agents may be prescribed. These drugs stimulate insulin secretion by beta cells and promote an increase in the number of insulin receptors per cell. In some cases, however, control may eventually require use of insulin.

✱ diabetic ketoacidosis complication of Type I diabetes due to decreased insulin intake. Marked by high blood glucose, metabolic acidosis, and, in advanced stages, coma. Ketoacidosis is often called diabetic coma.

Diabetic Ketoacidosis (Diabetic Coma)

Diabetic ketoacidosis is a serious, potentially life-threatening complication associated with Type I diabetes. It occurs when there is profound insulin deficiency coupled with increased glucagon activity. It may occur as the initial presentation of severe diabetes, as a result of patient noncompliance with insulin injections, or as the result of physiologic stress such as surgery or serious infection. Some of the major characteristics of diabetic ketoacidosis are listed in Tables 4-3 and 4-4.

Table 4-3 DIABETIC EMERGENCIES

Diabetic Ketoacidosis	Hyperglycemic Hyperosmolar Nonketotic (HHNK) Acidosis	Hypoglycemia
Common Causes	**Common Causes**	**Common Causes**
Cessation of insulin injections	Physiologic stress (such as infection or stroke) producing hyperglycemia and a noncompensated diuresis, modulated by both insulin and glucagon activity	Excessive administration of insulin
Physiologic stress (such as infection or surgery) that causes release of catecholamines, potentiating glucagon effects and blocking insulin effects		Excess insulin for dietary intake
		Overexertion, resulting in lowered blood glucose level
Signs and Symptoms	**Signs and Symptoms**	**Signs and Symptoms**
Polyuria, polydipsia, polyphagia	Polyuria, polydipsia, polyphagia	Weak, rapid pulse
Warm, dry skin and mucous membranes	Warm, dry skin and mucous membranes	Cold, clammy skin
Nausea/vomiting	Orthostatic hypotension	Weakness, uncoordination
Abdominal pain	Tachycardia	Headache
Tachycardia	Decreased mental function or frank coma	Irritable, agitated behavior
Deep, rapid respirations (Kussmaul's respirations)		Decreased mental function or bizarre behavior
Fruity odor on breath		Coma (severe cases)
Fever (if associated with infection)		
Decreased mental function or frank coma		
Management	**Management**	**Management**
Fluids, insulin as directed	Fluids, insulin as directed	Dextrose

Table 4-4 — DIAGNOSTIC SIGNS BY SYSTEM FOR DIABETIC EMERGENCIES

System	Diabetic Emergency		
	Diabetic Ketoacidosis	HHNK Coma	Hypoglycemia
Cardiovascular			
Pulse	Rapid	Rapid	Normal
Blood Pressure	Low	Normal to Low (may be affected by position, or orthostatic)	Normal
Respiratory			
Respiration rate	Exaggerated air hunger	Normal, unlabored	Normal or shallow
Breath odor	Acetone (sweet fruity)	None	None
Nervous			
Headache	Absent	None	Present
Mental state	Restlessness/ unconsciousness	Lethargy/ unconsciousness	Apathy, irritability/ unconsciousness
Tremors	Absent	Absent	Present
Convulsions	None	Possible	In late stages
Gastrointestinal			
Mouth	Dry	Dry	Drooling
Thirst	Intense	Excessive	Absent
Vomiting	Common	Common	Uncommon
Abdominal pain	Frequent	Common	Absent
Ocular			
Vision	Dim	Normal	Double vision (diplopia)

Pathophysiology Reread the discussion of ketosis in the prior section on Glucose Metabolism. Diabetic ketoacidosis reflects amplification of the same physiologic mechanisms as ketosis.

In the initial phase of diabetic ketoacidosis, profound hyperglycemia exists because of lack of insulin. Body cells cannot take in glucose. The compensatory mechanism for low glucose levels within cells, gluconeogenesis, only contributes more blood glucose. The consequent loss of glucose in the urine, accompanied by loss of water through osmotic diuresis, produces significant dehydration.

As the body switches to fat-based metabolism, the blood level of ketones rises. The ketone load accounts for the observed acidosis. By the time the characteristic decrease in pH from about 7.4 to about 6.9 has occurred, the patient is hours from death if left untreated.

Signs and Symptoms The onset of clinically obvious diabetic ketoacidosis is slow, lasting from 12 to 24 hours. In the initial phase, signs of diuresis appear, including increased urine production and dry, warm skin and mucous membranes. The individual often has excessive hunger and thirst, coupled with a progressive sense of general malaise. Volume depletion induces tachycardia and feelings of physical weakness.

As ketoacidosis develops, a major compensatory mechanism for acidosis appears: the rapid, deep breathing pattern termed *Kussmaul's respirations,* which helps expel carbon dioxide, CO_2, from the body (Figure 4-4). The breath itself may have a fruity or acetone-like smell as some blood acetone is expelled through the lungs. The blood profile not only includes hyperglycemia and acidic pH, but also electrolyte abnormalities. Low bicarbonate levels reflect loss of acid-base buffer via Kussmaul's respirations. Low potassium levels may be

The presence of a sweet, fruity odor on the patient's breath is a hallmark of diabetic ketoacidosis.

FIGURE 4-4 Kussmaul's respirations.

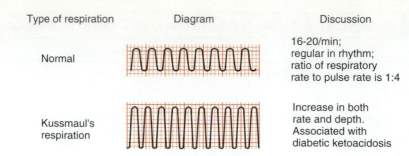

found secondary to diuresis, with marked hypokalemia increasing the risk for cardiac dysrhythmias or death. Over time, mental function declines and frank coma may occur. A fever is not characteristic of ketoacidosis. If present, it is a signal of infection.

Assessment and Management The approach used with the patient suffering from diabetic ketoacidosis is essentially the same as with any other patient who has mental impairment or is unconscious. First, complete your initial assessment of airway, breathing, and circulation. Then complete a focused history and physical exam. Look for a Medic-Alert bracelet and/or insulin in the refrigerator. Obtain a history from any bystanders. The sweet, fruity odor of ketones occasionally can be detected in the breath. If possible, complete the rapid test for blood glucose level (Procedure 4-1). It is not uncommon for patients with ketoacidosis to have blood glucose levels well in excess of 300 mg/dL.

Focus field management on maintenance of the ABCs and fluid resuscitation to counteract dehydration. In such cases, draw a red top tube (or the tube specified by local protocols) of blood. Following blood sampling, administer one to two liters of normal saline per protocol. If transport time is lengthy, the medical direction physician may request intravenous or subcutaneous administration of regular insulin.

If the blood glucose level cannot be quickly determined, draw a red top tube of blood for analysis and start an IV of normal saline. Following this, administer 50 ml (25 grams) of 50 percent dextrose solution. The additional glucose load will not adversely affect the ketoacidotic patient because it is negligible compared with the quantity present in the body. If the patient were hypoglycemic, however, the additional glucose might be sufficient to protect brain cells from damage. If the patient is a known alcoholic, consider administering 100 mg of thiamine.

Expedite transport to an appropriate facility for definitive therapy.

Hyperglycemic Hyperosmolar Nonketotic (HHNK) Coma

Hyperglycemic hyperosmolar nonketotic (HHNK) coma is a serious complication associated with Type II diabetes. Typically, both insulin and glucagon activity are present. HHNK coma develops when two conditions occur: Sustained hyperglycemia causes osmotic diuresis sufficient to produce marked dehydration, and water intake is inadequate to replace lost fluids. Dialysis, high-osmolarity feeding supplements, infection, and certain drugs can also be associated with development of HHNK coma. Some characteristics of HHNK coma are listed in Tables 4-3 and 4-4.

* **hyperglycemic hyperosmolar nonketotic (HHNK) coma** complication of type II diabetes due to inadequate insulin activity. Marked by high blood glucose, marked dehydration, and decreased mental function. Often mistaken for ketoacidosis.

Pathophysiology As sustained hyperglycemia develops, glucose spills into the urine, causing osmotic diuresis and resultant dehydration. The level of hyperglycemia is often much higher than the levels seen in ketoacidosis (up to 1000 mg/dL). However, insulin activity in patients with HHNK coma prevents significant production of ketone bodies. Inadequate fluid replacement results in characteristic signs and symptoms.

The mortality rate for HHNK coma is higher than that for ketoacidosis, ranging from 40 to 70 percent. The higher mortality rate may be due to the lack of early signs and symptoms that bring patients with ketoacidosis to the attention of family or health care professionals. The mortality rate of HHNK is also high because it primarily affects the elderly.

Signs and Symptoms The onset of HHNK coma is even slower than that of ketoacidosis, with development often occurring over several days. Early signs include increased urination and increased thirst. Subsequent volume depletion can result in orthostatic hypotension when the patient gets out of bed, along with other signs such as dry skin and mucous membranes as well as tachycardia. The patient may become lethargic, confused, or enter frank coma. Kussmaul's respirations are rarely seen because of the lack of acidosis.

Assessment and Management The approach used with the patient suffering from HHNK coma is essentially the same as with any other patient who has mental impairment or is unconscious. It is often difficult in the field to distinguish diabetic ketoacidosis from HHNK coma. Therefore, the prehospital treatment of both emergencies is identical (see earlier discussion of management of ketoacidosis) and transportation should be expedited.

Hypoglycemia (Insulin Shock)

Hypoglycemia, or low blood glucose, is a medical emergency. It can occur when a patient takes too much insulin, eats too little to match an insulin dose, or overexerts and uses almost all available blood glucose. As the period of hypoglycemia lengthens, the risk rises that brain cells will be permanently damaged or killed due to lack of glucose. You have learned that brain cells can adapt to use fats as an energy source. Note, however, that this adaptation requires hours to develop, and the switch to fat-based metabolism cannot correct any damage already incurred. This is why every second counts in treating hypoglycemia.

Pathophysiology Hypoglycemia, or insulin shock, reflects high insulin and low blood glucose. Regardless of the reason for low blood sugar, insulin causes almost all remaining blood glucose to be taken up by cells. Because of the high level of insulin, glucagon may be ineffective in raising blood glucose levels. In prolonged fasts, almost half the glucose normally produced through gluconeogenesis is of renal origin. This activity is stimulated by epinephrine. Diabetic patients with kidney failure may be predisposed to hypoglycemia because of lack of renal gluconeogenesis.

Signs and Symptoms The signs and symptoms of hypoglycemia are many and varied. Altered mental status is the most important. Recall the case study that opened this chapter. Mark, who was hypoglycemic, was confused as the police officer spoke to him. In the earliest stages of hypoglycemia, the patient may appear restless or impatient or complain of hunger. As blood glucose falls lower, he may display inappropriate anger (even rage) or display a bizarre behavior. Sometimes

✱ **hypoglycemia** deficiency of blood glucose.

Hypoglycemia is a true medical emergency that requires prompt intervention to prevent permanent brain injury.

Hypoglycemia virtually never occurs outside the setting of diabetes mellitus.

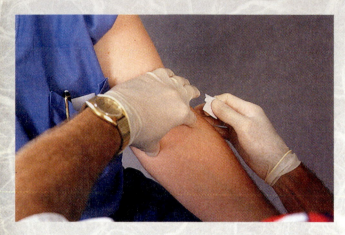

4-1a   Choose a vein, and prep the site.

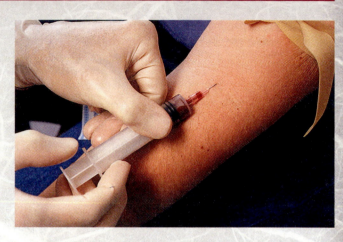

4-1b   Perform the venipuncture.

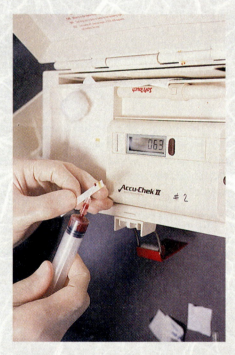

4-1c   Place a drop of blood on the reagent strip.
Activate the timer.

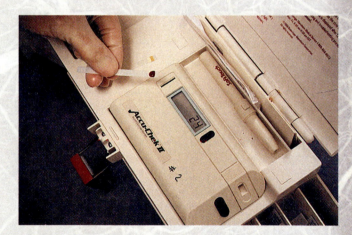

4-1d   Wait until the timer sounds.

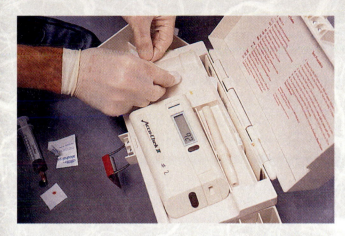

4-1e Wipe the reagent strip.

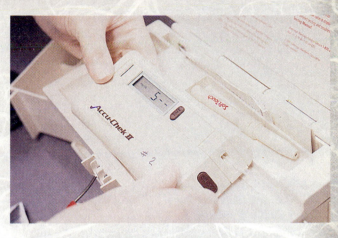

4-1f Place the reagent strip in the glucometer.

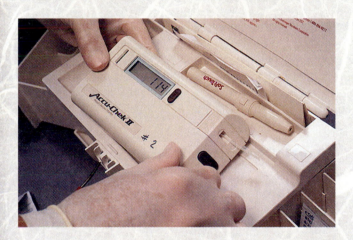

4-1g Read the blood glucose level.

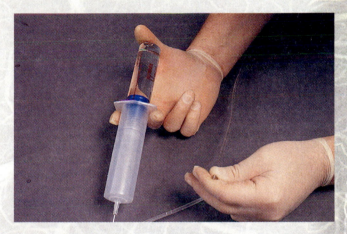

4-1h Administer 50 percent dextrose intravenously, if the blood glucose level is less than 80 mg.

* hypoglycemic seizure seizure that occurs when brain cells aren't functioning normally due to low blood glucose.

*All ALS vehicles **must** have the capability of rapidly determining a patient's blood glucose level.*

* hyperthyroidism excessive secretion of thyroid hormones resulting in an increased metabolic rate.

* thyrotoxicosis condition that reflects prolonged exposure to excess thyroid hormones with resultant changes in body structure and function.

* hypothyroidism inadequate secretion of thyroid hormones resulting in a decreased metabolic rate.

* myxedema condition that reflects long-term exposure to inadequate levels of thyroid hormones with resultant changes in body structure and function.

* Graves' disease endocrine disorder characterized by excess thyroid hormones resulting in body changes associated with increased metabolism; primary cause of *thyrotoxicosis*.

the patient may be placed in police custody for such behavior or be involved in an automobile accident.

Physical signs may include diaphoresis and tachycardia, both of which Mark showed. If blood glucose falls to a critically low level, the patient may have a **hypoglycemic seizure** or become comatose.

In contrast to diabetic ketoacidosis, hypoglycemia can develop quickly. A clear change in mental status can occur without warning. Always consider hypoglycemia when encountering a patient with bizarre behavior. See Tables 4-3 and 4-4 for additional information.

Assessment and Management In suspected cases of hypoglycemia, perform the initial assessment quickly. Look for a Medic-Alert bracelet. If possible, determine the blood glucose level. Because of the urgency of this emergency, most paramedic units need to have the capability to perform this task or to rush a blood sample along with the patient.

If the blood glucose level is less that 60 mg/dL, draw a red top tube of blood and start an IV of normal saline. Next, administer 50 to 100 milliliters (25 to 50 grams) of 50 percent dextrose intravenously. If the patient is conscious and able to swallow, complete glucose administration with orange juice, sugared sodas, or commercially available glucose pastes.

If blood glucose cannot be obtained and the patient is unconscious, start an IV of normal saline and administer 50 to 100 milliliters (25 to 50 grams) of 50 percent dextrose. Expedite transport to a medical facility. If you suspect alcoholism, also administer 100 mg of thiamine.

When an IV cannot be started, hypoglycemic patients may improve following the administration of glucagon. This is a much slower process and will only work if there are adequate stores of glycogen available. Glucagon must be reconstituted immediately prior to administration. A dose of 0.5 to 1.0 mg intramuscularly is usually adequate.

DISORDERS OF THE THYROID GLAND

You are more likely to see thyroid dysfunction as part of the medical history than as an emergency. However, you may see patients with acute complications of thyroid disorders. The most common of these are:

- **Hyperthyroidism**—the presence of excess thyroid hormones in the blood.
- **Thyrotoxicosis**—a condition that reflects prolonged exposure of body organs to excess thyroid hormones, with resultant changes in structure and function. Thyrotoxicosis is generally caused by *Graves' disease.*
- **Hypothyroidism**—the presence of inadequate thyroid hormones in the blood.
- **Myxedema**—a condition that reflects long-term exposure to inadequate levels of thyroid hormones, with resultant changes in structure and function.

Graves' Disease

Over 95 percent of cases of thyrotoxicosis are due to **Graves' disease.** Roughly 15 percent of Graves' disease patients have a close relative with Graves', which suggests a strong hereditary role in predisposition to the disorder. In addition,

Graves' disease is about six times more common in women than in men, with on-set typically in young adulthood (20s and 30s).

Pathophysiology Graves' disease has an autoimmune origin. Autoantibodies are generated that stimulate thyroid tissue to produce excessive amounts of thyroid hormones. The resultant changes in organ function are either responses to excess thyroid hormones or responses to the autoantibodies themselves.

Signs and Symptoms Signs and symptoms of Graves' disease include agitation, emotional changeability, insomnia, poor heat tolerance, weight loss despite increased appetite, weakness, dyspnea, and tachycardia or new-onset atrial fibrillation in the absence of a cardiac history. Nervous system symptoms tend to be more common in younger adults, whereas serious cardiovascular symptoms tend to predominate in older individuals. Prolonged reaction of orbital tissues with the pathological thyroid-stimulating autoantibodies can cause exophthalmos (protrusion of the eyeballs), whereas interaction of autoantibodies with thyroid tissue often produces diffuse goiter (a generally enlarged thyroid gland) (Figure 4-5).

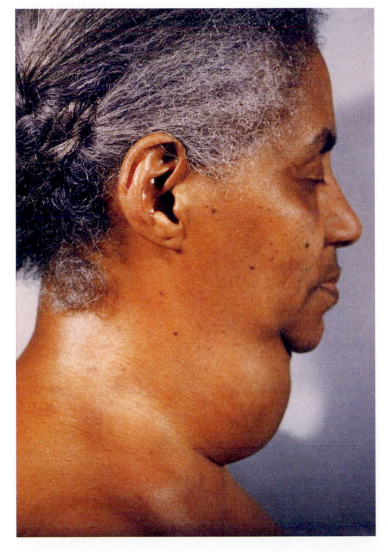

FIGURE 4-5 Generalized enlargement of the thyroid gland (goiter).

Assessment and Management Cardiac dysfunction is probably the most likely context within which an emergency call may arise from thyrotoxicosis (usually caused by Graves' disease, as noted earlier). Use of β-adrenergic blockers such as propranolol may temporarily reduce cardiac stress, but make sure the patient does not have heart failure before considering use. Glucocorticoid therapy (namely, dexamethasone) is sometimes helpful in quickly reducing the level of circulating T_4.

Thyrotoxic Crisis ("Thyroid Storm")

* **thyrotoxic crisis** toxic condition characterized by hyperthermia, tachycardia, nervous symptoms, and rapid metabolism; also known as *thyroid storm*.

Thyrotoxic crisis, or "thyroid storm," is a life-threatening emergency that can be fatal within as few as 48 hours if untreated. It is usually associated with severe physiologic stress (e.g., trauma, infection), less often with psychological stress. You may also encounter thyroid storm secondary to overdose of thyroid hormone in a hypothyroid individual.

Pathophysiology The mechanisms underlying thyrotoxic crisis are poorly understood. An acute increase in the levels of thyroid hormones does not appear to be the cause. It is more likely that thyroid storm is caused by a shift of thyroid hormone in the blood from the protein-bound (biologically inactive) to the free (biologically active) state.

Signs and Symptoms The signs and symptoms associated with thyrotoxic crisis reflect the patient's extreme hypermetabolic state and increased activity of the sympathetic nervous system. The syndrome is characterized by high fever (106°F/41°C or higher), irritability, delirium or coma, tachycardia, hypotension, vomiting, and diarrhea. A less severe presentation may also occur, with slight fever and marked lethargy.

Assessment and Management In the presence of the above-mentioned signs and symptoms of thyrotoxic crisis, field management is largely focused on supportive care: oxygenation, ventilatory assistance, fluid resuscitation, and cardiac monitoring. Glucocorticoids and β-adrenergic blockers may be helpful. Transport should be expedited for definitive therapy that blocks the high blood levels of thyroid hormones.

Hypothyroidism and Myxedema

Hypothyroidism can be congenital or acquired. Both sexes can be affected. The recent increase in incidence of hypothyroidism in middle-aged women may reflect better diagnostics, a true rise in incidence, or both. Advanced myxedema in middle-aged and elderly individuals is the condition you are most likely to see as part of a medical emergency, so we will focus most attention on myxedema and the uncommon complication of myxedema coma.

* **myxedema coma** life-threatening condition associated with advanced myxedema, with profound hypothermia, bradycardia, and electrolyte imbalance.

Pathophysiology Hypothyroidism creates a low metabolic state, and early signs reflect poor organ function and poor response to challenges such as exercise or infection. Over time, untreated severe hypothyroidism causes the additional sign of myxedema: a thickening of connective tissue in the skin and other tissues, including the heart. Patients with myxedema may progress into a hypothermic, stuporous state called **myxedema coma,** which can be fatal if respiratory depression occurs. Triggers for progression include infection, trauma, a cold environment, or exposure to central nervous system depressants such as alcohol or certain drugs.

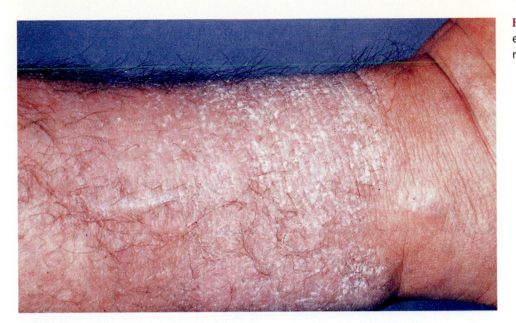

FIGURE 4-6 Doughy, edematous skin typical of myxedema.

Signs and Symptoms Early signs of hypothyroidism may be subtle. Symptoms may be as slight as fatigue and slowed mental function attributed falsely to aging. Typically, patients with hypothyroidism or myxedema show lethargy, cold intolerance, constipation, decreased mental function, or decreased appetite with increased weight. In addition, the relaxation stage of deep tendon reflexes (DTRs) is slowed. The classic appearance of myxedema is an unemotional, puffy face, thinned hair, enlarged tongue, and pale, cool skin that looks and feels like dough (Figure 4-6). Myxedema coma may be difficult to identify. Note if the history is consistent with hypothyroidism, and look for the physical appearance of myxedema. Other signs include profound hypothermia (temperatures as low as 75°F/24°C are not uncommon), low amplitude bradycardia, and carbon dioxide retention.

Assessment and Management The presence of the described signs and symptoms may alert you to the possible presence of myxedema. Keep in mind that heart failure due to the combination of age, atherosclerosis, and myxedematous enlargement is not uncommon, so focus on maintenance of ABCs and close monitoring of cardiac and pulmonary status. Most patients with myxedema coma require intubation and ventilatory assistance. Active rewarming is contraindicated due to risk of cardiac dysrhythmias and cardiovascular collapse secondary to vasodilatation. Although IV access is important, limit fluids because fluid and electrolyte imbalance is common. Expedite transport to an appropriate facility for definitive treatment.

DISORDERS OF THE ADRENAL GLANDS

Two disorders of the adrenal cortex can play a part in medical emergencies or complicate responses to trauma. **Cushing's syndrome** is caused by excessive adrenocortical activity. In contrast, **Addison's disease** is caused by deficient adrenocortical activity. Reread the earlier section where we discussed the anatomy and physiology of the adrenal glands to remind yourself how critical these hormones are to metabolic processes and to salt and water balance.

While most patients experiencing myxedema coma require intubation and ventilatory assistance, active rewarming is contraindicated due to risk of cardiac dysrhythmias and cardiovascular collapse secondary to vasodilation.

* **Cushing's syndrome** pathological condition resulting from excess adrenocortical hormones. Symptoms may include changed body habitus, hypertension, vulnerability to infection.

* **Addison's disease** endocrine disorder characterized by adrenocortical insufficiency. Symptoms may include weakness, fatigue, weight loss, hyperpigmentation of skin and mucous membranes.

Hyperadrenalism (Cushing's Syndrome)

Cushing's syndrome is a relatively common disorder of the adrenals. It usually affects middle-aged persons, with women affected more often than men. Excess cortisol can be due to abnormalities in the anterior pituitary or adrenal cortex. It can also be due to treatment with glucocorticoids, such as prednisone. Check the history to note any steroid treatment for nonendocrine conditions such as COPD, asthma, and cancer or rheumatologic disorders.

Pathophysiology Long-term exposure to excess glucocorticoids, primarily cortisol, produces numerous changes. Metabolically, cortisol is an antagonist to insulin. Gluconeogenesis is prominent, with profound protein catabolism. The body's handling of fats is altered: Atherosclerosis and hypercholesterolemia are common. Over time, diabetes mellitus also may develop. Cortisol's mineralo-corticoid activity causes sodium retention and increased blood volume. Increased vascular sensitivity to catecholamines occurs, and this may also be a contributor to hypertension. Potassium loss through the kidneys may cause hypokalemia. Cortisol's anti-inflammatory and immunosuppressive properties predispose to infection.

Signs and Symptoms Regardless of the cause, the presenting signs and symptoms are the same. The earliest sign is weight gain, particularly through the trunk of the body, face, and neck. A "moon-faced" appearance often develops (Figure 4-7). The accumulation of fat on the upper back is occasionally referred to as a "buffalo hump." Skin changes are also very common and may be an early clue to potential problems. These include thinning to an almost transparent appearance, a tendency to bruise easily, delayed healing from even minor wounds, and development of facial hair among women (hirsutism). Mood swings and impaired memory or concentration are also common.

Assessment and Management Although it is unlikely you will see a patient with acute hyperadrenal crisis, you are likely to encounter patients who exhibit signs and symptoms of Cushing's syndrome. Remember that these patients have

FIGURE 4-7   Facial features of Cushing's syndrome.

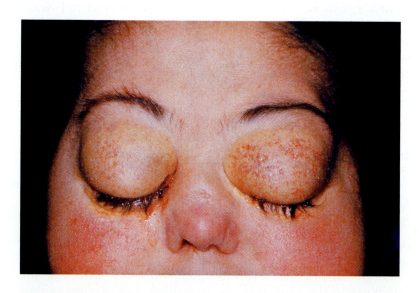

a higher incidence of cardiovascular disease, including hypertension and stroke. Pay particular attention to skin preparation when starting IV lines because of skin fragility and susceptibility to infection. Observations indicative of Cushing's syndrome should be noted in your report and relayed to hospital staff.

Adrenal Insufficiency (Addison's Disease)

Addison's disease is due to cortical destruction. Addison's has become less common as former leading causes of Addison's, such as tuberculosis, have come under control. Currently, over 90 percent of Addison's disease cases are due to autoimmune disease. As with Graves' disease, another autoimmune disorder, heredity plays a prominent role in predisposition. In fact, patients with Addison's are more likely than average to have other autoimmune disorders, including Graves' disease. Persons with Addison's may be tipped into metabolic failure called **Addisonian crisis** by acute stresses such as infection or trauma. Be alert for this potentially life-threatening emergency.

* Addisonian crisis form of shock associated with adrenocortical insufficiency and characterized by profound hypotension and electrolyte imbalances.

Pathophysiology Destruction of the adrenal cortex results in minimal production of all three classes of hormones: glucocorticoids, mineralocorticoids, and androgens. Low mineralocorticoid activity is key to the changes of Addison's: It causes major disturbances in water and electrolyte balance. Increased sodium excretion in urine causes low blood volume, and potassium retention can cause hyperkalemia and ECG changes. Note that many cases of adrenal insufficiency are due to therapy with steroids such as prednisone. Such therapy can completely suppress normal adrenal function, and sudden cessation of the drug may trigger symptoms of Addison's disease or even an Addisonian crisis, with cardiovascular collapse.

Signs and Symptoms Addison's disease is characterized by changes related to low corticosteroid activity: progressive weakness, fatigue, decreased appetite, and weight loss. Hyperpigmentation of the skin and mucous membranes, particularly in sun-exposed areas, is also characteristic.

You should include Addisonian crisis in your list of possible causes of unexplained cardiovascular collapse, particularly if the history suggests primary Addison's or Addison's secondary to drug therapy. Many patients will have gastrointestinal problems such as vomiting or diarrhea, which will exacerbate electrolyte imbalances, low blood volume, and hypotension and increase the potential for cardiac dysrhythmias.

Assessment and Management The patient may reveal the presence of Addison's disease during the history, or the signs and symptoms just discussed may lead you to suspect the presence of Addison's. Focus emergency management on maintenance of the ABCs and close monitoring of cardiac and oxygenation status as well as blood glucose level. Hypoglycemia poses its own threat. Assess blood glucose levels and administer 25–50 grams of 50% dextrose to patients with blood glucose levels less than 50 mg/dL or those with altered mental status. Obtain a baseline 12-lead ECG to check for dysrhythmias related to electrolyte imbalance. Be aggressive in fluid resuscitation. Follow your local protocol or contact medical direction for specific orders based on your patient's presentation. Expedite transport to an appropriate facility for definitive treatment.

SUMMARY

In conjunction with the nervous system, the endocrine system regulates body functions. The vast majority of endocrine emergencies involve complications of diabetes mellitus such as hypoglycemia or ketoacidosis. Other endocrine emergencies tend to be rare and will more likely be part of the history rather than the emergency. In the field, you should always suspect diabetes when patients present with unexplained changes in mental status. Hypoglycemia, the most urgent diabetic emergency, must be quickly treated to prevent serious nervous system damage. When the exact type of diabetic emergency is undetermined, treat for hypoglycemia. Keep in mind that treatment of diabetic ketoacidosis is primarily a hospital procedure.

YOU MAKE THE CALL

It's a beautiful Sunday afternoon in spring. You and your partner are dispatched for an "unknown medical emergency" in a residential neighborhood. Within four minutes you are on scene with a 23-year-old female who complains of extreme weakness and dizziness when she sits up or attempts to stand. She reports that over the past 48 hours she has had a fever (103°F) and abdominal pain, accompanied by nausea, vomiting, diarrhea, and loss of appetite. Blood pressure is 82/66 mmHg, pulse is 110 beats per minute, and respirations are 26 per minute and labored. Her skin is very pale but hot to the touch. Her mucous membranes are dry. Bilateral lung sounds are clear and equal. Pulse oximetry is 95 percent. ECG shows sinus tachycardia with peaked T waves and no ectopy. Glucometer reads "low" (< 50 mg/dL).

When obtaining her history you learn from her husband that she has had severe asthma since age eight and is routinely managed with albuterol (Ventolin), cromolyn (Intal), and prednisone (Deltasone). She had not had any problems for several months, but over the past two weeks she was treated for bronchitis with antibiotics. She reports that she finished the antibiotics three days before. However, on further questioning you find out that she has not had any prednisone for four days. It seems that she ran out of prednisone but did not refill the prescription because she was feeling so much better. She intended to refill it tomorrow when she had a follow-up appointment with her doctor.

1. What is your first priority?
2. What additional intervention is needed?
3. What do you suspect is the likely cause of her signs and symptoms?
4. Should you transport this patient to the hospital or could her husband take her in their private vehicle?

See Suggested Responses at the back of this book.

FURTHER READING

Bledsoe, Bryan E. "Dealing With Diabetic Emergencies." *JEMS* 16(12) (December 1991): 40–50.

Greenspan, Francis S. and Gordon J. Strewler. *Basic & Clinical Endocrinology.* 5th ed. New York: McGraw Hill, 1997.

Leske, Jane Stover. "Hyperglycemic Hyperosmolar Nonketotic Coma." *Journal of Emergency Nursing,* 10 (3) (May/June 1984): 145–150.

McCance, Kathryn L. and Sue E. Huether. *Pathophysiology: The Biologic Basis for Disease in Adults and Children.* 3rd ed. St. Louis, Missouri: C. V. Mosby Company, 1998.

Tortora, Gerard J. and Sandra Reynolds Grabowski. *Principles of Anatomy and Physiology.* 9th ed. New York: John Wiley & Sons, 1999.

ON THE WEB

Visit Brady's Paramedic Website at www.bradybooks.com/paramedic.

CHAPTER 5

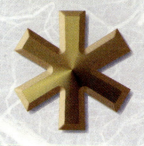

Allergies and Anaphylaxis

Objectives

After reading this chapter, you should be able to:

1. Describe the incidence, morbidity and mortality of anaphylaxis. (p. 347)
2. Identify the risk factors most predisposing to anaphylaxis. (p. 347)
3. Discuss the anatomy and physiology of the organs and structures related to anaphylaxis. (pp. 347–349)
4. Describe the prevention of anaphylaxis and appropriate patient education. (pp. 357–358)
5. Discuss the pathophysiology of allergy and anaphylaxis. (p. 347)

6. Describe the common routes of substance entry into the body. (pp. 350–351)
7. Define allergic reaction, anaphylaxis, antigen, antibody and natural and acquired immunity. (pp. 346–349)
8. List common antigens most frequently associated with anaphylaxis. (pp. 347–348)
9. Discuss human antibody formation. (pp. 347–349)

Continued

Objectives Continued

10. Describe the physical manifestations of anaphylaxis. (pp. 351–354, 356–357)
11. Identify and differentiate between the signs and symptoms of an allergic reaction and anaphylaxis. (p. 356)
12. Explain the various treatment and pharmacological interventions used in the management of allergic reactions and anaphylaxis. (pp. 354–357)

13. Correlate abnormal findings in assessment with the clinical significance in the patient with an allergic reaction or anaphylaxis. (pp. 351–354)
14. Given several pre-programmed and moulaged patients, provide the appropriate assessment, care and transport for the allergic reaction and anaphylaxis patient. (pp. 346–358)

CASE STUDY

Cherokee Nation EMS is dispatched to a clinic on the outskirts of town for a medical emergency. Upon arrival at the scene, paramedics are met by clinic staff who direct them to a treatment room. The nurse practitioner reports that a 39-year-old male had received an immunization injection approximately 15 minutes earlier. Immediately after the injection, the man developed a red rash and generalized itching. This quickly progressed to obvious hives, wheezing, and associated dyspnea. As the reaction worsened, the patient became hoarse, more dyspneic, and hypotensive. A nurse was now administering supplemental oxygen while another clinic employee was setting up an intravenous infusion.

Initial assessment reveals an alert 39-year-old Native American male in marked distress. His airway is open, but there is marked stridor and audible wheezing. The carotid pulse is rapid and weak. Paramedics quickly remove the nasal cannula placed by the clinic staff and place a nonrebreather oxygen mask. The airway kit is opened in case rapid endotracheal intubation is required.

Steve Williams, the lead paramedic, begins a more detailed assessment while his partner, Beth White Cloud, begins to search for a vein to catheterize.

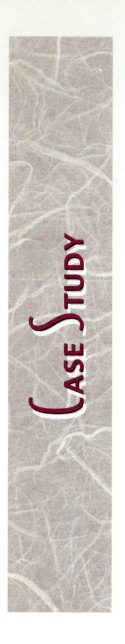

The patient is diaphoretic and has urticarial lesions on the trunk and extremities. In addition, he is tachypneic with a weak and thready pulse. The blood pressure is 88/50 mmHg, the pulse is 120 beats per minute, respirations are 32 breaths per minute, and oxygen saturation is 100 percent on the nonrebreather.

While Beth places the IV, Steve administers 0.4 milligrams of epinephrine 1:1,000 subcutaneously per system standing orders. Within approximately two minutes, the patient's stridor begins to improve and respirations slow. Beth completes placement of the IV and secures it with tape and tincture of benzoin because of the patient's marked diaphoresis. Beth administers 50 milligrams of diphenhydramine (Benadryl) intravenously. Steve prepares a pre-fill of epinephrine 1:10,000 for intravenous administration in case the patient does not improve.

Within five minutes, significant improvement is noted. In fact, it appears that most of the urticarial lesions have cleared. The patient's respiratory rate is down to 22 breaths per minute, but the patient's heart rate is up to 136 beats per minute, which the paramedics attribute to the epinephrine. A repeat blood pressure is 100/74 mmHg. Steve opens the IV infusion and administers a 500 milliliter fluid bolus.

The patient continues to improve and is moved to the ambulance for transport to the emergency department. Upon arrival, the patient is assessed by Stephen Johnston, M.D. Dr. Johnston orders the administration of an intravenous corticosteroid and additional IV fluids. The patient is observed for two hours and discharged symptom-free. A phone call to the clinic reveals that the patient received a tetanus immunization. In reviewing the case, Dr. Johnston learns from the patient that he had a similar reaction with a prior tetanus immunization but failed to relay this information to the clinic staff.

✱ **allergic reaction** an exaggerated response by the immune system to a foreign substance.

✱ **anaphylaxis** an unusual or exaggerated allergic reaction to a foreign protein or other substance. Anaphylaxis means the opposite of "phylaxis" or protection.

Anaphylaxis is the most severe form of allergic reaction and is often life threatening.

INTRODUCTION

An **allergic reaction** is an exaggerated response by the immune system to a foreign substance. Allergic reactions can range from mild skin rashes to severe, life-threatening reactions that involve virtually every body system. The most severe type of allergic reaction is called **anaphylaxis.** Anaphylaxis is a life-threatening emergency that requires prompt recognition and specific treatment by paramedics. The emergency treatment of anaphylaxis is one area of prehospital care where advanced life support measures often mean the difference between life and death. Anaphylaxis can develop within seconds and cause death just minutes after exposure to the offending agent. Fortunately, there are several emergency medications available that can reverse the adverse effects of anaphylaxis.

The first complete description of anaphylaxis was reported in 1902 by Portier and Richet. Portier and Richet were French immunologists who were attempting to immunize dogs against the toxin of the deadly sea anemone (sea flower). They were injecting small, non-lethal quantities of the toxin into the animals in hopes of stimulating immunity to the toxin. However, when the animals received secondary injections of sub-lethal quantities of the toxin, at a time when it might be expected that they would be immune, the dogs developed shock and died. Richet called this dramatic and unexpected phenomenon *anaphylaxis*, which means the opposite of "phylaxis" or protection.

Anaphylaxis results from exposure to a particular substance that sets off a biochemical chain of events that can ultimately lead to shock and death. The exact incidence of anaphylaxis is unknown. However, an estimated 400–800 deaths annually in the United States are attributed to anaphylaxis. Injected penicillin and bee and wasp *(Hymenoptera)* stings are the two most common causes of fatal anaphylaxis. Approximately 100–500 deaths per year are attributed to the parenteral administration of penicillin. Approximately 25–40 persons die each year from *hymenoptera* stings. Fortunately, the incidence of anaphylaxis appears to be declining. This is presumably due to better recognition and treatment, as well as the availability of numerous potent antihistamines.

PATHOPHYSIOLOGY

The immune system is the principal body system involved in allergic reactions. However, other body systems are also affected by an allergic reaction. These include *the cardiovascular system, the respiratory system, the nervous system,* and *the gastrointestinal system,* among others. To fully appreciate the complexity of allergic and anaphylactic reactions, it is first necessary to review the anatomy and physiology of the immune system as it relates to the immune response.

THE IMMUNE SYSTEM

The **immune system** is a complicated body system responsible for combating infection. Components of the immune system can be found in the blood, the bone marrow, and the lymphatic system.

The **immune response** is a complex cascade of events that occurs following activation by an invading substance, or **pathogen.** The goal of the immune response is the destruction or inactivation of pathogens, abnormal cells, or foreign molecules such as **toxins.** The body can accomplish this through two mechanisms, cellular immunity and humoral immunity. **Cellular immunity** involves a direct attack of the foreign substance by specialized cells of the immune system. These cells physically engulf and deactivate or destroy the offending agent. **Humoral immunity,** on the other hand, is much more complicated. Humoral immunity is basically a chemical attack of the invading substance. The principal chemical agents of this attack are **antibodies,** also called **immunoglobulins (Igs).** Antibodies are a unique class of chemicals that are manufactured by specialized cells of the immune system called *B cells.* There are five different classes of antibodies: IgA, IgD, IgE, IgG, and IgM.

The humoral immune response begins with exposure of the body to an antigen. An **antigen** is defined as any substance capable of inducing an immune response (Table 5-1). Most antigens are proteins. Following exposure to an antigen, antibodies are released from cells of the immune system. These antibodies attach themselves to the invading substance to facilitate removal of that substance from the body by other cells of the immune system.

If the body has never been exposed to a particular antigen, the response of the immune system is different than if it has been previously exposed to the particular antigen. The initial response to an antigen is called the **primary response.**

* *Hymenoptera* any of an order of highly specialized insects such as bees and wasps.

* **immune system** the body system responsible for combating infection.

* **immune response** complex of events within the body that works toward the destruction or inactivation of pathogens, abnormal cells, or foreign molecules.

* **pathogen** a disease-producing agent or invading substance.

* **toxin** any poisonous chemical secreted by bacteria or released following destruction of the bacteria.

* **cellular immunity** immunity resulting from a direct attack of a foreign substance by specialized cells of the immune system.

* **humoral immunity** immunity resulting from attack of an invading substance by antibodies.

* **antibody** principal agent of a chemical attack of an invading substance.

* **immunoglobulin** alternative term for antibody.

* **antigen** any substance that is capable, under appropriate conditions, of inducing a specific immune response.

* **primary response** initial, generalized response to an antigen.

Table 5-1	AGENTS THAT MAY CAUSE ANAPHYLAXIS

Antibiotics and other drugs

Foreign proteins (e.g., horse serum. Streptokinase)

Foods (nuts, eggs, shrimp)

Allergen extracts (allergy shots)

Hymenoptera stings (bees, wasps)

Hormones (Insulin)

Blood Products

Aspirin

Non-steroidal anti-inflammatory drugs (NSAIDs)

Preservatives (sulfiting agents)

X-ray contrast media

Dextran

✱ secondary response response by the immune system that takes place if the body is exposed to the same antigen again; in secondary response, antibodies specific for the offending antigen are released.

✱ natural immunity genetically predetermined immunity that is present at birth; also called *innate immunity.*

✱ acquired immunity immunity that develops over time and results from exposure to an antigen.

✱ naturally acquired immunity immunity that begins to develop after birth and is continually enhanced by exposure to new pathogens and antigens throughout life.

✱ induced active immunity immunity achieved through vaccination given to generate an immune response that results in the development of antibodies specific for the injected antigen; also called *artificially acquired immunity.*

Following exposure to a new antigen, several days are required before both the cellular and humoral components of the immune system respond. Generalized antibodies (IgG and IgM) are first released to help fight the antigen.

At the same time, other components of the immune system begin to develop antibodies specific for the antigen. These cells also develop a *memory* of the particular antigen. If the body is exposed to the same antigen again, the immune system responds much faster. This is called the **secondary response.** As a part of the secondary response, antibodies specific for the offending antigen are released. Antigen-specific antibodies are much more effective in facilitating removal of the offending antigen than the generalized antibodies released during the primary response.

Immunity may be either *natural* or *acquired*. **Natural immunity,** also called *innate immunity,* is genetically predetermined. It is present at birth and has no relation to previous exposure to a particular antigen. All humans are born with some innate immunity.

Acquired immunity develops over time and results from exposure to an antigen. Following exposure to a particular antigen, the immune system will produce antibodies specific for the antigen. This protects the organism as subsequent exposure to the same antigen will result in a vigorous immune response. **Naturally acquired immunity** normally begins to develop after birth and is continually enhanced by exposure to new pathogens and antigens throughout life. For example, a child contracts chicken pox (varicella) at age 18 months. Following the infection, the child's immune system creates antibodies specific for the varicella virus. Repeated exposure to the varicella virus usually will not result in another infection. In fact, it is not unusual for a patient exposed to varicella to develop lifelong immunity to the infection.

Induced active immunity, also called *artificially acquired immunity,* is designed to provide protection from exposure to an antigen at some time in the future. This is achieved through vaccination and provides relative protection against serious infectious agents. In vaccination, an antigen is injected into the body so as to generate an immune response. This results in the development of antibodies specific for the antigen and provides protection against future infection. Most vaccines contain antigenic proteins from a particular virus or bacterium. Later, when the individual is actually exposed to the pathogen, the immune response will be vigorous and will often be enough to prevent the infection from developing.

An example of a vaccine commonly used is the DPT (diphtheria/pertussis/tetanus) vaccine. This vaccine contains antigenic proteins from the bacteria that cause diphtheria, whooping cough, and tetanus. The vaccine is administered at several intervals during the first five years of life. It provides protection against infection from these bacteria. Some vaccinations will impart lifelong immunity while others must be periodically followed with a "booster dose" to assure continued protection.

Acquired immunity can be either *active* or *passive*. **Active immunity** occurs following exposure to an antigen and results in the production of antibodies specific for the antigen. Most vaccinations result in the development of active immunity. However, it takes some time for a patient to develop specific antibodies. In certain cases, it is necessary to administer antibodies to provide protection until the active immunity can kick in. The administration of antibodies is referred to as **passive immunity.** There are two types of passive immunity. *Natural passive immunity* occurs when antibodies cross the placental barrier from the mother to the infant so as to provide protection against embryonic or fetal infections. *Induced passive immunity* is the administration of antibodies to an individual to help fight infection or prevent diseases. An example of the clinical use of both active and passive immunity is the regimen used for the prevention of tetanus.

Most persons who are from developed countries have typically received some form of tetanus vaccination during their life. These persons typically have some antibodies to tetanus and often need nothing more than a tetanus booster. However, some persons have never received any sort of tetanus vaccination. When these persons seek treatment for a tetanus-prone wound, they must receive prophylaxis for tetanus in addition to care for their wound. This is best achieved by the provision of both passive and active immunity. To provide immediate protection, the patient is administered antibodies specific for tetanus (tetanus immune globulin (TIG) Hypertet®). Then, they are administered a tetanus vaccination (Td or Dt). The tetanus immune globulin (TIG) provides passive immunity until such time as the body's immune system can respond to the tetanus vaccination with the development of antibodies specific for tetanus. This should be followed by periodic tetanus boosters until such time as the patient's immunization program is complete.

ALLERGIES

The initial exposure of an individual to an antigen is referred to as **sensitization.** Sensitization results in an immune response. Subsequent exposure induces a much stronger secondary response. Some individuals can become hypersensitive (overly sensitive) to a particular antigen. **Hypersensitivity** is an unexpected and exaggerated reaction to a particular antigen. In many instances, hypersensitivity is used synonymously with the term **allergy.** There are two types of hypersensitivity reactions, delayed and immediate.

Delayed Hypersensitivity

Delayed hypersensitivity is a result of *cellular immunity* and therefore does not involve antibodies. Delayed hypersensitivity usually occurs in the hours and days following exposure and is the sort of allergy that occurs in normal people. Delayed hypersensitivity most commonly results in a skin rash and is often due to exposure to certain drugs and chemicals. The rash associated with poison ivy is an example of delayed hypersensitivity.

✳ **active immunity** acquired immunity that occurs following exposure to an antigen and results in the production of antibodies specific for the antigen.

✳ **passive immunity** acquired immunity that results from administration of antibodies either from mother to the infant across the placental barrier (natural passive immunity) or through vaccination (induced passive immunity).

✳ **sensitization** initial exposure of a person to an antigen that results in an immune response.

✳ **hypersensitivity** an unexpected and exaggerated reaction to a particular antigen. It is used synonymously with the term *allergy.*

✳ **allergy** a hypersensitive state acquired through exposure to a particular allergen.

✳ **delayed hypersensitivity reaction** a hypersensitivity reaction that takes place after the elapse of some time following reexposure to an antigen. Delayed hypersensitivity reactions are usually less severe than immediate reactions.

Immediate Hypersensitivity

* **immediate hypersensitivity reaction** a hypersensitivity reaction that occurs swiftly following reexposure to an antigen. Immediate hypersensitivity reactions are usually more severe than delayed reactions. The swiftest and most severe of such reactions is anaphylaxis.

* **allergen** a substance capable of inducing allergy of specific hypersensitivity. Allergens may be protein or non-protein, although most are proteins.

When people use the term "allergy" they are usually referring to **immediate hypersensitivity** reactions. Examples of immediate hypersensitivity reactions include hay fever, drug allergies, food allergies, eczema, and asthma. Some persons have an allergic tendency. This allergic tendency is usually genetic, meaning it is passed from parent to child and is characterized by the presence of large quantities of IgE antibodies. An antigen that causes release of the IgE antibodies is referred to as an **allergen.** Common allergens include:

- Drugs
- Foods and food additives
- Animals
- Insects (*Hymenoptera* stings) and insect parts
- Fungi and molds
- Radiology contrast materials

Allergens can enter the body through various routes. These include oral ingestion, inhalation, topically, and through injection or envenomation (Figure 5-1). The vast majority of anaphylactic reactions result from injection or envenomation.

Parenteral penicillin injections are the most common cause of fatal anaphylactic reactions. Insect stings are the second most frequent cause of fatal

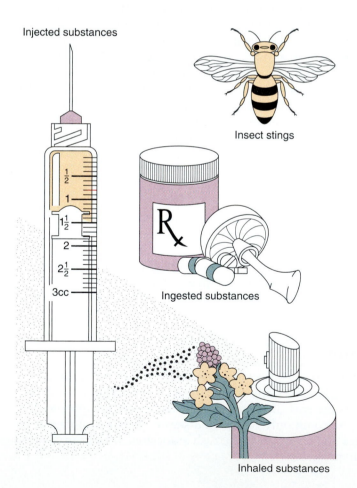

FIGURE 5-1 Anaphylactic reactions can result from a variety of causes.

Injected substances

Insect stings

Ingested substances

Inhaled substances

anaphylactic reactions. Insects in the order *Hymenoptera* are the most frequent offending insects. There are three families in this order: fire ants *(Formicoidea)*; wasps, yellow jackets, and hornets *(Vespidae)*; and the honey bees *(Apoidea)*. All produce a unique venom, although there are similar components in each. Honey bees often will leave their stinger embedded in the victim following a sting.

Following exposure to a particular allergen, large quantities of IgE antibodies are released. These antibodies attach to the membranes of **basophils** and **mast cells**—specialized cells of the immune system which contain chemicals that assist in the immune response. When the allergen binds to IgE attached to the basophils and mast cells, these cells release histamine, heparin, and other substances into the surrounding tissues. Histamine and other substances are stored in *granules* found within the basophils and mast cells. In fact, because of this feature, basophils and mast cells are often called *granulocytes*. The process of releasing these substances from the cells is called *degranulation*. This release results in what people call an *allergic reaction* which can be very mild or very severe.

The principal chemical mediator of an allergic reaction is histamine. **Histamine** is a potent substance that causes bronchoconstriction, increased intestinal motility, vasodilation, and increased vascular permeability. Increased vascular permeability causes the leakage of fluid from the circulatory system into the surrounding tissues. A common manifestation of severe allergic reactions and anaphylaxis is angioneurotic edema. **Angioneurotic edema**, also called *angioedema,* is marked edema of the skin and usually involves the head, neck, face, and upper airway. Histamine acts by activating specialized histamine receptors present throughout the body.

There are two classes of histamine receptors. H_1 receptors, when stimulated, cause bronchoconstriction and contraction of the intestines. H_2 receptors cause peripheral vasodilation and secretion of gastric acids. The goal of histamine release is to minimize the body's exposure to the antigen. Bronchoconstriction decreases the possibility of the antigen entering through the respiratory tract. Increased gastric acid production helps destroy an ingested antigen. Increased intestinal motility serves to move the antigen quickly though the gastrointestinal system with minimal absorption of the antigen into the body. Vasodilation and capillary permeability help remove the allergen from the circulation where it has the potential to do the most harm.

ANAPHYLAXIS

Anaphylaxis usually occurs when a specific allergen is injected directly into the circulation. This is the reason anaphylaxis is more common following injections of drugs and diagnostic agents and following bee stings. When the allergen enters the circulation, it is distributed widely throughout the body. The allergen interacts with both basophils and mast cells, resulting in the massive dumping of histamine and other substances associated with anaphylaxis. The principal body systems affected by anaphylaxis are the cardiovascular system, the respiratory system, the gastrointestinal system, and the skin. Histamine causes widespread peripheral vasodilation as well as increased permeability of the capillaries. Increased capillary permeability results in marked loss of plasma from the circulation. People sustaining anaphylaxis can actually die from circulatory shock.

Also released from the basophils and mast cells is a substance called **slow-reacting substance of anaphylaxis (SRS-A)**. This causes spasm of the bronchial smooth muscle, resulting in an asthma-like attack and occasionally asphyxia. SRS-A potentiates the effects of histamine, especially on the respiratory system.

* **basophil** type of white blood cell that participates in allergic responses.

* **mast cell** specialized cell of the immune system which contains chemicals that assist in the immune response.

* **histamine** a product of mast cells and basophils that causes vasodilation, capillary permeability, bronchoconstriction, and contraction of the gut.

* **angioneurotic edema** marked edema of the skin that usually involves the head, neck, face, and upper airway; a common manifestation of severe allergic reactions and anaphylaxis.

* **slow-reacting substance of anaphylaxis (SRS-A)** substance released from basophils and mast cells that causes spasm of the bronchiole smooth muscle, resulting in an asthma-like attack and occasionally asphyxia.

ASSESSMENT FINDINGS IN ANAPHYLAXIS

The signs and symptoms of anaphylaxis begin within 30–60 seconds following exposure to the offending allergen. In a small percentage of patients the onset of signs and symptoms may be delayed over an hour. The signs and symptoms of anaphylaxis (Table 5-2) can vary significantly. The severity of the reaction is often related to the speed of onset. Reactions that develop very quickly tend to be much more severe.

A rapid and focused assessment is crucial to the early detection and treatment of anaphylaxis. Patients suffering an anaphylactic reaction often have a sense of impending doom. This sense of impending doom is often followed by development of additional signs and symptoms.

If the patient's condition permits, a brief history should be gathered, including previous allergen exposures and reactions. If possible, try to determine how quickly symptoms started and how severe they were.

Next, quickly evaluate the patient's level of consciousness. Upper airway problems, including laryngeal edema, may result in the patient being unable to

Table 5-2	CLINICAL PRESENTATION OF ALLERGIES AND ANAPHYLAXIS
Skin	
Flushing	
Itching	
Hives	
Swelling	
Cyanosis	
Respiratory System	
Respiratory difficulty	
Sneezing, coughing	
Wheezing, stridor	
Laryngeal edema	
Laryngospasm	
Bronchospasm	
Cardiovascular System	
Vasodilation	
Increased heart rate	
Decreased blood pressure	
Gastrointestinal System	
Nausea and vomiting	
Abdominal cramping	
Diarrhea	
Nervous System	
Dizziness	
Headache	
Convulsions	
Tearing	

speak. As the emergency progresses, the patient will become restless. As cardio-vascular collapse continues, the patient will exhibit a decreased level of consciousness. If untreated, this may continue to unresponsiveness.

As noted earlier, a common manifestation of anaphylaxis is angioneurotic edema, involving the face and neck. Laryngeal edema is also a frequent complication and can threaten the airway. Initially, laryngeal edema will cause a hoarse voice. As the edema worsens, the patient may develop stridor. Finally, this all may lead to complete airway obstruction from either massive laryngeal edema, laryngospasm, or pharyngeal edema, or a combination of any of these.

The respiratory system is significantly involved in an anaphylactic reaction. Initially, the patient will become tachypneic. Later, as lower airway edema and bronchospasm develop, respirations will become labored as evidenced by retractions, accessory muscle usage, and prolonged expirations. Wheezing, resulting from bronchospasm and edema of the smaller airways, is a common manifestation and may be so pronounced that it can be heard without the aid of a stethoscope. Ultimately, anaphylaxis can result in markedly diminished lung sounds, which reflect decreased air movement and hypoventilation.

The skin is typically involved early in severe allergic reactions and anaphylaxis. Generally, a fine red rash will appear diffusely on the body. As histamine is released, fluid will diffuse from leaky capillaries, resulting in urticaria. **Urticaria,** also called "hives," is a wheal and flare reaction characterized by red, raised bumps which may appear and disappear across the body (Figure 5-2). As cardiovascular collapse and dyspnea progresses, the patient will become diaphoretic. This may, if untreated, progress to cyanosis and pallor.

The effect of histamine on the gastrointestinal system is pronounced. Initially, the patient may note a rumbling sensation in the abdomen as gastrointestinal motility increases. On physical examination, this may be evident as hyperactive bowel sounds. Later, nausea, vomiting, and diarrhea develop as the body tries to rid itself of the offending allergen.

The vital signs will vary depending on the severity and stage of the severe allergic or anaphylactic reaction. Initially there will be an increase in both the heart and respiratory rate. As airway edema and dyspnea occurs, the respiratory rate can fall—an ominous finding. The blood pressure will fall when significant capillary leakage and peripheral vasodilation occurs. This will often result in a reflex tachycardia as the body attempts to compensate for the fall in blood pressure. Very late in anaphylaxis the heart rate will fall. This too should be considered a very ominous sign.

State of the art advanced prehospital care of anaphylaxis includes use of all available monitoring devices. These include the cardiac monitor, the pulse oximeter, and, if the patient is intubated, an end-tidal carbon dioxide detector.

✱ **urticaria** the raised areas, or wheals, that occur on the skin, associated with vasodilation due to histamine release; commonly called "hives."

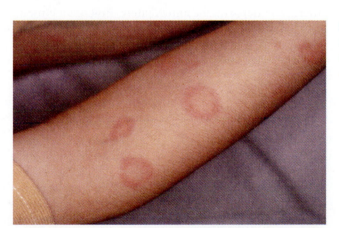

FIGURE 5-2 Hives are red, itchy blotches, sometimes raised, that often accompany an allergic reaction.

As anaphylaxis progresses, the end-tidal carbon dioxide level may climb due to the development of both respiratory and metabolic acidosis, which results in increased carbon dioxide elimination.

MANAGEMENT OF ANAPHYLAXIS

When responding to a patient with an anaphylactic reaction, first assure that the scene is safe to approach. The presence of chemicals or patrolling bees can pose a risk to EMS personnel as well as to the patient and bystanders. If the patient is still in contact with the agent causing the reaction, he should be moved a safe distance away. Honey bees often leave their stinger behind during a sting. If present, the stinger should be removed by scraping the skin with a fingernail or scalpel blade.

Always consider the possibility of trauma in anaphylaxis. If there is any suspicion of coincidental trauma, stabilize the cervical spine. It is not uncommon for people to fall or otherwise injure themselves as they try to escape from wasps and bees. The signs and symptoms of trauma may be masked by the signs and symptoms of anaphylaxis.

PROTECT THE AIRWAY

Position the patient and protect the airway. Administer oxygen via a nonrebreather mask. If the patient is hypoventilating or apneic, initiate ventilatory assistance. If an airway problem is detected, first apply basic airway maneuvers such as head positioning or the modified jaw-thrust maneuver. Use oropharyngeal and nasopharyngeal airways with caution as they can cause laryngospasm. If the patient is having severe airway problems, consider early endotracheal intubation to prevent complete occlusion of the airway. It is important to remember that the glottic opening may be smaller than expected due to laryngeal edema. Also, the larynx will be very irritable, and any manipulation of the airway may lead to laryngospasm. Ideally, the most experienced member of the crew should perform endotracheal intubation, as only one attempt may be possible. Have available equipment for placement of a surgical airway, such as a needle cricothryotomy, in case it is needed.

Establish an IV as soon as possible with a crystalloid solution such as lactated Ringer's or normal saline. Remember that patients suffering anaphylaxis are volume depleted due to histamine-mediated third spacing of fluid. If the patient is hypotensive, administer fluids wide open. If time allows, place a second IV line.

ADMINISTER MEDICATIONS

The primary treatment for anaphylaxis is pharmacological. If the necessary drugs cannot be administered in the field, then the patient should be transported to the emergency department immediately. Emergency medications used in the treatment of anaphylaxis include oxygen, epinephrine, antihistamines, corticosteroids, and vasopressors. Occasionally, inhaled beta agonists, such as albuterol, may be required.

Oxygen Oxygen is always the first drug to administer to a patient with an anaphylactic reaction. Administer high-concentration oxygen with a nonrebreather mask or similar device. If mechanical ventilation is required, attach supplemental oxygen to assure as high an oxygen delivery as possible.

Epinephrine is the primary drug for management of anaphylaxis.

Epinephrine The primary drug for use in treatment of severe allergic reactions and anaphylaxis is epinephrine. Epinephrine is a sympathetic agonist. It causes an increase in heart rate, an increase in the strength of the cardiac contractile force, and peripheral vasoconstriction. It can also reverse some of the bronchospasm associated with anaphylaxis. Epinephrine also reverses much of the capillary permeability caused by histamine. It acts within minutes of administration. In severe anaphylaxis, characterized by hypotension and/or severe airway obstruction, administer epinephrine 1:10,000 intravenously. Epinephrine 1:10,000 contains 1 milligram of epinephrine in 10 milliliters of solvent. The standard adult dose is 0.3–0.5 mg; child dose is 0.01 mg/kg. The effects of intravenous epinephrine wear off in 3–5 minutes, so repeat boluses may be required. In severe cases of sustained anaphylaxis, medical direction may order the preparation and administration of an epinephrine drip.

Antihistamines Antihistamines are second-line agents in the treatment of anaphylaxis. They should only be given following the administration of epinephrine. Antihistamines block the effects of histamine by blocking histamine receptors. They do not displace histamine from the receptors. They only block additional histamine from binding. They also help reduce histamine release from mast cells and basophils. Most antihistamines are non-selective and block both H_1 and H_2 receptors. Others are more selective for either H_1 or H_2 receptors.

Diphenhydramine (Benadryl) is probably the most frequently used antihistamine in the treatment of allergic reactions and anaphylaxis. It is non-selective and acts on both H_1 and H_2 receptors. The standard dose of diphenhydramine is 25–50 milligrams intravenously or intramuscularly. It should be administered slowly when given intravenously. The pediatric dose of diphenhydramine is 1–2 milligrams per kilogram of body weight. Other non-selective antihistamines frequently used are hydroxyzine (Atarax, Vistaril) and promethazine (Phenergan). Hydroxyzine is a potent antihistamine, but it can only be administered intramuscularly. Promethazine can be administered intravenously or intramuscularly, but does not appear to be as potent as diphenhydramine.

Selective histamine blockers have been available for the last 15–20 years. These are primarily H_2 blockers and are used to treat ulcer disease. Blockage of the H_2 receptors decreases gastric acid secretion. However, H_2 receptors are also present in the peripheral blood vessels. Administration of H_2 blockers conceivably will reverse some of the vasodilation associated with anaphylaxis. The two most frequently used H_2 blockers are cimetadine (Tagamet) and ranitidine (Zantac). Typically, 300 milligrams of cimetadine or 50 milligrams of ranitidine are administered by slow intravenous push (over 3–5 minutes). (Some recent studies have questioned the effectiveness of H_2 blockers in the treatment of allergic reactions and anaphylaxis). Also, these agents are considered more expensive than the non-selective antihistamines.

Corticosteroids Corticosteroids are important in the treatment and prevention of anaphylaxis. Although they are of little benefit in the initial stages of treatment they help suppress the inflammatory response associated with these emergencies. Commonly used corticosteroids include methylprednisolone (Solu-Medrol), hydrocortisone (Solu-Cortef), and dexamethasone (Decadron).

Vasopressors Severe and prolonged anaphylactic reactions may require the use of potent vasopressors to support blood pressure. Use these medications in conjunction with first line therapy and adequate fluid resuscitation. Commonly used agents include dopamine, norepinephrine, and epinephrine. These medications are prepared as infusions and are continuously administered to support blood pressure and cardiac output.

Beta Agonists Many patients with severe allergic reactions and anaphylaxis will develop bronchospasm, laryngeal edema, or both. In these cases, an inhaled beta agonist can be useful. The most frequently used beta agonist in prehospital care is albuterol (Ventolin, Proventil). Although usually used in the treatment of asthma, these agents will help reverse some of the bronchospasm and laryngeal edema associated with anaphylaxis. Give the adult patient 0.5 milliliters of albuterol in 3 milliliters of normal saline via a hand-held nebulizer. Children should receive 0.2–0.5 milliliters of albuterol based on their weight. Other beta agonists, such as metaproterenol (Alupent) and isoetharine (Bronkosol) may be used instead of albuterol.

Other Agents Other drugs occasionally used in the treatment of anaphylaxis include aminophylline and cromolyn sodium. Aminophylline is a bronchodilator unrelated to the beta agonists. It can be administered by slow intravenous infusion to treat the bronchospasm associated with anaphylaxis. Although cromolyn sodium (Intal) is not used in the treatment of allergic reactions and anaphylaxis, it is used in their prevention. Cromolyn sodium helps to stabilize the membranes of the mast cells, thus reducing the amount of histamine and other mediators released when these cells are stimulated.

OFFER PSYCHOLOGICAL SUPPORT

A severe allergic or anaphylactic reaction is a harrowing experience for the patient. Although it is essential to work fast, prehospital crews should provide the patient emotional support and explain the treatment regimen. Caution patients about the potential side effects of administered medications. For example, epinephrine will often cause a rapid heart rate, anxiety, and tremulousness. Likewise, the antihistamines may cause a dry mouth, thirst, and sedation. Careful explanation and emotional support will help allay patient anxiety and apprehension.

ASSESSMENT FINDINGS IN ALLERGIC REACTION

Many patients you will be called to treat will be suffering from forms of allergic reaction less severe than anaphylaxis. An allergic reaction, as contrasted with an anaphylactic reaction, will have a more gradual onset with milder signs and symptoms and the patient will have a normal mental status (Table 5-3).

Table 5-3	SIGNS AND SYMPTOMS OF ALLERGIC AND ANAPHYLACTIC REACTIONS
Mild Allergic Reaction	**Severe Allergic Reaction or Anaphylaxis**
Onset: Gradual	*Onset:* Sudden (30-60 seconds but can be more than an hour after exposure)
Skin/Vascular system: Mild flushing, rash, or hives	*Skin/vascular system:* Severe flushing, rash, or hives; angioneurotic edema to the face and neck
Respiration: Mild bronchoconstriction	*Respiration:* Severe bronchoconstriction (wheezing), laryngospasm (stridor), breathing difficulty
GI system: Mild cramps, diarrhea	*GI system:* Severe cramps, abdominal rumbling, diarrhea, vomiting
Vital signs: Normal to slightly abnormal	*Vital signs:* Increased pulse early, may fall in late/severe case; increased respiratory rate early, falling respiratory rate late; falling blood pressure late
Mental status: Normal	*Mental status:* Anxiety, sense of impending doom, may decrease to confusion and to unconsciousness
	Other Clues: Symptoms occur shortly after exposure to parenteral penicillin, *Hymenoptera* sting (fire ant, wasp, yellow-jacket, hornet, bee), or ingestion of foods to which patient is allergic such as nuts or shellfish
	Ominous signs: Respiratory distress, signs of shock, falling respiratory rate, falling pulse rate, falling blood pressure

Note: Not all signs and symptoms will be present in every case.

MANAGEMENT OF ALLERGIC REACTIONS

Common manifestations of mild (non-anaphylactic) allergic reactions include itching, rash, and urticaria. Patients with simple itching and non-urticarial rashes may be treated with antihistamines alone. In addition to antihistamines, epinephrine is often necessary for the treatment of urticaria.

Any patient suffering an allergic reaction who exhibits dyspnea or wheezing should receive supplemental oxygen. This should be followed by subcutaneous epinephrine 1:1,000. Lesser allergic reactions that are not accompanied by hypotension or airway problems can be adequately treated with epinephrine 1:1,000 administered subcutaneously (Figure 5-3). Epinephrine 1:1,000 contains 1 milligram of epinephrine in 1 milliliter of solvent. When administered into the subcutaneous tissue, the drug is absorbed more slowly and the effect prolonged. The subcutaneous dose is the same as the intravenous dose (0.3–0.5 milligram). The subcutaneous route should not be used in severe anaphylaxis. Many physicians prefer to give epinephrine 1:1,000 intramuscularly, because this has a faster rate of onset although a shorter duration of action.

PATIENT EDUCATION

Many severe allergic and anaphylactic reactions are preventable. Persons with history of anaphylactic reactions should be educated about recognition and treatment. They should wear some sort of identification device, such as a Medic-Alert bracelet, which will alert paramedics to their condition in the event they are unresponsive. Also, many patients can initiate emergency anaphylactic treatment at home with epinephrine delivery systems such as the EpiPen.

The severity of an allergic reaction can be diminished in certain cases through a process called *desensitization*. In these cases, physicians begin therapy by administering an extremely small amount of the allergen which causes the patient's anaphylactic reaction. The quantity of the allergen present in the injection is

Many severe allergic and anaphylactic reactions are preventable. Persons with history of anaphylactic reactions should be educated about recognition and treatment.

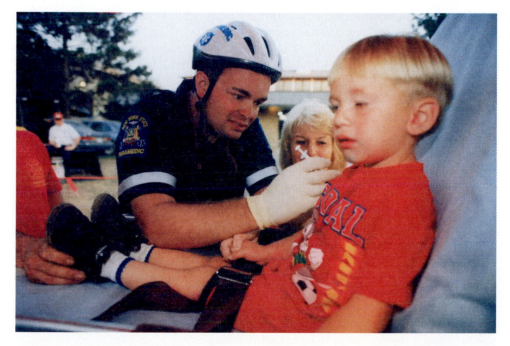

FIGURE 5-3 Epinephrine being administered to a pediatric patient.

gradually increased to a point where the body's immune response to the allergen is blunted and anaphylactic reactions are averted.

Paramedics often keep reference cards for anaphylactic patients living in their service area so that they can quickly identify them, their allergy, and their prehospital treatment history.

SUMMARY

Fortunately, severe allergies and anaphylaxis are uncommon. However, when they do occur, they can progress quickly and result in death in minutes. The central physiological action in anaphylaxis is the massive release of histamine and other mediators. Histamine causes bronchospasm, airway edema, peripheral vasodilation, and increased capillary permeability. The prehospital treatment of anaphylaxis is intended to reverse the effects of these agents.

The primary, and most important, drug used in the treatment of anaphylaxis is epinephrine. Epinephrine helps reverse the effects of histamine. It also supports the blood pressure and reverses detrimental capillary leakage. Following the administration of epinephrine, potent antihistamines should be used to block the adverse effects of the massive histamine release. Inhaled beta agonists are useful in cases of severe bronchospasm and airway involvement. Intravenous fluid replacement is crucial in preventing hypovolemia and hypotension.

The key to successful prehospital management of anaphylaxis is prompt recognition and treatment.

YOU MAKE THE CALL

You are assigned to a hospital-based EMS service that serves a beach town on the Gulf coast. At 1420 you are dispatched to an "injured person" on the beach just outside the Suntide III building. You and your partner are in a four-wheel-drive ambulance stationed only minutes from the call. You turn off Gulf Boulevard onto the beach access road and are able to pull up to a crowd of people on the beach.

You determine the scene is safe and leave the ambulance with your jump kit and a monitor. The patient is a young male lying supine on the beach, softly moaning. He is in obvious distress. A rapid assessment reveals the patient is breathing, has a rapid, thready pulse, and is alert but anxious and slightly agitated. He reports that he and his newlywed wife were taking a leisurely walk along the beach. He accidentally stepped on a dead "hardhead" saltwater catfish that a fisherman had discarded on the beach. The sharp dorsal fin had penetrated the patient's tennis shoe. He immediately developed a burning pain in his foot. Shortly thereafter, he became weak and dizzy and developed trouble breathing.

The patient is in moderate distress with audible wheezing. Your partner and you notice the presence of hives on the patient's chest and back. A quick look at the dead fish confirms that it is a saltwater catfish locally referred to as a "hardhead." You know that these fish have a toxin that can cause pain and burning. However, the reactions to such an injury are usually localized and this patient is certainly having a more generalized reaction.

1. What is the most likely explanation of the patient's emergency?
2. How would you treat this patient?
3. Should the local marine institute be advised of a potentially toxic strain of hardhead catfish?

See Suggested Responses at the back of this book.

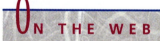

FURTHER READING

Atkinson, T.P. and M.A. Kaliner. "Anaphylaxis." *The Medical Clinics of North America*. 6:4 (July, 1992).

Barrett, James T. *Textbook of Immunology: An Introduction to Immunochemistry and Immunobiology,* 4th ed. Saint Louis, MO: C.V. Mosby Company, 1983. [out of print search or library]

Bledsoe, Bryan E., Dwayne Clayden, and Frank J. Papa. *Prehospital Emergency Pharmacology,* 4th ed. Upper Saddle River, NJ: Brady/Prentice Hall, 1996.

"Dyspnea, Respiratory Distress, and Respiratory Failure" in Dalton, Alice L., Daniel Limmer, Joseph J. Mistovich, and Howard A. Werman. *Advanced Medical Life Support: A Practical Approach to Adult Medical Emergencies.* Upper Saddle River, NJ: Brady/Prentice Hall, 1999.

Guyton, Arthur C. *Textbook of Medical Physiology,* 9th ed. Philadelphia, PA: W.B. Saunders Company, 1996.

"Hypoperfusion (Shock)" in Dalton, Alice L., Daniel Limmer, Joseph J. Mistovich, and Howard A. Werman. *Advanced Medical Life Support: A Practical Approach to Adult Medical Emergencies.* Upper Saddle River, NJ: Brady/Prentice Hall, 1999.

Portier, P. and C. Richet. "De l'action anphylactique de certains venins." *CR Soc Biol (Paris)*. 6:170 (1902).

Runge, J.W., et. al. "Histamine Antagonists in the Treatment of Acute Allergic Reactions." *Annals of Emergency Medicine*. 21 (March 1992).

Salomone, J. A. "Anaphylaxis and Acute Allergic Reactions" in Tintinalli, J. E., et. al. *Emergency Medicine: A Comprehensive Study Guide,* 4th ed. New York, NY: McGraw-Hill, 1996.

Yunginger, J.W. "Anaphylaxis." *Current Problems in Pediatrics*. (March 1992).

ON THE WEB

Visit Brady's Paramedic Website at www.bradybooks.com/paramedic.

CHAPTER 6

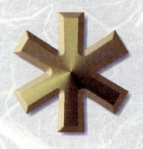

Gastroenterology

Objectives

After reading this chapter, you should be able to:

1. Describe the incidence, morbidity and mortality of gastrointestinal emergencies. (p. 363)

2. Identify the risk factors most predisposing to gastrointestinal emergencies. (p. 363)

3. Discuss the anatomy and physiology of the organs and structures related to gastrointestinal diseases. (pp. 368–369, 376)

4. Discuss the pathophysiology of abdominal inflammation and its relationship to acute pain. (pp. 363–365)

5. Define somatic, visceral, and referred pain as they relate to gastroenterology. (pp. 363–365)

6. Differentiate between hemorrhagic and nonhemorrhagic abdominal pain. (pp. 364–365, 367)

7. Discuss the signs and symptoms and differentiate between local, general, and peritoneal inflammation relative to acute abdominal pain. (pp. 363–365)

8. Describe the questioning technique and specific questions when gathering a focused history in a patient with abdominal pain. (pp. 365–367)

9. Describe the technique for performing a comprehensive physical examination on a patient

Continued

Objectives Continued

complaining of abdominal pain. (p. 367)

10. Discuss the pathophysiology, assessment findings, and management of the following gastroenterological problems:
    - Upper gastrointestinal bleeding (pp. 369–370)
    - Lower gastrointestinal bleeding (pp. 376–377)
    - Acute gastroenteritis (pp. 372–373)
    - Colitis (pp. 377–378)
    - Gastroenteritis (pp. 373–374)
    - Diverticulitis (pp. 380–381)
    - Appendicitis (pp. 385–386)
    - Ulcer disease (pp. 374–376)
    - Bowel obstruction (pp. 382–385)
    - Crohn's disease (pp. 378–380)
    - Pancreatitis (p. 388)
    - Esophageal varices (pp. 370–372)
    - Hemorrhoids (pp. 381–382)
    - Cholecystitis (pp. 386–388)
    - Acute hepatitis (pp. 389–390)

11. Differentiate between gastrointestinal emergencies based on assessment findings. (pp. 365–367)

12. Given several preprogrammed patients with abdominal pain and symptoms, provide the appropriate assessment, treatment, and transport. (pp. 363–390)

CASE STUDY

George Kastner and his partner, Stephanie Emrick, are working a twelve-hour shift on Sunday morning when they are dispatched Code 3 to an "unknown medical emergency" in an affluent section of the city. They arrive on scene within five to six minutes.

The house is well off the road, hidden by a row of large pine trees. As George and Stephanie are transferring their equipment from the truck to the cot, a woman runs from the house, panic stricken. She screams, "I think he's dead! There's blood all over the bathroom!" The woman identifies herself only as the victim's wife and begins to cry uncontrollably. Since George and Stephanie do not know the circumstances, they decide it will be safer to have police officers enter the house first. Stephanie radios dispatch, requesting the police and an additional advanced life support unit.

Deputy Sheriff Marcus Eliot arrives within a few moments. Almost immediately after entering the house, he screams for George and Stephanie to hurry inside.

In the house, they find their patient lying face down in a pool of blood. With BSI already on, Stephanie takes C-spine stabilization. Then she and George log roll the victim onto his back. Their initial assessment reveals a

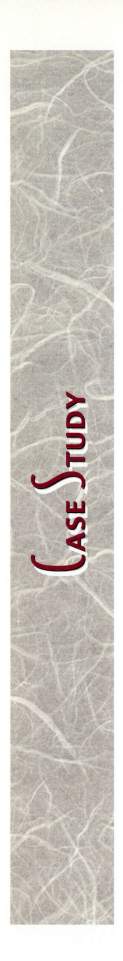

middle-aged man who has shallow, gurgling respirations. His radial pulse is extremely rapid, weak, and barely palpable. They find no external hemorrhages to account for the pool of blood.

George and Stephanie's first concern is the patient's compromised airway. They size an oropharyngeal airway and attempt to insert it with the help of a tongue depressor. Their patient still has a gag reflex and begins to vomit. Stephanie has the suction ready, and George begins to suction copious amounts of bright red blood. When the patient takes a shallow breath they fear that he will aspirate the blood. Unable to control the hemorrhage, they decide to intubate to control the patient's airway and prevent aspiration.

The second crew arrives and paramedic Nicia Logan begins to search for a vein for intravenous access. Her partner, Anthony Rivera, readies the cot for removal.

The patient's intact gag reflex inhibits George's initial attempts at intubation, so he decides to perform rapid sequence intubation. He administers Anectine and midazolam and successfully intubates the patient with a 7.5 mm tube. Nicia and Anthony administer a 500 cc fluid bolus of 0.9% NaCl.

His airway secured, they move the patient to the truck and begin rapid transport to the hospital. En route, George reassesses the patient: respirations are 18, assisted with 100% oxygen via a bag-valve unit; breath sounds are diminished, with rales in the bases. The cardiac monitor reveals sinus tachycardia at 124 beats per minute without ectopy. Blood pressure is 78/42. Stephanie radios ahead to the hospital, giving a full report on the patient and the seriousness of his status.

The emergency department staff readies the resuscitation bay with the rapid transfuser and pages the surgical resident on call. When George and Stephanie wheel the patient through the door, the emergency department team immediately recognizes the patient as one they see regularly. He has been diagnosed with severe portal hypertension from alcoholic-induced hepatic failure. They begin resuscitation as the surgical resident performs an upper endoscopic examination, which reveals a bleeding esophageal varix at the junction of the patient's esophagus and his stomach. The emergency physician places a central line for hemodynamic monitoring and volume fluid resuscitation. Then the staff hurries the patient to the operating room for emergency surgery.

After George and Stephanie complete their charting and restock the unit, they stop by the emergency desk to chat with the attending physician. She tells them that increased portal pressure and forceful retching probably caused the varix to tear. She explains the injury's pathophysiology and assures George and Stephanie that their actions probably saved the patient's life.

INTRODUCTION

Gastrointestinal emergencies account for over 500,000 emergency visits and hospitalizations every year, approximately 5 percent of all visits to the emergency department. Of that number, more than 300,000 are due to gastrointestinal bleeding. These figures will probably increase as more and more people treat themselves with over-the-counter medications and delay seeing a physician until their symptoms become severe. Perhaps more important, the numbers will rise as the general population ages. In the last few years the number of patients over 60 years of age included in these statistics has risen from approximately three percent to more than 45 percent.

GENERAL PATHOPHYSIOLOGY, ASSESSMENT, AND TREATMENT

Gastrointestinal (GI) emergencies usually result from an underlying pathologic process that can be predicted by evaluating numerous risk factors. These risk factors are commonly known to physicians; most are self-induced by patients. They include excessive alcohol consumption, excessive smoking, increased stress, ingestion of caustic substances, and poor bowel habits. The wide variety of risk factors and potential causes requires the emergency care provider to complete a thorough focused history and physical examination before making a field diagnosis, along with assessing the seriousness of the emergency and the need for any prevention strategy to minimize organ damage.

GENERAL PATHOPHYSIOLOGY

Pain is the hallmark of the acute abdominal emergency. The three main classifications of abdominal pain are visceral, somatic, and referred. **Visceral pain** originates in the walls of hollow organs such as the gallbladder or appendix, in the capsules of solid organs such as the kidney or liver, or in the visceral peritoneum. Three separate mechanisms can produce this pain—inflammation, distention (being stretched out or inflated), and ischemia (inadequate blood flow). Because these processes progress at varying rates, they likewise can cause varying intensities, characteristics, and locations of pain.

Inflammation, distention, and ischemia all transmit a pain signal from visceral afferent neural fibers back to the spinal column. Because the nerves enter the spinal column at various levels, visceral pain usually is not localized to any one specific area. Instead, it is often described as very vague or poorly localized, dull, or crampy. The body most often responds to this vague pain with sympathetic stimulation that causes nausea and vomiting, diaphoresis, and tachycardia.

Organs that consist of hollow viscera can frequently cause visceral pain, e.g., the gallbladder (cholecystitis) and the small and large intestines. Many hollow organs first cause visceral pain when they become distended and then cause a different, more specific type of pain (somatic pain, described below) when they rupture or tear. For example, appendicitis initially presents with vague periumbilical abdominal pain that is classified as visceral. If the appendix ruptures it can spill its contents into the peritoneal cavity, causing bacterial **peritonitis** and generating somatic pain. Various microbes associated with pelvic inflammatory diseases can also cause bacterial peritonitis.

Somatic pain, as contrasted to visceral pain, is a sharp type of pain that travels along definite neural routes (determined by the dermatomes, or tissue blocks, present during embryonic development) to the spinal column (Figure 6-1).

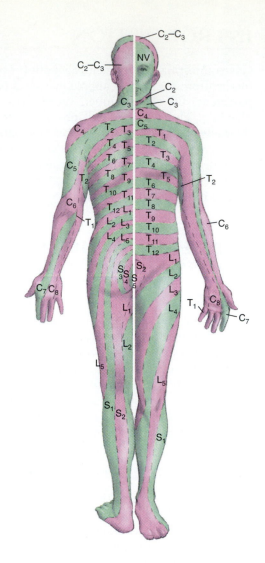

FIGURE 6-1. Dermatome chart. Somatic pain follows neural routes determined by the dermatomes to the spinal column.

* **referred pain** pain that originates in a region other than where it is felt.

Because these routes are clearly defined, the pain can be localized to a particular region or area. As previously noted, bacterial and chemical irritations of the abdomen commonly cause somatic pain. Bacterial irritation can originate from a perforated or ruptured appendix or gallbladder. Chemical irritation of the abdomen can result from leakage of acidic juices from a perforated ulcer or from an inflamed pancreas. Whether the cause is bacterial or chemical, the resulting peritonitis can lead to sepsis and even death. The degree of pain is initially proportional to the spread of the irritant through the abdominal cavity. Somatic pain allows the examiner to locate the specific area of irritation, providing valuable information.

The third type of pain, referred pain, is not a true pain-producing mechanism. As its name implies, **referred pain** originates in a region other than where it is felt. Many neural pathways from various organs pass through or over regions where the organ was formed during embryonic development. For example, the afferent neural pathways that originate in the diaphragm enter the spinal column at the cervical enlargement at the fourth cervical vertebra. Therefore, patients who have an inflammation or injury of the diaphragm often feel pain in their necks or shoulders. One of the most significant hemorrhagic emergencies, the dissecting abdominal aortic artery, produces referred pain felt between the shoulder blades. Some common nonhemorrhagic emergencies are associated with referred-pain patterns, too. Appendicitis often presents with periumbilical pain, whereas pneumonia can cause pain below the lower margin of the rib cage.

GENERAL ASSESSMENT

Your assessment of a patient who complains of abdominal discomfort or whom you suspect of having an abdominal pathology is similar to a trauma assessment with an expanded history. Do not approach the patient until you and your partner have determined the scene to be free and clear of any apparent dangers. Always take appropriate body substance isolation measures, including gloves, eyewear, mask, and disposable body gown to prevent contamination. As you approach the patient, survey the scene for potential evidence of your patient's problem. Medication bottles, alcohol containers, ashtrays, and buckets with emesis or sputum, for instance, can provide valuable information.

Scene Size-up and Initial Assessment

As you approach, look for mechanisms of injury to help determine whether the call is medical or trauma. If you suspect trauma, always immobilize the cervical spine as you assess the adequacy of the patient's airway and his level of responsiveness. In the vast majority of medical patients you can check responsiveness and airway patency by asking the patient his name and chief complaint (why he called the ambulance today) and noting the answers. You can further evaluate the rate, depth, and quality of the patient's respirations fairly rapidly and without great difficulty. As you evaluate the respiratory functions, quickly palpate a pulse and check skin color, temperature, and circulation, including signs of bleeding and capillary refill. If you discover a life-threatening condition during the initial assessment, treat it and then rapidly continue the assessment to identify any other life threats.

History and Physical Exam

Once you have completed the initial assessment and dealt with any life threats, conduct the focused history and physical examination. Your ability to obtain a history from the patient will depend on his level of responsiveness. In some cases, you may detect deterioration of the patient's mental status over time as you take the history.

History An accurate and thorough history can provide invaluable information. After you conduct the SAMPLE history (*s*ymptoms, *a*llergies, *m*edications, *p*ast medical history, *l*ast oral intake, and *e*vents), you can take a more thorough, focused history, exploring the chief complaint, the history of the present illness, the past medical history, and the current health status. The history of the present illness and the past medical history will be especially helpful in sorting the multitude of signs and symptoms and piecing together a clear picture of the underlying pathophysiology.

> *The history of the present illness and the past medical history will be especially helpful in piecing together a clear picture of the underlying gastrointestinal pathophysiology.*

   History of the present illness   Your OPQRST-ASPN history for gastrointestinal patients should address the following specific concerns:

- *Onset.* When did the pain first start? Was the onset very sudden or gradual? Sudden onsets of abdominal pain are generally caused by perforations of abdominal organs or capsules. Gradual onset of pain usually is associated with the blockage of hollow organs.

- *Provocation/Palliation.* What makes the pain worse? What makes the pain better? If the pain lessens when the patient draws his legs up to his chest or lies on his side, it usually indicates peritoneal inflammation, which is often of GI origin. If walking relieves the pain, the cause may be in the GI or urinary systems—perhaps an obstruction of the gallbladder or a stone caught in the renal pelvis or ureter.

- *Quality.* How would you describe the pain: dull, sharp, constant, intermittent? Localized, tearing pain is usually associated with the rupture of an organ. Dull, steadily increasing pain may indicate a bowel obstruction. Sharp pain, particularly in the flank, may indicate a kidney stone.

- *Region/radiation.* Does the pain travel to any other part of your body? Radiated pain, or pain that seems to change location, is common because it involves the same neural routes as referred pain. Pain referred to the shoulder or neck is usually associated with an irritation of the diaphragm, such as happens with cholecystitis.

- *Severity.* On a scale of 1 to 10, with 10 representing the worst pain possible, how would you rate the pain you are feeling now? The severity of pain usually worsens as the pathology (ischemia, inflammation, or stretching) of the organ advances.

- *Time.* When did the pain first start? Estimation of the pain's time of onset is important to determine its possible causes. Any abdominal pain lasting over six hours is considered a surgical emergency and needs to be evaluated in the emergency department.

- *Associated Symptoms.* Have you experienced any associated nausea and or vomiting with the discomfort? If yes, try to determine the content, color, and smell of the vomitus. Ask if the vomitus contained any bright red blood, "coffee grounds," or clots. Determining if your patient has an active gastrointestinal bleed is imperative.

  Have you experienced any changes in bowel habits—constipation or diarrhea—associated with this discomfort/pain? Question the patient further to determine if there have been any changes in feces such as a tarry, foul-smelling stool. Changes in bowel morphology, color, or smell can be the only indication of such conditions as a lower GI hemorrhage, gastritis, or bleeding diverticula.

  Have you had an associated loss of appetite or weight loss? Patients who have an acute abdomen usually have an associated loss of appetite.

- *Pertinent Negatives.* The absence of symptoms associated with GI function or the presence of symptoms related to urinary function may mean the problem originates in the urinary system. Pain in the lowest part of the abdomen, the pelvis, can be due to problems in the reproductive system. Last, remember that an inferior myocardial infarction (MI) can irritate the diaphragm and generate its referred-pain pattern. Be sure to check for cardiovascular history when this pain pattern (pain in shoulder and/or neck area) is present.

Keep in mind the information that your SAMPLE history gave you about your patient's last oral intake. It can help you to differentiate the possible causes of your patient's pain if the problem is in the GI system.

Not all abdominal emergencies result in abdominal pain. Some may cause chest pain. This, typically, is referred pain. Common gastrointestinal emergencies that can cause chest pain include: gastroesophageal reflux, gastric ulcers, duodenal ulcers, and, in some cases, gall bladder disease. When confronted by a patient with chest pain, always consider the gastrointestinal system as a possible cause.

Past medical history   Have you ever experienced this same type of pain or discomfort before? If the patient answers yes, then investigate whether he saw a physician for the problem and how it was diagnosed. Commonly, patients have been treated for the complaint in the past and the pain is a flare-up of an old problem.

Physical Examination While you are conducting the history you can also begin the physical examination. Your patient's general appearance and posture strongly suggest his apparent state of health and the severity of his complaint. Usually patients with severe abdominal pathology lie as still as possible, often in the fetal position. They do not writhe around on the floor or cry out, because doing so increases the pain. You also should continually monitor the patient's level of consciousness for any subtle changes that indicate early signs of shock.

Take a complete set of vital signs to establish a baseline for further evaluation and treatment. These include pulse, respiratory rate, blood pressure, and pulse oximetry. You can also ascertain additional important information such as body temperature.

Visually inspect the abdomen before palpating it, auscultating it, or moving the patient. Remove the patient's clothing as necessary to freely visualize the entire abdomen. Distention of the abdomen may be an ominous sign. It can be caused by a build-up of free air due to an obstruction of the bowel. If the distention is caused by hemorrhage, the patient has lost a large amount of his circulating volume, for the abdomen can hold from four to six liters of fluid before any noticeable change in abdominal girth occurs. Other signs of fluid loss include periumbilical ecchymosis (**Cullen's sign**) and ecchymosis in the flank (**Grey-Turner's sign**).

Auscultating the abdomen usually provides little helpful information because bowel sounds are heard throughout this area. If you auscultate the abdomen, you must do so before palpating it. Listen for at least two minutes in each quadrant, beginning with the quadrant farthest from the affected area and auscultating the affected area last. Like auscultation, percussion requires a quiet environment and an experienced clinician. It too provides little or no useful information and, therefore, is not routinely performed in the field.

Palpating the abdomen, on the other hand, can give you a plethora of information. It can define the area of pain and identify the associated organs. Before palpating, ask the patient to point to where he is experiencing the most discomfort. Then work in reverse order, palpating that area last. Palpate the abdomen with a gentle pressure, feeling for muscle tension or its absence, as well as for masses, pulsations, and tenderness beneath the muscle. If you identify a pulsating mass, stop palpating at once; the increase in pressure may cause the affected blood vessel or organ to rupture.

GENERAL TREATMENT

Once you have completed the initial assessment and the focused history and physical examination, you can address treatment and transport. Your highest priority when treating a patient with abdominal pain is to secure and maintain his airway, breathing, and circulation. Be prepared to suction the airway of vomitus and blood. High-flow oxygenation and aggressive airway management may be indicated, depending on your patient's status. Monitor circulation by placing the patient on a cardiac monitor and frequently assessing his blood pressure. Measurement of the hematocrit will give an indirect measure of blood loss.

Establish a large-bore IV line in patients who complain of abdominal discomfort for use if emergency blood transfusion becomes necessary. You can use the IV for pharmacological intervention or to replace volume lost to hemorrhage or dehydration. In general, the need to avoid masking any abdominal pain for further evaluation will limit your pharmacological interventions to palliative agents such as antiemetics. Place the patient in a comfortable position and provide emotional reassurance based on your field assessment, any conversation with hospital staff or

Usually patients with severe abdominal pathology lie as still as possible, often in the fetal position.

Distention of the abdomen may be an ominous sign.

* **Cullen's sign** ecchymosis in the periumbilical area.

* **Grey-Turner's sign** ecchymosis in the flank.

If you auscultate the abdomen, you must do so before palpating it.

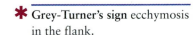

Palpating the abdomen can give you a plethora of information.

Your highest priority when treating a patient with abdominal pain is to secure and maintain his airway, breathing, and circulation.

Persistent abdominal pain lasting longer than six hours always requires transport.

Content Review

THE GASTROINTESTINAL SYSTEM

GI tract
Liver
Gallbladder
Pancreas
Appendix

Content Review

THE UPPER GI TRACT

Mouth
Esophagus
Stomach
Duodenum

family, and knowledge of estimated transport time. Keep your voice and actions quiet and collected. Calm, as well as anxiety, are transmitted easily to patients and family. How you transport the patient will depend on his physiological status. Normally, gentle but rapid transport is sufficient. Remember that persistent abdominal pain lasting longer than six hours is classified as a surgical emergency and always requires transport. In all cases, be sure to maintain monitoring of mental status and vital signs and to give nothing by mouth. Bring vomitus to the emergency department for evaluation.

SPECIFIC ILLNESSES

The gastrointestinal (GI) tract is essentially one long tube divided structurally and functionally into different parts (Figure 6-2). Three other organs, the liver, gallbladder, and pancreas, are intimately associated with it, as is the small structure called the vermiform appendix, which protrudes from the first portion of the large intestine. Collectively, these organs are called the GI, or digestive, system. The GI system converts food into nutrient molecules that individual cells can use, and it excretes solid wastes from the body.

UPPER GASTROINTESTINAL DISEASES

For convenience, clinicians often divide the GI tract broadly into the upper and lower GI tracts. The upper GI tract consists of the mouth, esophagus, stomach, and duodenum, the latter being the first part of the small intestine. Physical digestion of

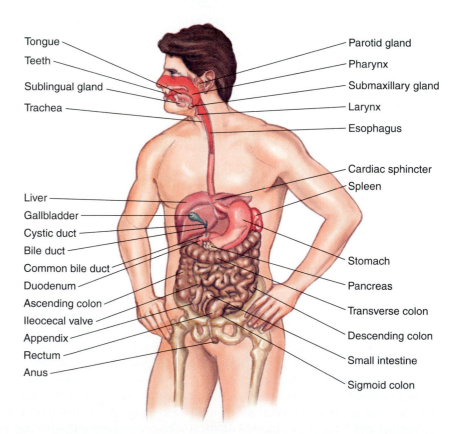

FIGURE 6-2. The gastrointestinal tract is one long tube divided structurally and functionally into different parts.

food and some chemical digestion take place here. As food passes through the lower GI tract, consisting of the remainder of the small intestine and the large intestine, nutrients are absorbed into the blood and solid wastes are formed and excreted.

Upper Gastrointestinal Bleeding

Upper gastrointestinal bleeding can be defined as bleeding within the gastrointestinal tract proximal to the **ligament of Treitz,** which supports the duodenojejunal junction, the point where the first two sections of the small intestine (the duodenum and the jejunum) meet.

Upper gastrointestinal bleeds account for over 300,000 hospitalizations per year. The mortality rate has remained fairly steady at approximately 10 percent over the past years. Many factors contribute to this high mortality. First, the number of patients who treat their symptoms with home remedies and over-the-counter medications is increasing rapidly. Many of these patients come under medical care only when their disease has caused significant damage, such as large-scale hemorrhage from an ulcerated lesion. Second, the overall age of the population is increasing. The infirmities of age and its greater likelihood of coexisting illnesses, such as hypertension, atherosclerosis, diabetes, and substance abuse (including abuse of medications), make this older population more vulnerable to the effects of upper gastrointestinal bleeds. The mortality rate is highest in those over 60 years of age. One prevention strategy for the field is to check for such coexisting problems, especially in elderly patients, and to treat accordingly. In particular, look at the history and physical for evidence of tobacco or alcohol use, or both.

The six major identifiable causes of upper GI hemorrhage, in descending order of frequency, are peptic ulcer disease, gastritis, variceal rupture, **Mallory-Weiss syndrome** (esophageal laceration, usually secondary to vomiting), esophagitis, and duodenitis. Peptic ulcer disease accounts for approximately 50 percent of upper GI bleeds, with gastritis accounting for an additional 25 percent. Overall, irritation or erosion of the gastric lining of the stomach causes more than 75 percent of upper GI bleeds. Most cases of upper GI bleeding are chronic irritations or inflammations that cause minimal discomfort and minor hemorrhage. Physicians can manage these conditions on an outpatient basis; however, if a peptic ulcer erodes through the gastric mucosa, if the esophagus is lacerated in Mallory-Weiss syndrome, or if varices (often secondary to alcoholic liver damage) rupture, an acute-onset, life-threatening, and difficult-to-control hemorrhage can result.

Upper GI bleeds may be obvious, or they may present quite subtly. Most often patients will complain of some type of abdominal discomfort ranging from a vague burning sensation to an upset stomach, gas pain, or tearing pain in the upper quadrants. Because blood severely irritates the GI system, most cases present with nausea and vomiting. If the bleeding is in the upper GI tract, the patient may experience **hematemesis** (bloody vomitus) or, if it passes through the lower GI tract, **melena.** The partially digested blood will turn the stool black and tarry. For melena to be recognizable, approximately 150 cc of blood must drain into the GI tract and remain there for from five to eight hours. Blood in emesis may be bright red (new, fresh blood) or look like coffee grounds (old, partially digested blood).

Upper GI bleeding may be light or it may be brisk and life threatening. Patients who suffer a rupture of an esophageal varix or a tear or disruption in the esophageal or gastric lining may vomit copious amounts of blood. These hemorrhages can cause the classic signs and symptoms of shock, including alteration in mental status, tachycardia, peripheral vasoconstriction, diaphoresis (sweating producing pale, cool, clammy skin), and hemodynamic instability. Besides shock, the vomitus itself can compromise the airway, resulting in impaired respirations, aspiration, and ultimately, respiratory arrest.

* **upper gastrointestinal bleeding** bleeding within the gastrointestinal tract proximal to the ligament of Treitz.

* **ligament of Treitz** ligament that supports the duodenojejunal junction.

Content Review

MAJOR CAUSES OF UPPER GI HEMORRHAGE

- Peptic ulcer disease
- Gastritis
- Varix rupture
- Mallory-Weiss tear
- Esophagitis
- Duodenitis

* **Mallory-Weiss tear** esophageal laceration, usually secondary to vomiting.

If an ulcer erodes through the gastric mucosa, if the esophagus tears, or if varices rupture, an acute, life-threatening, and difficult-to-control hemorrhage can result.

* **hematemesis** bloody vomitus.

* **melena** dark, tarry, foul smelling stool indicating the presence of partially digested blood.

Content Review

UPPER GI DISEASES
Esophageal varices
Acute gastroenteritis
Gastroenteritis (chronic)
Peptic ulcers

A frequently employed clinical indicator is the tilt test, which indicates if the patient has orthostatic hypotension (a 10-mmHg change in blood pressure or a 20-bpm change in heart rate when the patient rises from supine to standing). Hypotension suggests a decreased circulating volume. The human body can compensate for a circulating volume deficit of approximately 15 percent before clinical indicators such as the tilt test show positive results. Thus, those patients whose systolic blood pressure drops 10 mmHg or whose heart rate increases 20 bpm or more need aggressive fluid resuscitation.

When evaluating the patient and his laboratory values, remember that the hematocrit might be within normal ranges when the patient is in the early phase of an acute hemorrhage. The key prevention strategy is to identify subtle indicators and treat the condition before it worsens. More general complaints include malaise, weakness, syncopal (fainting) and near-syncopal (lightheaded) spells, tachycardia, and indigestion.

Your patient's general appearance may be the best indicator of his condition's severity. Because the hemorrhage is internal and histories are often misleading, you must perform a thorough physical examination. The patient may present doubled over in pain or lying very still. The latter is usually an ominous sign that any movement causes extreme pain. If you place the patient supine, be alert to the possibility of vomitus compromising the airway. Patients with a history of GI problems may have scars from past surgeries.

Examination in cases of suspected hemorrhage may be very helpful. Abdominal inspection may show symmetric distention or bulging in one region of the abdomen. Ecchymosis may be present if much blood has been lost into the abdominal cavity. If auscultation is subsequently performed, bowel sounds may be absent if the bleeding is severe or they may be hyperactive if the bleeding is minimal.

Prehospital treatment of an upper gastrointestinal bleed centers on maintaining a patent airway, oxygenation, and circulatory status. Place the patient in the left lateral recumbent or high semi-Fowler's position to prevent aspiration. To maximize the remaining hemoglobin molecules' carrying capability, administer high-flow oxygenation via a nonrebreather mask to all patients with a suspected gastrointestinal bleed.

Establish two large-bore (14–16 gauge) IVs in any patient whom you suspect of having a gastrointestinal bleed. Start one with blood tubing for possible transfusion and one with volume-replacement 0.9% NaCl. Base fluid resuscitation on the patient's condition and response to the treatment. In general you can administer a 20 cc/kg fluid bolus to begin treating hemorrhagic hypovolemia.

Once the patient reaches the emergency department, treatment may include gastric decompression and lavage with a nasogastric tube, further fluid/blood resuscitation, endoscopy, **Sengstaken-Blakemore tube** placement, antacid and histamine antagonist administration, or immediate surgery.

Esophageal Varices

An **esophageal varix** is a swollen vein of the esophagus. Often these varices rupture and hemorrhage. When they do, the mortality rate is over 35 percent.

The cause of esophageal varices usually is an increase in **portal** pressure (portal hypertension). The blood flows from the abdominal organs, through the portal vein, and into the liver, where nutrients are absorbed into liver tissue and numerous compounds are detoxified and returned to the blood. From the liver, blood courses directly into the inferior vena cava through the hepatic veins. Blood flow through the liver ordinarily encounters little, if any, resistance. Damage to that organ, however, can impede circulation, causing blood to back up into the left gastric vein and, from there, into the esophageal veins. The dramat-

* **Sengstaken-Blakemore tube** three-lumen tube used in treating esophageal bleeding.

* **esophageal varix** swollen vein of the esophagus.

When varices rupture and hemorrhage, the mortality rate is over 35 percent.

* **portal** pertaining to the flow of blood into the liver.

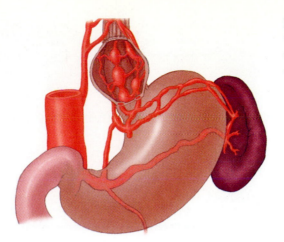

ically higher pressure in these normally low-pressure pathways causes the esophageal veins to dilate and emerge from their sheaths (to evaginate, or "out-pocket"). These small evaginations are called esophageal varices (Figure 6-3). As they become engorged, the varices continue to dilate outward under extreme pressure until they rupture, causing massive hemorrhage. They may also erode through the submucosal layer and directly into the esophagus.

The primary causes of esophageal varices are the consumption of alcohol and the ingestion of caustic substances. Alcoholic liver cirrhosis accounts for two-thirds of cases of esophageal varices. Over time, alcohol consumption can cause a degenerative process known as **cirrhosis** of the liver. Cirrhosis results in fatty deposits and fibrosis in the liver parenychmal tissue, thus obstructing portal blood flow. Consequently, esophageal varices are common in the United States and the Western Hemisphere in general, where the alcohol consumption rate is high. In fact, cirrhosis is one of the leading causes of death in the Western Hemisphere. Caustic substances such as battery acid or drain cleaners can erode the esophagus from the inside out, causing hemorrhage of a vessel. Caustic ingestion, along with variceal formation due to viral hepatitis and erosive esophagitis accounts for the remaining one-third of cases of esophageal varices.

* **cirrhosis** degenerative disease of the liver.

Patients suffering from leaking or ruptured esophageal varices often present initially with painless bleeding and signs of hemodynamic instability. They may complain of hematemesis with bright red blood, dysphagia (difficulty swallowing), and a burning or tearing sensation as the varices continue to bleed, irritating the lining of the esophagus. The hematemesis can be very forceful and copious if the hemorrhage is large. Clotting time increases because the high portal pressure backs up blood into the spleen, destroying platelets. The patient may exhibit the classic signs of shock, including an increased pulse, increased respirations, and cool, clammy, diaphoretic skin, possibly associated with an altered level of consciousness and hypotension.

Because paramedics cannot tamponade the bleeding in the prehospital setting, your care should focus on aggressive airway management, intravenous fluid resuscitation, and rapid transport to the emergency department. Airway management is a top priority. You may need to suction emesis frequently and diligently from the airway. Orotracheal intubation also may be needed to maintain airway patency. To maximize oxygenation, administer high-flow oxygen via a nonrebreather mask. If the patient shows signs and symptoms of shock, place him in

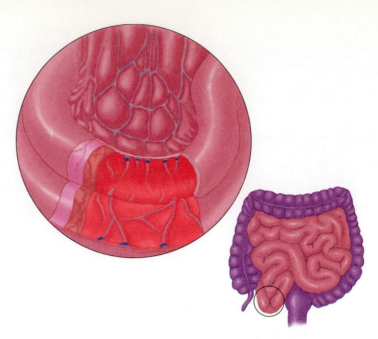

FIGURE 6-4. Mucosal surfaces of GI tract.

Prehospital placement of nasogastric tubes should be avoided in cases of suspected esophageal varices.

* **acute gastroenteritis** sudden onset of inflammation of the stomach and intestines.

the shock position and begin fluid resuscitation. If the patient continues to hemorrhage, management in the emergency department might include the use of a Sengstaken-Blakemore tube to tamponade the bleeding, endoscopic cauterization, or sclerotherapy (injection of a thrombus-forming drug into the vein itself).

Acute Gastroenteritis

Acute gastroenteritis is defined as inflammation of the stomach and intestines with associated sudden onset of vomiting and/or diarrhea. It affects from three to five million people yearly worldwide and affects approximately 20 percent of all hospitalized patients. The pathologic inflammation causes hemorrhage and erosion of the mucosal and submucosal layers of the gastrointestinal tract (Figure 6-4). This inflammation and erosion can in turn damage the villi inside the intestine, which absorb water and nutrients. The water that healthy villi normally would absorb now moves through the bowel at an increased rate. Dehydration secondary to diarrhea is a common cause of death in developing nations but is seen far less frequently in the United States. Adequate volume replacement is your major prehospital prevention strategy to minimize the likelihood of hypovolemia, or even possible hypovolemic shock.

Individuals who abuse alcohol and tobacco are at high risk for gastritis (inflammation of the stomach) and gastroenteritis (inflammation of the stomach and intestines). A wide variety of chemical agents and incidents can lead to acute gastritis. One of the most common is the use of nonsteroidal anti-inflammatory drugs such as aspirin, which break down the mucosal surfaces of the stomach and GI tract. Other causes include excessive alcohol intake and tobacco use; alcohol and nicotine have the same irritating effect on the mucosa as nonsterodial anti-inflammatory drugs. Stress, chemotherapeutic agents, and the ingestion of acidic or alkalotic agents can also cause acute gastroenteritis. Both systemic infection (salmonellosis) and infection from ingested pathogens (staphylococcus) can cause infectious acute gastroenteritis.

As the name implies, the onset of acute gastroenteritis is rapid and usually severe. The swift movement of fluid through the gastrointestinal tract causes multiple problems. First, and most obvious, diarrhea is almost always associated with this condition. Approximately 7–9 liters of fluid (secretions and ingested fluids) normally move through the GI tract every 24 hours. Of that, less then 2 percent, or approximately 100 ml, is lost in the stool. With acute gastroenteritis, the GI tract expels the fluid that normally would be absorbed. This fluid loss leads to dehydration, which can cause severe hypovolemia in pediatric, geriatric, and previously compromised patients. Besides appearing watery, the stool might show either melena or **hematochezia**, the latter bright red blood from erosion of the lining of the lower GI tract. Along with the changes in stool, patients may have bouts of hematemesis, fever, nausea and vomiting, and general malaise. Due to dehydration and hemorrhage, the patient can be hemodynamically unstable; the exam may show hypotension, tachycardia, and pale, cool, and clammy skin. The patient may appear restless or show decreased mental status. If dehydration is severe, he can develop chest pain and cardiac dysrhythmias from electrolyte disturbances. The patient may complain of widespread and diffuse abdominal pain that is not specific to any one region. Visible distention is relatively unlikely unless significant gas has built up within the intestines; palpation will probably reveal tenderness throughout the abdomen.

* **hematochezia** bright red blood in the stool.

Treatment for acute gastroenteritis is mainly supportive and palliative. Keep the patient positioned with head forward or face to the side to minimize the likelihood of aspiration should vomiting occur. Be prepared to clear the airway of vomit or secretions. Maintaining adequate oxygenation is also a high priority. When there is no significant blood loss, the circulatory system's oxygen-carrying capabilities remain intact. You can establish adequate supplemental oxygenation with a nasal cannula at 2–4 lpm. Rehydration is the next step in treating your patient. If he is conscious and alert, oral fluid rehydration may be appropriate. The easiest and quickest route, however, is IV fluid administration. In the prehospital setting, the fluid of choice is either 0.9% NaCl or lactated Ringer's solution to replace the patient's circulating volume. In-hospital treatment will switch the fluid to D_5/LR or D_5/NS to replace electrolytes. Pharmacological treatment can involve antiemetics such as prochlorperazine (Compazine) or promethazine (Phenergan). Additional replacement of electrolytes such as potassium may be needed. Offer emotional support during transport. Exercise extreme caution and use BSI throughout patient contact to prevent any spread of infectious disease.

Gastroenteritis

Gastroenteritis, is inflammation of gastrointestinal mucosa marked by long-term mucosal changes or permanent mucosal damage. Unlike acute gastroenteritis, gastroenteritis is due primarily to microbial infection. The most prevalent pathogen in the United States is the *Helicobacter pylori* bacillus. Other bacteria that can cause gastroenteritis include *Escherichia coli, Klebsiella pneumoniae, Enterobacter, Campylobacter jejuni, Vibrio cholerae, Shigella,* and *Salmonella.* Many of these bacteria can be found as part of normal enteric flora, and effective vaccination against pathogenic strains has not been possible. *Shigella* and *Salmonella* are not part of the normal spectrum of intestinal flora. Viral pathogens include the Norwalk virus and rotavirus. Among the parasitic causes are the protozoa *Giardia lamblia, Cryptosporidium parvum,* and *Cyclosporidium cayetenis.*

* **gastroenteritis** nonacute inflammation of the gastrointestinal mucosa.

Most cases of gastroenteritis are viral. Patients with bacterial gastroenteritis tend to be considerably more ill than those with viral gastroenteritis.

All of these microbes and their associated gastric disorders are far more common in underdeveloped countries. They are transmitted via the fecal-oral route or through infected food or water. Fecal-oral transmission can occur whenever people practice poor personal hygiene or food handling techniques. Local water supplies can become contaminated during natural disasters that disrupt normal water distribution and sewage treatment practices. In such instances, people from outside the endemic area may be more vulnerable to infection than is the local population. *Cyclosporidium* infection reportedly can be contracted by swimming in contaminated water.

Gastroenteritis patients commonly present with nausea and vomiting, fever, diarrhea, abdominal pain, cramping, anorexia (loss of appetite), lethargy, and in severe cases, shock. Usually the intensity of signs and symptoms reflects the degree of microbial contamination. On the other hand, infection with *H. pylori*, the most common infectious gastroenteritis in the United States, often presents with common signs such as heartburn, abdominal pain, and on endoscopic examination, gastric ulcers.

When in contaminated conditions, be sure to decontaminate the drinking water or use a different water source; when in doubt about the reliability of the water, drink only beverages that have been brisk boiled or disinfected. Make sure proper sanitation and preparation of foods is maintained. Handwashing and BSI will protect most EMS providers and prevent transmitting the organism further. To avoid transmitting the disease to patients, health care providers should not work when they are ill.

Prehospital treatment involves protecting yourself and the patient from further contamination, monitoring the ABCs, and transport. Medical treatment of infectious gastroenteritis will require identification of the offending organism. Some of the causative microorganisms are sensitive to antibiotics, but for most the patient will be supported while the disease takes its natural path.

Peptic Ulcers

Peptic ulcers are erosions caused by gastric acid (Figure 6-5). They can occur anywhere in the gastrointestinal tract; terminology is based on the portion of the GI tract affected. Duodenal ulcers most frequently occur in the proximal portion of the duodenum; gastric ulcers occur exclusively in the stomach. Overall, peptic ulcers occur in males four times more frequently than in females, and duodenal ulcers occur from two to three times more frequently than do gastric ulcers. Current statistics place the number of peptic ulcers at 4–5 million, with approximately 500,000 new cases diagnosed yearly. Those patients who are more likely to have gastric ulcers are over 50 years old and work in jobs requiring physical activity. Their pain usually increases after eating or with a full stomach and they usually have no pain at night. Duodenal ulcers are more common in patients from 25 to 50 years old who are executives or leaders under high stress. There is also some familial tendency toward duodenal ulcer, suggesting genetic predisposition. Patients with duodenal ulcers commonly have pain at night or whenever their stomach is empty. Thus, it is important in taking the focused history to get family history and a reliable estimate of the patient's last oral intake. Measurement of hematocrit may substantiate any suspicions of chronic or acute hemorrhage.

Nonsteroidal anti-inflammatory medications (aspirin, Motrin, Advil, Naprosyn), acid-stimulating products (alcohol, nicotine), or *Helicobacter pylori* bacteria are the most common causes of peptic ulcers. To help break down food boluses, the stomach secretes hydrochloric acid. One of the enzymes that control this secretion is pepsinogen. The hydrochloric acid helps to convert pepsinogen into its active form, pepsin. Between them, the pepsin and the hydrochloric acid can make the digestive enzymes very irritating to the GI tract's mucosal lining. Ordinarily, mucous gland secretions protect the stomach's mucosal barrier from these irritants. But when nonsteroidal anti-inflammatory medications, acid stimulators, or *H. pylori* damage the barrier, the mucosa is exposed to the highly acidic fluid, and peptic ulcers result. Prostaglandin, an important locally acting hormone, decreases the stimulation for blood flow through the gastric mucosa, thus

Helicobacter pylori is associated with gastric and duodenal ulcers.

* **peptic ulcer** erosion caused by gastric acid.

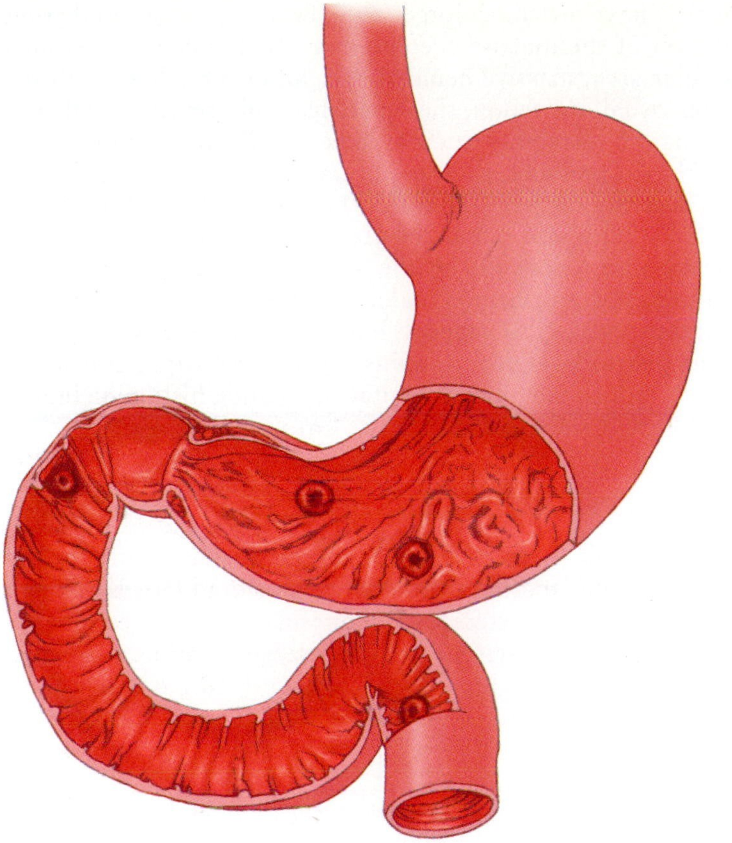

FIGURE 6-5. Peptic ulcer.

allowing its further destruction. Treatment strategies in the prehospital setting focus on antacid treatment and support of any complications such as hemorrhage.

The recent discovery that *Helicobacter pylori* bacteria appear in over 80 percent of gastric and duodenal ulcers has enabled physicians to treat the disease by eliminating its cause with antacids and antibiotics, rather than merely treating its symptoms. Definitive treatment includes tamponade of any bleed, possibly by surgical resection, and antibiotic therapy along with histamine blockers and antacids. If medical therapy fails and the problem persists, it may require surgical resection of the vagus nerve (vagotomy) to reduce the stimulation for acid secretion.

A blocked pancreatic duct can also contribute to duodenal ulcers. As chyme passes through the pyloric sphincter from the stomach into the duodenum, the pancreas secretes an alkalotic solution laden with bicarbonate ions that neutralize the acidic hydrogen ions in the chyme. If the pancreatic duct is blocked, however, the acidic chyme can cause ulcerations throughout the intestine. One other cause of duodenal ulcers is **Zollinger-Ellison syndrome,** in which an acid-secreting tumor provokes the ulcerations.

* **Zollinger-Ellison syndrome** condition that causes the stomach to secrete excessive amounts of hydrochloric acid and pepsin.

Findings on clinical examination of a patient with peptic ulcer can vary. Chronic ulcers can cause a slow bleed with resulting anemia. Visual inspection of the abdomen is usually helpful only if significant hemorrhage has occurred, in which case the same signs of ecchymosis and distention are found as in other causes of upper GI bleeding. On palpation, pain may be localized or diffuse. These patients often have relief of pain after eating or coating their GI tract with a liquid such as milk.

Acute, severe pain is probably due to a rupture of the ulcer into the peritoneal cavity causing hemorrhage. Depending on the ulcer's location, the patient may have hematemesis or may have melena-colored stool. Bouts of nausea and vomiting due to the irritation of the mucosa are common. If the ulcer has eroded through a highly vascular area, massive hemorrhage can occur. Along with the signs of hemorrhage on visual inspection, these patients will appear very ill and have signs of hemodynamic instability such as pale, cool, and clammy skin, tachycardia, decreased blood pressure, and possibly, altered mental status. Most patients will lie still to decrease the pain. They may have surgical scars from previous ulcer repair. Bowel sounds will usually be absent.

Treatment for peptic ulcers depends on the severity of the patient's pain. Those who have abdominal pain or hemodynamic instability may require comfortable positioning and psychological support, high-flow oxygen, IV access for fluid resuscitation and pharmacological administration, and rapid transport. Common medications to reduce the mucosal irritation include histamine blockers such as Zantac and Pepcid and antacids such as Carafate.

LOWER GASTROINTESTINAL DISEASES

The lower GI tract consists of the jejunum and ileum of the small intestine and the entire large intestine, the rectum, and the anus. As digestive fluid moves through the small intestine (approximately 6 meters long), nutrients are absorbed into the blood. Water is absorbed and solid wastes formed in the large intestine, also called the large bowel or colon, which is roughly 1.5 meters long (Figure 6-2).

Lower GI Bleeding

Lower gastrointestinal bleeding is defined as bleeding in the GI tract distal to the ligament of Treitz. Lower GI hemorrhages most frequently occur in conjunction with chronic disorders and anatomic changes associated with advanced age. The most common cause is diverticulosis, which is most prevalent in elderly people. Other causes are colon lesions (cancer or benign polyps), rectal lesions (hemorrhoids, anal fissures, anal fistulas), and inflammatory bowel disorders such as ulcerative colitis and Crohn's disease. These chronic disorders and diverticulosis rarely result in a massive hemorrhage such as that which can occur in the esophagus or stomach.

Your assessment of patients with suspected lower GI bleeds will be identical to your assessment of those with suspected upper GI bleeds. After you complete your initial assessment and treat all life-threatening conditions, you can conduct your focused history and physical examination. First, ask the patient whether this is a new complaint or a chronic problem. If a chronic problem, check the abdomen visually for scars from previous surgery. Frequent complaints with lower GI bleeding include cramping pain that may be described as like a muscle cramp or like gas pain, nausea and vomiting, and changes in stool. Melenic stool usually indicates a slow GI bleed. If the stool contains bright red blood, the hemorrhage either is very large (thus passing through the intestines before melenic change can occur) or has occurred in the distal colon. In the latter case, hemorrhoids or rectal fissures are possible causes. The abdominal exam will show findings similar to those for a bleeding peptic ulcer. If the abdomen has the distention or ecchymosis characteristic of significant hemorrhage, check for signs of early shock such as pale, cool, and clammy skin, tachycardia, decreased blood pressure, and possibly, altered mental status. Because most patients with lower GI bleeds have not lost significant amounts of blood, they will present with hemodynamic stability, including warm dry skin, on physical exam.

How you manage the patient with a lower GI bleed will depend on his physiological status. Watch his airway and oxygenation status closely. If hypoventilation or inadequate respirations develop, administer high-flow oxygenation via a nonrebreather mask or positive pressure ventilation. Establish IV access and fluid resuscitation based on your patient's hemodynamic status. If you find a

* **lower gastrointestinal bleeding** bleeding in the gastrointestinal tract distal to the ligament of Treitz.

Lower gastrointestinal bleeding is usually chronic and rarely results in exsanguinating hemorrhage.

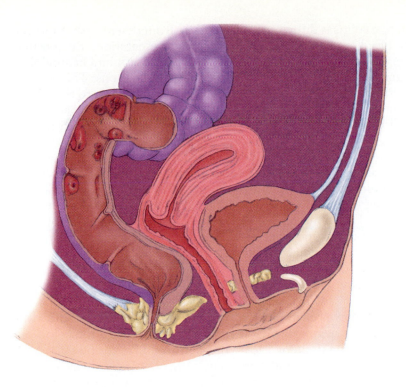

FIGURE 6-6. Ulcerative colitis. As ulcers heal, granular tissue replaces the ulcerations, thickening the mucosa.

drop in hematocrit along with other signs of significant blood loss be especially sure that one IV line is of sufficiently large bore for emergency transfusion. Place him in a comfortable position, offer psychological support, and transport him for further examination. If hemodynamic instability develops during transport, consider use of the pneumatic anti-shock garment (PASG) if directed in local protocols.

Ulcerative Colitis

Ulcerative colitis is classified as an idiopathic inflammatory bowel disorder (IBD), that is, one of unknown origin. The inflammatory (ulcerative) process creates a continuous length of chronic ulcers in the mucosal layer of the colon; extension of the ulcers into the submucosal layer is uncommon. As ulcers heal, granular tissue replaces the ulcerations, thickening the mucosa (Figure 6-6). Approximately 75 percent of all ulcerative colitis involves the rectum or rectosigmoid portion of the large intestine. The inflammatory process usually starts in the rectum and then extends proximally into the colon, sometimes affecting the entire large intestine. If it spreads throughout the entire colon it is called **pancolitis**; if limited to the rectum, it is called **proctitis**.

Though ulcerative colitis is relatively unusual in Africa or Asia, its occurrence in the Western Hemisphere is increasing rapidly. In the United States, more than ten thousand new cases are diagnosed each year. It most frequently strikes people between the ages of 20 and 40 years. While researchers have not found a specific pathogen or cause of ulcerative colitis, they have determined many different contributing factors—psychological, allergic and other immunological, toxic, environmental, immunological, and infectious. Current research has found that the release of cytokines can cause an overwhelming inflammatory response in the submucosa much like the release of histamines during anaphylaxis.

Content Review

LOWER GI DISEASES
Ulcerative colitis
Crohn's disease
Diverticulitis
Hemorrhoids
Bowel obstruction

* **pancolitis** ulcerative colitis spread throughout the entire colon.

* **proctitis** ulcerative colitis limited to the rectum.

Acute ulcerative colitis is difficult to differentiate from other causes of lower gastrointestinal bleeding. Because of its insidious presentation, diagnosing, tracking, and treating ulcerative colitis may require hematocrit and hemoglobin results, guaiac analyses of the stool, and endoscopic examinations. The severity of ulcerative colitis's signs and symptoms is usually related directly to the extent and severity of current inflammation in the colon. In patients with mild signs and symptoms, the disease often is isolated in one distal segment of the GI tract. Severe presentations, on the other hand, normally involve the entire colon.

Typically, ulcerative colitis presents as a recurrent disorder with occasional bloody diarrhea or stool containing mucus. Accompanying the stool abnormalities are **colicky** abdominal pain (cramping), nausea and vomiting, and occasionally, fever (suggesting infection) or weight loss (suggesting severe or longer-term colonic dysfunction). The cramping is usually limited to the lower quadrants, depending on the extent of colonic involvement, and it occurs when hypertrophic muscles lying beneath the submucosa prevent the colon from stretching in response to pressure from its contents. These patients will typically appear restless due to abdominal discomfort but will not show signs of hemodynamic instability (that is, skin will be warm and dry rather than cool and clammy).

More severe cases may present with bloody diarrhea and intense colicky abdominal pain, electrolyte derangements due to fluid loss through the colon, ischemic damage to the colon itself, or, eventually, perforation of the bowel. Often these patients present with signs and symptoms of hypovolemic shock such as pale, cool, clammy skin, hypotension, and tachycardia. Such patients with advanced disease and ongoing hemorrhage may have distention or ecchymosis on the skin and may show guarding of the lower quadrants during the physical examination. Significant hemorrhage is common in patients with ulcerative colitis.

Your management of the patient with ulcerative colitis will depend on his physiological status. If he presents with signs and symptoms of hypovolemic shock, administer high-flow oxygen and circulatory support including intravenous access and fluid resuscitation. If your patient has bouts of nausea and vomiting, you must diligently manage his airway to prevent aspiration of vomitus. Additional management may include antiemetics and antispasmodic medications. Transport any patient who presents with lower GI bleeding or colicky pain to the emergency department for diagnostic evaluation.

Crohn's Disease

Crohn's disease, along with ulcerative colitis, is the other idiopathic inflammatory bowel disorder in humans. It is more common in the Western Hemisphere, with from 20,000 to 30,000 new cases reported annually in the United States. This disease, which strongly tends to run in families, is most prevalent among white females, those under frequent stress, and in the Jewish population.

Unlike ulcerative colitis, which affects the large intestine, Crohn's disease can occur anywhere from the mouth to the rectum. Between 35 and 45 percent of less severe cases involve the small intestine only; approximately 40 percent involve the colon itself. Severe cases of Crohn's disease may involve any portion of the GI tract, causing a variety of problems ranging from diarrhea to intestinal and perianal abscesses and fistulas (the latter, abnormal passages connecting two internal organs or different lengths of intestine). Complete intestinal obstruction, a surgical emergency, can also occur. Significant lower GI bleeding, on the other hand, is rare with Crohn's disease.

As the pathologic inflammation begins, it damages the innermost layer of tissue, the mucosa. Granulomas then form and further break down the mucosal and submucosal layers. The affected section of intestinal wall eventually becomes rubbery and nondistendable due to hypertrophy and fibrosis of the muscles underlying

---

 colic acute pain associated with cramping or spasms in the abdominal organs.

Patients with ulcerative colitis are at increased risk of developing colon cancer.

Transport any patient who presents with lower GI bleeding or colicky pain to the emergency department for diagnostic evaluation.

 Crohn's disease idiopathic inflammatory bowel disorder associated with the small intestine.

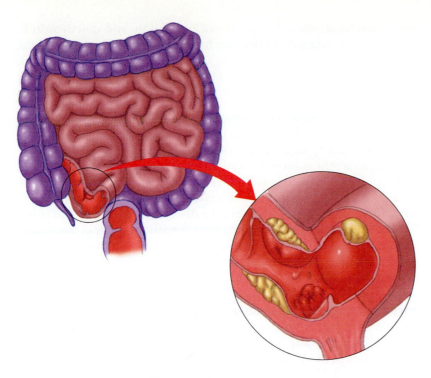

FIGURE 6-7. Crohn's disease. The intestinal wall eventually becomes rubbery and nondistendable due to hypertrophy and fibrosis of the muscles underlying the submucosa.

the submucosa (Figure 6-7). The patchwork-quilt formation of granulomas, fibrosis, and hypertrophy also decreases the intestine's internal diameter, resulting in fissures (incomplete tears) in the mucosa and possibly deeper into the submucosa as food boluses pass through. If a tear extends into the blood vessels in the submucosal layer, small bleeds result. The same pathologic pattern of ulceration and scarring can lead to creation of fistulas, most commonly between lengths of small intestine, or to obstruction of the small bowel. Increased suppressor T-lymphocyte activity suggests an immune-mediated role in the inflammatory process.

Crohn's patients' clinical presentations can vary drastically as the disease progresses, and prehospital diagnosis is difficult or next to impossible. Common signs and symptoms include GI bleeding, recent weight loss, intermittent abdominal cramping/pain, nausea and vomiting, diarrhea, and fever. Onset of a flareup in disease activity is usually rapid, often requiring a visit to the emergency department or physician's office. Abdominal pain cannot be localized to any specific quadrant since the disease can affect any portion of the small intestine and often affects more than one. The physical exam is also nonspecific and nonlocalized, with diffuse tenderness the most commonly found sign. Absence of bowel sounds in a patient with Crohn's disease strongly suggests intestinal obstruction, a surgical emergency.

Because the vast majority of patients with Crohn's disease are hemodynamically stable, prehospital treatment is largely palliative. Your management depends on the patient's physiological status. If he has bouts of nausea and vomiting you must diligently manage the airway to prevent aspiration of vomitus. Additional management may include antiemetics and antispasmodic medications. Particularly if he presents with signs and symptoms of obstruction or significant hemorrhage, administer high-flow oxygenation and circulatory support including

Prehospital diagnosis of Crohn's disease is next to impossible because the patient's clinical presentations can vary drastically as the disease progresses.

intravenous access and fluid resuscitation. As always, calmly and quietly inform the patient of all measures taken and offer psychological support en route to the emergency facility.

Diverticulitis

✱ **diverticulitis** inflammation of diverticula.

✱ **diverticulosis** presence of diverticula, with or without associated bleeding.

✱ **diverticula** small outpouchings in the mucosal lining of the intestinal tract.

Diverticulitis is a relatively common complication of diverticulosis. **Diverticulosis** a condition characterized by the presence in the intestine of **diverticula,** small outpouchings of mucosal and submucosal tissue that push through the outermost layer of the intestine, the muscle. Colonic diverticula are far more common in developed countries such as the United States and increase markedly in prevalence with increased age. They are present in more than half of patients over 60 years of age. Diverticulitis is an inflammation of diverticula secondary to infection. Unlike diverticulosis, it is symptomatic; patients will complain of lower left-sided pain (because most diverticula are in the sigmoid colon); exam and testing will show fever and an increased white blood cell count.

The pathogenesis of an acquired diverticulum is twofold. First, stool passes sluggishly through the colon, a condition associated with the relatively low fiber diets common in developed countries. The colon responds with muscle spasms that increase bulk movement by raising the pressure on the contents inside the colon and pushing the fecal material forward. Second, the outermost layer of colon tissue is made up of fibrous bands of muscle wrapped around one another. Among them are muscles called the teniae coli. Nerves and blood vessels enter the colon through small openings within the teniae coli. These openings become weakened with age, and the increased pressure of muscle spasms can cause the inner layers of tissue, the mucosa and submucosa, to herniate through the openings, forming diverticula (Figure 6-8).

These diverticula commonly trap small amounts of fecal material, including sunflower seeds, popcorn fragments, okra seeds, sesame seeds, and others. The entrapped feces may allow bacteria other then the normal flora to grow and cause an infection. The problem is compounded when the diverticula become inflamed, causing diverticulitis. Complications secondary to diverticulitis include possible

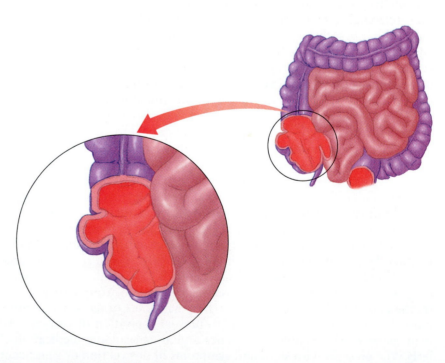

FIGURE 6-8. Diverticulosis.

hemorrhage or larger perforations of the colon wall through which the infected fecal contents can spill into the peritoneal cavity and cause peritonitis.

The most common presentation of diverticulitis is colicky pain associated with a low-grade fever, nausea and vomiting, and tenderness upon palpation. The pain is usually localized to the lower left side because the sigmoid colon is involved in 95 percent of reported cases. Thus diverticulitis is often called left-sided appendicitis. If the diverticula begin to bleed significantly, the usual signs and symptoms associated with severe lower GI bleeding may be present: cool, clammy skin, tachycardia, and diaphoresis. Bleeding diverticula can also result in bright red and bloody feces (hematochezia) because of their close proximity to the rectum. Patients may additionally complain of the perception that they cannot empty their rectums, even after defecation.

Prehospital treatment for diverticulitis is mainly supportive. Measures to counter hypovolemic shock will only be needed when significant hemorrhage has occurred. Monitor the patient's airway and oxygenation and provide supplemental oxygen if needed. Establish intravenous access and begin fluid resuscitation if the patient is hemodynamically unstable. Antiemetics (Phenergan or Vistaril) may comfort the patient. Treatment in the hospital includes antibiotic therapy, endoscopy, and radiological tests to locate the diverticula. Long-term treatment includes implementing a high fiber diet to stimulate daily bowel movements.

Hemorrhoids

Hemorrhoids are small masses of swollen veins that occur in the anus (external) or rectum (internal) (Figure 6-9). They frequently develop during the fourth decade of life. Most hemmorhoids are idiopathic (of unknown cause), although they can

The most common presentation of diverticulitis is colicky pain—usually on the lower left side—associated with a low-grade fever, nausea and vomiting, and tenderness upon palpation.

The presence of diverticuli in the colon is common in the elderly. Some patients with diverticuli will develop bleeding, while others will develop an infection (diverticulitis).

* **hemorrhoid** small mass of swollen veins in the anus or rectum.

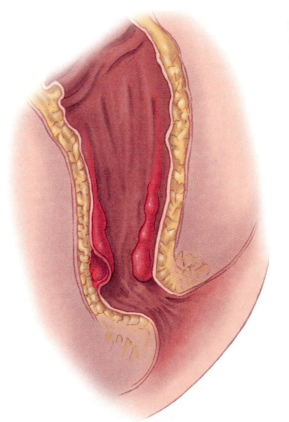

FIGURE 6-9. Hemorrhoids are small masses of swollen veins.

result from pregnancy or protal hypertension. External hemorrhoids often result from lifting a heavy object. Other causes of hemorrhoids include straining at defecation and a diet low in fiber. Overall, hemorrhoids are very common, particularly in persons over the age of 50 years. Their morbidity is low in most cases; one marked exception is in alcoholic patients with cirrhosis of the liver.

Internal hemorrhoids most often involve the inferior hemorrhoidal plexus and vasculature. They commonly bleed during the process of defecation due to straining and then thrombose into closed state again. External hemorrhoids result from thrombosis of a vein, often following lifting or straining, causing bright red bleeding with a bowel movement. The increased venous pressure sometimes causes the vessels to erode and bleed spontaneously, which increases the risk of infection. Rarely do hemorrhoids cause a significant hemorrhage.

Patients with hemorrhoids commonly call for emergency care because of bright red bleeding and pain on defecation. Physical assessment usually reveals a hemodynamically stable patient with relatively normal appearance (warm, dry skin, perhaps with slight tachycardia consistent with anxiety) who bleed with defecation. Visual examination of the stool may reveal gross bleeding. Treatment for hemorrhoids depends on the patient's condition. Most frequently, emotional reassurance and transport are all that is needed; however, you should remain alert to the possibility that the bleeding could be from a lower GI bleed, potentially resulting in uncontrolled hemorrhage. Either significant hemorrhage or bleeding hemorrhoids in an alcoholic patient warrant closer monitoring and transport for immediate follow-up.

Bowel Obstruction

Bowel obstructions are blockages of the hollow space, or lumen, within the small and large intestines. Obstructions can be either partial or complete. An obstructed bowel segment can be catastrophic if not rapidly diagnosed and treated. Of this malady's many different causes, **hernias, intussusception, volvulus,** and **adhesions** are the four most frequent, accounting for over 70 percent of all reported cases (Figure 6-10). Other common causes are foreign bodies, gallstones, tumors, adhesions from previous abdominal surgery, and bowel **infarction.** The most common location for obstructions is the small intestine, due to its smaller diameter and its greater length, flexibility, and mobility.

The obstruction may be chronic, as with tumor growth or adhesion progression, or its onset may be sudden and acute, as with obstruction by a foreign body. Chronic obstruction usually results in a decreased appetite, fever, malaise, nausea and vomiting, weight loss, or if rupture occurs, peritonitis. Acute-onset pain may follow ingestion of a foreign body. Pain might also be due to a strangulated hernia, one that has rotated through the muscle wall of the abdomen such that blood flow is suddenly cut off (the herniated tissue has been "strangulated") and ischemia, or even infarction, of tissue occurs. Patients with bowel obstruction will frequently vomit, with the vomitus often containing a significant amount of bile. Severe bowel obstructions may result in the patient's vomiting material that looks and smells like feces. All of these findings suggest a bowel obstruction.

These patients present with diffuse visceral pain, usually poorly localized to any one specific location. They may be hemodynamically unstable due to necrosis within an organ, and you may see signs and symptoms of shock (pale, cool, clammy skin, tachycardia, alterations in level of consciousness, and hypotension). Visual inspection may reveal distention, peritonitis, or free air within

---

Rarely do hemorrhoids cause a massive hemorrhage.

✷ **bowel obstruction** blockage of the hollow space within the intestines.

An obstructed bowel segment can be catastrophic if not rapidly diagnosed and treated.

✷ **hernia** protrusion of an organ through its protective sheath.

✷ **intussusception** condition that occurs when part of an intestine slips into the part just distal to itself.

✷ **volvulus** twisting of the intestine on itself.

✷ **adhesion** union of normally separate tissue surfaces by a fibrous band of new tissue.

✷ **infarction** area of dead tissue caused by lack of blood.

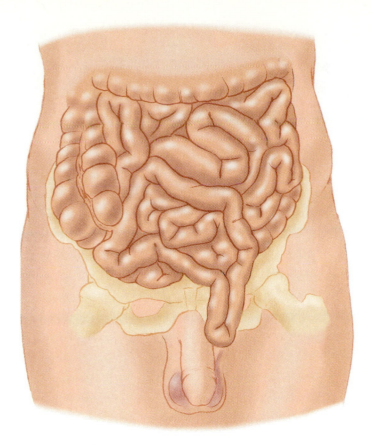

FIGURE 6-10a.   Intestinal hernia.

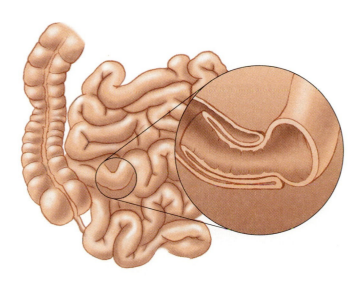

FIGURE 6-10b.   Intestinal intussusception.

FIGURE 6–10c. Intestinal volvulus.

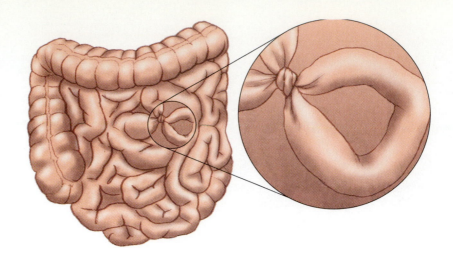

FIGURE 6–10d. Intestinal adhesion.

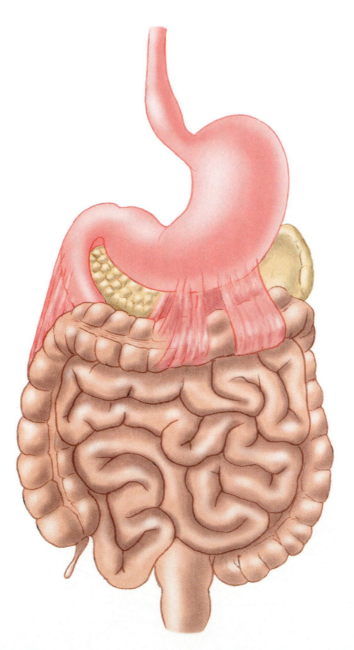

the abdomen secondary to rupture of a strangulated segment of intestine. Look for scars left from previous surgery, as well as for the ecchymosis indicating that significant hemorrhage has occurred into the abdominal cavity. In the earliest phase of acute obstruction, bowel sounds may be present as a high-pitched obstruction sound. In most cases, however, bowel sounds will be greatly reduced or absent. Palpation will reveal tenderness. Be careful to palpate very lightly if you suspect obstruction, as additional pressure may bring about rupture of the obstructed segment.

The treatment for a patient with an obstructed bowel is based on physiological and psychological support during expedited transport to an appropriate facility. Measures include airway management, oxygenation via a nonrebreather mask at 15 lpm, position of comfort or shock position, and fluid resuscitation to prevent shock.

ACCESSORY ORGAN DISEASES

As you learned earlier in this chapter, the GI tract has three closely associated organs, the liver, gallbladder, and pancreas, as well as the small structure called the vermiform appendix. Accessory organ emergencies can arise in all four locations.

Appendicitis

Appendicitis is an inflammation of the vermiform appendix, located at the junction of the large and small intestines (the ileocecal junction). Appendicitis occurs in approximately 10 to 20 percent of the population in the United States, and it is most common in young adults. Acute appendicitis is the most common surgical emergency you will encounter in the field, mostly in older children and young adults. There are no particular risk factors.

The appendix has no known anatomic or physiologic function; most of its tissue is lymphoid in type. It lies just inferior to the ileocecal valve and the first section of the ascending colon. Depending on the individual patient, it may be in the retroperitoneal, pelvic, or abdominal cavity. The appendix can become inflamed, and if left untreated it can rupture, spilling its contents into the peritoneal cavity and setting up peritonitis.

The pathogenesis of appendicitis is most often due to obstruction of the appendiceal lumen by fecal material. The shape and location of the appendix make it particularly vulnerable to obstruction by feces or other material such as food particles or tumor. This inflames the lymphoid tissue and often leads to bacterial or viral infection that ulcerates the mucosa. The inflammation also causes the appendix's internal diameter to expand, which can block the appendicular artery and cause thrombosis. With its blood supply cut off, the appendix becomes ischemic, and infarction and necrosis of tissue follows. At this point the vessel walls often weaken to the point of rupture, spilling the appendiceal contents into the peritoneal cavity.

Appendicitis is frequently misdiagnosed due to the wide variety of signs and symptoms that can accompany it. Mild or early appendicitis causes diffuse, colicky pain often associated with nausea and vomiting and sometimes a low-grade fever. Often the pain is initially located in the periumbilical region. Due to appendiceal blockage, the patient usually loses his appetite. As the appendix continues to dilate the pain will localize in the right lower quadrant. A common site of pain is **McBurney's point**, 1½ to 2 inches above the anterior iliac crest along a direct line from the anterior crest to the umbilicus (Figure 6-11). Once the appendix ruptures the pain becomes diffuse due to development of peritonitis.

* **appendicitis** inflammation of the vermiform appendix at the juncture of the large and small intestines.

Appendicitis is evaluated in the emergency department and eventually treated in the operating room more frequently than any other abdominal emergency.

* **McBurney's point** common site of pain from appendicitis, one to two inches above the anterior iliac crest in a direct line with the umbilicus.

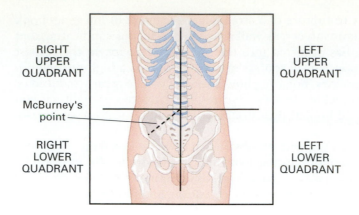

Physical assessment will find a patient who appears to be in discomfort. The abdominal exam will reveal tenderness or guarding around the umbilicus or right lower quadrant. Do not repeatedly palpate for rebound tenderness. The pressure that this procedure exerts can cause an inflamed appendix to rupture.

Prehospital care for appendicitis includes placing the patient in a position of comfort, giving psychological support, diligently managing his airway to prevent aspiration, establishing intravenous access, and transporting him. In most cases the appendix will not have ruptured, and the patient will remain hemodynamically stable. Monitor as you would for bowel obstruction, and treat any complications such as tachycardia or other signs of shock as they arise.

Cholecystitis

Cholecystitis is an inflammation of the gallbladder. Cholelithiasis (the formation of gallstones), which causes 90 percent of cholecystitis cases, occurs in approximately 15 percent of the adult population in the United States, with over one million new cases diagnosed annually. There are two types of gallstones, cholesterol-based and bilirubin-based. Cholesterol-based stones are far more common and are associated with a specific risk profile: obese, middle-aged women with more than one biological child.

Definitive treatment of acute cholecystitis includes antibiotic therapy, laparoscopic surgery, lithotripsy (ultrasound treatment to break up the stones), and surgery if the other, less invasive, therapies fail. With the advent of laparoscopic surgery, mortality has fallen to less then 1 percent, with an overall morbidity of approximately 6 percent.

Cholecystitis caused by gallstones can be chronic or acute. (Figure 6-12). The liver produces bile, the primary vehicle for removing cholesterol from the body. The bile travels down the common bile duct to empty into the small intestine at the sphincter of Oddi. The sphincter of Oddi opens when chyme exits the stomach through the cardiac sphincter. When the sphincter of Oddi closes, the flow of bile backs up into the gallbladder via the cystic duct. The bile remains in the gallbladder until the sphincter of Oddi opens again.

The bile can become supersaturated and calculi—stone-like masses based on bilirubin, cholesterol, or both—form. These calculi travel down the cystic duct, frequently lodging in the common bile duct. When they obstruct the flow of bile, gallbladder inflammation and irritation result. The bile salts subsequently attack the mucosal membrane lining the gallbladder, leaving the underlying epithelial tissue without protection. Prostaglandins are also released, further irritating the epithelial

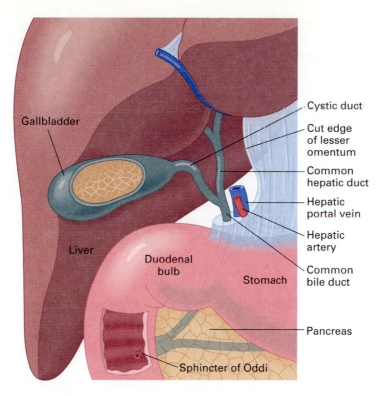

Figure 6-12. The gallbladder is located below the liver.

wall. As irritation continues, the inflammation grows, increasing intraluminal pressure and ultimately reducing blood flow to the epithelium.

Other causes of cholecystitis include acalculus cholecystitis (cholecystitis without associated stones) and chronic inflammation caused by bacterial infection. Acalculus cholecystitis usually results from burns, sepsis, diabetes, and multiple organ failure. Chronic cholecystitis resulting from a bacterial infection (*Escherichia coli* and enterococci) presents with an inflammatory process similar to cholelithiasis.

An inflamed gallbladder usually causes an acute attack of upper right quadrant abdominal pain. The inflammation can cause an irritation of the diaphragm with referred pain in the right shoulder. If the gallstones are lodged in the cystic duct, the pain may be colicky, due to expansion and contraction of the duct. Often the pain occurs after a meal that is high in fat content because of the secondary release of bile from the gallbladder. The right subcostal region may be tender because of abdominal muscle spasms. Patients may experience extreme pain as the epithelium in the gallbladder erodes away. Sympathetic stimulation because of the pain may cause pale, cool, clammy skin. If peritonitis occurs, the skin may be warm due to increased blood flow to the inflamed peritoneum. Nausea and vomiting are common, due to cystic duct spasm.

Visual inspection may reveal scars from previous gallstone surgeries, but distention and ecchymosis are rarely seen. Palpation may reveal either diffuse right-sided tenderness or point tenderness under the right costal margin, a positive **Murphy's sign.**

Prehospital treatment of the patient with acute cholecystitis is mainly palliative. Place the patient in the position of comfort, maintain his ABCs, ensuring

Gallbladder pain is located in the right upper quadrant or epigastrium and is collicky in nature. The problem tends to recur unless surgery is performed.

* **Murphy's sign** pain caused when an inflamed gallbladder is palpated by pressing under the right costal margin.

adequate oxygenation, and finally establish intravenous access. Pain medications commonly used include meperidine (Demerol) and butorphanol (Stadol). Morphine is contraindicated because it is believed to cause spasms of the cystic duct.

Pancreatitis

Pancreatitis is an inflammation of the pancreas. Its four main categories, based on cause, are metabolic, mechanical, vascular, and infectious. Metabolic causes, specifically alcoholism, account for approximately 80 percent of all cases; consequently, pancreatitis is widespread in the United States, due to the high incidence of alcoholism. Mechanical obstructions caused by gallstones or elevated serum lipids account for another 9 percent. Vascular injuries caused by thromboembolisms or shock, along with infectious diseases, account for the remaining 11 percent. Overall mortality in acute pancreatitis is relatively high, approximately 30–40 percent, mainly due to accompanying sepsis and shock, which lead to multisystem organ failure. In acute pancreatitis, the rate of serious morbidity and mortality has been found to be 14 percent in patients with fewer than three positive findings. The mortality rate exceeded 95 percent when there were three or more positive findings.

The vast bulk of the pancreas's tissue is arranged in glandular structures called *acini* (singular, *acinus*). These cells produce digestive enzymes that empty into the duodenum at the ampulla of Vater, near the junction with the stomach. The other function of the pancreas is endocrine: A small amount of tissue located in isolated islets of tissue secretes the hormones insulin and glucagon. Frequently, gallstones leaving the common bile duct become lodged at the ampulla of Vater and obstruct the pancreatic duct. These obstructions back up pancreatic digestive enzymes into the pancreatic duct and the pancreas itself. The digestive enzymes inflame the pancreas and cause edema, which reduces blood flow, as in the pathogenesis of acute appendicitis. In turn, the decreased blood flow causes ischemia and, finally, acinar destruction. This is often called acute pancreatitis based on rapidity of onset.

Acinar tissue destruction causes a second form of pancreatitis, chronic pancreatitis. Acinar tissue destruction commonly occurs due to chronic alcohol intake, drug toxicity, ischemia, or infectious diseases. Alcohol ingestion results in the deposit of platelet plugs in the acinar tissue. The plugs disrupt the enzymes' flow from the pancreas. When digestive juices back up into the pancreas from the ampulla of Vater, the digestive enzymes can become activated and begin to digest the pancreas itself. Morphologically this autodigestion appears as lesions and fatty tissue changes on the pancreas.

As tissue digestion continues, the lesion can erode and begin to hemorrhage. This acute exacerbation of pancreatitis causes intense abdominal pain. Its intensity reflects the number of lesions affected or the degree of acinar tissue death. The pain can be localized to the left upper quadrant or may radiate to the back or the epigastric region. Most patients experience nausea followed by uncontrolled vomiting and retching that can further aggravate the hemorrhage. Visual inspection may reveal previous surgical scars for lesion removal; ecchymosis and swelling of the left upper quadrant may also be present due to hemorrhage or significant organ edema. The patient will appear acutely ill with diaphoresis, tachycardia, and possible hypotension if massive hemorrhaging is involved.

Prehospital treatment is supportive and aimed at maintaining the ABCs by providing high flow oxygenation and establishing intravenous access. Fluid resuscitation with crystalloid may be warranted if the patient appears hemodynamically unstable. Definitive treatment involves gastric intubation and suctioning for emesis control, diagnostic peritoneal lavage, antibiotic therapy, fluid resuscitation, and surgery to remove the blockage.

Acute pancreatitis is most often due to alcohol abuse or gallstones.

Content Review

CAUSES OF ACUTE PANCREATITIS

Alcohol abuse
Gallstones
Elevated serum lipids (cholesterol and triglycerides)
Drug-induced

Content Review

PANCREATITIS (MILD) SIGNS AND SYMPTOMS

Epigastric pain
Abdominal distention
Nausea/vomiting
Elevated amylase and lipase

Content Review

PANCREATITIS (SEVERE) SIGNS AND SYMPTOMS

Refractory hypotensive shock
Blood loss
Respiratory failure

Hepatitis

Hepatitis involves any injury to hepatocytes (liver cells) associated with an inflammation or infection. Due to its wide range of potential causes, hepatitis has a high mortality rate. Five viruses—hepatitis types A, B, C, D, and E—are the disease's most common causes, resulting in five different kinds of hepatitis that together account for 60–70 percent of all cases. Alcoholic hepatitis, which arises from alcoholic cirrhosis, rather than an infectious agent, is responsible for another 20–30 percent. Trauma and other diseases account for the remaining 10 percent. Factors that increase the risk of contracting hepatitis include, to name a few, crowded, unsanitary living conditions, poor personal hygiene that invites oral-fecal transmission, exposure to blood borne pathogens, and chronic alcohol intake. (Specific risk factors are associated with the different types of hepatitis—A, B, C, D, and E.)

The liver is in the upper right abdominal quadrant. A very vascular organ, it filters and detoxifies blood returning from the abdomen and certain abdominal organs. Its other important functions include synthesizing fatty acids, converting glucose to glycogen, and helping to remove toxic products such as ammonia from the body. Any of the viral pathogens, alcoholic exposure, or trauma can injure the hepatocytes, causing inflammation and, possibly, chronic liver disease. Whatever its cause the results are usually similar. The changes in the liver include enlargement and hypertrophy, fatty changes, loss of architecture, and appearance of lesions and spontaneous hemorrhages. The symptoms' severity can range from mild to complete liver failure and death.

Of the five types of viral hepatitis, hepatitis A (HAV) is probably the best known. Commonly referred to as infectious hepatitis, (HAV) spreads by the oral-fecal route. The disease is self-limiting, usually lasting between two and eight weeks. It rarely causes severe hepatic injury and, thus, has a very low mortality rate. Hepatitis B (HBV), known as "serum hepatitis," is transmitted as a blood borne pathogen that can stay active in bodily fluids outside the body for days. With well over 310 million carriers worldwide, HBV is an epidemic. Its effects may be only minimal, but they can also range to severe liver ischemia and necrosis. Hepatitis C (HCV) is caused by the pathogen most commonly responsible for spreading hepatitis through blood transfusions. Hepatitis C is marked by chronic and often debilitating damage to the liver. Hepatitis D (HDV) is a less common disorder because its pathogen is dormant until activated by HBV. Hepatitis E (HEV) is a waterborne infection that has caused epidemics in Africa, Mexico, and other third-world nations. Its mortality rate for pregnant women is high.

Patients with hepatitis commonly present with symptoms relative to the severity of their disease. Usually they complain of upper right quadrant abdominal tenderness, not relieved by antacids, food, or positioning. They may lose their appetite and become anorexic, usually losing weight. The decrease in bile production changes their stool to a clay color, and increased bilirubin retention causes jaundice, a yellow coloring of the skin, and scleral icterus, a yellowing of the white of the eyes. Other signs and symptoms include severe nausea and vomiting, general malaise, photophobia, pharyngitis, and coughing.

Physical examination will reveal a sick patient, possibly with a jaundiced appearance. Depending on the patient's severity, his positioning can range from standing up and walking around to lying in a fetal position with his knees drawn to his chest. Pain may present in the right upper quadrant or the right shoulder (referred from diaphragmatic irritation). Fever may be secondary to infection or to tissue necrosis. Inspection may yield nonspecific findings. Palpation may reveal an enlarged liver. Skin color and temperature can range from warm and dry

With well over 310 million carriers worldwide, HBV is an epidemic.

Be wary of HIV, but fear hepatitis B and C. Do not forget to use personal protective equipment (PPE) and body substance isolation (BSI) precautions.

If you suspect hepatitis, you must consider carefully any pharmacological administration because the liver breaks down many active drug metabolites.

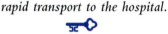

(due to the infection) to cool, clammy, and diaphoretic if a hepatic lesion has ruptured and begun to bleed.

Prehospital treatment is mainly palliative. Secure the ABCs and establish intravenous access for fluid resuscitation or antiemetic administration. You must carefully consider any pharmacological administration because the liver breaks down many active drug metabolites. Definitive treatment involves antiviral and anti-inflammatory medications and symptomatic treatment.

Several large fire departments on the Eastern Seaboard of the United States have experienced increased rates of hepatitis C in their personnel. So always take precautions and work closely with your department infection control officer.

SUMMARY

The key to successful treatment of gastrointestinal ailments is prompt recognition, treatment, and rapid transport to the hospital.

Abdominal pain can originate from a wide variety of causes, either from the abdominal organs or from areas outside of the abdominal cavity. The prehospital management priorities for the abdominal patient are to establish and maintain his airway, breathing, and circulation. The differential diagnosis can include a multitude of causes that usually cannot be identified without laboratory and radiographic analysis. Airway management is of paramount importance, since patients frequently suffer from severe bouts of nausea and vomiting. Be prepared to turn the patient onto his side if necessary to clear large amounts of vomitus from the airway. Oxygenation usually can be adequately stabilized by placing the patient on high flow oxygen via a nonrebreather mask. Fluid loss, hemorrhage, or sepsis may compromise the circulatory status. You should initiate fluid resuscitation for the hemodynamically unstable patient in the field, but never delay transport. Patients who have abdominal pain lasting over six hours should always be evaluated by a physician. The key to successful treatment of gastrointestinal ailments is prompt recognition, treatment, and rapid transport to the hospital.

YOU MAKE THE CALL

You are working your third straight day. The tones in the ambulance bay go off and the call comes through: "Medic 22 respond to 727 McCluer Road for a man down." You and your partner find the road on the map and leave the station.

When you arrive on the scene, it appears to be free of danger. At the door a woman meets you. She says she found her husband slumped over in the bathroom. You enter the bathroom and find an approximately 30-year-old male patient, extremely pale and diaphoretic, sitting on the toilet. As you begin your assessment, the patient tells you he feels light-headed and then passes out.

1. What are your first steps in caring for this patient?
2. What are some of the possible causes for the patient's condition?
3. What information would you attempt to ascertain from the patient's wife?
4. What physical clues might you identify in this situation?

See Suggested Responses at the back of this book.

FURTHER READING

Cotran, R.S., V. Kumar, T. Collins. *Robbins Pathological Basis of Disease.* 6th ed. Philadelphia: W.B. Saunders, 1998.

Dalton, A., et al. *Advanced Medical Life Support.* Upper Saddle River, N.J.: Brady, 1998.

Guyton, A. and J. Hall. *Textbook of Medical Physiology.* 9th ed. Philadelphia: W.B. Saunders, 1996.

Rosen, P., et al. *Emergency Medicine Concepts and Clinical Practice.* St. Louis: Mosby, 1998.

Taylor, M. *Gastrointestinal Emergencies.* 2nd ed. Baltimore: Williams and Wilkins, 1997.

Tintinalli, J.G. Kelen, J.S. Stapczynski. *Emergency Medicine: A Comprehensive Study Guide.* 5th ed. New York: McGraw-Hill, 1999.

ON THE WEB

Visit Brady's Paramedic Website at www.bradybooks.com/paramedic.

CHAPTER 7

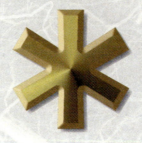

Urology and Nephrology

Objectives

After reading this chapter, you should be able to:

1. Describe the incidence, morbidity, mortality, and risk factors predisposing to urologic and nephrologic emergencies. (pp. 395–396, 409, 413, 419, 421)
2. Discuss the anatomy and physiology of the organs and structures related to urologic and nephrologic diseases. (pp. 396–403)
3. Define referred pain and visceral pain as they relate to urology. (p. 404)
4. Describe the questioning technique and specific questions the paramedic should use when gathering a focused history in a patient with abdominal pain. (pp. 405–406)
5. Describe the technique for performing a comprehensive physical examination of a patient complaining of abdominal pain. (pp. 406–408)
6. Define acute renal failure. (p. 409)
7. Discuss the pathophysiology of acute renal failure. (pp. 409–411)
8. Recognize the signs and symptoms related to acute renal failure. (pp. 411–412)
9. Describe the management of acute renal failure. (pp. 412–413)
10. Integrate pathophysiological principles and assessment findings to

Continued

Objectives Continued

formulate a field impression and implement a treatment plan for the patient with acute renal failure. (pp. 409–413)

11. Define chronic renal failure. (p. 413)
12. Discuss the pathophysiology of chronic renal failure. (pp. 413–414)
13. Recognize the signs and symptoms related to chronic renal failure. (pp. 414–416)
14. Describe the management of chronic renal failure. (pp. 416–419)
15. Integrate pathophysiological principles and assessment findings to formulate a field impression and implement a treatment plan for the patient with chronic renal failure. (pp. 413–419)
16. Define renal dialysis. (pp. 416–419)
17. Discuss the common complications of renal dialysis. (pp. 417–418)
18. Define renal calculi. (p. 419)
19. Discuss the pathophysiology of renal calculi. (p. 419)
20. Recognize the signs and symptoms related to renal calculi. (p. 420)
21. Describe the management of renal calculi. (p. 421)
22. Integrate pathophysiological principles and assessment findings to formulate a field impression and implement a treatment plan for the patient with renal calculi. (pp. 419–421)
23. Define urinary tract infection. (p. 421)
24. Discuss the pathophysiology of urinary tract infection. (pp. 421–422)
25. Recognize the signs and symptoms related to urinary tract infection. (pp. 422–423)
26. Describe the management of a urinary tract infection. (p. 423)
27. Integrate pathophysiological principles and assessment findings to formulate a field impression and implement a treatment plan for the patient with a urinary tract infection. (pp. 421–423)
28. Apply epidemiology to develop prevention strategies for urologic and nephrologic emergencies. (pp. 396, 409)
29. Integrate pathophysiological principles to the assessment of a patient with abdominal pain. (pp. 404–408)
30. Synthesize assessment findings and patient history information to accurately differentiate between pain of a urologic or nephrologic emergency and that of another origin. (pp. 404–408)
31. Develop, execute, and evaluate a treatment plan based on the field impression made in the assessment. (pp. 403–423)

Case Study

Shortly after midnight Rachel Gutierrez and Jack White receive a call that a man has fallen in his bathroom and cannot get up. As they arrive at the house, they are met by a young woman who identifies herself as Amy Jackson, the patient's wife and the person who called 911 for help. She says she woke up hearing her husband, David, yelling from the bathroom that he needed help. As the three go up the steps, they can hear a man calling, "Hurry up. This pain is awful."

Rachel and Jack see an athletic looking man in pajamas lying in the bathroom and moaning. He is pale, sweating profusely, and restlessly moving over the floor. When Rachel asks about the pain, he says "It's in my lower back. On the right. I can't move, it's so bad. And I have to pee. Help me." Rachel gets a urine bottle while Jack introduces himself quietly to David and begins the assessment. Jack helps David to void and then checks the bottle. The urine is reddish yellow. Jack looks for a vein to start an IV line, and Rachel asks David about the pain. He answers that the same spot in his back hurt a bit after dinner, but he was in a lot of pain when he woke up and tried to go to the bathroom. David says his brother had a kidney stone last year. "Could this be one? Am I going to die?" Rachel answers that it might be a kidney stone and that they will take care of him and get him to a hospital. Then she asks more questions quietly, trying to find out if his urination pattern had been normal before he got up, and whether he has ever had bloody urine or been told he had any kind of urinary system trouble before. Jack completes the physical exam, and Rachel reports vital signs of blood pressure 140/90, pulse 150, and respirations 36/min. After an IV line is established and an oxygen mask is in place, Rachel and Jack help the patient onto the stretcher and out to the ambulance.

David stays in the Emergency Room for almost 24 hours, medicated with meperidine to relieve pain and with an IV drip to keep him well hydrated and move fluid through his kidneys. An IVP shows complete obstruction midway down the right ureter with what appears to be a radiopaque stone. His urine is intermittently bloody, and all samples are screened for stones. Finally David passes a visible stone, and with his pain easing back to an ache, he sleeps a bit before going home.

INTRODUCTION

The **urinary system** performs a number of vital functions. It maintains blood volume and the proper balance of water, electrolytes, and pH (acid-base balance). It ensures that key substances such as glucose remain in the bloodstream, yet it also removes a variety of toxic wastes from the blood. It plays a major role in arterial blood-pressure regulation. In addition, the urinary system controls development of red blood cells, or erythrocytes.

The body eliminates water and other substances removed from blood in the form of the fluid **urine.** The kidneys' regulation of water and other important substances in blood is an example of homeostasis, the body's ability to maintain an appropriate internal environment despite changing conditions. Metabolism, the intracellular processes that generate the energy and materials necessary for cell growth and repair, also creates many waste products. For example, significant amounts of ammonia form in the liver when amino acids are broken down in gluconeogenesis, a process that produces glucose between meals. Ammonia is highly toxic to body cells, particularly brain cells. Liver cells convert the ammonia into **urea,** a less toxic compound. The kidneys remove urea efficiently from the blood and pass it into the urine. Moreover, the urinary system eliminates many foreign chemicals such as drug metabolites.

The urinary system in women is physically distinct from the reproductive system: they share no structures. (Chapters 13 and 14 discuss medical emergencies related to the female reproductive system.) In contrast, the urinary system in men does share some structures with the reproductive system. For instance, both urine and the male reproductive fluid are eliminated from the body through the opening at the tip of the penis. Consequently, the term **genitourinary system** is often used with men. The urinary and reproductive systems' proximity in women and their shared structures in men are due to the common embryonic origin of their tissues.

The most significant medical disorders involving the urinary system affect the kidneys and kidney function. **Nephrology** (from the Greek *nephros,* kidney) is the medical specialty devoted to kidney disorders. **Urology** is the surgical specialty devoted to care of the entire urinary system in women and the genitourinary system in men. We will use nephrology and nephrologic (or the preferred adjective, **renal,** from the Latin *renes,* kidneys) to refer to conditions primarily affecting the kidneys. We will use urology and urologic to refer to conditions that significantly affect other parts of the urinary or genitourinary systems.

Renal and urologic disorders are common, affecting about 20 million Americans. Many disorders are very serious. More than 50,000 Americans die annually from kidney disease. More than 250,000 Americans suffer from the most severe form of long-term kidney failure, **end-stage renal failure.** They require either **dialysis,** a process that artificially performs the most important kidney functions, or **kidney transplantation,** implantation of a kidney from another person, to survive. The leading causes of end-stage renal failure are poorly controlled diabetes mellitus (both type I and type II) and uncontrolled or inadequately controlled hypertension.

Among acute, or sudden-onset, disorders, **renal calculi,** or kidney stones, are very common. More than 500,000 Americans are treated for kidney stones each year. Infections are also common, and they may have different causes in women and men. A woman complaining of burning pain on urination probably has an infection in the urinary system. Men with the same chief

* **urinary system** the group of organs that produces urine, maintaining fluid and electrolyte balance for the body.

* **urine** the fluid made by the kidney and eliminated from the body.

* **urea** waste derived from ammonia produced through protein metabolism.

* **genitourinary system** the male organ system that includes reproductive and urinary structures.

* **nephrology** the medical specialty dealing with the kidneys.

* **urology** the surgical specialty dealing with the urinary/genitourinary system.

* **renal** pertaining to the kidneys.

* **end-stage renal failure** an extreme failure of kidney function due to nephron loss.

* **dialysis** a procedure that replaces some lost kidney functions.

* **kidney transplantation** implantation of a kidney into a person without functioning kidneys.

* **renal calculi** kidney stones.

complaint may have an infection that arose in the urinary system or as a sexually transmitted disease. Noncancerous enlargement of the prostate gland, or **benign prostatic hypertrophy,** affects about 60 percent of men by age 50 and about 80 percent by age 80. If prostatic hypertrophy obstructs urine flow, a medical emergency involving sharp pain and inability to urinate results.

All of these conditions, as well as others described later, are sufficiently common that you will see them in the field. In any case where existing kidney function may be jeopardized, prehospital care includes **preventive strategies,** or steps to minimize the likelihood of any further loss of function. Our discussion of assessment and management will cover these procedures.

ANATOMY AND PHYSIOLOGY

The urinary system contains four major structures, the kidneys, ureters, urinary bladder, and urethra (Figure 7-1). First we will discuss the structures and functions of the urinary system, focusing on the kidneys. Then we will cover the additional structures of the male genitourinary system.

KIDNEYS

The left kidney lies in the upper abdomen behind the spleen, and the right kidney lies behind the liver. These locations correspond to the left and right areas of the small of the back, or the **flanks.** A healthy **kidney** in a young adult is about the size of a fist and contains about one million **nephrons,** the microscopic structures that produce urine. With aging comes a normal loss of nephrons—ten percent per

* **benign prostatic hypertrophy** a noncancerous enlargement of the prostate associated with aging.

* **preventive strategy** a management plan to minimize further damage to vital tissues.

* **flanks** the part of the back below the ribs and above the hip bones.

* **kidney** an organ that produces urine and performs other functions related to the urinary system.

* **nephron** a microscopic structure within the kidney that produces urine.

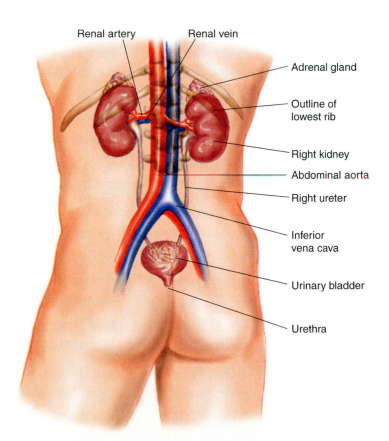

Renal artery   Renal vein

Adrenal gland

Outline of lowest rib

Right kidney

Abdominal aorta

Right ureter

Inferior vena cava

Urinary bladder

Urethra

FIGURE 7-1. Anatomy of the female urinary system, posterior view.

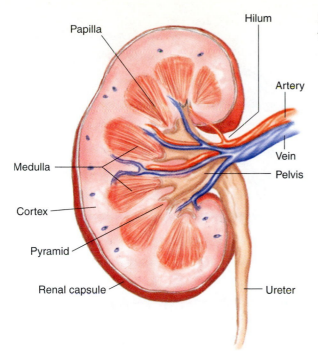

Papilla

Hilum

Artery

FIGURE 7-2. Cross section of the kidney.

Vein

Medulla

Pelvis

Cortex

Pyramid

Renal capsule

Ureter

* **hilum** the notched part of the kidney where the ureter and other structures join kidney tissue.

* **cortex** the outer tissue of an organ such as the kidney.

* **medulla** the inner tissue of an organ such as the kidney.

* **pyramid** the visible tissue structures within medulla of kidney.

* **papilla** the tip of a pyramid; it juts into the hollow space of the kidney.

* **renal pelvis** the hollow space of the kidney that junctions with a ureter.

* **glomerulus** a tuft of capillaries from which blood is filtered into a nephron.

* **Bowman's capsule** the hollow, cup-shaped first part of the nephron tubule.

* **proximal tubule** the part of the tubule beyond Bowman's capsule.

* **descending loop of Henle** the part of the tubule beyond the proximal tubule.

* **ascending loop of Henle** the part of the tubule beyond the descending loop of Henle.

* **distal tubule** the part of the tubule beyond the ascending loop of Henle.

* **collecting duct** the larger structure beyond the distal tubule into which urine drips.

decade of life after age 40—so you should always be alert to the possibility of compromised kidney function in elderly patients.

Gross and Microscopic Anatomy of the Kidney

The renal artery and vein, as well as nerves, lymphatic vessels, and the ureter, pass into the kidney through the notched region called the **hilum.** The tissue of the kidney itself is visibly divided into an outer region, the **cortex,** and an inner region, the **medulla.** Medullary tissue is divided into fan-shaped regions, or **pyramids.** Each pyramid ends in a portion of tissue called the **papilla,** which projects into the hollow space of the **renal pelvis** (Figure 7-2). The spaces of the pelvis come together at the origin of the ureter. Urine forms in the cortical and medullary tissue of the kidney and leaves the kidney through the renal pelvis and ureter.

The functional unit of the kidney, the nephron, forms urine (Figure 7-3). Each nephron consists of a tubule divided into structurally different portions and capillaries that form a complex net of vessels covering the surface of the tubule. Blood that has entered the kidney through the renal artery flows through successively smaller vessels until it reaches a **glomerulus,** a cluster of capillaries surrounded by **Bowman's capsule,** the cup-shaped, hollow structure that is the first part of the nephron. Water and chemical substances enter the tubule through Bowman's capsule. After passage through successive parts of the tubule—the **proximal tubule, descending loop of Henle, ascending loop of Henle,** and **distal tubule**—urine drips into the **collecting duct** before entering the renal pelvis and ureter.

Kidney Physiology

The physiology of the kidneys is one of the most complex topics in human physiology. Its explanation often requires several book chapters. You may wish to reread the section on kidneys in your physiology book before reading further in this chapter, or you may wish to keep the textbook handy in case you need more detail on a topic.

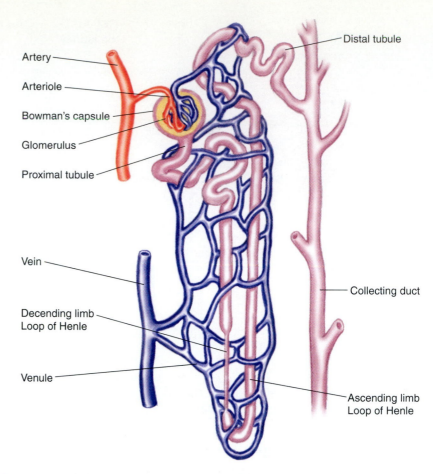

Artery
Arteriole
Bowman's capsule
Glomerulus
Proximal tubule
Vein
Decending limb Loop of Henle
Venule
Distal tubule
Collecting duct
Ascending limb Loop of Henle

FIGURE 7-3. Anatomy of the nephron.

✱ **glomerular filtration** the removal from blood of water and other elements, which enter the nephron tubule.

✱ **reabsorption** the movement of a substance from a nephron tubule back into the blood.

✱ **secretion** the movement of a substance from the blood into a nephron tubule.

✱ **filtrate** the fluid produced in Bowman's capsule by filtration of blood.

✱ **glomerular filtration rate (GFR)** the volume per day at which blood is filtered through capillaries of the glomerulus.

Overview of Nephron Physiology Forming and eliminating urine are the basis for two of the kidneys' major functions: (1) maintaining blood volume with proper balance of water, electrolytes, and pH and (2) retaining key compounds such as glucose while excreting wastes such as urea. A third function, controlling arterial blood pressure, relies both on urine formation and on a second mechanism that does not involve urine production. Last, kidney cells regulate erythrocyte development, but this process does not involve urine formation in any way.

Urine is produced through the interactions among capillary blood flowing over the nephron tubule, the fluid flowing inside the tubule, and the capillary and tubular cells themselves. Three general processes are involved in formation of urine: **glomerular filtration, reabsorption** of substances from the renal tubule into blood, and **secretion** of substances from blood into the renal tubule.

The first step in urine formation is filtration of blood. As blood flows through the capillaries of the glomerulus, water and numerous chemical materials are filtered out of the blood and into Bowman's capsule. Normally, the only blood elements that are not freely filtered into the capsule are blood cells and the plasma proteins, all of which are too large to pass through the pores formed by cell junctions in the capillary walls. Consequently, the fluid formed in the capsule—the **filtrate**—roughly resembles blood plasma except for the absence of proteins.

The rate at which blood is filtered, the **glomerular filtration rate (GFR)**, averages 180 liters/day, the equivalent of 60 complete passages of blood plasma through the glomerular filters. This remarkable efficiency underlies the kidneys' ability to excrete toxic or foreign substances such as urea or drug metabolites so quickly that the substances do not accumulate in the blood.

Filtration is a nonselective process based primarily on molecular size (electrical charge is a secondary factor), and it is essential to urine formation. In contrast, reabsorption of substances into the blood and secretion of substances into the renal tubule are highly selective processes. Almost all elements of filtrate are handled independently of the other elements. The processes of reabsorption and secretion are essential to forming urine with the correct composition and volume to compensate for current body conditions, that is, to maintain homeostasis.

Reabsorption and secretion involve intercellular transport, the movement of a molecule across a cell membrane to either enter or exit a cell. Like other intercellular transport processes, they occur in one of three ways: simple diffusion, facilitated diffusion, or active transport. Both simple and facilitated diffusion are passive processes: neither requires the cell to spend energy. In **simple diffusion**, molecules small enough to pass through a cell membrane randomly move into and out of the cell. Because net movement is always from the region of higher concentration to that of lower concentration, simple diffusion leads toward equalization of molecular concentration on both sides of the membrane. Water molecules always move by simple diffusion. **Osmosis** is the process in which water molecules move so that the concentrations of particles dissolved in water (or **osmolarity**) approach equivalence on both sides of a membrane. A solution with a higher concentration than another solution is **hyperosmolar** to the other; a solution with a lower, more dilute concentration is **hypo-osmolar** to the other.

In **facilitated diffusion**, molecules still move from the region of higher concentration to that of lower concentration. However, a molecule-specific carrier in the membrane acts as a tunnel and speeds the molecules' movement through the membrane. The body cells' normal handling of glucose is an example of this process. When insulin binds to a glucose-specific carrier in the cell membrane, glucose can pass into the cell ten times faster than when insulin is not bound to the carrier.

Active transport is the only process that can produce a net movement of molecules from a region of lower concentration to one of higher concentration. This uphill movement against the concentration gradient is possible because energy is spent to drive the action of the molecule-specific carrier in the membrane. Active transport processes are vital to renal tubular physiology because they allow for the precise balance of reabsorption and secretion that results in independent, homeostatic handling of electrolytes and other substances such as glucose.

Tubular Handling of Water and Electrolytes Tubular handling of water and electrolytes including sodium (Na^+), potassium (K^+), hydrogen (H^+), and chloride (Cl^-) is the basis for control of blood volume and maintenance of electrolyte balance, including pH. As you recall, Na^+ is the dominant cation in the body's extracellular fluids, including blood, whereas K^+ is the dominant cation in intracellular fluid. Appropriate retention of Na^+ in the body, along with osmotic retention of water, is key to maintaining blood volume. Selective retention of K^+ and H^+, along with anions such as Cl^-, maintains the balance of blood electrolytes and blood pH.

Filtrate formed in Bowman's capsule enters the proximal tubule (see Figure 7-3). The cells of the proximal tubule have an extensive brush border that maximizes contact between cell membrane and filtrate. They also have high concentrations of molecule-specific carriers in their membranes and maintain a high level of metabolic activity, producing energy that can support active transport. Under normal conditions, about 65 percent of filtered Na^+ and Cl^-

---

* **simple diffusion** the random motion of molecules from an area of high concentration to an area of lower concentration.

* **osmosis** the diffusion pattern of water in which molecules move to equalize concentrations on both sides of a membrane.

* **osmolarity** the measure of a substance's concentration in water.

* **hyperosmolar** a solution that has a concentration of the substance greater than that of a second solution.

* **hypo-osmolar** a solution that has a concentration of the substance lower than that of a second solution.

* **facilitated diffusion** a form of molecular diffusion in which a molecule-specific carrier in a cell membrane speeds the molecule's movement from a region of higher concentration to one of lower concentration.

* **active transport** movement of a molecule through a cell membrane from a region of lower concentration to one of higher concentration; movement requires energy consumption within the cell.

Table 7-1	HORMONES THAT AFFECT TUBULAR HANDLING OF WATER AND KEY ELECTROLYTES	
Hormone	**Target Tissue**	**Effect(s)**
Aldosterone	Distal tubule, collecting duct	Increase in reabsorption of Na^+, Cl^-, and water
		Increase in secretion of K^+
Angiotensin II	Proximal tubule	Increase in reabsorption of Na^+, Cl^-, and water
		Increase in secretion of H^+
Antidiuretic Hormone (ADH)	Distal tubule, collecting duct	Increase in reabsorption of water
Atrial Natriuretic Hormone (ANH)	Distal tubule, collecting duct	Decrease in reabsorption of Na^+ and Cl^-

Note: Aldosterone, ADH, and ANH are discussed in detail in "Endocrinology," Chapter 4 of this book; angotensin II is discussed in "Cardiology," Chapter 2.

Table derived from Arthur C. Guyton and John E. Hall, *Textbook of Medical Physiology,* 9th ed. (Philadelphia: W.B. Saunders Company, 1996).

is reabsorbed in the proximal tubule, along with osmotic reabsorption of about the same percentage of filtered water. Reabsorption takes place by both passive and active transport processes. Much of the active Na^+ reabsorption is coupled with secretion of H^+ into the tubule; H^+ secretion raises the pH of the arterial-derived blood flowing in capillaries surrounding the tubule. Further handling of H^+ as the filtrate moves through the tubule determines the pH both of the venous blood leaving the kidneys and of the urine excreted from the body.

As filtrate moves through the next part of the nephron, the loop of Henle, its volume and composition change further. Simple diffusion is the dominant process in the first part of the loop. By the time filtrate has moved through the descending limb of the loop, roughly another 20 percent of the filtrate's original water load has been reabsorbed. The cells of the second, ascending limb of the loop of Henle are normally virtually impermeable to water; however, passive and active reabsorption of significant amounts of electrolytes occurs in the same part of the tubule. This reabsorption of electrolytes without reabsorption of water produces a relatively dilute fluid that may exit the collecting duct as dilute urine. Healthy kidneys can produce urine with an osmolarity as low as one-sixth the osmolar concentration of blood plasma, an action termed **diuresis.** A number of hormones alter tubular handling of water and electrolytes (Table 7-1). Some increase the permeability of the distal tubule, collecting duct, or both, so that far more water is reabsorbed. **Antidiuresis,** the result of this hormonal activity, can form a very concentrated urine with an osmolarity as high as four times that of plasma.

The ability of healthy kidneys to handle significant swings in water and electrolyte intake is remarkably large. Studies have shown that an individual can increase his sodium intake to ten times the average amount or decrease it to roughly one-tenth the average, and the kidneys will still compensate properly. Blood volume and sodium content will change only modestly from their baseline, normal levels.

Tubular Handling of Glucose and Urea Glucose and urea represent substances that the kidneys handle in opposite fashion. Critical substances such as glucose are retained in the body, and wastes such as urea are excreted.

✱ **diuresis** formation and passage of a dilute urine, decreasing blood volume.

✱ **antidiuresis** formation and passage of a concentrated urine, preserving blood volume.

Glucose is freely filtered into Bowman's capsule as an element of filtrate. Normally, glucose is completely reabsorbed through an active transport process by the time filtrate leaves the proximal tubule. The body's absolute retention of glucose is usually maintained until the blood glucose level reaches about 180 mg/dL; above that level, glucose begins to be lost in urine. This pattern, in which glucose is completely reabsorbed until a ceiling, or threshold level of blood glucose is reached, is due to saturation of the active-transport process responsible for reabsorption of glucose. At excessively high blood glucose levels, so much glucose enters the filtrate that the proximal tubule's transport capacity to reabsorb it is insufficient. When this occurs, as in uncontrolled diabetes mellitus type I, the body loses not only glucose but also large amounts of water through **osmotic diuresis.**

Urea, a waste product, is also freely filtered into Bowman's capsule. However, tubular handling of this small molecule is very different from that of glucose. Urea is passively reabsorbed throughout most of the tubule, and about half of the filtered load will remain in urine. Thus, the kidneys' ability to excrete urea efficiently depends on the glomerular filtration rate, or GFR. If blood passes through the glomerular capillaries at an adequate rate, the net result of filtration and passive reabsorption will keep the blood level from rising toward a toxic level. The blood urea nitrogen test, or BUN, directly measures blood concentration of urea and is an indirect indicator of GFR. **Creatinine,** another waste product of metabolism, has larger molecules than urea and is not reabsorbed. Because all of the filtered creatinine will be eliminated in urine, the blood concentration of creatinine is a direct indicator of GFR.

Control of Arterial Blood Pressure The kidneys regulate systemic arterial blood pressure in several ways. Over the long term, they control the body's balance of water and electrolytes, thus maintaining blood volume at a healthy level. In addition, juxtaglomerular cells, specialized cells adjacent to glomerular capillary cells, respond to low blood pressure by releasing an enzyme called **renin.** Within seconds of its release renin produces significant amounts of the active hormone angiotensin I. As angiotensin I flows through the lungs, angiotensin converting enzyme (ACE) produces angiotensin II, the powerful vasoconstrictor that immediately raises arterial blood pressure. Angiotensin II acts both on kidney tubular cells (Table 7-1) and on adrenal cells, causing the latter to secrete aldosterone. The renin-angiotensin system's maintenance of blood pressure, as well as its role in hypertension, are covered in detail in Volume 1, Chapters 8 and 9, "Pathophysiology" and "Pharmacology."

Control of Erythrocyte Development The kidneys produce 90 percent of the body's **erythropoietin,** a hormone that regulates the rate at which erythrocytes mature in bone marrow. The exact mechanism that produces erythropoietin is unclear. The impact of renal tissue death, however, is clear and profound; the nonkidney sources of erythropoietin can produce only about one-third to one-half the red cell mass (measured as hematocrit) needed by the body.

URETERS

Urine drains from the renal pelvis into the **ureter,** the long duct that runs from the kidney to the urinary bladder (Figure 7-1). Each ureter is about 25 cm long, and like the kidney, is located in the retroperitoneum of the abdomen. A thin muscular layer in the ureters' walls limits their ability to distend in response to internal pressure. The ureters' nerves derive from renal, gonadal, or hypogastric nerve trunks. The microscopic structure of the ureters and the nature of their nerve supply are important in understanding the symptoms caused by kidney stones caught in a ureter.

* **osmotic diuresis** greatly increased urination and dehydration that results when high levels of glucose cannot be reabsorbed into the blood from the kidney tubules and the osmotic pressure of the glucose in the tubules also prevents water reabsorption.

* **creatinine** a waste product caused by metabolism within muscle cells.

BUN and creatinine are both important indications of renal function.

* **renin** an enzyme produced by kidney cells that plays a key role in controlling arterial blood pressure.

* **erythropoietin** a hormone produced by kidney cells that stimulates maturation of red blood cells.

* **ureter** a duct that carries urine from kidney to urinary bladder.

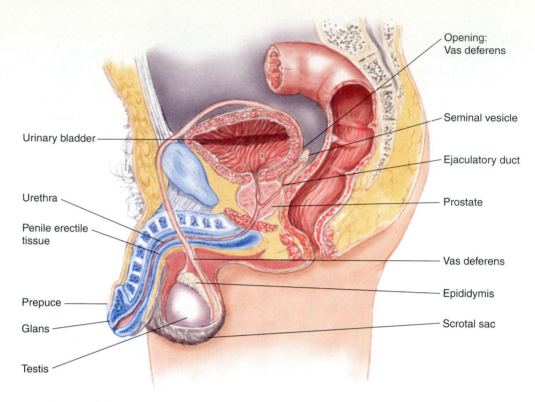

Labels on figure:
Opening: Vas deferens
Seminal vesicle
Ejaculatory duct
Prostate
Vas deferens
Epididymis
Scrotal sac
Urinary bladder
Urethra
Penile erectile tissue
Prepuce
Glans
Testis

FIGURE 7-4. Anatomy of the male genitourinary system.

URINARY BLADDER

✳ **urinary bladder** the muscular organ that stores urine before its elimination from the body.

The **urinary bladder,** the anteriormost organ in the pelvis of both men and women, stores urine. The muscular bladder usually contains at least a small amount of urine, which produces its roughly spherical shape. The bladder neck, through which urine passes during urination, is held in place by ligaments. In women, connective tissue loosely attaches the bladder's posterior wall to the anterior vaginal wall. In men, the bladder's wall bladder is structurally continuous with the prostate gland (Figure 7-4).

URETHRA

✳ **urethra** the duct that carries urine from the bladder out of the body; in men, it also carries reproductive fluid (semen) to the outside of the body.

The **urethra** is the duct that carries urine from the bladder to the exterior of the body. In women, the urethra is only about 3 to 4 cm long and opens to the external environment via a small orifice just anterior to that of the vagina. In men, the urethra is about 20 cm long and ends at the tip of the penis. The female urethra's shortness is probably one reason the female urinary system is more vulnerable to bacterial infection from environmental (largely skin) sources. Because the male urethra carries both urine and male reproductive fluid, it can be an entry way for sexually transmitted diseases.

TESTES

✳ **testes** male sex organs.

✳ **sperm cell** male reproductive cell.

The **testes** (singular, *testis*), are the primary male reproductive organs. They produce both the hormones responsible for sexual maturation and **sperm cells,** male sex cells. The testes lie outside of the abdomen in a muscular sac called the **scrotum.** Normal scrotal temperature is about 2–3°C lower than abdominal temperature, which is critical for development of sperm.

EPIDIDYMIS AND VAS DEFERENS

Sperm cells pass from the testis into the **epididymis,** a small sac where they are stored. Each testis with its paired epididymis is palpable inside the scrotum (Figure 7-4). Sperm are channeled from the epididymis into the **vas deferens,** a muscular duct that carries them into the pelvis and through the substance of the prostate gland to its opening into the urethra. Sperm cells mix with special fluid before passing into the urethra for ejaculation, elimination from the body.

PROSTATE GLAND

The **prostate gland** surrounds the male urinary bladder neck, and the first part of the urethra runs through its tissue. The prostate gland is a major source of the fluid that combines with sperm to form **semen,** the ejaculated male reproductive fluid. In emergency care, the prostate is probably most important in its role as part of the urinary system. Because the first part of the urethra passes through the prostate, any enlargement of the prostate that narrows or obstructs the urethra can block urine flow and create a possible medical emergency.

PENIS

The **penis** is the male organ of copulation. Its spongy internal tissues fill with blood to produce penile erection. The skin covering the end of the penis, the foreskin, is often surgically removed in infancy through **circumcision;** the difference in appearance will be noticeable after you have treated a number of male patients.

GENERAL MECHANISMS OF NONTRAUMATIC TISSUE PROBLEMS

Both traumatic and nontraumatic problems can affect the urinary system, particularly the kidneys. The kidneys' retroperitoneal location protects them relatively well against injury. Nontraumatic renal and urologic disorders result from four general mechanisms: inflammatory or immune-mediated disease, infectious disease, physical obstruction, or hemorrhage. Traumatic renal and urologic disorders are discussed in Volume 4, *Trauma Emergencies.* We will discuss nontraumatic disorders later in this chapter.

GENERAL PATHOPHYSIOLOGY, ASSESSMENT, AND MANAGEMENT

As you learned in Chapter 6, abdominal emergencies are common. Because of many gastrointestinal (GI) and urologic emergencies' similar presentation, you may have difficulty determining the source of an abdominal problem when pain is the sole complaint. You can often find clues to the eventual diagnosis when you take a focused history and perform the focused physical exam. Before reading further, you may want to review the discussion of GI pathophysiology, assessment, and management in Chapter 6.

* **scrotum** a muscular sac outside of the abdominal cavity that contains the testes, epididymi, and vas deferens.

* **epididymis** a saclike duct adjacent to a testis that stores sperm cells.

* **vas deferens** the duct that carries sperm cells from epididymis to the urethra.

* **prostate** a gland that surrounds the male bladder neck and the first portion of urethra; it produces fluid that mixes with sperm to make semen.

* **semen** male reproductive fluid.

* **penis** the male organ of copulation.

* **circumcision** the surgical removal of the foreskin of the penis.

Content Review

MECHANISMS OF NONTRAUMATIC UROLOGIC DISORDERS

- Inflammatory or immune-mediated disease
- Infectious disease
- Physical obstruction
- Hemorrhage

Because of many gastrointestinal and urologic emergencies' similar presentation, you may have difficulty determining the source of an abdominal problem when pain is the sole complaint.

PATHOPHYSIOLOGIC BASIS OF PAIN

The nerve fibers that carry pain messages to the brain are triggered by different stimuli. Some are triggered when damage to the epithelial lining of an organ exposes the underlying tissue layer, where the nerve endings are located. Others respond to stretching forces generated when an organ is inflamed or enlarged by internal hemorrhage or obstruction.

Causes of Pain

Bacterial infection damages the epithelial tissue that lines structures such as the urethra and urinary bladder. This damage causes pain that often worsens when urine flows over the affected tissue during urination. Bacteria normally found on the skin can cause infections in women. In men, the same symptom, pain on voiding, is often due to a sexually transmitted disease such as gonorrhea. Distention of a ureter by a renal calculus (kidney stone) causes a sharp pain that may ease or worsen when the stone shifts position inside the ureter.

Types of Pain

The most common types of pain in urologic emergencies are visceral and referred. **Visceral pain** usually arises in hollow structures such as the ureters, urinary bladder, and urethra, or the vas deferens or epididymis in males. Its chief characteristic, an aching or crampy pain felt deep within the body and poorly localized, is due to the relatively low number of nerve fibers in the involved structures. Visceral pain can also be the initial presentation of urinary tract infection or of renal calculi. **Referred pain** is felt in a location other than its site of origin. This occurs when afferent nerve fibers carrying the pain message merge with other pain-carrying fibers at the junction with the spinal cord. If that junction has far more nerve fibers from one or more other locations than from the site of origin, the brain may perceive the pain as coming from those locations rather than the affected one. Pyelonephritis, inflammation associated with kidney infection, is not only associated with pain in the flank, the skin surface closest to the kidney, but sometimes with pain in the neck or shoulder. The referred pain originates in diaphragmatic irritation due to kidney inflammation, but the brain perceives the pain as coming from the area of the neck or shoulder.

ASSESSMENT AND MANAGEMENT

Do not try to pinpoint the cause of abdominal pain in the field.

The assessment steps are the same for all abdominal emergencies. Do not try to pinpoint the cause of abdominal pain in the field; diagnosis is often difficult even in the hospital setting. However, you do need to do an assessment to detect and manage life-threatening conditions such as shock and to provide historical and physical information that will be helpful in the hospital.

Scene Size-Up

Blood always calls for personal protective equipment and proper sample handling on your part.

During scene size-up, look for evidence of a traumatic versus medical cause and for signs of a life-threatening situation, perhaps an observer performing CPR or the presence of blood. Remember to employ personal protective equipment and proper handling.

Initial Assessment

Initial assessment of the patient concentrates on the ABCs of airway, breathing, and circulation, as well as on patient disability (for example, signs of agitation and confused mental state). If the patient is conscious and responsive, ask for the chief complaint.

Focused History

Information about Pain. When the chief complaint is pain or involves pain, initial questions should elicit information about the timing, character, and associated symptoms of the pain. The OPQRST template is useful for beginning your questions.

- *Onset* When did the pain start, and what were you doing at the time? Visceral pain often arises gradually, with the patient first aware of vague discomfort and only later aware of pain.

- *Provocation/Palliation* What makes the pain worse or better? Increased pain on urination, particularly in light of a fever or history of fever, suggests urinary/genitourinary tract infection. Pain associated with the inability to urinate, particularly in elderly men, points toward urethral obstruction due to prostatic enlargement. Improvement with knees drawn up to the chest points toward peritonitis, whereas improvement with walking may indicate a kidney stone that moved into a less painful position.

- *Quality* What is the pain like? Visceral pain is frequently described as dull or crampy; because many urinary-system structures are hollow, visceral pain is common in these emergencies. Vague discomfort followed by a change to sharp pain localized in the flank, for instance, may indicate ureteral obstruction due to a kidney stone that has moved.

- *Region/Radiation* Where is the pain located, or do you feel pain in several places? Does the pain seem to move from one part of your body to another? Listen for patterns of referred pain such as pain in the lower back and the neck or shoulder, as well as changes in perception of pain on movement of a limb or whole body. In postpubertal women, be sure to ask for menstrual history, particularly if menstrual-like cramps are described or blood is present in the perineal area. (For more on gynecologic and obstetrical emergencies, see Chapters 13 and 14.)

- *Severity* Where is the pain on a scale of 1 to 10? Has the intensity changed over time, and if so, how? Sudden changes to sharp pain, particularly when associated with decreased responsiveness and early signs of shock, may indicate rupture of an internal organ such as the appendix in appendicitis or the fallopian tube in an ectopic pregnancy. Most urologic problems will not show this pattern of abrupt and significant shift in severity and type of pain.

- *Time* How long ago did the pain start? Is it constant or does it come and go? Remember that any case of abdominal pain lasting about 6 hours or longer is considered a surgical emergency until proven otherwise, and the patient should be transported to an appropriate facility. Pelvic visceral pain of long duration and unchanging intensity, particularly if associated with signs suggesting urinary-tract origin such as fever and increased pain on urination, suggests a medical case rather than a surgical one, but you still may need to transport the patient to the hospital. When confronted with an acute abdomen (sudden onset of severe abdominal pain), always err on the side of considering it a potential surgical emergency.

- *Previous history of similar event* Some urologic emergencies such as renal calculus and infection may recur. This makes it especially important to elicit any history of a similar event, the diagnosis at the time, and the treatment given. Because increased risk for renal calculi is genetic in some cases, listen for a history of family members similarly affected.

- *Nausea/Vomiting* As you learned in Chapter 6, severe pain is often associated with autonomic nervous system discharge producing the signs of nausea, possibly with vomiting, along with profuse sweating, clammy skin, and rapid heart rate. Remember that such a presentation does not necessarily indicate that the problem is in the GI system. For instance, the severe pain of a kidney stone can cause this presentation.

- *Changes in bowel habits and stool* Frequent stools, especially if they are diarrheal or contain signs of blood (either melena or hematochezia), suggest a problem in the GI system. Recent constipation may not be relevant except in the context of physical findings.

- *Weight loss* Significant weight loss over a very short period (hours or days) almost always reflects water loss, and signs of dehydration will be evident. Longer-term weight loss may suggest chronic illness or GI dysfunction. Be sure to ask about conditions including diabetes, cardiovascular disease, and cancer, as well as medications and medication changes.

- *Last oral intake* The timing and content of the last meal may indicate an acute, progressive problem (a normal appetite, normal meal) or exacerbation of a long-standing one (poor appetite, small meal). Ask explicitly about fluid intake, because patients may not consider beverages to be food. The timing of the last oral intake is also important if the patient will be undergoing general anesthesia for a surgical procedure.

- *Chest pain* Chest pain, particularly left-sided, does not necessarily indicate a myocardial infarction (MI). Assess whether the pain pattern suggests angina (for example, chest pain associated with radiation to jaw and left arm). Also remember that patients with long-standing or severe diabetes may not show the typical pain pattern of an MI due to diabetic neuropathy (nerve damage), but signs of ischemia may appear on an ECG.

Focused Physical Examination

The focused examination includes forming an overall impression as well as examining the abdomen. Remember that you will not be able to diagnose most cases of abdominal pain in the field. Your job is to gather the historical and physical evidence that can be used in the hospital and to make sure the patient is supported before and during transport.

During the focused history and physical exam, your job is to gather the historical and physical evidence that can be used in the hospital and to make sure the patient is supported before and during transport.

Appearance In general, any person with significant pain, particularly pain of some duration, will appear uncomfortable. A patient may show discomfort by rigidly maintaining the position of least pain or by constantly pacing if walking helps ease the pain.

Posture Lying with knees drawn to chest suggests peritonitis, which is often of GI origin. Relief with walking suggests visceral pain; kidney stones may shift position during walking, easing the sharp pain. Check visually if the patient who is walking is upright or favoring one side. Someone who looks feverish and walks hunched up, leaning to one side, and complaining of back pain may have a pyelonephritis (kidney infection).

Level of Consciousness In the absence of fever, acute-onset decreases in responsiveness often suggest hemorrhage and evolution of hypovolemic shock. Hemorrhage is far more often tied to GI or reproductive (namely, obstetric) emergencies than to urinary system problems. You may see a decreased level of consciousness in sick patients who are undergoing dialysis, the artificial technique that replaces some vital kidney functions, including maintenance of electrolyte balance and removal of wastes. Try to determine if the change in responsiveness is acute or chronic, which may suggest a new problem or an aggravation of preexistent problems.

Apparent State of Health Patients with chronic illness, whether or not it originates in the urinary system, often look ill even without an acute problem. Extreme thinness, pale skin or mucous membranes, or the presence of home health equipment such as a bedside toilet, dialysis machine, or an oxygen tank all suggest chronic problems. In significant emergency states, the patient will usually not be tidy and neatly dressed. If he is, this may suggest that the emergency occurred suddenly, as with a hemorrhage or painful passage of a stone.

Skin Color Pale, dry, cool skin and mucous membranes may suggest chronic anemia such as that found in persons with chronic renal failure. Pale clammy skin suggests severe pain or shock, whereas flushed, dry skin may accompany fever.

Examination of the Abdomen The four components of the abdominal exam are inspection, auscultation, percussion, and palpation.

Always inspect the abdomen first. Note any ecchymotic discoloration or distention, as well as any surgical or traumatic scars. Most nephrologic and urologic emergencies will not show acute abnormalities on exam, whereas a number of GI emergencies will. Auscultation rarely produces a positive finding because bowel sounds are almost always present. Absence of bowel sounds, however, is important and suggests a GI emergency such as bowel obstruction.

Percussion and palpation may be more useful in the field. Percussion of the abdomen or other involved areas may produce clues to the origin of a urologic problem. Pain induced by percussion of the flanks, especially when accompanied by fever, strongly suggests pyelonephritis, or kidney infection. Pain on percussion just above the pelvic rim of the abdomen, especially when accompanied by fever and an increased urge to void, suggests cystitis, bladder infection. Constant, sharp pain increased by percussion of the affected flank may indicate where a kidney stone has lodged in a ureter.

Pain on percussion of the costovertebral angle (CVA—where the last rib meets the lumbar vertebrae) is known as Lloyd's sign and is indicative of pyelonephritis (infection of the kidney and renal pelvis).

In postpubescent girls and women, abdominal palpation may reveal pregnancy if you feel the firm, muscular mass of the gravid uterus above the pelvic rim. A ruptured ectopic pregnancy is possible when palpation increases pain in the lower quadrant, particularly when accompanied by evidence of hemorrhage or early shock. A vaginal exam is rarely indicated in the field; however, you should check for blood or other discharge at the urethral or vaginal openings. In all cases, ask the patient for the date of her last menstrual period.

Palpation of the lower abdomen may help diagnose acute urinary obstruction in older men due to prostatic enlargement. If enough urine has been retained, you will feel a large (up to roughly the size of a two-liter bottle), painful, fluctuant mass above the pelvic rim of the abdomen. This represents the distended bladder. The male abdominal exam should also include inspection of the penis and scrotum. Purulent discharge from the penis may indicate a sexually transmitted disease (STD). Palpation of the scrotum may detect a testicular mass (remember that testicular cancer is far more common in younger men—the opposite of the age risk for prostatic cancer). Palpable nontesticular masses may be painful (infectious epididymitis) or nonpainful (varicocele, a noninfectious swelling of the epididymis). Ask relevant questions, such as whether swelling has been present for some time (as occurs with a varicocele) or is of recent onset (epididymitis).

Assessment Tools A hematocrit may detect significant or chronic bleeding. If blood is present in underwear or on the perineum itself, consider obtaining a small amount of material from the rectum or penile opening or opening of the vagina to be checked for visible blood or occult bleeding. The latter may help to localize the affected system.

Vital Signs Temperature is important because fever suggests an infectious process. If you found high blood pressure, increased heart rate, or both during the ABC assessment, put those findings into context with other impressions from the exam. For instance, both heart rate and blood pressure commonly increase in someone with severe pain. On the other hand, it is also important to find out the patient's usual readings, if either he or a bystander can tell you. Uncontrolled chronic hypertension is one of the two most common causes of nephron damage and chronic renal failure (with the other cause being diabetes mellitus).

Management and Treatment Plans

Management of the patient with abdominal pain includes general and case-specific elements.

Airway, Breathing, Circulation Field management always starts with the ABCs—airway, breathing, and circulation. Be sure to maintain an open airway and use high-flow oxygen by mask. Be prepared for vomiting in any patient with severe pain, whether or not it is likely of genitourinary origin. Circulatory support is also vital, especially when there is any indication of hemorrhage, dehydration, or shock or the patient appears to have any compromise of renal function. Monitor blood pressure closely, and monitor cardiac status with ECG per local protocol or discussion with medical direction.

In cases of abdominal pain, use analgesics as sparingly as possible.

Pharmacological Interventions Consider placing a large bore IV line for volume replacement or drug administration. Where possible, use a needle of sufficiently large bore for any emergency blood transfusion. In almost all cases involving abdominal pain, the question of **analgesics**, pain-relieving medications, will arise. The positive aspects of analgesic use are that the patient is more comfortable during transport and that pain- or stress-induced tachycardia, hypertension, or both may be abated. On the other hand, analgesics may mask the problem's signs and symptoms, making it very difficult to accurately gauge progression of the pathologic process. Use analgesics as sparingly as possible; local protocol or discussion with medical direction may be advisable.

Nonpharmacological Interventions Remember that patients with an acute abdominal problem are possible surgical cases. Thus, nothing should be given by mouth. Administer fluid or medication only by IV or IM routes. Monitor vital signs closely and look for any change in level of consciousness. Be sure the patient is in a position of relative comfort, but also ensure that the position minimizes risk of aspiration if vomiting occurs.

Transport Considerations Each patient with abdominal pain of greater than 6 hours is considered a surgical emergency until hospital evaluation proves otherwise. Rapidly yet gently transport all such patients. During transportation, talk quietly to the patient, both to calm him and to keep him informed of time until arrival or other pertinent matters. All of your actions, both with the patient and any family or friends in the ambulance, should reflect caring and competence.

RENAL AND UROLOGIC EMERGENCIES

You must know how to respond properly and quickly to each major type of urinary or genitourinary emergency. Prevention strategies, procedures that minimize further loss of any existing kidney function, are vital. Most of this discussion focuses on renal emergencies, those affecting the kidneys. The leading causes of kidney failure are diabetes mellitus (both types) and uncontrolled or inadequately controlled hypertension. Add to that profile the fact that nephron number decreases with age, and you have the general profiles of patients most at risk for significant problems affecting kidney function: older patients, those with diabetes or chronic hypertension, or those with more than one risk factor.

We will discuss three renal emergencies—acute renal failure, chronic renal failure, and renal calculi (kidney stones). We will also discuss one urologic disorder, urinary tract infection, which can affect any or all parts of the urinary/genitourinary system.

ACUTE RENAL FAILURE

Acute renal failure (ARF) is a sudden (often over a period of days) drop in urine output to less than 400–500 ml per day, a condition called **oliguria**. Output may literally fall to zero, a condition called **anuria**. ARF is not uncommon among severely ill, hospitalized patients. It is less common in the field. Noting ARF in the prehospital setting is vital because the condition may be reversible, dependent upon the cause and extent of damage associated with the disorder. Overall mortality is roughly 50 percent, in part because the condition usually appears in significantly injured or ill persons.

Pathophysiology

The three types of ARF are prerenal, renal, and postrenal. The distinct initial pathophysiology of each type determines both the severity of ARF and the likelihood for reversal and preserving renal function. The three types' common point is their clinical presentation: sudden-onset oliguria or anuria. You may wish to reread the summary of kidney physiology before reading about the pathophysiology for each type of ARF.

Prerenal ARF Prerenal ARF begins with dysfunction before the level of the kidney; that is, with insufficient blood supply to the kidneys, or hypoperfusion. Prerenal ARF not only accounts for the highest proportion of ARF cases—40 to 80 percent—but is also often reversible through restoration of proper perfusion. These factors make it extremely important to know conditions associated with increased risk of renal hypoperfusion and to treat the patient quickly and properly. Problems that can trigger prerenal ARF include some common field conditions: hemorrhage, heart failure (MI or CHF), sepsis, and shock (Table 7-2). These triggers decrease renal blood supply through a drop in blood volume, blood pressure, or both. In addition, any anomaly directly affecting blood flow into the kidneys (such as thrombosis of a renal artery or vein) can trigger prerenal ARF through an increase in renal vascular resistance. When renal vascular resistance becomes higher in the renal vessels than in systemic vessels, blood is effectively shunted away from the kidneys.

Normally, the kidneys receive about 20 to 25 percent of cardiac output. This high level of perfusion is essential to sustaining a GFR sufficient to maintain blood volume and composition and to clear wastes such as urea and creatinine from the bloodstream. As GFR drops, less urine forms, and the bloodstream retains water, electrolytes, and wastes such as urea and creatinine. Because the retained electrolytes include H^+ and K^+, metabolic acidosis and hyperkalemia may appear.

Content Review

PATIENTS MOST AT RISK FOR SIGNIFICANT KIDNEY PROBLEMS
- Older patients
- Patients with diabetes
- Patients with chronic hypertension
- Patients with more than one risk factor

Content Review

MOST COMMON RENAL EMERGENCIES
- Acute renal failure
- Chronic renal failure
- Renal calculi

* **acute renal failure (ARF)** the sudden-onset of severely decreased urine production.

* **oliguria** decreased urine elimination to 400-500 ml or less per day.

* **anuria** no elimination of urine.

Content Review

CAUSES OF ARF
- Prerenal
- Renal
- Postrenal

* **prerenal acute renal failure** ARF due to decreased blood perfusion of kidneys.

Table 7-2   CAUSES OF PRERENAL, RENAL, AND POSTRENAL ACUTE RENAL FAILURE (ARF)

Prerenal ARF	Renal ARF	Postrenal ARF
Hypovolemia (hemorrhage, dehydration, burns)	Small vessel/glomerular damage (vasculitis—often immune-mediated, acute glomerulonephritis, malignant hypertension)	Abrupt obstruction of both ureters (secondary to large stones, blood clots, tumor)
Cardiac failure (myocardial infarction, congestive heart failure, valvular disease)	Tubular cell damage (acute tubular necrosis—either ischemic or secondary to toxins)	Abrupt obstruction of the bladder neck (secondary to benign prostatic hypertrophy, stones, tumor, clots)
Cardiovascular collapse (shock, sepsis)	Interstitial damage (acute pyelonephritis, acute allergic interstitial reactions)	Abrupt obstruction of the urethra (secondary to inflammation, infection, stones, foreign body)
Renal vascular anomalies (renal artery stenosis, or thrombosis, embolism of renal vein)		

Note: ARF secondary to transplant rejection is considered an immune-mediated form of renal ARF.

If hypoperfusion is prolonged or worsens in degree, two things happen. First, GFR decreases still further, and less filtrate means still less urine formation. Second, the nephron tubular cells become ischemic and active reabsorption and secretion decrease or cease. All of these metabolic effects of decreased nephron function further stress the body, particularly the cardiovascular system, and increase the likelihood that tubular ischemia will advance toward tubular cell death. At this point, the process is renal ARF, not prerenal.

Renal ARF   In **renal ARF**, the pathologic process is within the kidney tissue, or renal parenchyma, itself. Three different processes cause renal ARF. The first is injury to small blood vessels (or **microangiopathy**) or glomerular capillaries; the second is injury to tubular cells; the third is inflammation or infection in the interstitial tissue surrounding nephrons (Table 7-2).

Microangiopathy and glomerular injury both result in obstruction of these minute vessels that are a vital part of the blood vessel-tubule structure of the nephron; consequently, nephron function is lost. Microangiopathy and glomerular injury are often immune-mediated and may be associated with systemic immune-mediated diseases such as diabetes mellitus type I and systemic lupus erythematosus. In these cases, ARF involves both preexistent and ongoing (that is, chronic and acute) nephron destruction.

Tubular cell death, or **acute tubular necrosis,** can follow prerenal ARF or can develop directly due to toxin deposition. Along with heavy metals and miscellaneous inorganic and organic compounds, a number of medications (including some antibiotics and cisplatin, an anticancer agent) can cause acute tubular necrosis.

Interstitial nephritis, a chronic inflammatory process also commonly due to toxic compounds including drugs (antibiotics, nonsteroidal anti-inflammatory drugs, diuretics), can also result in renal ARF.

Postrenal ARF   The third form of ARF, **postrenal ARF,** originates in a structure distal to the kidney—the ureters, bladder, or urethra. In its earliest phase (before urine has backed up into the kidneys, shutting down further urine formation), postrenal ARF is reversible simply by removing the obstruction that is preventing elimination of urine. Urinary-tract obstruction causes fewer than 5 percent of ARF cases, but like prerenal ARF, it is important to identify be-

✳ **renal ARF (renal acute renal failure)** ARF due to pathology within the kidney tissue itself.

✳ **microangiopathy** a disease affecting the smallest blood vessels.

✳ **acute tubular necrosis** a particular syndrome characterized by the sudden death of tubular cells.

✳ **interstitial nephritis** an inflammation within the tissue surrounding the nephrons.

✳ **postrenal acute renal failure** ARF due to obstruction distal to the kidney.

cause the odds of reversal are good. If obstruction is not cleared, renal ARF may develop secondary to nephron and interstitial injury caused by renovascular obstruction.

Because both ureters must be blocked simultaneously for postrenal ARF to develop (assuming two kidneys are present), it is probably the least likely cause of the cases you will see. Far more common will be obstruction of the bladder neck or of the urethra.

Regardless of probable cause, treat ARF aggressively in the field so the patient will have the best chance for recovery.

Assessment

The focused history will often provide clues to the severity and duration of ARF. For instance, if the patient complains of inability to void for a number of hours associated with a feeling of painful bladder fullness, the cause may simply be acute obstruction at the bladder neck or urethra. In contrast, a patient with poor mentation may be unable to give a coherent history, and a family member will tell you that the patient has felt increasingly ill for several days and has not urinated at all within the past twelve hours or so. Questions likely to provide useful information include the following:

- *When was the decrease or absence of urine first noticed, and has there been any observed change in output since the problem was first noted? What was the patient's previous output?* The last question may be useful because patients with chronic renal failure due to inadequate renal function can develop ARF as a complication.

- *Has the patient noted development of edema (swelling) in the face, hands, feet, or torso? How about feelings of heart palpitations or irregular rhythm? Has a family member or friend noticed decreased mental function, lethargy, or overt coma?* If the patient continued to consume fluids after ARF developed, retention of water and Na^+ can lead to visible edema in a relatively short time. Retention of K^+ can lead to hyperkalemia, a condition that can be lethal, especially in a person with previously compromised heart function. Increasingly poor mentation can be a sign of metabolic acidosis.

The focused physical examination may be helpful in assessing the degree of ARF present, the antecedent condition, and any immediate threats to life. Impaired mentation or clear decreases in consciousness in a person with previously good mental function suggest severe ARF and a potential threat to life. In a patient without evidence of shock, cardiovascular findings may include hypertension due to fluid retention, tachycardia, and ECG evidence of hyperkalemia (Figure 7-5). If shock triggered the ARF or has developed more recently, profound hypotension may be present, accompanied by tachycardia and hyperkalemia.

General visual inspection will usually show pale, cool, moist skin; if shock is not present, these findings may still represent homeostatic shunting of blood to the internal organs, including the kidneys. Look for edema in face, hands, and feet (Figure 7-6). Examination of the abdomen will reveal very different findings dependent on the cause of ARF. As with any abdominal complaint, look for scars, ecchymosis, and distention. If the abdomen is distended, note whether the swelling is symmetric. Palpate for pulsing masses, which may indicate an abdominal aortic aneurysm. Auscultation is rarely helpful in renal and urological emergencies, and bowel sounds may be muffled if ascites (fluid

Impaired mentation or clear decreases in consciousness in a person with previously good mental function suggest severe ARF and a potential threat to life.

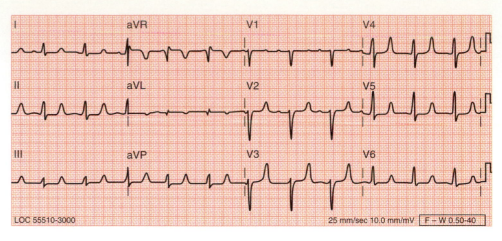

FIGURE 7-5. ECG with signs of hyperkalemia.

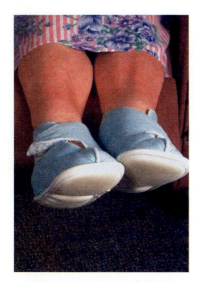

FIGURE 7-6. Edema of the feet consistent with fluid retention in acute renal failure.

> *Because ARF can lead to life-threatening metabolic derangements, monitoring and supporting the ABCs is vital.*

within the abdomen) is present. Percussion and palpation findings will depend on the trigger condition.

A hematocrit may be useful if either acute hemorrhage or chronic anemia is suspected (the latter common in patients with cancer or chronic renal failure). Urinalysis can offer useful information very quickly. Proteinuria and glycosuria (urinary protein and glucose, respectively) suggest renal dysfunction. In some infections, notably pyelonephritis, the urine may contain so many white blood cells that they form a visible sediment in the specimen.

Renal function is clinically evaluated by laboratory analysis of the blood. Two frequently used indicators of renal function are the blood urea nitrogen (BUN) level and the serum creatinine. An elevation in either of these two values points toward renal insufficiency or failure. Usually, the ratio of BUN to creatinine (BUN/creatinine ratio) should be less than 20. A BUN/creatinine ratio greater than 20 indicates prerenal or postrenal problems, while a BUN/creatinine ratio of 20 or less indicates a renal problem.

Management

Because ARF can lead to life-threatening metabolic derangements, monitoring and supporting the ABCs is vital. Use high-flow oxygen to maximize breathing efficiency; couple this with circulatory supports such as positioning with head down and legs up to assist blood flow to the brain and internal organs and IV fluid resuscitation (bolus followed by drip) if hypovolemia is present. Patients who undergo peritoneal dialysis may benefit from fluid lavage of the abdomen; consult with medical direction to see if this is an option. Monitor ECG readings closely and adjust supports per local protocol or discussion with medical direction.

The chief prevention strategies are protecting fluid volume and cardiovascular function, as indicated by some of the steps previously noted, and eliminating or reducing exposure to any nephrotoxic agents or medications. If you are unsure whether an antibiotic, analgesic, or other drug is nephrotoxic and you are not in a position to check, discontinue the medication until the patient is at the appropriate care facility.

During transportation, be sure to talk quietly to the patient, both to calm him and to keep him informed of time until arrival or other pertinent matters. As

Table 7-3	CAUSES OF CHRONIC RENAL FAILURE
Type of Tissue Injury	**Examples**
Microangiopathy, glomerular injury	Systemic hypertension, diabetes mellitus, atherosclerosis, glomerulonephritis, systemic lupus erythematosus
Tubular cell injury	Nephrotoxins including analgesics and heavy metals, stones, obstruction at bladder neck or urethra
Interstitial injury	Infections including pyelonephritis, tuberculosis

Note: Congenital disorders resulting in CRF include polycystic disease and renal hypoplasia.

always, your actions should reflect caring competence. Even if the patient is confused or comatose, you should still address him respectfully as you perform procedures and avoid saying anything you do not want him to hear.

CHRONIC RENAL FAILURE

Chronic renal failure (CRF) is inadequate kidney function due to permanent loss of nephrons. Usually, at least 70 percent of the nephrons (healthy norm, 1 million per kidney) must be lost before significant clinical problems develop and the diagnosis is made. Metabolic instability does not occur until about 80 percent or more of nephrons are destroyed. When this point of dysfunction is reached, an individual is said to have developed **end-stage renal failure,** and must have either dialysis or a kidney transplant to survive. Anuria is not necessarily present in either CRF or end-stage renal failure.

* **chronic renal failure** permanently inadequate renal function due to nephron loss.

Together, diabetes mellitus and hypertension cause more than half of all cases of end-stage renal failure. The death toll from CRF is high: More than 250,000 Americans have end-stage renal failure, and more than 50,000 die yearly from kidney disease. Roughly 30,000 new cases of CRF are diagnosed each year. The number of donor kidneys available in recent years has been sufficient for only about one-third of the persons on the waiting list to receive a kidney.

Pathophysiology

The three pathologic processes that initiate the nephron damage of CRF are the same as those underlying renal ARF: microangiopathy or glomerular capillary injury, tubular cell injury, and inflammation or infection in interstitial tissue (Table 7-3). Although the cause of initial nephron destruction is different for each of the three pathological processes, the same cycle of ongoing nephron damage becomes established: Functional nephrons adapt by increasing glomerular filtration primarily (through decreased vascular resistance in glomerular vessels and hypertrophy of capillary vessels) and by increasing tubular reabsorption and secretion secondarily (through cellular hypertrophy and functional adaptation of tubular cells). After a time, the compensatory changes damage these nephrons, leading to their destruction and initiating adaptive changes in additional, functional nephrons. Most of the damage seems to affect the glomeruli. Under the microscope, surviving nephrons often show dilated, abnormal glomeruli, and nonfunctional nephrons have heavily scarred glomeruli or no visible glomeruli, only sclerotic tissue.

This characteristic loss of nephrons, or **reduced nephron mass,** is also visible at the level of gross anatomy as shrunken, scarred kidneys, or **reduced renal mass.** Physiologically, each of the kidney's four major functions is highly disturbed or absent, depending upon the degree of renal failure:

- *Maintenance of blood volume with proper balance of water, electrolytes, and pH.* In CRF, active transport in the tubules decreases significantly or ceases. Filtrate simply passes through the tubules, leading to characteristic **isosthenuria,** the inability to concentrate or dilute urine. As overall GFR falls over time, retention of Na^+ and water increases, causing a high-volume stress on the cardiovascular system. Retention of K^+ can lead to dangerous hyperkalemia, and retention of H^+ can lead to equally dangerous metabolic acidosis. Hypocalcemia is also common. It results from several causes, including renal retention of phosphate ions (with higher levels of serum phosphate facilitating Ca^{++} absorption into bone) and lack of renal production of Vitamin D.

- *Retention of key compounds such as glucose with excretion of wastes such as urea.* Glucose and other substances that normally are actively reabsorbed are also lost in urine as filtrate flows passively through the nephron. Any hypoglycemic effect is overshadowed, however, by the significant hyperglycemic effect (**glucose intolerance**) in most patients due to cellular resistance to insulin. The wastes urea and creatinine accumulate in blood almost in direct proportion to the number of nephrons lost. In fact, the general syndrome of signs and symptoms caused by severe CRF is termed **uremia,** for this characteristic buildup of blood urea.

- *Control of arterial blood pressure.* The renin-angiotensin loop is disrupted; even small amounts of renin can lead to severe hypertension. Hypertension may also develop due to retention of Na^+ and water. Cardiac decompensation, with hypotension and tachycardia, can develop suddenly, especially if cardiac function has been independently impaired.

- *Regulation of erythrocyte development.* Because erythropoietin is no longer produced in normal quantities (or at all, in some end-stage patients), chronic anemia develops. Anemia is another cardiac stressor, and it can contribute to cardiac failure.

Assessment

During the focused history and physical exam, you will probably find many characteristics of uremia in patients with CRF and end-stage disease. Table 7-4 lists some of these signs and symptoms, which affect nearly every organ system. Many of the listed problems can precipitate shock or other major physiologic instability; this is one reason you must always be alert when dealing with patients with CRF or end-stage disease, even when they initially appear stable. In addition, this list is by no means exhaustive. Kidney failure affects almost every organ and major function in the body.

The focused history will typically show GI symptoms such as anorexia and nausea, sometimes with vomiting. The patient's mentation as he speaks is an important clue to CNS impairment. Signs may be as subtle as anxiety or mood swings or as immediately serious as seizures or coma.

Always be alert for shock or other major physiologic instability when dealing with CRF or end-stage disease, even when the patient initially appears stable.

Table 7-4	COMMON ELEMENTS OF UREMIC SYNDROME	
System	**Pathophysiology**	**Clinical Sign/Symptom**
Fluid/Electrolyte	Water/Na^+ retention	Edema, arterial hypertension[1]
	K^+ retention	Hyperkalemia[1]
	H^+ retention	Metabolic acidosis
	PaO_2 retention	Hyperphosphatemia/hypocalcemia[1]
Cardiovascular/Pulmonary	Fluid volume overload	Ascites, pulmonary edema
	Arterial hypertension	Congestive heart failure, accelerated atherosclerosis
	Dysfunctional fat metabolism; retention urea, other wastes	Pericarditis
Neuromuscular		
Central Nervous System	Retention urea, other wastes	Headache, sleep disorders, impaired mentation, lethargy, coma, seizures
Skeletal Muscle	Retention urea, other wastes; hypocalcemia	Muscular irritability and cramps, muscle twitching
Gastrointestinal (GI)	Retention urea, other wastes	Anorexia, nausea, vomiting
	Impaired hemostasis	Peptic ulcer, GI bleeding
Endocrine-Metabolic	Low vitamin D, other factors	Osteodystrophy
	Cellular resistance to insulin	Glucose intolerance
	Mechanisms unclear	Poor growth and development, delayed sexual maturation[2]
Dermatologic	Chronic anemia	Pallor skin, mucous membranes
	Retention urea, pigments	Jaundice, uremic frost
	Clotting disorders	Ecchymoses, easy bleeding
	Secondary hyperparathyroidism	Pruritus, scratches
Hematologic	Lack of renal erythropoeitin	Chronic anemia
	Impaired platelet function and prothrombin consumption	Impaired hemostasis, with easy bleeding, bruising; splenomegaly
Immunologic	Lymphopenia, general leukopenia	Vulnerability to infection

[1]Although relatively uncommon, fluctuations to the other extreme (example, hypokalemia) may occur if oral intake is poor over prolonged period or during or after dialysis treatment.

[2]Primarily seen in children, adolescents, young adults.

Your general impression before the focused physical exam is likely to note marked abnormalities. Skin will typically be pale, moist, and cool. Scratches and ecchymoses are common skin changes associated with CRF. Mucous membranes may also be very pale, dependent on the degree of anemia. Jaundice may be present, dependent on the degree of retention of urea and other pigmented metabolic wastes. A skin condition called uremic frost appears when excessive amounts of urea are eliminated through sweat. As the sweat dries, a white 'frosty' dust of urea may appear on the skin.

The major organ systems often show significant abnormalities on direct examination (Table 7-4). Because of the failure of vital urinary system functions, cardiovascular stress can be enormous. Either hypertension or hypotension may occur, dependent on the degree of fluid retention (retention detectable as peripheral edema or pulmonary edema) and the level of cardiac function; tachycardia is common with both presentations. ECG findings may include a dysrhythmia secondary to hyperkalemia. Metabolic acidosis, when present, compounds the effects of hyperkalemia. Pericarditis is also common, and a rub may be heard on chest auscultation. Neuromuscular abnormalities, in addition to impaired mentation, include muscle cramps and "restless legs syndrome," as well as muscle twitching or tonic-clonic or other forms of seizure.

Your abdominal exam will reveal many abnormalities. The challenge is to begin separating (by exam and history) chronic findings from those of recent onset or aggravated by the emergency that led to your call. For instance, you know that ecchymoses on the abdomen or flank may suggest acute hemorrhage. You may find a patient with ecchymoses scattered over the body surface. Look for evidence of new abdominal ecchymoses versus older bruises or a clear history of recent onset as signs of a current problem. Be sure to note abdominal contour, including the presence of symmetric distention or localized bulges, scars, and ecchymoses before the exam and to clearly document the pre-exam appearance. Findings on auscultation, percussion, and palpation will depend on the presenting problem.

The hematocrit and urinalysis generally have less value in CRF than in ARF. A hematocrit is useful only if you know the patient's baseline value, and recent changes in the amount of urinary output may be more significant than the content. The exceptions are blood (red blood cells) in urine, which is always a significant finding on dipstick analysis, and visible amounts of white blood cells, which suggest significant infection.

Management

Immediate Management As with ARF, CRF can lead to life-threatening complications, so monitoring and supporting the ABCs is vital. Use high-flow oxygen to maximize breathing efficiency. Couple this with circulatory supports such as positioning with the head down and the legs up to support blood flow to the brain and internal organs. Consider a small IV bolus for fluid resuscitation if hypovolemia is evident. Indications for fluid lavage (in peritoneal dialysis patients) are the same as those for patients with ARF. Monitor the ECG readings closely and adjust supports according to your local protocol or discussion with medical direction.

The chief prevention strategies are regulation of fluid volume and cardiovascular function and major electrolyte disturbances (for example, use of a vasopressor in hypotension and administration of bicarbonate for partial correction of acidosis, respectively) and elimination or reduction of exposure to any nephrotoxic agents or medications. Although uncommon, severe swings in electrolyte levels may occur during and after dialysis, so be cautious about replacement measures in the field in these patients. Err on the side of conservative treatment except for clearly life-threatening complications. If you are unsure whether a drug is nephrotoxic and you are not in a position to check, discontinue it until the patient is at the emergency department.

Expedite transportation to an appropriate facility in the same manner appropriate for patients with ARF. Be sure to talk quietly to the patient, both to calm him and to keep him informed of the time until arrival or other pertinent matters. If the patient is confused, ask short orientation questions periodically to assess lucidity and level of consciousness.

Long-term Management **Renal dialysis,** the artificial replacement of some of the kidney's most critical functions, is a fact of life for most patients with CRF and end-stage disease. Although dialysis is necessary for survival, it is not without risk.

In CRF emergencies, the challenge is to separate chronic findings from those of recent onset or aggravated by the emergency that led to your call.

In CRF, err on the side of conservative treatment except for clearly life-threatening complications.

* **renal dialysis** artificial replacement of some critical kidney functions.

One risk that you have already learned about is the possibility of physiologically destabilizing shifts in blood volume and composition and arterial blood pressure.

Dialysis was first developed about 30 years ago. Since then, two different technologies, hemodialysis and peritoneal dialysis, have been refined. Both rely on the same physiologic principles: osmosis and equalization of osmolarity across a semipermeable membrane such as that of the renal nephron. (You may wish to reread the explanation of osmosis in this chapter's physiology section before reading further.) In dialysis, the patient's blood flows past a semipermeable membrane that has a special cleansing fluid on the other side that is hypo-osmolar to blood for a number of impurities (such as urea, creatinine) and critical substances (such as Na^+, K^+, H^+). As the blood flows over the membrane, these substances in blood move into the hypo-osmolar solution, called the **dialysate,** and their concentrations in blood are thus reduced. The effect of dialysis is to temporarily lessen or eliminate volume overload and toxically high blood concentrations of electrolytes, urea, and other substances.

In **hemodialysis** (*hemo*=blood, *dia*=across, *lysis*=separation), the patient's blood is passed through a machine that contains an artificial membrane and the dialysate solution. Vascular access is required in order to achieve the necessary blood flow of 300 to 400 ml/minute. Often, a superficial, internal fistula is created surgically by anastamosing an artery and vein in the lower forearm. If the required healthy artery and vein are not available, surgeons can insert a special vascular graft made of artificial material between an artery and vein (Figure 7-7). If creating such a fistula is not possible, an indwelling catheter may need to be placed in the internal jugular vein. Because hemodialysis can be performed in settings including outpatient clinics and at home, you may see patients both between and during hemodialysis sessions. The three most common complications relate to vascular access. Two of the three complications are bleeding from the needle puncture site and local

✱ **dialysate** the solution used in dialysis that is hypo-osmolar to many of the wastes and key electrolytes in blood.

✱ **hemodialysis** a dialysis procedure relying on vascular access to the blood and on an artificial membrane.

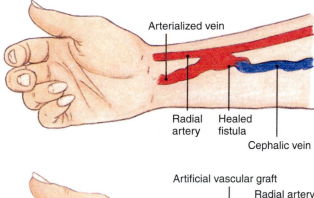

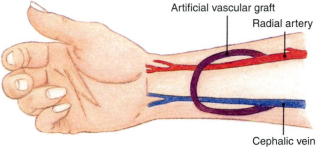

FIGURE 7-7. Vascular access for hemodialysis. (a) arteriovenous fistula; (b) artificial graft between artery and vein.

FIGURE 7-8. Peritoneal
dialysis.

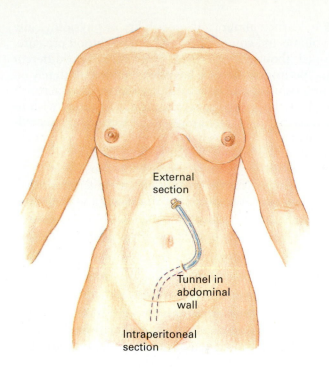

External
section

Tunnel in
abdominal
wall

Intraperitoneal
section

✳ peritoneal dialysis a dialysis
procedure relying on the peritoneal membrane as the semipermeable membrane.

infection. The third is the narrowing or closing of the internal fistula. Under
normal flow conditions, the internal fistula will have a palpable thrill (vibration), or bruit, due to the relatively high-volume turbulent flow from artery
into vein. If the fistula narrows significantly or closes, however, this vibration
is lost. The leading complications that require hospitalization are thrombosis,
infection, and aneurysm development. They are particularly common in patients with grafts of artificial material.

Peritoneal dialysis uses the peritoneal membrane within the patient's abdomen as the semipermeable dialysis membrane, and dialysate solution is introduced and removed from the abdominal cavity via an indwelling catheter
(Figure 7-8). This simpler technique, which used to be significantly less effective than hemodialysis, has been improved greatly in recent years. Currently,
many patients practice either chronic peritoneal lavage (intermittent cycles in
which dialysate is introduced, allowed to remain for an extended period, and
then removed) or continuous peritoneal lavage (in which dialysate is introduced via a closed system that allows the patient to remain ambulatory during dialysis). Peritoneal dialysis avoids some of the risk of fluid and electrolyte
shifts seen during hemodialysis, but its success requires additional physical
characteristics (such as healthy vasculature around the peritoneum). The most
common complication is infection in the catheter, the abdominal tunnel containing the catheter, or the peritoneum itself. The incidence of peritonitis is
about one episode per year, so you may find its signs in these patients.

Both forms of dialysis have complications not related to vascular access in
common. They include hypotension, shortness of breath, chest pain, and neurologic abnormalities ranging from headache to seizure or coma. If the patient is
hypotensive, check for dehydration, hemorrhage, or infection. Shortness of
breath and chest pain may reflect cardiac dysrhythmias (often secondary to hyperkalemia) or may be without identifiable cause. Be aware that these patients,
many of whom have cardiac compromise, are at higher risk for ischemia or MI

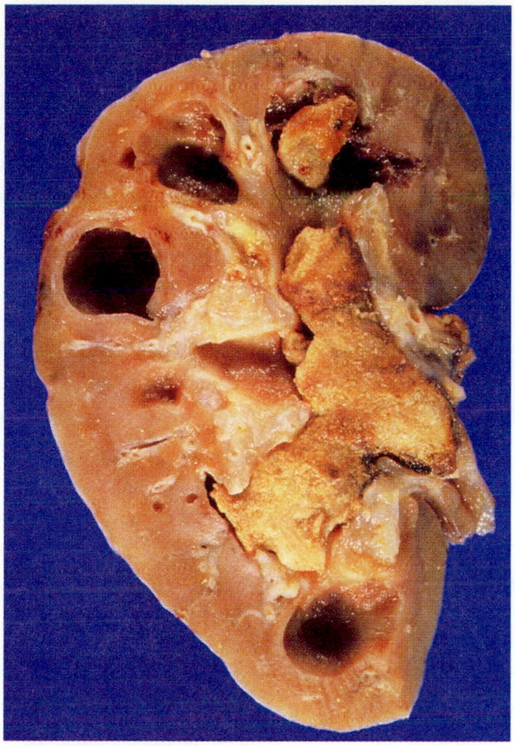

FIGURE 7-9. Sectioned kidney with kidney stones.

during these periods. Neurologic abnormalities may occur before, during, or after treatment. In most cases they represent neurotoxicity of accumulated blood urea; in some cases rapid removal of urea from blood causes an osmotic diuresis from brain tissue with a resulting increase in intracranial pressure. Benzodiazepines may be useful in patients who develop seizures.

RENAL CALCULI

Kidney stones, or *renal calculi* (singular, *calculus*), represent crystal aggregation in the kidney's collecting system (Figure 7-9). This condition is also called nephrolithiasis (from Greek *lithos,* stone). Kidney stones affect about 500,000 persons each year. Brief hospitalization is common due to the severity of pain as a stone travels from the renal pelvis, through the ureter, to the bladder, and is eliminated in urine. If necessary, additional inpatient treatment may include shock-wave lithotripsy, a procedure that uses sound waves to break large stones into smaller ones. Overall morbidity and mortality are low, however, unless a complication such as hemorrhage or urinary-tract obstruction results. Stones form more commonly in men than women, although the ratio varies for types of stones with different compositions. Certain stones also occur in familial patterns, suggesting hereditary factors. Another risk factor for calculus formation is immobilization due to surgery or injury, with the latter including immobilization secondary to paraplegia or other paralysis syndromes that involve the absence of motor impulses, sensation, or both. Last, the use of certain medications, including anesthetics, opiates, and psychotropic drugs, increases the risk for stones.

Kidney stones occur more frequently in summer and fall.

Pathophysiology

Stones may form in metabolic disorders such as gout or primary hyperparathyroidism, which produce excessive amounts of uric acid and calcium, respectively. More often, they occur when the general balance between water conservation and dissolution of relatively insoluble substances such as mineral ions and uric acid is lost and excessive amounts of the insolubles aggregate into stones. The problem boils down to "too much insoluble stuff" and urine "too concentrated," a situation that may more likely arise with change in diet, climate, or physical activity.

Stones consisting of calcium salts (namely, calcium oxalate and calcium phosphate) are by far the most common. These compounds are found in from 75 to 85 percent of all stones. Calcium stones are from two to three times more common in men than in women, and the average age at onset is between 20 and 30 years. Their formation frequently runs in families, and anyone who has had a calcium stone is at fairly high risk to form another within two to three years.

Struvite stones (chemically denoted $MgNH_4PO_4$) are also common, representing about 10 to 15 percent of all stones. The pathophysiology of struvite stones differs from that of calcium stones. Their formation is associated with chronic urinary tract infection (UTI) or frequent bladder catheterization. The association with bacterial UTI makes struvite stones much more common in women than in men. These stones can grow to fill the renal pelvis, producing a characteristic "staghorn" appearance on X-rays.

Far less common are stones made of uric acid or cystine. Uric acid stones form more often in men than in women and tend to occur in families; about half of all patients with uric acid stones have gout. Cystine stones are the least common. They are associated with excess levels of cystine in filtrate and are probably due at least in part to hereditary factors, as they often run in families.

Assessment

The focused history almost always centers on pain. (Kidney stones are generally conceded to be among the most painful of human medical conditions.) Typically, the patient first notes discomfort as a vague, visceral pain in one flank. Within 30 to 60 minutes it progresses to an extremely sharp pain that may remain in the flank or migrate downward and anteriorly toward the groin. Migrating pain indicates that the stone has passed into the lowest third of the ureter. Stones that lodge in the lowest part of the ureter, within the bladder wall, often cause characteristic bladder symptoms such as frequency during the day or during the night (nocturia), urgency, and painful urination. Because these latter three symptoms far more frequently suggest bladder infection, making the probable diagnosis may be difficult, particularly in women. Visible hematuria is not uncommon in urine specimens taken during passage of a stone. Fever, however, is not typical unless infection is present. Whenever kidney stones are suspected, be sure to get the patient's personal medical history and family history, because both will often provide useful information.

The physical exam will almost always reveal someone who is very uncomfortable. The patient may be agitated or physically restless; walking sometimes reduces the pain. Vital signs will vary with level of discomfort, with highest blood pressure and heart rate associated with greatest pain. Skin will typically be pale, cool, and clammy. Abdominal examination may be difficult, depending on the patient's ability to remain still. First inspect the abdomen for contour and symmetry. Auscultation and percussion are generally useful only in ruling out GI conditions. Palpation results will vary and may depend, in part, on whether pain is so great that muscle guarding is present, making palpation of underlying structures impossible.

Whenever kidney stones are suspected, be sure to get the patient's personal medical history and family history.

Many male patients with kidney stones present with testicular pain on the affected side.

Management

As always, management begins with the ABCs. Positioning should center on comfort, but be prepared for vomiting due to the severe pain, especially if the patient's last meal was within several hours. Consider analgesia en route to the hospital, according to your local protocol and your perception of the patient's condition. Use narcotics cautiously if a GI condition is at all possible or if mentation is impaired. If the pain is in the initial, intermittent, colicky phase, consider coaching pain management through breathing techniques similar to those used for women in labor. An IV line is useful for volume replacement or drug administration. The usual prevention strategy, if kidney function is adequate, is IV fluid to promote urine formation and movement through the system. Transport is the same as that for other abdominal conditions, i.e., position of comfort and supportive care.

Parenteral narcotic analgesics or ketorolac (Toradol) should be considered for the patient with renal colic.

URINARY TRACT INFECTION

Urinary tract infection, or UTI, affects the urethra, bladder, or kidney, as well as the prostate gland in men. UTIs are extremely common, accounting for over 6 million office visits yearly. Almost all UTIs start with pathogenic colonization of the bladder by bacteria that enter through the urethra. Thus, females in general are at higher risk because of their relatively short urethra. Other groups at risk for UTI are paraplegic patients or patients with nerve disruption to the bladder, including some diabetic persons. Any condition that promotes **urinary stasis** (incomplete urination with urine remaining in the bladder that may serve as nutrition for pathogens) places a person at higher risk. Pregnant women often have urinary stasis due to pressure from the gravid uterus. People with neurological impairment (some patients with spina bifida or with diabetic neuropathy, for example) also tend to have urinary stasis, which predisposes them to infection. The use of instrumentation in patients who require bladder catheterization places them at even higher risk of UTIs.

Morbidities such as scarring, abscesses, or eventual development of CRF are most likely in persons with anatomic abnormalities of the urinary system or chronic calculi (the latter acting as a focus for continuing infection and inflammation), those who are immunocompromised, or those who have renal disease due to diabetes mellitus or another condition.

* **urinary tract infection (UTI)** an infection, usually bacterial, at any site in the urinary tract.

* **urinary stasis** a condition in which the bladder empties incompletely during urination.

Pathophysiology

UTIs are generally divided into those of the lower urinary tract, namely, urethritis (urethra), cystitis (bladder), and prostatitis (prostate gland), and those of the upper urinary tract, pyelonephritis (kidney).

Lower UTIs are far more common than upper UTIs, for two reasons. First, seeding of infection via the bloodstream is rare. Second, asymptomatic bacterial colonization of the urethra, especially in females, is very common, and can predispose a person to infection by other, pathogenic bacteria.

In females, infection may begin when Gram-negative bacteria normally found in the bowel (that is, the enteric flora) colonize the urethra and bladder. Symptomatic **urethritis,** inflammation secondary to urethral infection, is very uncommon. More often you will see joint symptomatic infection of the urethra and bladder (urethritis and **cystitis,** respectively). Sexually active females are at higher risk, which may be attributed to use of contraceptive devices or agents, to the introduction of enteric flora during intercourse, or both. Recently, homosexually active men who engage in anal sex have also been found to be at higher risk for bacterial cystitis, possibly due to introduction of enteric bacterial flora during

* **urethritis** an infection and inflammation of the urethra.

* **cystitis** an infection and inflammation of the urinary bladder.

intercourse. In any case, sexually active persons who suffer from urinary stasis are at even higher risk for infection. Persons who urinate after intercourse might lower their risk because voiding eliminates some bacteria. The pathophysiology for persons using bladder catheterization probably differs only in that pathogenic bacteria are introduced directly into the bladder via the catheter. In general, the likelihood that active cystitis will develop, that antibiotic treatment will clear such infections, and that reinfection will occur are all determined by the interplay of the pathogen's virulence, the size of its colony, its sensitivity to antibiotic treatment, and the strength of the host's local and systemic immune functions.

Prostatitis, inflammation of the prostate gland, in our context, denotes inflammation secondary to bacterial infection, as well as any general inflammatory condition. Men with acute bacterial prostatitis, the closest parallel to acute cystitis in women, also tend to show evidence of joint urethritis, and the same bowel flora tend to be involved. The major difference between acute bacterial prostatitis and acute cystitis is the much lower incidence of prostatitis among men who do not require bladder catheterization.

Upper UTIs usually evolve from infection that spreads upward into the kidney. **Pyelonephritis** is an infectious inflammation of the renal parenchyma: nephrons, interstitial tissue, or both. Acute pyelonephritis is ten times more common in women than in men. Its incidence is highest in pregnancy and during periods of sexual activity, reflecting the epidemiology of lower UTIs. If the infection of pyelonephritis persists, intrarenal or perinephric abscesses may occur, but these complications are uncommon. **Intrarenal abscesses** form within the renal parenchyma. If they rupture and spill their contents into the adjacent fatty tissue, **perinephric abscesses** may result. From 20 to 60 percent of patients who develop perinephric abscesses have a clear predisposing factor such as renal calculi, anatomic abnormalities of the kidney, history of urologic surgery or injury, or diabetic renal disease.

Urinary tract infections may be community-acquired or nosocomial. Among **community-acquired infections,** Gram-negative enteric bacteria predominate. In fact, *E. coli* accounts for roughly 80 percent of infections in persons without the complicating factors of bladder catheterization, renal calculi, or anatomic abnormalities. In **nosocomial infections,** cases acquired in an inpatient setting or related to catheterization, *Proteus, Klebsiella,* and *Pseudomonas* are commonly identified. Less common, but still important, are sexually transmitted pathogens (among women and men) such as *Chlamydia* and *N. gonorrhoeae.* Fungi such as *Candida* are rarely seen except in catheterized or immunocompromised patients or patients with diabetes mellitus.

Assessment

The focused history of lower UTI typically centers on three symptoms: painful urination, frequent urge to urinate, and difficulty in beginning and continuing to void. Pain often begins as visceral discomfort that progresses to severe, burning pain, particularly during and just after urination. The evolution of pain corresponds roughly to the degree of epithelial damage caused by the pathogen. In both men and women, pain is often localized to the pelvis and perceived as in the bladder (in women) or bladder and prostate (in men). The patient may complain of a strong or foul odor in the urine. Many women will give a history of similar episodes, which may or may not have been diagnosed or treated. Patients with pyelonephritis are more likely to feel generally ill or feverish. They typically complain of constant, moderately severe or severe pain in a flank or lower back (just under the rib cage). Pain may be referred to the shoulder or neck. The triad of urgency, pain, and difficulty may or may not be present or included in the past history.

✳ **prostatitis** infection and inflammation of the prostate gland.

✳ **pyelonephritis** an infection and inflammation of the kidney.

✳ **intrarenal abscess** a pocket of infection within kidney tissue.

✳ **perinephric abscess** a pocket of infection in the layer of fat surrounding the kidney.

✳ **community-acquired infection** an infection occurring in a non-hospitalized patient who is not undergoing regular medical procedures, including the use of instruments such as catheters.

✳ **nosocomial infection** an infection acquired in a medical setting.

On physical exam, patients with UTI appear restless and uncomfortable. Typically, patients with pyelonephritis appear more ill and are far more likely to have a fever. Skin will often be pale, cool, and moist (in lower UTI) or warm and dry (in febrile upper UTI). Vital signs will vary with the degree of illness and pain, but in an otherwise healthy individual they should not be far from the norms. Inspect and auscultate the abdomen to document findings, but neither procedure is likely to be very useful, as visible appearance and bowel sounds are usually within normal limits. Percussion and palpation will probably reveal painful tenderness over the pubis in lower UTI and at the flank in upper UTI. Lloyd's sign, tenderness to percussion of the lower back at the costovertebral angle (CVA), indicates pyelonephritis.

The patient with acute pyelonephritis will usually appear quite ill. The patient with cystitis, on the other hand, will be uncomfortable but will not appear toxic.

Management

UTI management should center on the ABCs and circulatory support. If pain is severe, help the patient to a comfortable position, but consider the risk of aspiration during vomiting. Analgesics should be considered as with renal calculi; they will probably be needed only for severely painful cases of pyelonephritis. Consider nonpharmacological pain management with breathing and relaxation techniques. The best prevention technique is hydration to increase blood flow through the kidneys and to produce a more dilute urine. In many cases, this is better accomplished by IV administration, which eliminates the risk of vomiting and satisfies the guidelines for possible surgical cases. Expedite transport to an appropriate facility.

SUMMARY

The urinary system (1) maintains blood volume and the proper balance of water, electrolytes, and pH; (2) enables the blood to retain key substances such as glucose and removes a variety of toxic wastes from the blood; (3) plays a major role in regulation of arterial blood pressure; and (4) controls maturation of red blood cells. Kidney nephrons produce urine. Homeostasis through urine production is responsible for the first two functions and assists in the third, regulating blood pressure, by producing renin, the enzyme through which blood pressure is controlled. Other kidney cells produce erythropoietin, the hormone that stimulates red blood cell maturation.

Renal and urologic emergencies typically present as an acute abdomen. The most common are acute renal failure (ARF), chronic renal failure (CRF, with the subset of end-stage renal disease), and renal calculi. Both ARF and CRF may present with life-threatening complications and impaired function of other systems. Be prepared for apparently stable patients to acutely develop destabilizing complications (often, cardiovascular). Urinary tract infections, or UTIs, are divided into those of the lower urinary tract (urethra, bladder, and prostate in men) and those of the upper urinary tract (kidney). Both types of infection can present with considerable pain, but pyelonephritis is the more serious, with fever likely and complications including abscesses possible.

Because renal function is often lowered in the elderly and in persons with hypertension or diabetes, consider it potentially impaired in all of these patients. The best prevention strategies are to minimize the likelihood of prerenal failure by protecting blood volume and blood pressure and to investigate possible postrenal urinary tract obstruction.

Shortly after dinner, you're called to an "unknown medical" case in a nearby apartment complex. You are met by a middle-aged woman who introduces herself as the person who called in the emergency. She tells you she is worried about her neighbor, whom she describes as an elderly gentleman who has been on his own since his wife died. She is concerned tonight that he seemed very shaky on his feet when she brought dinner for him and his speech did not make sense when she asked if he was all right. She says he normally speaks "like an educated gentleman."

A thin, elderly man opens the door. He is neatly dressed in shirt and pants but is pale and shaky. As he says he is fine and starts to close the door, you introduce yourselves and ask if you may come in and check to be sure he is all right. He reluctantly agrees. When you ask about his health, he says the doctor told him he had the flu and he was supposed to take it easy. He seems worried about your approval and repeats that he is fine. He cannot tell you the day of the week or his apartment number, and he sits down, trembling slightly. You note that his skin is cool and dry, and the inside of his mouth seems dry when he speaks. While your partner takes his vital signs, you ask about his problems with the flu. He says he had diarrhea for a few days but it is better. When you ask if he has eaten, he says he cannot remember but he knows he made tea to take his pills. He shows you a bottle of antibiotic capsules and one of a diuretic. He thinks there might be some other bottles in the kitchen. He mentions he might stop taking the water pills because he is not making water any more. When you ask him about that, he says he slept all day and did not need to go to the bathroom. Your partner reports blood pressure of 80/60, heart rate of 130 beats per minute, and labored respirations of 28 per minute. He also notes that the heartbeat seems somewhat irregular.

The patient says he will go to the hospital, but only if he can "finish dressing" and have his neighbor drive him.

1. What is your first management priority?
2. What risk factors, if any, might the patient have for a renal complication to his condition? Which renal complication, if any?
3. Should you agree to the neighbor's driving the patient to the hospital after he finishes dressing? If not, why?

See Suggested Responses at the back of this book.

FURTHER READING

Braunwald, Eugene, et. al., eds. *Harrison's Principles of Internal Medicine.* 14th ed. New York: McGraw-Hill, 1999.

Chandrasoma, Parakrama and Clive R. Taylor. *Concise Pathology.* 3rd ed. Stamford, Connecticut: Appleton & Lange, 1998.

Guyton, Arthur C. and John E. Hall. *Textbook of Medical Physiology.* 9th ed. Philadelphia: W.B. Saunders, 1996.

McCance, K.L. and S.E. Heuther. *Pathophysiology: The Biologic Basis for Disease in Adults and Children.* 3rd ed. St. Louis: Mosby, 1998.

ON THE WEB

Visit Brady's Paramedic Website at www.bradybooks.com/paramedic.

CHAPTER 8

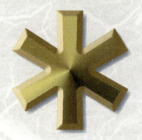

Toxicology and Substance Abuse

Objectives

After reading this chapter, you should be able to:

1. Describe the incidence, morbidity, and mortality of toxic and drug abuse emergencies. (p. 429)
2. Identify the risk factors most predisposing to toxic emergencies. (p. 429)
3. Discuss the anatomy and physiology of the organs and structures related to toxic emergencies. (pp. 430–431)
4. Describe the routes of entry of toxic substances into the body. (pp. 430–431)
5. Discuss the role of Poison Control Centers in the United States. (pp. 429–430)
6. Discuss the pathophysiology, assessment findings, need for rapid intervention and transport, and management of toxic emergencies. (pp. 429–468)
7. List the most common poisonings, pathophysiology, assessment findings, and management of poisoning by ingestion, inhalation, absorption, injection, and overdose. (pp. 430–468)
8. Define the following terms:
   a. Substance or drug abuse (p. 461)
   b. Substance or drug dependence (p. 461)
   c. Tolerance (p. 461)
   d. Withdrawal (p. 462)
   e. Addiction (p. 461)
9. List the most commonly abused drugs (both by chemical name and by street names). (pp. 464–465)
10. Describe the pathophysiology, assessment findings, and management of commonly used drugs. (pp. 438–452, 461–468)
11. List the clinical uses, street names, pharmacology, assessment findings, and management for patients who

Continued

have taken the following drugs or been exposed to the following substances:

a. Cocaine (pp. 462–463, 464)
b. Marijuana and cannabis compounds (p. 465)
c. Amphetamines and amphetamine-like drugs (pp. 463, 465)
d. Barbiturates (pp. 463, 464)
e. Sedative-hypnotics (p. 465)
f. Cyanide (pp. 438–439)
g. Narcotics/opiates (p. 464)
h. Cardiac medications (pp. 442–443)
i. Caustics (pp. 443–444)
j. Common household substances (pp. 443–444)
k. Drugs abused for sexual purposes/sexual gratification (p. 463)
l. Carbon monoxide (p. 439)
m. Alcohols (p. 463–468)
n. Hydrocarbons (pp. 444–445)
o. Psychiatric medications (pp. 445–448)
p. Newer anti-depressants and serotonin syndromes (p. 447)
q. Lithium (pp. 447–448)
r. MAO inhibitors (p. 446)
s. Non-prescription pain medications (1) Nonsteroidal antiinflammatory agents (2) Salicylates (3) Acetaminophen (pp. 448–450)
t. Theophylline (p. 450)
u. Metals (pp. 450–451)
v. Plants and mushrooms (pp. 452–453)

12. Discuss common causative agents or offending organisms, pharmacology, assessment findings, and management for a patient with food poisoning, a bite, or a sting. (pp. 451–461)

13. Given several scenarios of poisoning or overdose, provide the appropriate assessment, treatment, and transport. (pp. 428–468)

CASE STUDY

Paramedics rush to their vehicle as a call comes in to Rescue 190. Rescue 190 is staffed by paramedics Kevin Lucia, Charles Wright, and David Schrodt. Dispatch reports an unconscious person at 1301 North 7th street. The address seems very familiar. As the paramedics turn the corner and approach the residence they immediately remember this location. They have been called here many times in the past to attend to a chronically depressed young woman who has trouble coping with stressful situations. David reports that the crew from another shift was there four days ago.

Inside they find the young woman unresponsive and lying on the floor beside the sofa. She was found like this by her boyfriend, who states that she called him at work two hours ago crying that "she just couldn't take it anymore." On the floor beside her is an empty bottle of acetaminophen (Tylenol) and an empty bottle of nortriptyline (Pamelor), a tricyclic antidepressant. There is a pharmacy receipt on the floor showing that the bottles were just purchased today. Because of this, the paramedics have to assume that the bottles were full. The smell of alcohol pervades the air. A quick look around the scene reveals several empty bottles of an expensive wine on the sofa table.

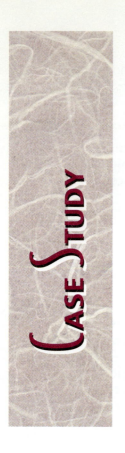

CASE STUDY

Initial assessment shows that the young woman is unresponsive but alive. Respirations are slow and shallow. She is tachycardiac with weak pulses. The paramedics intubate her and begin mechanical ventilation. They then establish an IV and place the various monitors. A focused history from the patient's boyfriend provides no additional information. The police arrive and start to interrogate the boyfriend in an adjacent room. Kevin and Charles complete a rapid medical assessment. The only noteworthy findings are multiple shallow scars across both wrists.

The paramedics quickly transport the patient to the hospital, remembering to bring all bottles of medicines (full and empty) found at the scene. The patient does not seem to improve while en route. Shortly after arrival at the emergency department, the patient has a grand mal seizure that requires intravenous diazepam for treatment. The patient continues to deteriorate despite aggressive medical intervention. She does not regain consciousness and is eventually transferred to the ICU. She dies in ICU forty-eight hours later from cardiac dysrhythmias and hepatic failure. Her physicians hope to learn the cause of death from an autopsy performed by the hospital's pathologist. Results should be known in several weeks.

INTRODUCTION

* **toxicology** study of the detection, chemistry, pharmacological actions, and antidotes of toxic substances.

* **toxin** any chemical (drug, poison, or other) that causes adverse effects on an organism that is exposed to it.

Toxicology is the study of **toxins** (drugs and poisons) and antidotes and their effects on living organisms. Toxicological emergencies result from the ingestion, inhalation, surface absorption, or injection of toxic substances that then exert their adverse effects on the body's tissues and metabolic mechanisms. Theoretically all toxicological emergencies can be classified as poisoning. However, in this discussion, the term *poisoning* will be used to describe exposure to non-pharmacological substances. The term *overdose* will be used to describe exposure to pharmacological substances, whether the overdose is accidental or intentional. Substance abuse, although technically a form of poisoning, will be addressed separately.

In this chapter we will discuss various aspects of toxicological emergencies as they apply to prehospital care. We will establish general treatment guidelines for each type of toxic exposure, then address the specific issues surrounding some of the more common substances involved. Because the field of toxicology is rapidly changing, it is virtually impossible for a paramedic to remain up to date on treatment guidelines for each type of toxic exposure. Specific treatment should be supervised by medical direction in association with a Poison Control Center. This plan ensures that the patient receives the most current level of care available.

EPIDEMIOLOGY

Over the years, the occurrence of toxicological emergencies has continued to increase in number and severity. The following figures reveal the high potential for toxic substance involvement on an EMS call.

- The American Association of Poison Control Centers estimates over 4 million poisonings occur annually.
- Ten percent of all emergency department visits and EMS responses involve toxic exposures.
- Seventy percent of accidental poisonings occur in children under the age of 6 years.
- A child who has experienced an accidental ingestion has a 25 percent chance of another, similar ingestion within one year.
- Eighty percent of all attempted suicides involve a drug overdose.

Although over half of all poisonings occur in children aged 1–5, they are generally accidental and relatively mild, accounting for only ten percent of hospital admissions for poisoning and only five percent of the fatalities. EMS personnel must be aware that more serious poisonings, especially in children older than 5, may represent intentional poisoning by parents or caretakers. Unfortunately, poisoning due to drug experimentation and suicide attempts are also becoming a common consideration in older children.

Adult poisonings and overdoses, although less frequent, account for 90 percent of hospital admissions for toxic substance exposure. They also account for 95 percent of the fatalities in this category. Most adult poisonings and overdoses are intentional. Intentional poisonings and overdoses can be due to illicit drug use, alcohol abuse, attempted suicide, and "suicidal gesturing" in which the patient is making a cry for help but may miscalculate and take a type or amount of toxin that does actually cause injury. More rarely, intentional poisoning can result from attempted homicide or chemical warfare. Accidental poisonings are increasingly caused by exposure to chemicals and toxins on the farm or in the industrial workplace. More often they are the result of idiosyncratic (individual hypersensitivity) reactions or dosage errors when taking prescribed medications, but these usually do not require medical attention.

POISON CONTROL CENTERS

Poison Control Centers have been set up across the United States and Canada to assist in the treatment of poison victims and to provide information on new products and new treatment recommendations. They are usually based in major medical centers and teaching hospitals and serve a large population. Almost all Poison Control Centers now have computer systems to rapidly access information.

Poison Control Centers are usually staffed by physicians, toxicologists, pharmacists, nurses, or paramedics with special training in toxicology. These experts provide information to callers 24 hours a day, seven days a week. They update information regularly and offer the most current treatment guidelines.

Memorize the number of the nearest Poison Control Center and access it routinely. There are several advantages to this. First, the Poison Control Center can help you immediately determine potential toxicity based on the type of agent,

Memorize the number of the nearest Poison Control Center and access it routinely for information regarding a poisoning or overdose.

Content Review

ROUTES OF TOXIC
EXPOSURE

• Ingestion
• Inhalation
• Surface absorption
• Injection

amount and time of exposure, and physical condition of the patient. Second, the most current, definitive treatment can sometimes be started in the field. Finally, the Poison Control Center can notify the receiving hospital of current treatment and recommendations even before arrival of the patient.

ROUTES OF TOXIC EXPOSURE

In order to have a destructive effect, poisons must gain entrance into the body. The four portals of entry are *ingestion, inhalation, surface absorption,* and *injection.* It is important to note that, regardless of the portal of entry, toxic substances have both immediate and delayed effects.

INGESTION

Ingestion is the most common route of entry for toxic exposure. Frequently ingested poisons include:

- Household products
- Petroleum-based agents (gasoline, paint)
- Cleaning agents (alkalis and soaps)
- Cosmetics
- Drugs (prescription, non-prescription, illicit)
- Plants
- Foods

Immediate toxic effects of ingestion of corrosive substances, such as strong acids or alkalis, can involve burns to the lips, tongue, throat, and esophagus. Delayed effects result from absorption of the poison from the gastrointestinal tract. Most absorption occurs in the small intestine, with only a small amount being absorbed from the stomach. Some poisons may remain in the stomach for up to several hours, because the intake of a large bolus of poison can retard absorption. Aspirin ingestion is a classic example of this. When a patient ingests a large number of aspirin tablets, the tablets can bind together to form a large bolus that is difficult to remove or break down.

INHALATION

Inhalation of a poison results in rapid absorption of the toxic agent through the alveolar-capillary membrane in the lungs. Inhaled toxins can irritate pulmonary passages, causing extensive edema and destroying tissue. When these toxins are absorbed, wider systemic effects can occur. Causative agents can appear as gases, vapors, fumes, or aerosols. Common inhaled poisons include:

- Toxic gases
- Carbon monoxide
- Ammonia
- Chlorine
- Freon
- Toxic vapors, fumes, or aerosols
- Carbon tetrachloride
- Methyl chloride
- Tear gas

It is important to remember that toxic substances have both immediate and delayed effects.

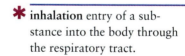

* **ingestion** entry of a substance into the body through the gastrointestinal tract.

* **inhalation** entry of a substance into the body through the respiratory tract.

- Mustard gas
- Nitrous oxide

SURFACE ABSORPTION

Surface absorption is the entry of a toxic substance through the skin or mucous membranes. This most frequently occurs from contact with poisonous plants such as poison ivy, poison sumac, and poison oak. Many toxic chemicals may also be absorbed through the skin. **Organophosphates,** often used as pesticides, are easily absorbed through dermal contact.

INJECTION

Injection of a toxic agent under the skin, into muscle, or into a blood vessel results in both immediate and delayed effects. The immediate reaction is usually localized to the site of the injection and appears as red, irritated, edematous skin. An allergic or anaphylactic reaction can also appear (see Chapter 5). Later, as the toxin is distributed throughout the body by the circulatory system, delayed systemic reactions can occur.

Other than intentional injection of illicit drugs, most poisonings by injection result from the bites and stings of insects and animals. Most insects that can sting and bite belong to the class *Hymenoptera,* which includes honey bees, hornets, yellow jackets, wasps, and fire ants. Only the females in this group can sting. In addition, spiders, ticks, and other arachnids, such as scorpions, are notorious for causing poisonings by injection. Higher animals that bite and sting include snakes and certain marine animals. Marine animals with venomous stings include jellyfish (especially the Portuguese man-of-war), stingrays, anemones, coral, hydras, and certain spiny fish.

GENERAL PRINCIPLES OF TOXICOLOGIC ASSESSMENT AND MANAGEMENT

Although specific protocols for managing toxicological emergencies may vary, certain basic principles apply to most situations. Keep in mind the importance of recognizing the poisoning promptly. Have a high index of suspicion if circumstances suggest involvement of a toxin in the emergency.

SCENE SIZE-UP

Always begin assessment with a thorough evaluation of the scene. Take note of where you are and who is around you. Be alert for any potential danger to you, the rescuer. Remember, despite your natural urge to immediately assess and treat the patient, if you are incapacitated you will not be able to help anyone and you will become a patient yourself. In toxicological emergencies there are specific hazards to keep in mind.

- Patients who are suicidal may have the potential for violence. They are often intoxicated, may act irrationally, and will not always be cooperative or happy to see you. Therefore, look for signs of overdose such as empty pill bottles and used needles or other drug paraphernalia. Never put your hand blindly into a patient's pocket as it may contain used needles.

* **surface absorption** entry of a substance into the body directly through the skin or mucous membrane.

* **organophosphates** phosphorus-containing organic chemicals.

* **injection** entry of a substance into the body through a break in the skin.

- Chemical spills and hazardous material emergencies can quickly incapacitate any individuals who are nearby. Make sure you have the proper clothing and equipment needed for the particular emergency. Distribute this gear to rescuers who have been trained in their use.

INITIAL ASSESSMENT

After the scene size-up, perform the standard initial assessment. Form a general impression and quickly assess mental status. Assessment of the ABCs is critical in toxicological emergencies because airway and respiratory compromise are common complications. This can be due to direct airway injury, pulmonary injury, profuse secretions, or decreased respiratory effort secondary to altered mental status. After assessing the ABCs, set a transport priority for the patient.

HISTORY, PHYSICAL EXAM, AND ONGOING ASSESSMENT

For responsive patients, start by obtaining a history. It is important to find out not only what toxin the patient was exposed to but when the exposure took place, since toxic effects develop over time. Then proceed to a focused physical exam with full vital signs. With unresponsive patients, start with a rapid head-to-toe exam. Be alert for signs of trauma inconsistent with the suspected intoxication. Then proceed to obtain a history from relatives or other bystanders. Relay this information to the local Poison Control Center. They will advise you on the most current protocol for treatment. Be aware of your local policy, which will outline whether you can initiate this protocol or whether you must first contact on-line medical direction. Never delay supportive measures or immediate transport to the hospital based on a delay in contacting or obtaining information from the Poison Control Center.

A detailed physical exam can be performed en route if time and the patient's condition permit. Ongoing assessment is essential for these patients. Poisoned patients can deteriorate suddenly and quickly. Repeat the initial assessment and vitals and re-evaluate every five minutes for critical/unstable patients and every fifteen minutes for stable patients.

TREATMENT

Decontamination

Once you have initiated supportive treatment (airway control, breathing assistance, and IV fluids), proceed to a mode of treatment that is specific to toxicological emergencies: decontamination. **Decontamination** is the process of minimizing toxicity by reducing the amount of toxin absorbed into the body. There are three steps to decontamination.

✱ **decontamination** the process of minimizing toxicity by reducing the amount of toxin absorbed into the body.

1. *Reduce intake of toxin.* This means that you must remove a person from an environment where they are inhaling toxic fumes, or you must properly remove a stinger and sac from someone stung by a bee. A classic example involves a person who has had organophosphates spilled on him. The patient's clothes must be removed and the skin cleaned with soap and water to reduce absorption of the toxins.
2. *Reduce absorption of toxin once in the body.* This usually applies to ingested toxins, which wait in the stomach and intestines while the body absorbs them into the blood stream.

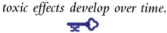

Content Review

PRINCIPLES OF DECONTAMINATION
- Reduce intake
- Reduce absorption
- Enhance elimination

In the past, syrup of ipecac was used to induce vomiting in order to empty the stomach. **Use of syrup of ipecac is no longer acceptable.** Studies consistently show that the use of syrup of ipecac to induce emesis reduces absorption by only 30 percent. This still leaves 70 percent of the toxin to be absorbed and cause injury. Vomiting also limits the use of other oral agents that are more effective for decontamination (e.g., activated charcoal) or oral antidotes (e.g., N-Acetylcysteine). There is also an increased risk of aspiration with vomiting, which makes induction of vomiting a procedure with minimal usefulness and high risk. Although ipecac may have some minor role in home management of some pediatric poisonings, it has generally become an obsolete treatment.

Gastric lavage ("pumping the stomach") has also been found to be of limited use. This process involves passing a tube into the stomach and repeatedly filling and emptying the stomach with water or saline in hopes of removing the ingested poison. Most studies have shown that gastric lavage removes almost no poisons from the stomach unless it is initiated within one hour of the ingestion. Possible complications, such as aspiration or perforation, make this procedure a risk without much benefit. Except in limited situations with ingestions of highly toxic substances that do not bind to charcoal and for which there is no antidote, gastric lavage has become an uncommon decontamination procedure.

* **gastric lavage** removing an ingested poison by repeatedly filling and emptying the stomach with water or saline via a gastric tube; also known as "pumping the stomach."

The most effective and widely used method of reducing absorption of toxins is **activated charcoal.** Because of its extremely large surface area, it can adsorb, or bind, molecules from the offending toxin and prevent their absorption into the bloodstream.

* **activated charcoal** a powder, usually pre-mixed with water, that will adsorb (bind) some poisons and help prevent them from being absorbed by the body.

3. *Enhance elimination of toxin.* Cathartics, such as sorbitol (often mixed with activated charcoal), increase gastric motility, thereby shortening the amount of time toxins stay in the gastrointestinal tract to be absorbed. Cathartics must be used cautiously, since there is controversy regarding their effectiveness. Cathartics should not be used in pediatric patients because of the potential to cause severe electrolyte derangements.

Whole bowel irrigation is another method of enhancing elimination. Using a gastric tube, polyethylene glycol electrolyte solution is administered continuously at 1–2 L/hr until the rectal effluent is clear or objects recovered. This technique seems effective with few complications and is therefore gaining popularity. Its availability, however, is limited to a few centers.

* **whole bowel irrigation** administration of polyethylene glycol continuously at 1–2 L/hr through a nasogastric tube until the effluent is clear or objects are recovered.

* **antidote** a substance that will neutralize a specific toxin or counteract its effect on the body.

Antidotes

Finally, if indicated, the appropriate antidote should be administered. An **antidote** is a substance that will neutralize a specific toxin or counteract its effect on the body. There are not many antidotes (Table 8-1), and they will rarely be 100 percent effective. Most poisonings will not require the administration of an antidote.

The specific actions you take when dealing with toxicological emergencies will be dictated by consultation with medical direction, by protocols obtained from the Poison Control Center, and by your local policy and procedures on initiating these protocols.

Specific actions in a toxicological emergency will be dictated by consultation with medical direction, protocols from the Poison Control Center, and local policy on initiating these protocols.

Table 8-1   ANTIDOTES FOR TOXICOLOGICAL EMERGENCIES

Toxin	Antidote	Adult Dosage (Pediatric Dosage)
Acetaminophen	N-Acetylcysteine	Initial: 140 mg/kg
Arsenic	*see* Mercury, Arsenic, Gold	
Atropine	Physostigmine	Initial: 0.5–2 mg IV
Benzodiazepines	Flumazenil	Initial: 0.2 mg q 1 min to total of 1–3 mg
Carbon Monoxide	Oxygen	
Cyanide	Amyl nitrite	Inhale crushed pearl for 30 seconds, then oxygen for 30 seconds
	then sodium nitrite	10 mL of 3% sol'n over 3 min IV (Pediatric: 0.33 mL/kg)
	then sodium thiosulfate	50 mL of 25% sol'n over 10 min IV (Pediatric: 1.65 mL/kg)
Ethylene glycol	Fomepizole (or as methyl alcohol)	Initial: 15 mg/kg IV
Gold	*see* Mercury, Arsenic, Gold	
Iron	Defroxamine	Initial: 10–15 mg/kg/hr IV
Lead	Edetate calcium disodium	1 amp/250 mL D5W over 1 hr
	or Dimercaptosuccinic acid (DMSA)	250 mg PO
Mercury, Arsenic, Gold	BAL (British anti-Lewisite)	5 mg/kg IM
	DMSA	250 mg PO
Methyl alcohol	Ethyl alcohol +/− dialysis	1 mL/kg of 100% ethanol IV
Nitrates	Methylene blue	0.2 mL/kg of 1% sol'n IV over 5 min
Opiates	Naloxone	0.4–2.0 mg IV
Organophosphates	Atropine	Initial: 2–5 mg IV
	Pralidoxime (Protopam)	Initial: 1 g IV

SUICIDAL PATIENTS AND PROTECTIVE CUSTODY

Involve law enforcement early in any possible suicide case.

Before leaving a suicidal patient who claims to have been "just kidding," consider the legal ramifications. You may be charged later with patient abandonment. At the same time, be aware of protective custody laws in your state. Always involve law enforcement personnel in these cases and involve them early. Only law enforcement personnel can place a patient in protective custody and ultimately consent to treatment.

INGESTED TOXINS

Poisoning by ingestion is the most common route of poisoning you will encounter in prehospital care. It is essential to initiate the following principles of assessment and treatment promptly.

Assessment

It takes time for an ingested toxin to make its way from the gastrointestinal system into the circulatory system. Therefore, you need to find out not only what was ingested but when it was ingested. Following are some general guidelines for managing patients who have ingested toxins as well as information about specific substances.

History Begin your history by trying to find out the type of toxin ingested, the quantity of the toxin, the time elapsed since ingestion, and whether the patient took any alcohol or other potentiating substance. Also ask the patient about drug habituation or abuse and underlying medical illnesses and allergies. Remember that in cases of poisoning, inaccuracies creep into nearly half the histories because of drug-induced confusion, patient misinformation, or deliberate patient attempts at deception.

The following questions will help you to develop a relevant history.

In cases of poisoning, histories are often unreliable because of drug-induced confusion, patient misinformation, or deliberate deception.

- What did you ingest? (Obtain pill containers and any remaining contents, samples of the ingested substance, or samples of vomitus. Bring them with the patient to the emergency department.)
- When did you ingest the substance? (Time is critical for decisions regarding lab tests and the use of gastric lavage and/or antidotes.)
- How much did you ingest?
- Did you drink any alcohol?
- Have you attempted to treat yourself (including inducing vomiting)?
- Have you been under psychiatric care? If so, why? (Answers may indicate a potential for suicide.)
- What is your weight?

Physical Examination Because the history can be unreliable, the physical examination is extremely important. It has two purposes: (1) to provide physical evidence of intoxication and (2) to find any underlying illnesses that may account for the patient's symptoms or that may affect the outcome of the poisoning. As you complete the initial assessment and rapid physical exam, pay attention to the following patient features:

- *Skin.* Is there evidence of cyanosis, pallor, wasting, or needle marks? Flushing of the skin may indicate poisoning with an anticholinergic substance. Staining of the skin may occur from chronic exposure to mercuric chloride, bromine, or similar chemicals.
- *Eyes.* Constriction or dilation of the pupils can occur with various types of poisons (e.g., marijuana, methamphetamines, narcotics). Ask about impaired vision, blurring of vision, or coloration of vision.
- *Mouth.* Look for signs of caustic ingestion, presence of the gag reflex, the amount of salivation, any breath odor, or the presence of vomitus.
- *Chest.* Breath sounds may reveal evidence of aspiration, atelectasis, or excessive pulmonary secretions.
- *Circulation.* Cardiac examination may give clues as to the type of toxin ingested. For example, the presence of tachydysrhythmias (e.g., from methamphetamine) or bradydysrhythmias (e.g., from organophosphates) may suggest specific toxins.
- *Abdomen.* Abdominal pain may result from poisoning by salicylates, methyl alcohol, caustics, or botulism toxin.

You can frequently expect to encounter patients who have ingested more than one toxin. This may be the result of a suicide attempt or of experimentation with illicit drugs. Such multiple ingestions present a diagnostic and therapeutic dilemma. Signs and symptoms may be inconsistent with a single diagnosis, and attempted treatment may produce unexpected results. A common example of this is the "speedball" (heroin mixed with cocaine). If the narcotic overdose is treated, the rescuer is often presented with a patient who is now in a cocaine-induced catecholamine crisis (tachycardia, hypertension, seizures). In such cases, or if you cannot identify what the patient has ingested, consult medical direction and/or the Poison Control Center according to your local protocols.

Management

Maintaining airway, breathing, and circulation is top priority in treating a poisoned patient. Preventing aspiration must be one of your major objectives.

Prevent Aspiration As previously discussed, initiation of supportive measures (maintaining airway, breathing, and circulation) is top priority in the treatment of the poisoned patient. Aspiration is a frequent complication of poisoning, resulting from an altered level of consciousness and a decreased gag reflex. Preventing aspiration must be one of your major objectives. If insertion of an endotracheal tube is necessary, nasotracheal intubation is preferred in patients who have a gag reflex.

Poisoning is a situation where rapid sequence intubation (RSI) may be required (see Volume 1, Chapter 13). It is not uncommon to encounter a patient with altered mental status who is vomiting. The prevention of aspiration is a primary concern, but attempts at endotracheal intubation fail because the patient will "clamp down" his teeth. In these situations, it is often prudent to use RSI to quickly control and maintain the airway. This is far superior to waiting for the patient to deteriorate to the point where an endotracheal tube can be placed without the aid of neuromuscular blockers. Remember, most poisoning patients will have compromised respiration or circulation, so routinely give high-flow oxygen.

Administer Fluids and Drugs Once you have assured the ABCs, establish intravenous access. An IV of lactated Ringer's or normal saline at a to-keep-open rate is recommended for all potentially dangerous ingestions. In addition to volume replacement with a crystalloid solution, conduct cardiac monitoring and repeat assessments, including frequent monitoring of vital signs.

Many EMS systems still utilize an empiric therapeutic regimen for comatose patients consisting of $D_{50}W$, naloxone (Narcan), and thiamine (Vitamin B_1). This so-called "coma cocktail" should not be used. Instead, treatment should be guided by objective patient information obtained on scene. If immediate determination of blood glucose levels is available (glucometer and chemstrips), withhold the administration of $D_{50}W$ until determination of hypoglycemia is made. If indicated, use 25–50 g of $D_{50}W$ IV push. If narcotic intoxication is suspected (respiratory depression or pinpoint pupils), give 1–2 mg of naloxone IV push. Naloxone reverses the effects of narcotic intoxication. If chronic alcoholism is suspected, consider administration of 100 mg of thiamine IV to address possible encephalopathy. Do not give these medications empirically!

Follow these supportive measures with the decontamination procedures outlined earlier. Often, decontamination is performed in the emergency department rather than on scene or during transport. This also applies to the use of most antidotes. There are exceptions, of course, and each case needs to be treated individually. Consult the Poison Control Center and medical direction according to your local protocols.

Do Not Induce Vomiting As mentioned earlier, induction of vomiting is no longer an accepted routine intervention for patients who have ingested toxins. It is still important to contact the Poison Control Center about this, since, in rare cases of pediatric ingestion, induction of vomiting may play some role. However, for the overwhelming majority of cases, inducement of vomiting is not required and may even be contraindicated.

INHALED TOXINS

Toxic inhalations can be self-induced or the result of accidental exposure from such sources as house fires or industrial accidents. Commonly abused inhaled toxins include: paint (and other hydrocarbons), Freon, propellants, glue, amyl nitrite, butyl nitrite, and nitrous oxide. The general guidelines for assessment and management of toxicological emergencies apply to inhaled toxins, but the following provides some specifics.

Assessment

Inhaled toxic substances produce signs and symptoms primarily in the respiratory system. These symptoms are particularly severe in patients who have inhaled chemicals and propellants concentrated in paper or plastic bags. Patients who inhale paint or propellants are often referred to as "huffers." Look for the presence of paint on the upper or lower lip. "Huffers," who report it to be more potent, often prefer gold paint. The presence of paint on the upper or lower lips should alert you to the possibility of inhalant abuse. The sniffing of paint, propellants, or hydrocarbons has become an epidemic problem in many developing countries. This is particularly true in the lower socioeconomic groups, most notably the legions of street children in Latin and South America. "Huffing" can lead to serious, irreversible brain damage. As the toxins are inhaled, oxygen is gradually displaced from the respiratory system, producing a relative hypoxia. Signs and symptoms of aerosol inhalation include:

- *Central nervous system:* dizziness, headache, confusion, seizures, hallucinations, coma
- *Respiratory:* tachypnea, cough, hoarseness, stridor, dyspnea, retractions, wheezing, chest pain or tightness, rales or rhonchi
- *Cardiac:* dysrhythmias

Management

Your first priority in the case of toxin inhalation is to remove the patient from the source as soon as it is safe to do so. Then follow these guidelines:

- Safely remove the patient from the poisonous environment. In doing so, take the following essential precautions:
  - Wear protective clothing.
  - Use appropriate respiratory protection.
  - Remove the patient's contaminated clothing.
- Perform the initial assessment, history, and physical exam.
- Initiate supportive measures.
- Contact the Poison Control Center and medical direction according to your local protocols.

Your first priority in any inhalation emergency is personal safety, then removal of the patient from the toxic environment.

SURFACE-ABSORBED TOXINS

Many poisons, including organophosphates, cyanide, and other toxins, can be absorbed through the skin and mucous membranes.

Assessment and Management

Signs and symptoms of absorbed poisons can vary depending on the toxin involved. See the discussion of specific toxins in the sections that follow. Whenever you suspect absorption of a toxin (especially cyanide or organophosphates), take the following steps:

Your first priority in any surface-absorbed poisoning emergency is personal safety, then removal of the patient from the toxic environment.

- Safely remove the patient from the poisonous environment. It is essential that you follow these guidelines:
  - Wear protective clothing.
  - Use appropriate respiratory protection.
  - Remove the patient's contaminated clothing.
  - Perform the initial assessment, history, and physical exam.
  - Initiate supportive measures.
  - Contact the Poison Control Center and medical direction according to your local protocols.

SPECIFIC TOXINS

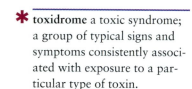
toxidrome a toxic syndrome; a group of typical signs and symptoms consistently associated with exposure to a particular type of toxin.

To recognize and implement the proper procedure in a given poisoning, you must be familiar with the signs and symptoms that a particular toxin will trigger. Often, you may not be able to identify the exact toxin a patient has been exposed to, but usually a group of toxins will have very similar manifestations and effects and will require similar interventions. Similar toxins with similar signs and symptoms are organized into **toxidromes** (toxic syndromes), which make remembering the details of their effects much simpler. Study the toxidromes listed in Table 8-2.

The following sections address specific toxins commonly encountered. While the standard toxicological emergency procedures, discussed earlier, apply to all of these toxins, pay close attention to variations in treatment. Variations include specific procedures you must perform in a particular case or a poisoning in which an antidote is available or immediately necessary. Management of injected toxins, drug overdose, and substance abuse will be covered later in the chapter.

CYANIDE

Cyanide can enter the body by a variety of routes. It is present in many commercial and household items that can be either ingested or absorbed—rodenticides, silver polish, and fruit pits and seeds (apricots, cherries, pears, and so on). It also can be inhaled, especially in fires that release cyanide from products containing nitrogen. A roomful of burning plastics, silks, or synthetic carpeting can also be a roomful of cyanide-filled smoke. Cyanide also forms in patients on long-term sodium nitroprusside therapy. Suicidal patients have been known to take cyanide salt. Regardless of the entry route, cyanide is an extremely fast-acting toxin. Once cyanide enters the body, it acts as a *cellular asphyxiant*. It inflicts its damage by inhibiting an enzyme vital to cellular use of oxygen.

Signs and Symptoms

Signs and symptoms of cyanide poisoning include:

- A burning sensation in the mouth and throat
- Headache, confusion, combative behavior

- Hypertension and tachycardia followed by hypotension and further dysrhythmias
- Seizures and coma
- Pulmonary edema

Management

First safely remove the patient from the source of exposure. To prevent inhalation, always wear breathing equipment when entering the scene of a fire. Initiate supportive measures immediately. Follow this with the cyanide antidote kit (Figure 8-1). This kit contains amyl nitrite ampules, a sodium nitrite, and a sodium thiosulfate solution. Adding nitrites to blood converts some hemoglobin to *methemoglobin*, which allows cyanide to bind to it. Thiosulfate then binds with the cyanide to form thiocyanate, a nontoxic substance readily excreted renally. Because cyanide is rapidly toxic, you must administer the cyanide antidote kit without delay. If your unit carries this kit, familiarize yourself with its contents and use.

CARBON MONOXIDE

Carbon monoxide (CO) is an odorless, tasteless gas that is often the byproduct of incomplete combustion. Because of its chemical structure, it has more than 200 times the affinity of oxygen to bind with the red blood cell's hemoglobin (producing carboxyhemoglobin). Once this molecule has bound with hemoglobin, it is very resistant to removal and causes an effective hypoxia. Because of the variability of the signs and symptoms, people usually ignore CO poisoning until very toxic levels occur. Common circumstances for CO poisoning include improperly vented heating systems or the use of a small barbecue to heat a house or camper. Symptoms of early poisoning are very similar to those of the flu. Be alert for CO poisoning in multiple patients living together in a poorly heated and vented space, having "flulike" symptoms.

Signs and Symptoms

Signs and symptoms of CO poisoning include:

- Headache
- Nausea, vomiting
- Confusion or other altered mental status
- Tachypnea

Management

Because of the difficulty in removing CO from hemoglobin, definitive treatment is often performed in a hyperbaric chamber (Figure 8-2). In this specially designed environment, oxygen under several atmospheres of pressure surrounds the body. This increases oxygenation of available hemoglobin. In field settings, take the following supportive steps:

- Ensure safety of rescue personnel.
- Remove the patient from the contaminated area.
- Begin immediate ventilation of the area.
- Initiate supportive measures. High-flow oxygen by nonrebreather is critical in this setting.

Table 8-2 TOXIC SYNDROMES

Toxidromes	Toxin	Signs and Symptoms
Anticholinergic	**Belladonna alkaloids** Atropine (hyoscyamine) Belladonna alkaloid mixtures: belladonna leaf, fluid extract, tincture Homatropine Methscopolamine Methylatropine nitrate Plants: *Atropa belladonna, Datura stramonium, Hyoscyamus niger, Amanita muscaria* or *pantherina* Scopolamine (l-hyoscine) **Synthetic anticholinergics** Adiphenine Isopropamide Pipenzolate Anisotropine Mepenzolate Piperiodolate Cyclopentolate Methantheline Poldine Dicyclomine Methixene Propantheline Diphemanil Oxyphenonium Thiphenamil Eucatropine Oxyphencyclimine Tridihexethyl Glycopyrrolate Pentapiperide Tropicamide Hexocyclium **Incidental anticholinergics** Antihistamines Benactyzine Phenothiazines Tricyclic antidepressants	Dry skin and mucous membranes Thirst Dysphagia Vision blurred for near objects Fixed dilated pupils Tachycardia Sometimes hypertension Rash, like scarlet fever Hyperthermia, flushing Urinary urgency and retention Lethargy Confusion to restlessness, excitement Delirium, hallucinations Ataxia Seizures Respiratory failure Cardiovascular collapse
Acetylcholinesterase inhibition	**Organophosphates** TEPP OMPA Dipterex Chlorthion Di-Syston Co-ral Phosdrin Parathion Methylparathion Malathion Systox EPN Diazinon Guthion Trithion	Sweating, constricted pupils, lacrimation, excessive salivation, wheezing, cramps, vomiting, diarrhea, tenesmus, bradycardia *or* tachycardia, hypotension *or* hypertension, blurred vision, urinary incontinence Striated muscle: cramps, weakness, twitching, paralysis, respiratory failure, cyanosis, arrest Sympathetic ganglia: tachycardia, elevated blood pressure CNS effects: anxiety, restlessness ataxia, seizures, insomnia, coma, absent reflexes, Cheyne-Stokes respirations, respiratory and circulation depression
Cholinergic	Acetylcholine Betel nut Methacholine *Area catechu* Bethanechol Muscarine Carbachol Pilocarpine *Clitocybe dealbata* *Pilocarpus species*	Sweating, constricted pupils, lacrimation, excessive salivation, wheezing, cramps, vomiting, diarrhea, tenesmus, bradycardia *or* tachycardia, hypotension *or* hypertension, blurred vision, urinary incontinence

Toxidromes	Toxin			Signs and Symptoms
Extrapyramidal	Acetophenazine Butaperazine Carphenazine Chlorpromazine Haloperidol	Mesoridazine Perphenazine Piperacetaxine Promazine	Thioridazine Thiothixene Trifluoperazine Triflupromazine	Parkinsonian Dysphagia, eye muscle spasm, rigidity, tremor, neck spasm, shrieking, jaw spasm, laryngospasm
Hemoglobinopathies	Carbon monoxide Methemoglobin			Headache, nausea, vomiting, dizziness, dyspnea, seizures, coma, death Cutaneous blisters, gastroenteritis Epidemic occurrence with carbon monoxide Cyanosis, chocolate blood with non-functional hemoglobin
Metal fume fever	Fumes of oxides of: Brass Cadmium Copper Zinc	Iron Magnesium Mercury	Nickel Titanium Tungsten	Chills, fever, nausea, vomiting, muscular pain, throat dryness, headache, fatigue, weakness, leukocytosis, respiratory disease
Narcotic	Alphaprodine Anileridine Codeine Cyclazocine Dextromethorphan Dextromoramide Diacetylmorphine Dihydrocodeine Dihydrocodeinone Dipipanone Diphenoxylate (Lomotil)	Ethylmorphine Ethoheptazine (meperidene metabolite) Fentanyl Heroin Hydromorphone Levorphanol Meperidine Methadone Metopon Morphine	Normeperidene Opium Oxycodone Oxymorphone Pentazocine Phenazocine Piminodine Propoxyphene Racemorphan	CNS depression Pinpoint pupils Slowed respirations Hypotension Response to naloxone Pupils may be dilated and excitement may predominate Normeperidine: tremor, CNS excitation, seizures
Sympathomimetic	Aminophylline Amphetamines Caffeine Catha edulus (Khat) Cocaehylene Cocaine Dopamine	Ephedrine Epinephrine Fenfluramine Levarterenol Metaraminol Methamphetamine Methcathinone	Methylphenidate (Ritalin) Pemoline Phencyclidine Phenmetrazine Phentermine	CNS excitation Seizures Hypertension Hypotension with caffeine Tachycardia
Withdrawal	Alcohol Barbiturates Benzodiazepines Chloral hydrate	Cocaine Ethchlorvynol Glutethimide Meprobamate	Methaqualone Methyprylon Opiods Paraldehyde	Diarrhea, large pupils, piloerection, hypertension, tachycardia, insomnia, lacrimation, muscle cramps, restlessness, yawning, hallucinations Depression with cocaine

Adapted from Done AK. *Poisoning—A Systematic Approach for the Emergency Department Physician.* Presented Aug. 6–9, 1979, at Snowmass Village, CO, Symposium sponsored by Rocky Mountain Poison Center. Used by Permission.

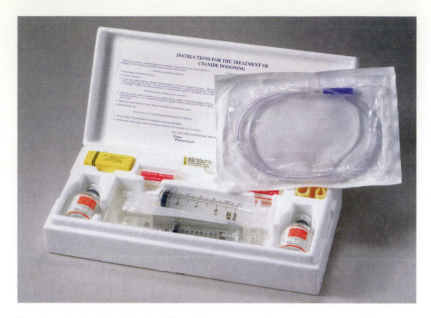

FIGURE 8-1   Cyanide antidote kit.

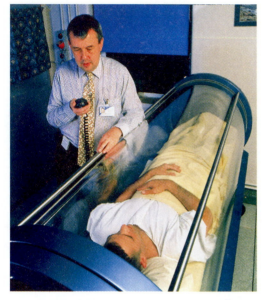

FIGURE 8-2   Hyperbaric chamber.

CARDIAC MEDICATIONS

The list of cardiac medications grows almost daily. Many classes of these drugs exist, including antidysrythmics, beta blockers, calcium channel blockers, glycosides, ACE inhibitors, and so on. Generally these medications regulate heart function by decreasing heart rate, suppressing automaticity, and/or reducing vascular tone. Overdoses of these drugs can be intentional but are more often due to errors in dosage.

Signs and Symptoms

In overdose quantities, signs and symptoms of cardiac medication poisoning include:

- Nausea and vomiting
- Headache, dizziness, confusion
- Profound hypotension
- Cardiac dysrhythmias (usually bradycardia)
- Heart conduction blocks
- Bronchospasm and pulmonary edema (especially beta blockers)

Management

Initiate standard toxicological emergency assessment and treatment immediately. Be aware that severe bradycardia may not respond well to atropine; therefore, you may need to use an external pacing device. Some cardiac medications do have antidotes that may help with severe adverse effects. These include calcium for calcium channel blockers, glucagon for beta blockers, and Digoxin-specific Fab (Digibind) for digoxin. Contact medical direction before giving these antidotes.

CAUSTIC SUBSTANCES

Caustic substances are either **acids** or **alkalis** (bases) that are found in both the home and the industrial workplace. Approximately 12,000 exposures occur annually with 150 major complications or deaths. Strong caustics can produce severe burns at the site of contact and, if ingested, cause tissue destruction at the lips, mouth, esophagus, and other areas of the gastrointestinal tract.

Strong *acids* have a pH less than 2. They are found in plumbing liquids such as drain openers and bathroom cleaners. Contact with strong acids usually produces immediate and severe pain. This is a result of tissue coagulation and necrosis. Often this type of contact injury will produce *eschar* at the burn site, which will act like a shield and prevent further penetration or damage to deeper tissues. If ingested, acids will cause local burns to the mouth and throat. Because of the rapid transit through the esophagus, the esophagus is not usually damaged. More likely, the stomach lining will be injured. Immediate or delayed hemorrhage can occur and may be associated with perforation. Pain is severe and usually due to direct injury and spasm from irritation. Absorption of acids into the vascular system will occur quite readily, causing a significant acidemia, which will need to be managed along with the direct local effects.

Strong *alkaline* agents typically have a pH greater than 12.5. They can be in solid or liquid form (such as in Drano or Liquid Plumber) and are routinely found around the house. These agents cause injury by inducing liquefaction necrosis. Pain is often delayed, which allows for longer tissue contact and deeper tissue injury before the exposure is even recognized. Solid alkaline agents can stick to the oropharynx or esophagus. This can cause perforation, bleeding, and inflammation of central chest structures. Liquid alkalis are more likely to injure the stomach because they pass quickly through the esophagus. Within 2–3 days of exposure, complete loss of the protective mucosal tissue can occur, followed by either gradual healing and recovery or further bleeding, necrosis, and stricture formation.

Signs and Symptoms

Signs and symptoms of caustic injury include:

- Facial burns
- Pain in the lips, tongue, throat, or gums
- Drooling, trouble swallowing
- Hoarseness, stridor, or shortness of breath
- Shock from bleeding, vomiting

Management

Assessment and intervention must be aggressive and rapid to minimize morbidity and mortality. Take precautions to prevent injury to rescuers. Initiate standard toxicological emergency assessment and treatment, but pay particular attention to establishing an airway. Injury to the oropharynx and larynx may make airway

* **acid** a substance that liberates hydrogen ions (H+) when in solution.

* **alkali** a substance that liberates hydroxyl ions (OH^-) when in solution; a strong base.

control and ventilation very difficult and may even require cricothyrotomy. Since caustics will not adsorb to activated charcoal, there is no indication to administer it. In the past, rescuers often gave water or milk to dilute any ingested caustics but there is controversy as to whether this is beneficial. Rapid transport to the emergency department is essential.

HYDROFLUORIC ACID

Hydrofluoric acid is used to clean glass in lab settings and for etching glass in art.

Hydrofluoric (HF) acid deserves special attention because it is extremely toxic and can be lethal despite the appearance of only moderate burns on skin contact. HF acid penetrates deeply into tissues and is inactivated only when it comes in contact with *cations* such as calcium. Calcium fluoride is formed by this inactivation and settles in the tissue as a salt. The removal of calcium from cells causes a total disruption of cell functioning and can even cause bone destruction as calcium is leeched out of the bones. Death has been reported from exposure of < 2.5% body surface area to a highly concentrated solution.

Signs and Symptoms

Signs and symptoms of HF acid exposure include:

- Burning at site of contact
- Trouble breathing
- Confusion
- Palpitations
- Muscle cramps

Management

Management includes:

- Ensure the safety of rescue personnel.
- Initiate supportive measures.
- Remove exposed clothing.
- Irrigate the affected area with water thoroughly.
- Immerse the affected limb in iced water with magnesium sulfate, calcium salts, or benzethonium chloride.
- Transport immediately for definitive care.

ALCOHOL

See the section on Alcohol Abuse later in this chapter.

HYDROCARBONS

Hydrocarbons are organic compounds composed of mostly carbon and hydrogen. They include such common recognizable names as kerosene, naphtha, turpentine, mineral oil, chloroform, toluene, and benzene. These chemicals are found in common household products such as lighter fluid, paint, glue, lubricants, solvents, and aerosol propellants. Toxicity from hydrocarbons can occur through any route, including ingestion, inhalation, or surface absorption.

Signs and Symptoms

Signs and symptoms of hydrocarbon poisoning will vary with the type and route of exposure but may include:

- Burns due to local contact
- Wheezing, dyspnea, hypoxia, and pneumonitis from aspiration/inhalation
- Headache, dizziness, slurred speech, ataxia (irregular and difficult-to-control movements), and obtundation (dulled reflexes)
- Foot and wrist drop with numbness and tingling
- Cardiac dysrhythmias

Management

Recent studies have shown that very few poisonings with hydrocarbons are serious, and less than one percent require physician intervention. If you know the exact chemical that the patient has been exposed to and the patient is asymptomatic, medical direction may suggest that the patient can be left at home. On the other hand, a few hydrocarbon poisonings can be very serious. Any patient who is symptomatic, does not know what he has taken, or who has taken a hydrocarbon that requires gastrointestinal decontamination (halogenated or aromatic hydrocarbons) must be treated using standard toxicological emergency procedures. Since charcoal will not bind hydrocarbons, this may be one of the few cases in which gastric lavage can be useful.

TRICYCLIC ANTIDEPRESSANTS

Tricyclic antidepressants were once commonly used to treat depression. Close monitoring was required because these medications have a narrow **therapeutic index,** meaning that a relatively small increase in dose can quickly lead to toxic effects. The very nature of their use, treating depression, presents a dilemma because the patients most seriously in need of treatment may also be the most likely to attempt to take an overdose. Deaths due to antidepressant overdose have dropped significantly in recent years since the development and rapid acceptance of safer agents unrelated to tricyclics. However, tricyclic antidepressants are still used for various clinical problems such as chronic pain or migraine prophylaxis and may still be responsible for more deaths due to intentional overdose than any other medication. Common agents include amitriptyline (Elavil), amoxapine, clomipramine, doxepin, imipramine, nortriptyline.

* therapeutic index the maximum tolerated dose divided by the minimum curative dose of a drug; the range between curative and toxic dosages; also called *therapeutic window.*

Signs and Symptoms

Signs and symptoms of tricyclic antidepressant toxicity include:

- Dry mouth
- Blurred vision
- Urinary retention
- Constipation

Late into an overdose, more severe toxicity may produce:

- Confusion, hallucinations
- Hyperthermia

- Respiratory depression
- Seizures
- Tachycardia and hypotension
- Cardiac dysrhythmias (heart block, wide QRS, *Torsades de pointes*)

Management

If you suspect a mixed overdose with benzodiazepines, do not *use Flumazenil, since it may precipitate seizures.*

Toxicity from tricyclic antidepressants requires immediate initiation of standard toxicological emergency procedures. Cardiac monitoring is critical since dysrhythmias are the most common cause of death. If you suspect a mixed overdose with benzodiazepines, do *not* use Flumazenil, since it may precipitate seizures. If significant cardiac toxicity occurs, sodium bicarbonate can be used as an additional therapy. Contact medical direction as necessary.

MAO INHIBITORS

Monoamine oxidase inhibitors (MAOIs) have been used, although rarely, to treat depression. Recently they have been used, on a limited basis, to treat obsessive-compulsive disorders. They are relatively unpopular because of a narrow therapeutic index, multiple-drug interactions, serious interactions with foods containing *tyramine* (for example, red wine and cheese), and high morbidity and mortality when taken in overdose. These drugs inhibit the breakdown of neurotransmitters such as norepinephrine and dopamine while increasing the availability of the components needed to make even more neurotransmitters. When taken in overdose, MAOIs can be extremely dangerous, although symptoms may not appear for up to 6 hours.

Signs and Symptoms

Signs and symptoms of MAOI overdose include:

- Headache, agitation, restlessness, tremor
- Nausea
- Palpitations
- Tachycardia
- Severe hypertension
- Hyperthermia
- Eventually bradycardia, hypotension, coma, and death occur

New MAOIs have recently entered the marketplace. These next-generation drugs are reversible, less toxic, and do not have the same reactions with food as the older MAOIs. Data is not yet available on the outcome of patients overdosing with these newer agents.

Management

No antidote exists for MAOI overdose because the inhibition is not reversible except with newer drugs. Therefore, institute standard toxicological emergency procedures as soon as possible. If necessary, give symptomatic support for seizures and hyperthermia using benzodiazepines. If vasopressors are needed, use norepinephrine.

NEWER ANTIDEPRESSANTS

In recent years, several new agents have been developed to treat depression. Because of their high safety profile in therapeutic and overdose amounts, these drugs have been widely accepted and have virtually replaced tricyclic antidepressants.

Recently introduced drugs include trazodone (Desyrel), bupropion (Wellbutrin), and the large group of very popular *selective serotonin re-uptake inhibitors*, or SSRIs, (Prozac, Luvox, Paxil, Zoloft). SSRIs prevent the re-uptake of serotonin in the brain, theoretically making it more available for brain functions. The true mechanism by which these drugs treat depression is unclear.

Signs and Symptoms

When these drugs are taken in overdose, usually the signs and symptoms are mild. Occasionally trazodone and buproprion will cause CNS depression and seizures, but deaths are very rare and have only been reported in mixed overdoses with multiple ingestions. More commonly, signs and symptoms of overdose with the newer antidepressant agents include:

- Drowsiness
- Tremor
- Nausea and vomiting
- Sinus tachycardia

SSRIs are now also associated with *serotonin syndrome*. This syndrome is caused by increased serotonin levels and is often triggered by increasing the dose of SSRI or adding a second drug such as Demerol, codeine, dextromethorphan (cough syrup), or other antidepressants. Signs and symptoms of serotonin syndrome include:

- Agitation, anxiety, confusion, insomnia
- Headache, drowsiness, coma
- Nausea, salivation, diarrhea, abdominal cramps
- Cutaneous piloerection, flushed skin
- Hyperthermia, tachycardia
- Rigidity, shivering, incoordination, myoclonic jerks

Management

Overdose with these new antidepressants is not as life threatening as with previous agents unless other drugs or alcohol are taken simultaneously. Consequently, treat overdoses with the standard toxicological emergency procedures. Also have the patient discontinue all serotonergic drugs and implement supportive measures. Benzodiazepines or beta blockers occasionally are used to improve patient comfort, but these are rarely given in the field.

LITHIUM

In the treatment of bipolar (manic-depressive) disorder, no other drug has been proven to be more effective than lithium. It is unclear how lithium exerts its therapeutic effect. However, like tricyclic antidepressants, lithium has a narrow therapeutic index which results in toxicity during normal use and in overdose situations.

Signs and Symptoms

Signs and symptoms of lithium toxicity include:

- Thirst, dry mouth
- Tremor, muscle twitching, increased reflexes
- Confusion, stupor, seizures, coma
- Nausea, vomiting, diarrhea
- Bradycardia, dysrhythmias

Management

Treat lithium overdose with mostly supportive measures. Use the standard toxicological emergency procedures, but remember that activated charcoal will not bind lithium and need not be given. Alkalinizing the urine with sodium bicarbonate and osmotic diuresis using mannitol may increase elimination of lithium, but severe toxic cases require hemodialysis.

SALICYLATES

Salicylates are some of the more common drugs taken in overdose, largely due to the fact that they are readily available over the counter. The most recognizable forms are aspirin, oil of wintergreen, and some prescription combination medications.

Aspirin in large doses can cause serious consequences. About 300 mg/kg is required to cause toxicity. In such amounts, salicylates inhibit normal energy production and acid buffering in the body. This results in a metabolic acidosis, which further injures other organ systems.

Signs and Symptoms

Signs and symptoms of salicylate overdose include:

- Rapid respirations
- Hyperthermia
- Confusion, lethargy, coma
- Cardiac failure, dysrhythmias
- Abdominal pain, vomiting
- Pulmonary edema, ARDS (adult respiratory distress syndrome)

Chronic overdose symptoms are somewhat less severe and do not tend to include abdominal complaints. It is difficult to distinguish chronic overdose from very early acute overdose or early overdose that has progressed past the abdominal irritation stage.

Management

In all cases, salicylate poisoning should be treated using standard toxicological emergency procedures. Activated charcoal definitely reduces drug absorption and should be used. If possible, find out the time of ingestion, since blood levels measured at the right time can indicate the expected degree of injury. Most symptomatic patients will require generous IV fluids and may need urine alkalinization with sodium bicarbonate. Severe cases may require dialysis.

ACETAMINOPHEN

Due to its few side effects in normal dosages, acetaminophen (e.g., paracetamol, Tylenol) is one of the most common drugs in use today. It is used to treat fever and/or pain and is a common ingredient in hundreds of over-the-counter preparations. It can be also obtained by prescription in combination with various other drugs.

In large doses, however, acetaminophen can be a very dangerous pharmaceutical. A dose of 150 mg/kg is considered toxic and may result in death due to injury to the liver. A highly reactive byproduct of acetaminophen metabolism is responsible for most adverse effects, but this is usually avoided by the body's detoxification system. When large amounts of acetaminophen enter the system, the detoxification system is overwhelmed and gradually depleted, leaving the toxic metabolite in the circulation to cause hepatic necrosis.

Signs and Symptoms

Signs and symptoms of acetaminophen toxicity appear in four stages.

Stage 1	½ hour to 24 hours	Nausea, vomiting, weakness, fatigue
Stage 2	24–48 hours	Abdominal pain, decreased urine, elevated liver enzymes
Stage 3	72–96 hours	Liver function disruption
Stage 4	4–14 days	Gradual recovery or progressive liver failure

Management

Treat acetaminophen overdose with standard toxicological emergency procedures. Find out the time of ingestion since blood levels taken at the right time can predict the potential for injury. An antidote called N-acetylcysteine (NAC, Mucomyst) is available and highly effective. However, NAC is usually administered based on clinical and laboratory studies and is rarely given in the prehospital setting.

OTHER NON-PRESCRIPTION PAIN MEDICATIONS

Non-steroidal anti-inflammatory drugs (NSAIDs) are another group of medications that are readily available and are often overdosed. Common examples include naproxen sodium, indomethacin, ibuprofen, and ketorolac (Toradol).

Signs and Symptoms

The presentation of toxicity caused by NSAIDs varies greatly but can include:

- Headache
- Ringing in the ears (tinnitus)
- Nausea, vomiting, abdominal pain
- Swelling of the extremities
- Mild drowsiness
- Dyspnea, wheezing, pulmonary edema
- Rash, itching

Management

There is no specific antidote for NSAID toxicity. Use general overdose procedures, including supportive care as soon as possible and transport to the emergency department for observation and any necessary symptomatic treatment.

THEOPHYLLINE

Theophylline belongs to a group of medications called xanthines. It is usually used for patients with asthma or COPD because of its moderate bronchodilation and mild anti-inflammatory effects. Like other drugs with a narrow therapeutic index and high toxicity, theophylline has become less popular recently and therefore is not implicated in as many overdose injuries as in the past.

Signs and Symptoms

Symptoms of theophylline toxicity include:

- Agitation
- Tremors
- Seizures
- Cardiac dysrhythmias
- Nausea and vomiting

Management

Theophylline can cause significant morbidity and mortality. In overdose situations, it is essential that you institute toxicological emergency procedures immediately. In fact, theophylline is on the small list of drugs that have significant *entero-hepatic circulation*. This means that multiple doses of activated charcoal over time will continuously remove more and more of the drug from the body. Treat any dysrhythmias according to ACLS procedures.

METALS

With the exception of iron, overdose of heavy metals is a rare occurrence. Other possible involved metals include lead, arsenic, and mercury. All metals affect numerous enzyme systems within the body and therefore present with a variety of symptoms. Some also have direct local effects when ingested and when accumulated in various organs.

Iron

The body only requires small amounts of iron on a daily basis to maintain a sufficient store for enzyme and hemoglobin production. Excess amounts are easily obtained from nonprescription supplements and multi-vitamins. Children have a tendency to accidentally overdose on iron by taking too many candy-flavored chewable vitamins containing iron. To determine the amount of iron ingested, you must calculate the amount of elemental iron present in the type of pill ingested. Symptoms occur when more than 20 mg/kg of elemental iron are ingested.

Signs and Symptoms Excess iron will cause gastrointestinal injury and possible shock from hemorrhage, especially if it forms *concretions* (lumps of iron formed when tablets fuse together after being swallowed). Patients with significant iron ingestions will often have visible tablets or concretions in the stomach or small intestine when x-rayed. Other signs and symptoms of iron ingestion include:

- Vomiting (often hematemesis), diarrhea
- Abdominal pain, shock
- Liver failure
- Metabolic acidosis with tachypnea
- Eventual bowel scarring and possible obstruction

Management It is essential to initiate standard toxicological emergency procedures immediately. Since iron tends to inhibit gastrointestinal motility, pills sit longer in the stomach and may possibly be easier to remove through gastric lavage. Because activated charcoal will not bind iron (or any metals), it should not be used. Deferoxamine, a chelating agent, may be used in iron overdose as an antidote since it binds to iron so that less is moved into cells and tissues to cause damage.

Lead and Mercury

Both lead and mercury are heavy metals found in varying amounts in the environment. Lead was often used in glazes and paints before the toxic potential of such exposure became apparent. Mercury is a contaminant from industrial processing but is also found in thermometers and temperature-control switches in most homes. Chronic and acute exposures are possible with both metals.

Signs and Symptoms Signs and symptoms of heavy metal toxicity include:

- Headache, irritability, confusion, coma
- Memory disturbance
- Tremor, weakness, agitation
- Abdominal pain

Management Chronic poisoning can cause permanent neurological injury, which makes it imperative that the proper agencies monitor heavy metal levels in the environment of a patient who has presented with toxicity. Learn to recognize the signs of heavy metal toxicity and institute standard toxicology emergency procedures as needed. Activated charcoal will not bind heavy metals but various chelating agents (DMSA, BAL, CDE) are available and may be used in definitive management in the hospital.

CONTAMINATED FOOD

Food poisoning is caused by a spectrum of different factors. For example, bacteria, viruses, and toxic chemicals notoriously produce varying levels of gastrointestinal distress. The patient may present with nausea, vomiting, diarrhea, and diffuse abdominal pain.

Bacterial food poisonings range in severity. Bacterial **exotoxins** (secreted by bacteria) or **enterotoxins** (exotoxins associated with gastrointestinal diseases, including food poisoning) cause the adverse GI complaints noted previously. Food contaminated with other bacteria such as *Shigella, Salmonella,* or *E. coli* can produce even more severe gastrointestinal reactions, often leading to electrolyte imbalance and hypovolemia. *Clostridium botulinum,* the world's most toxic poison, presents as severe respiratory distress or arrest. The incubation of this toxin can range from 4 hours to 8 days. Fortunately, botulism rarely occurs, except in cases of improper food storage methods such as canning.

✱ **exotoxin** a soluble poisonous substance secreted during growth of a bacterium.

✱ **enterotoxin** an exotoxin that produces gastrointestinal symptoms and diseases such as food poisoning.

A variety of seafood poisonings are a result of specific toxins found in dinoflagellate contaminated shellfish such as clams, mussels, oysters, and scallops and can produce a syndrome referred to as *paralytic shellfish poisoning*. This condition can lead to respiratory arrest in addition to standard gastrointestinal symptoms.

Increased fish consumption by North Americans has also increased the number of cases of poisonings from toxins found in many commonly eaten fish. *Ciguatera (bony fish) poisoning* most frequently turns up in fish caught in the Pacific Ocean or along the tropical reefs of Florida and the West Indies. Ciguatera normally takes 2–6 hours to incubate and may produce myalgia and paresthesia. *Scombroid (histamine) poisoning* results from bacterial contamination of mackerel, tuna, bonitos, and albacore. Both types of poisoning cause the common gastrointestinal symptoms. Scombroid poisoning will present with an immediate facial flushing as histamines cause vasodilation.

Signs and Symptoms

As mentioned above, signs and symptoms of food poisoning may include:

- Nausea, vomiting, diarrhea, abdominal pain
- Facial flushing, respiratory distress (with some seafood poisonings)

Management

Except for botulism, food poisoning is rarely life threatening. Treatment, therefore, is largely supportive. In suspected cases of food poisoning, contact poison control and medical direction, and take the following steps.

- Perform the necessary assessment.
- Collect samples of the suspected contaminated food source.
- Perform the following management actions:
  - Establish and maintain the airway.
  - Administer high-flow oxygen.
  - Intubate and assist ventilations, if appropriate.
  - Establish venous access.
- Consider the administration of antihistamines (especially in seafood poisonings) and antiemetics.

POISONOUS PLANTS AND MUSHROOMS

Plants, trees, and mushrooms contribute heavily to the number of accidental toxic ingestions. While the vast majority of plants are nontoxic, many of the popular decorative houseplants can present a danger to children, who frequently ingest non-food items. Most Poison Control Centers distribute pamphlets that identify toxic household plants. (These pamphlets will help "poison proof" the home.)

It is impossible to cover all the toxic plants and mushrooms. Few rescuers are trained as botanists, and they find it difficult to identify the offending material. Mushrooms are particularly difficult to identify from small pieces. Additionally, most people recognize mushrooms and other plants by common names rather than by the nomenclature of scientific species. A general approach is to obtain a sample of the plant, if possible. Try to find a full leaf, stem, and any flowers.

Since many ornamental plants contain irritating chemicals or crystals, examine the patient's mouth and throat for redness, blistering, or edema. Identify other abnormal signs during the focused physical exam.

Mushroom poisonings generally fall into two categories: people seeking edible mushrooms and accidental ingestions by children. Fortunately, few of the

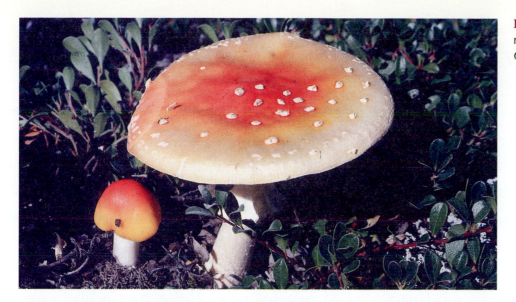

FIGURE 8-3 Poisonous mushrooms from *Amanita* and *Galerina* class.

many mushroom species possess extremely dangerous toxins. Toxic mushrooms fall into seven classes. *Amanita* and *Galerina* belong to the deadly *cyclopeptide* group (Figure 8-3). (*Amanita* accounts for over 90 percent of all deaths.) These mushrooms produce a poison that is extremely toxic to the liver, with a mortality rate of about 50 percent.

Signs and Symptoms

Signs and symptoms of poisonous plant ingestion include:

- Excessive salivation, lacrimation (secretion of tears), diaphoresis
- Abdominal cramps, nausea, vomiting, diarrhea
- Decreasing levels of consciousness, eventually progressing to coma

Management

For guidance on the treatment of plant poisonings, call the Poison Control Center. If contact cannot be made, use the procedures outlined under treatment of food poisoning earlier.

INJECTED TOXINS

Although we generally think of intentional or accidental drug overdoses as sources of injected poisons, the most common source for these poisonings is the animal kingdom. Bites and stings from a variety of insects, reptiles, and animals are among the most common injuries sustained by humans. Further injury can result from bacterial contamination or from a reaction produced by an injected substance.

GENERAL PRINCIPLES OF MANAGEMENT

The general principles of field management for bites and stings include:

- Protect rescue personnel—the offending organism may still be around.
- Remove the patient from danger of repeated injection, especially in the case of yellow jackets, wasps, or hornets.

In the case of a bite or sting, remember to protect rescue personnel. The offending organism may still be around.

- If possible, identify the insect, reptile, or animal that caused the injury and bring it to the emergency department along with the patient (if it can be done safely).
- Perform an initial assessment and rapid physical exam.
- Prevent or delay further absorption of the poison.
- Initiate supportive measures as indicated.
- Watch for anaphylactic reaction (see Chapter 5).
- Transport the patient as rapidly as possible.
- Contact the Poison Control Center and medical direction according to your local protocols.

INSECT BITES AND STINGS

Insect Stings

Many people die from allergic reactions to the stings from an order of insects known as *Hymenoptera*. As mentioned earlier, *Hymenoptera* includes wasps, bees, hornets, and ants. Only the common honeybee leaves a stinger. Wasps, yellow jackets, hornets, and fire ants sting repeatedly until removal from contact.

In most cases of insect bite, local treatment is all that is necessary. Unless an allergic reaction occurs, most patients will tolerate the isolated *Hymenoptera* sting.

Signs and Symptoms Signs and symptoms include:

- Localized pain
- Redness
- Swelling
- Skin wheal

Idiosyncratic reactions to the toxin may occur, resulting in a progressing localized swelling and edema. This is not an allergic reaction, however, if it responds well to an antihistamine such as diphenhydramine hydrochloride. The major problem resulting from a *Hymenoptera* sting is an allergic reaction or anaphylaxis. Signs and symptoms of allergic reaction include the following:

- Localized pain, redness, swelling, and a skin wheal
- Itching or flushing of the skin, rash
- Tachycardia, hypotension, bronchospasm, or laryngeal edema
- Facial edema, uvular swelling

Management For *Hymenoptera* stings, take the following supportive measures:

- Wash the area.
- Gently remove the stinger, if present, by scraping without squeezing the venom sac.
- Apply cool compresses to the injection site.
- Observe for and treat allergic reactions and/or anaphylaxis. (See Chapter 5.)

Brown Recluse Spider Bite

The brown recluse spider lives in the southern and midwestern states. It is found in large numbers in Tennessee, Arkansas, Oklahoma, and Texas. It has also been reported in Hawaii and California.

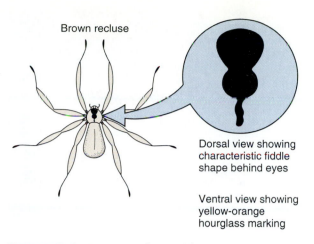

Brown recluse

Dorsal view showing characteristic fiddle shape behind eyes

Ventral view showing yellow-orange hourglass marking

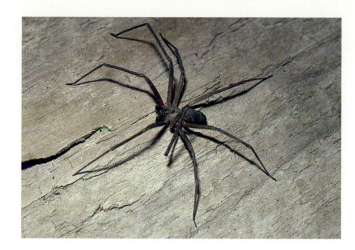

FIGURE 8-4   Brown recluse spider.

The brown recluse is about 15 mm in length. It generally lives in dark, dry locations and can often be found in and around the house. There is a characteristic violin-shaped marking on the back, giving the spider its nickname, "fiddleback spider" (Figure 8-4). Another identifying feature is the presence of six eyes (three pairs in a semicircle), instead of the eight eyes common to most spiders.

Signs and Symptoms Brown recluse spider bites are usually painless. Not uncommonly, bites occur at night while the patient sleeps. Most victims are unaware they have been bitten until the local reaction starts. Initially a small erythematous macule surrounded by a white ring forms at the site (Figure 8-5). This usually appears within a few minutes of the bite. Over the next eight hours localized pain, redness, and swelling develop. Tissue necrosis at the site occurs over days to weeks (Figure 8-6). Other symptoms include chills, fever, nausea and vomiting, joint pain and in severe situations, bleeding disorders (disseminated intravascular coagulation).

Management Treatment is mostly supportive. Since there is no antivenin, the emergency department treatment consists of antihistamines to reduce systemic reactions and possible surgical excision of necrotic tissue.

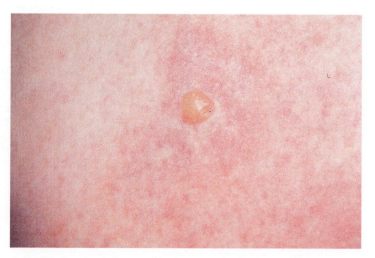

FIGURE 8-5   Brown recluse spider bite 24 hours after bite. Note the bleb and surrounding white halo. (Courtesy of Scott and White Hospital and Clinic.)

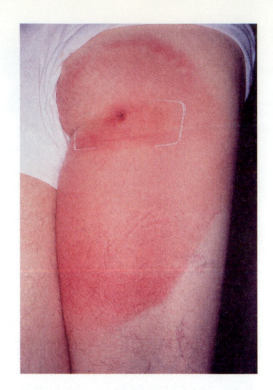

FIGURE 8-6   Brown recluse spider bite 4 days after the bite. Note the spread of erythema and early necrosis. (Courtesy of Scott and White Hospital and Clinic.)

Black Widow Spider Bites

Black widow spiders live in all parts of the continental United States. They are usually found in woodpiles or brush. The female spider is responsible for bites and can be easily identified by the characteristic orange hourglass marking on her black abdomen (Fig. 8-7). The venom of the legendary black widow is very potent, causing excessive neurotransmitter release at the synaptic junctions.

Signs and Symptoms   Signs and symptoms of black widow spider bites start as immediate localized pain, redness, and swelling. Progressive muscle spasms of all large muscle groups can occur and are usually associated with severe pain. Other systemic symptoms include nausea, vomiting, sweating, seizures, paralysis, and decreased level of consciousness.

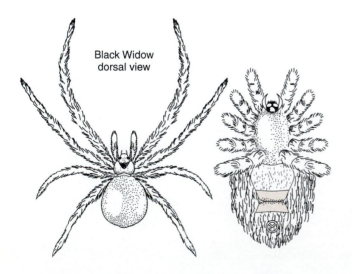

Black Widow
dorsal view

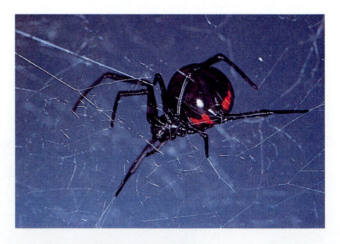

FIGURE 8-7   Black widow spider.

Management Prehospital treatment is mostly supportive. It is important to reassure the patient. IV muscle relaxants may be necessary for severe spasms. With physician order you may use diazepam (2.5–10 mg IV) or calcium gluconate (0.1–0.2/kg of 10 percent solution IV). Note that calcium chloride is not effective and should not be used. Since hypertensive crisis is possible, monitor blood pressure carefully. Antivenin is available, so transfer the patient to the emergency department as soon as possible.

Scorpion Stings

There are many species of scorpion in the United States (Figure 8-8). All can sting, causing localized pain, but only one, the bark scorpion, has caused fatalities. These arthropods live mostly in Arizona and adjacent areas of California, Nevada, New Mexico, and Texas. There have been no deaths in Arizona from scorpion stings since 1970.

Scorpions move mostly at night, hiding in the day under debris and buildings. The venom they inject is stored in a bulb at the end of the tail. If provoked the scorpion will sting with its tail, injecting only a small amount of poison.

Signs and Symptoms The bark scorpion's venom acts on the nervous system, producing a burning and tingling effect without much evidence of injury initially. Gradually this progresses to numbness. Systemic effects are more pronounced with slurred speech, restlessness (hyperactivity in 80 percent of children), muscle twitching, salivation, abdominal cramping, nausea and vomiting, and seizures.

Management Begin treatment by reassuring the patient. Apply a constricting band above the wound site no tighter than a watchband to occlude lymphatic flow only. Avoid the use of analgesics, which may increase toxicity and potentiate the venom's effect on airway control. Transport the patient to the emergency department if systemic symptoms develop. Antivenin is available but is an unlicensed goat-serum-derived product found in Arizona only. It can produce allergic or anaphylactic reactions and should be used only in severe cases.

SNAKEBITES

There are several thousand snakebites each year in the United States. Fortunately, these bites result in very few deaths. The signs and symptoms of snakebite depend upon the snake, the location of the bite, and the type and amount of venom injected.

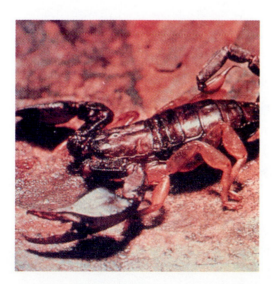

FIGURE 8-8 Scorpion.

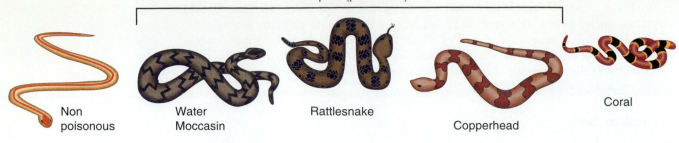

Pit Vipers (poisonous)

Non poisonous   Water Moccasin   Rattlesnake   Copperhead   Coral

FIGURE 8-9   Venomous snakes in the United States.

There are two families of poisonous snakes native to the United States (Figure 8-9). One family (*Crotalidae*) includes the pit vipers. Common pit vipers are cottonmouths (water moccasins), rattlesnakes, and copperheads. Pit vipers are so named because of the distinctive pit between the eye and the nostril on each side of the head. These snakes have elliptical pupils, two well-developed fangs, and a triangular-shaped head. Only the rattlesnake, the most common pit viper, has rattles on the end of its tail.

The second family of poisonous snakes is the *Elapidae*, or coral snake, which is a distant relative of the cobra. Several varieties of coral snakes are found in the United States, primarily in the southwest. Because it is a small snake and has small fangs, the coral snake cannot readily attach itself to a large surface, such as an arm or leg. The coral snake has round eyes, a narrow head, and no pit. It has characteristic yellow-banded red and black rings around its body. Several nonpoisonous snakes, such as the King Snake, mimic this coloration pattern. Keep in mind a helpful mnemonic: "red touch yellow, kill a fellow; red touch black, venom lack." This rhyme indicates the distinctive pattern of the coral snake—a pattern that signals danger.

Pit Viper Bites

Pit viper venom contains hydrolytic enzymes that are capable of destroying proteins and most other tissue components. These enzymes may produce destruction of red blood cells and other tissue components and may affect the body's blood clotting system within the blood vessels. This will produce infarction and tissue necrosis, especially at the site of the bite.

A severe pit-viper bite can result in death from shock within 30 minutes. However, most deaths from pit-viper bites occur from 6 to 30 hours after the bite, with 90% occurring within the first 48 hours.

Signs and Symptoms Signs and symptoms of pit viper bite include:

- Fang marks (often little more than a scratch mark or abrasion)
- Swelling and pain at the wound site
- Continued oozing at the wound site
- Weakness, dizziness, or faintness
- Sweating and/or chills
- Thirst
- Nausea and vomiting
- Diarrhea
- Tachycardia and hypotension

- Bloody urine and gastrointestinal hemorrhage (late)
- Ecchymosis
- Necrosis
- Shallow respirations progressing to respiratory failure
- Numbness and tingling around face and head (classic)

Management In treating a person who has been bitten by a pit viper, the primary goal is to slow absorption of the venom. Remember, about 25% of all rattlesnake bites are "dry" and no venom is injected. The amount of venom a pit viper injects varies significantly. It is helpful to try to classify the degree of envenomation:

Degree of Envenomation	Signs and Symptoms
None	None (either local or systemic)
Minimal	Swelling
	Pain
	No systemic symptoms
Moderate	Progressive swelling
	Mild systemic symptoms
	– paresthesias
	– nausea and vomiting
	– unusual tastes
	– mild hypotension
	– mild tachycardia
	– tachypnea
Severe	Swelling (spreading rapidly)
	Severe pain
	Systemic symptoms
	– altered mental status
	– nausea and vomiting
	– hypotension (systolic <80)
	– severe tachycardia
	– severe respiratory distress
	Blood oozes freely from puncture wounds

Antivenin is available for the various common pit vipers found in the United States. However, antivenin should only be considered for severe cases where there is marked envenomation as evidenced by severe systemic symptoms. In some cases, people become more ill from the antivenin than they do from the snakebite itself. Routine emergency treatment of pit viper bites includes the following steps:

- Keep the patient supine.
- Immobilize the limb with a splint.
- Maintain the extremity in a neutral position. Do not apply constricting bands.

Initiate supportive care using the following guidelines:

- Apply high-flow oxygen.
- Start IV with crystalloid fluid.
- Transport the patient to the emergency department for management, which may include the administration of antivenin.
- DO NOT apply ice, cold pack, or freon spray to the wound.
- DO NOT apply an arterial tourniquet.
- DO NOT apply electrical stimulation from any device in an attempt to retard or reverse venom spread.

Coral Snake Bites

The venom of the coral snake contains some of the enzymes found in pit viper venom. However, because of the presence of neurotoxin, coral snake venom primarily affects nervous tissue. The classic, severe coral snake bite will result in respiratory and skeletal muscle paralysis.

Signs and Symptoms After the bite of a coral snake, there may be no local manifestations or even any systemic effects for as long as 12–24 hours. Signs and symptoms of a coral snake bite include:

- Localized numbness, weakness, and drowsiness
- Ataxia
- Slurred speech and excessive salivation
- Paralysis of the tongue and larynx (produces difficulty breathing and swallowing)
- Drooping of eyelids, double vision, dilated pupils
- Abdominal pain
- Nausea and vomiting
- Loss of consciousness
- Seizures
- Respiratory failure
- Hypotension

Management Treatment in cases of suspected coral snake bites includes the following steps:

- Wash the wound with copious amounts of water.
- Apply a compression bandage and keep the extremity at the level of the heart.
- Immobilize the limb with a splint.
- Start an IV using crystalloid fluid.
- Transport the patient to the emergency department for administration of antivenin.
- DO NOT apply ice, cold pack, or freon sprays to the wound.
- DO NOT incise the wound.
- DO NOT apply electrical stimulation from any device in an attempt to retard or reverse venom spread.

MARINE ANIMAL INJECTION

Although most dangerous marine life prefer warm, tropical waters, some can be found in more northern waters. With the large number of people who flock to beaches and coastal recreation areas every year, the number of injuries from marine life has increased moderately. The most common encounters occur while the person is walking on the beach but can also happen while wading in shallow waters or scuba diving in deeper waters. Injection of toxins from marine life can result from stings of jellyfish and corals or from punctures by the bony spines of animals such as sea urchins and stingrays (Figure 8-10). All venoms of marine animals contain substances that produce pain out of proportion to the size of the injury. These poisonous toxins are unstable and heat sensitive. Heat will relieve pain and inactivate the venom.

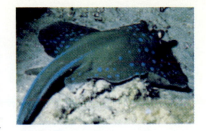

FIGURE 8-10   Stingray.

Both fresh water and salt water contain considerable bacterial and viral pollution. Therefore, secondary infection is always a possibility in injuries from marine animals. Particularly severe and life-threatening infections can be inflicted by a number of organisms. In all cases of marine-acquired infections, *Vibrio* species must be considered.

Signs and Symptoms Signs and symptoms of marine animal injection include:

- Intense local pain and swelling
- Weakness
- Nausea and vomiting
- Dyspnea
- Tachycardia
- Hypotension or shock (severe cases)

Management In suspected cases or marine animal injection, take the following steps:

- Establish and maintain the airway.
- Apply a constricting band between the wound and the heart no tighter than a watchband to occlude lymphatic flow only.
- Apply heat or hot water (110°–113°F).
- Inactivate or remove any stingers.

SUBSTANCE ABUSE AND OVERDOSE

Substance abuse, the use of a pharmacological substance for purposes other than medically defined reasons, is a very serious problem in our nation. Drugs are abused because they stimulate a feeling of euphoria in the abuser. Eventually, abusers begin to crave the feeling the drug gives them and therefore develop a *dependence* on the drug, also called **addiction.** An addiction exists when a person repeatedly uses and feels an overwhelming need to obtain and continue using a particular drug. Becoming accustomed to the use of the drug is called *habituation. Physiological dependence* is the resulting condition if removal of the drug causes adverse physical reactions. There can also be *psychological dependence,* in which use of the drug is required to prevent or relieve tension or emotional stress. With continued use, **tolerance** develops, which means that the abuser must use increasingly larger doses to get the same effect.

✱ **substance abuse** use of a pharmacological substance for purposes other than medically defined reasons.

✱ **addiction** compulsive and overwhelming dependence on a drug; an addiction may be physiological dependence, a psychological dependence, or both.

✱ **tolerance** the need to progressively increase the dose of a drug to reproduce the effect originally achieved by smaller doses.

Attempts to stop the drug can trigger a psychological or physical reaction known as **withdrawal**. Withdrawal reactions can be quite unpleasant and severe. In some cases (especially with alcohol), withdrawal can be severe enough to cause death. These reactions further strengthen the victim's dependence on the drug. At this point the abuser may begin to withdraw from regular activities. He may have conflicts with family, friends, and coworkers as his personality and priorities change. Often the abuser will be involved in criminal activities to support the habit. The abuser has formed an addiction at the point when the substance abuse begins to affect some part of his life. This includes affecting the abuser's health, work, or relationships. Also, the abuser begins to act in a manner so as to seek out the drug he abuses.

The National Institute on Drug Abuse performed a survey to estimate national use and exposure to illicit drugs. The results were astounding.

- 28 million Americans used illicit drugs at least once.
- 14.5 million use illicit drugs regularly.
- 20 million Americans have tried cocaine.
- 860,000 people use cocaine weekly.
- 11.6 million use marijuana regularly.
- 770,000 use hallucinogens such as PCP or LSD regularly.
- 2.5 million have used heroin.

The use of illicit drugs has fluctuated in recent years. Most recently, heroin has regained popularity, especially among middle to upper class teenagers and young adults. Beyond hurting themselves, substance abusers are 18 times more likely to be involved in criminal activities. These include violent crimes as well as theft to support drug habits. (The Secretary of Health and Human Services has estimated that cocaine is a $65 billion per year industry.)

In general terms, **drug overdose** refers to poisoning from a pharmacological substance, either legal or illegal. This can occur by accident, miscalculation, changes in the strength of a drug, suicide, polydrug use, or recreational drug usage. Many overdose emergencies seen in the field occur in the habitual drug abuser. It is most difficult to obtain a good history in these cases. However, if the paramedic is familiar with street-drug slang, a more accurate history may be obtained. It is imperative that the paramedic maintain a nonjudgmental attitude in these cases, even though this may be difficult.

The presentation of the drug overdose will vary based on the substance used. Management should be the same as for any ingested, inhaled, or injected poison. Poison control should be contacted for additional direction.

DRUGS OF ABUSE

Drugs Commonly Abused

Drugs of abuse are both common and dangerous. These drugs all have various signs and symptoms and require supportive treatment and general toxicological emergency management. Refer to Table 8-3 for further details on what you may find on assessment and the interventions required.

Remember these specific guidelines for patients who have taken the following drugs:

- *Alcohol*—May require thiamine and $D_{50}W$ for hypoglycemia.
- *Cocaine*—Benzodiazepines (diazepam) may be needed for sedation and to treat seizures. Beta blockers are absolutely contraindicated

because unopposed alpha receptor stimulation can cause cardiac ischemia, hypertension, and hyperthermia.

- *Narcotics/Opiates*—Naloxone is effective in reversing respiratory depression and sedation, but be careful, since it may trigger a withdrawal reaction in chronic opiate abusers.
- *Amphetamines*—Use benzodiazepines (diazepam) for seizures and in combination with haloperidol for hyperactivity.
- *Hallucinogens*—Use benzodiazepines for seizures and in combination with haloperidol for hyperactivity.
- *Benzodiazepines*—Use flumazenil to counteract adverse effects. Be careful not to trigger a withdrawal syndrome with seizures.
- *Barbiturates*—Forced diuresis and alkalinization of the urine improve elimination of barbiturates from the body.

Drugs Used for Sexual Purposes

There are a number of drugs that deserve mention as a separate category. These drugs are used to stimulate and enhance the sexual experience, but without medically approved indications for such use. *Ecstasy,* also called *MDMA,* is one such drug. Ecstasy is a modified form of methamphetamines and has similar, although milder effects. It is very popular in today's university and nightclub environments.

Use of Ecstasy initially causes anxiety, nausea, tachycardia, and elevated blood pressure, followed by relaxation, euphoria, and feelings of enhanced emotional insight. No definitive data exists as to whether the experience of sexual intercourse is improved. Studies show that prolonged use may cause brain damage. Some deaths from MDMA ingestion have been reported. These cases present with confusion, agitation, tremor, high temperature, and diarrhea. No specific treatment exists. Standard supportive measures should be initiated.

Rohypnol (Flunitrazepam) is another drug abused for sexual purposes. Illegal in the United States, it is commonly called the "date rape drug," since it can be secretly slipped into a woman's drink. This drug is a strong benzodiazepine like diazepam, lorazepan, and midazolam. The resulting sedation and amnesia allows the perpetrator to rape the victim. Treatment is the same as for any benzodiazepine, but consequences of the sexual assault require attention as well.

ALCOHOL ABUSE

Alcohol is the most common substance of abuse in the United States and most of the world. Almost 75 percent of Americans have at least one drink per year. The average American consumes 2.5 gallons of pure ethanol every year. Alcohol has been linked to 5 percent of deaths in the United States. Alcoholism costs over $100 billion per year due to lost work time and medical costs to treat complications and injuries. Alcoholism progresses in much the same way as drug dependence, discussed earlier.

PHYSIOLOGICAL EFFECTS

Alcohol (ethyl alcohol, or ethanol) depresses the central nervous system, potentially to the point of stupor, coma, and death. In patients with severe liver disease, metabolism of alcohol may become impaired, which increases the course and severity of intoxication. At low doses, alcohol has excitatory and stimulating effects, thus depressing inhibitions. At higher doses alcohol's depressive effect is more obvious.

Table 8-3 COMMON DRUGS OF ABUSE

Drug	Signs and Symptoms	Routes	Prehospital Management
Alcohol beer whiskey gin vodka wine tequila	CNS depression Slurred speech Disordered thought Impaired judgment Diuresis Stumbling gait Stupor Coma	Oral	ABCs Respiratory support Oxygenate Establish IV access Administer 100 mg thiamine IV ECG monitor Check glucose level Administer $D_{50}W$, if hypoglycemic
Barbiturates thiopental phenobarbital primidone	Lethargy Emotional lability Incoordination Slurred speech Nystagmus Coma Hypotension Respiratory depression	Oral IV	ABCs Respiratory support Oxygenate Establish IV access ECG monitor Contact Poison Control—may order bicarbonate

Cocaine
crack
rock
	Euphoria
	Hyperactivity
	Dilated pupils
	Psychosis
	Twitching
	Anxiety
	Hypertension
	Tachycardia
	Dysrhythmias
	Seizures
	Chest pain
		Snorting
		Injection
		Smoking (freebasing)
			ABCs
			Respiratory support
			Oxygenate
			ECG monitor
			Establish IV access
			Treat life-threatening
			    dysrhythmias
			Seizure precautions:
			    diazepam 5–10 mg

Narcotics
heroin
codeine
meperidine
morphine
hydromorphone
pentazocine
Darvon
Darvocet
methadone
	CNS depression
	Constricted pupils
	Respiratory depression
	Hypotension
	Bradycardia
	Pulmonary edema
	Coma
	Death
		Oral
		Injection
			ABCs
			Respiratory support
			Oxygenate
			Establish IV access
			*Administer 1–2 mg naloxone IV
			    or endotracheally as ordered by
			    medical direction until
			    respirations improve.
			Larger than average doses
			    (2–5 mg) have been used in
			    the management of Darvon
			    overdose and alcoholic
			    coma
			ECG monitor

*With the advent of the opiate antagonist naloxone, narcotic overdosage became easier to manage. It is possible to titrate this effective medication to increase respirations to normal levels without fully awakening the patient. In the case of narcotics addicts, this prevents hostile and confrontational episodes.

Abuse of and dependence on alcohol is called *alcoholism*. It is a major problem in our society, contributing to many highway traffic fatalities, drownings, burns, trauma, and drug overdoses.

Alcohol is completely absorbed from the stomach and intestinal tract in approximately 30 to 120 minutes after ingestion. Once absorbed, alcohol is distributed to all body tissues and fluids, with concentrations of alcohol in the brain rapidly approaching the alcohol level in the blood.

Drug	Signs and Symptoms	Routes	Prehospital Management
Marijuana grass weed hashish	Euphoria Dry mouth Dilated pupils Altered sensation	Smoked Oral	ABCs Reassure the patient Speak in a quiet voice ECG monitor if indicated
Amphetamines Benzedrine Dexedrine Ritalin "speed"	Exhilaration Hyperactivity Dilated pupils Hypertension Psychosis Tremors Seizures	Oral Injection	ABCs Oxygenate ECG monitor Establish IV access Treat life-threatening dysrhythmias Seizure precautions: diazepam 5–10 mg
Hallucinogens LSD STP mescaline psilocybin PCP**	Psychosis Nausea Dilated pupils Rambling speech Headache Dizziness Suggestibility Distortion of sensory perceptions Hallucinations	Oral Smoked	ABCs Reassure the patient "Talk down" the "high" patient Protect the patient from injury Provide a dark, quiet environment Speak in a soft, quiet voice Seizure precautions: diazepam 5–10 mg

**While PCP was originally an animal tranquilizer, it manifests hallucinogenic properties when used by humans. In addition to bizarre delusions, it can cause violent and dangerous outbursts of aggressive behavior. The rescuer is advised to remain safe when attempting to treat this type of overdose. PCP patients have been known to have almost superhuman strength and high pain tolerance.

Drug	Signs and Symptoms	Routes	Prehospital Management
Sedatives Seconal Valium Librium Xanax Halcion Restoril Dalmane Phenobarbital	Altered mental status Hypotension Slurred speech Respiratory depression Shock Bradycardia Seizures	Oral	ABCs Respiratory support Oxygenate Establish IV access ECG monitor Medical direction may order naloxone
Benzodiazepines* Valium Librium Xanax Halcion Restoril Dalmane Centrax Ativan Serax	Altered mental status Slurred speech Dysrhythmias Coma	Oral	ABCs Respiratory support Oxygenate Activated charcoal as ordered by medical Direction Establish IV access ECG monitor Contact poison control

***Deaths due to pure benzodiazepine ingestion are very rare. Minor toxicity ranges are 500–1,500 mg. A benzodiazepine antagonist (Romazicon) is available. IV dosage is 1–10 mg, or an infusion of 0.5 mg/hr. It may cause seizures in a benzodiazepine dependent patient.

Some alcoholics will drink methanol (wood alcohol) or ethylene glycol (a component of antifreeze) if ethanol is unavailable. Both are readily available and, when ingested, will be absorbed quickly from the gastrointestinal tract. Ingestion of these chemicals can cause blindness or death.

In addition, alcohol causes a peripheral vasodilator effect on the cardiovascular system, resulting in flushing and a feeling of warmth. In cold conditions, alcohol's dilation of the blood vessels results in an increased loss of body heat. The diuretic effect seen when large amounts of alcohol are ingested is due to the inhibition of *vasopressin,* which is the hormone responsible for the conservation of body fluids. Without vasopressin, an increase in urine flow occurs. The "dry mouth syndrome" experienced after alcohol consumption may be the result of alcohol-induced cellular dehydration.

In addition, methanol will also cause visual disturbances, abdominal pain, and nausea and vomiting even at low doses. In fact, death has been reported after ingestion of only 15 mL of a 40 percent solution. Occasionally patients will complain of headache or dizziness and may even present with seizures and obtundation. Ethylene glycol ingestion has similar symptoms, but the CNS effects such as hallucinations, coma, and seizures are more pronounced in the early stages.

GENERAL ALCOHOLIC PROFILE

Most alcoholics are not unkempt street people but are functional people at all levels of society who are able to mask their addiction.

The classic alcoholic portrayed in movies is an unkempt, continually intoxicated street person who is completely non-functional. Although alcoholics of this type exist, it would be a grave error to consider this the typical picture of someone dependent on alcohol. More commonly, alcoholism is characterized by impaired control over drinking, preoccupation with the drug ethanol, use of ethanol despite adverse consequences, and distortions in thinking, such as denial. This is the definition used by the National Council on Alcoholism and Drug Dependence. Obviously, this definition applies to many people, including many functional people at all levels of society who have masked their addiction well. Take note of these warning signs, which may indicate alcohol abuse:

- Drinks early in the day
- Prone to drink alone and secretly
- Periodic binges (may last for several days)
- Partial or total loss of memory ("blackouts") during period of drinking
- Unexplained history of gastrointestinal problems (especially bleeding)
- "Green tongue syndrome" (using chlorophyll-containing substances to disguise the odor of alcohol on the breath)
- Cigarette burns on clothing
- Chronically flushed face and palms
- Tremulousness
- Odor of alcohol on breath under inappropriate conditions

CONSEQUENCES OF CHRONIC ALCOHOL INGESTION

Alcohol has many deleterious effects on the body. Chronic abuse can be devastating, effecting every organ system as shown in Figure 8-11. Some of the more common effects include:

- Poor nutrition
- Alcohol hepatitis
- Liver cirrhosis with subsequent esophageal varices
- Loss of sensation in hands and feet
- Loss of cerebellar function (balance and coordination)
- Pancreatitis
- Upper gastrointestinal hemorrhage (often fatal)

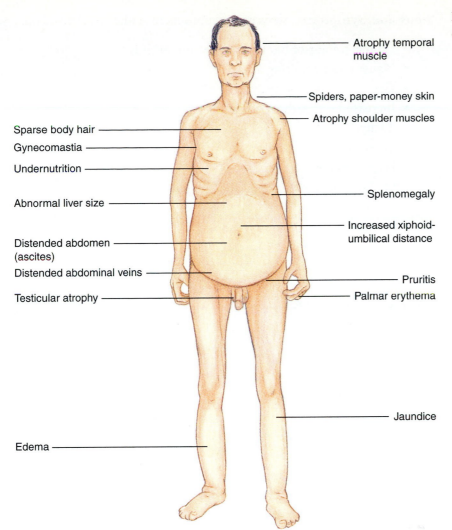

FIGURE 8-11 The chronic alcoholic.

Atrophy temporal muscle

Spiders, paper-money skin

Atrophy shoulder muscles

Sparse body hair

Gynecomastia

Undernutrition

Abnormal liver size

Splenomegaly

Increased xiphoid-umbilical distance

Distended abdomen (ascites)

Distended abdominal veins

Pruritis

Testicular atrophy

Palmar erythema

Jaundice

Edema

- Hypoglycemia
- Subdural hematoma (due to falls)
- Rib and extremity fractures (due to falls)

Keep in mind that conditions such as subdural hematomas, sepsis, and other life-threatening disease processes may mimic the signs and symptoms of alcohol intoxication. For example, diabetic ketoacidosis produces a breath odor that can easily be confused with the odor of alcohol.

Withdrawal Syndrome

The alcoholic may suffer a withdrawal reaction from either abrupt discontinuation of ingestion after prolonged use or from a rapid fall in blood-alcohol level after acute intoxication. Alcohol withdrawal can be potentially fatal. Withdrawal symptoms can occur several hours after sudden abstinence and can last up to 5 to 7 days. Seizures (sometimes called "rum fits") may occur within the first 24–36 hours of abstinence. **Delirium tremens (DTs)** usually develops on the second or third day of the withdrawal. Delirium tremens is characterized by a decreased level of consciousness during which the patient hallucinates and misinterprets nearby events. Seizures and delirium tremens are ominous signs. There is a significant mortality from delirium tremens. Medical direction may order diazepam in severe cases.

Conditions such as subdural hematomas, sepsis, and other diseases may mimic signs and symptoms of alcohol intoxication. For example, ketoacidosis produces an odor similar to alcohol on the breath.

✱ **delirium tremens (DTs)** disorder found in habitual and excessive users of alcoholic beverages after cessation of drinking for 48–72 hours. Patients experience visual, tactile, and auditory disturbances. Death may result in severe cases.

Signs and Symptoms Signs and symptoms of withdrawal syndrome include:

- Coarse tremor of hands, tongue, and eyelids
- Nausea and vomiting
- General weakness
- Increased sympathetic tone
- Tachycardia
- Sweating
- Hypertension
- Orthostatic hypotension
- Anxiety
- Irritability or a depressed mood
- Hallucinations
- Poor sleep

Do not underestimate alcohol intoxication as a toxic emergency.

Management Alcohol intoxication, whether acute or chronic, should not be underestimated as a toxic emergency problem. In cases of suspected alcohol abuse, take the following steps.

- Establish and maintain the airway.
- Determine if other drugs are involved.
- Start an IV using lactated Ringer's or normal saline.
- Chemstrip and administer 25 g of D50W if hypoglycemic.
- Administer 100 mg of thiamine intravenously or intramuscularly.
- Maintain a sympathetic attitude and reassure the patient of help.
- Transport to the emergency department for further care.

SUMMARY

Clearly, there is much to remember when dealing with toxicological emergencies. To effectively manage these situations you must focus on three things.

- *Recognize the poisoning promptly.* In other words, you must have a high index of suspicion when circumstances suggest a toxin may be involved.
- *Be thorough in your initial assessment and evaluation of the patient.* This will facilitate your efforts to identify the toxin and the measures needed to control the situation.
- *Initiate the standard treatment procedures required for all toxicological emergencies.* Beyond the usual concern for rescuer safety and rapid implementation of ABCs and supportive measures, consider the methods needed to minimize any further exposure to the toxin, decontaminate the patient from the toxins already involved, and finally administer any useful antidote if one exists for the particular toxin.

If you remember these three steps, you will be equipped to handle most toxicological emergencies promptly and efficiently.

YOU MAKE THE CALL

It is a beautiful sunny day in south Oshawa, where you and your partner Amit Shaw are polishing up your truck, Medic 24. A call comes in from central dispatch, sending you to 1502 Tom Sawyer Lane, the home of local pest-control guru Robert Walsh and his wife Leslie. As you pull into the driveway, Leslie is standing in front of the garage and motions you to come quickly. She informs you that her husband is very ill. He was packaging some of the new chemicals for work when he dropped the bottle onto the floor of the garage spilling it everywhere.

When you look into the garage, you see Rob sitting on a chair looking sweaty and weak and he is having some difficulty breathing. He has vomited twice. There is a strong, vaguely familiar odor (like the last time you sprayed your lawn for bugs) emanating from a big puddle in the back of the garage. As you complete your scene size-up, it becomes clear that quick intervention is needed. You spring into action.

1. What class of toxin are you dealing with?
2. What toxidrome (including signs and symptoms) will you expect to find when you make a further assessment of the patient?
3. What are your priorities in managing this situation?
4. Beyond standard supportive measures, what other intervention will help treat this patient?

See Suggested Responses at the back of this book.

FURTHER READING

Auerbach, Paul S., ed. *Wilderness Medicine: Mangement of Wilderness and Environmental Emergencies*, 3rd edition. St. Louis: Mosby Year Book, 1995.

Bledsoe, Bryan E., Dwayne Clayden, and Frank J. Papa. *Prehospital Emergency Pharmacology*, 4th ed. Upper Saddle River, NJ: Brady/Prentice Hall, 1996.

Braunwald, Fauci, et. al., eds. *Harrison's Principles of Internal Medicine Companion Handbook*, 14th ed. New York, NY: McGraw-Hill, 1999.

Cecil, Russel L., et. al. *Cecil Essentials of Medicine*, 4th ed. Philadelphia, PA: W.B. Saunders, 1997.

Goldfrank, Lewis R., ed. and Neal E. Flamenbau (contributor). *Goldfink's Toxicologic Emergencies*, 6th ed. New York: McGraw Hill, 1998.

Hantsch, Christina E., Donna L. Seger, and Tim Meredith. "New Thinking on Gastrointestinal Decontamination." *Pediatric Emergency Medicine Reports* (February 1998).

Mueller, P.D. and W.S. Korey. "Death by Ecstasy." *Annals of Emergency Medicine*. 32, No. 3 (September 1998).

Tintinalli, Judith E., et. al., eds. *Emergency Medicine: A Comprehensive Study Guide*, 5th ed. New York, NY: McGraw-Hill, 1999.

ON THE WEB

Visit Brady's Paramedic Website at www.bradybooks.com/paramedic.

CHAPTER 9

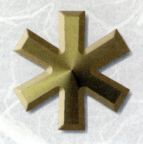

Hematology

Objectives

After reading this chapter, you should be able to:

1. Identify the anatomy and physiology of the hematopoietic system. (pp. 473–486)
2. Describe normal red blood cell (RBC) production, function, and destruction. (pp. 474–476)
3. Explain the significance of the hematocrit with respect to red cell size and number. (p. 476)
4. Explain the correlation of the RBC count, hematocrit, and hemoglobin values. (p. 476)
5. Identify the characteristics of the inflammatory process. (p. 480)
6. Identify the difference between cellular and humoral immunity. (pp. 479–480)
7. Identify alterations in immunologic response. (p. 480)
8. Describe the number, normal function, types and life span of leukocytes, platelets, white blood cells, and red blood cells. (pp. 473–481)

Continued

9. List the leukocyte disorders. (pp. 495–496)
10. Describe the components of the hemostatic mechanism. (pp. 481–483)
11. Describe the intrinsic and extrinsic clotting systems and the function of coagulation factors, platelets, and blood vessels necessary for normal coagulation. (pp. 481–483)
12. Identify blood groups. (pp. 484–485)
13. Describe how acquired factor deficiencies may occur. (pp. 497–498)
14. Define fibrinolysis. (p. 482)
15. Identify the components of physical assessment as they relate to the hematology system. (pp. 486–491)

16. Describe the pathology and clinical manifestations and prognosis associated with:
    - Anemia (pp. 492–493)
    - Leukemia (pp. 495–496)
    - Lymphomas (p. 496)
    - Polycythemia (p. 494)
    - Disseminated intravascular coagulopathy (p. 499)
    - Hemophilia (pp. 497–498)
    - Sickle cell disease (pp. 493–494)
    - Multiple myeloma (p. 499)
17. Given several preprogrammed patients with hematological problems, provide the appropriate assessment, management, and transport. (pp. 472–499)

CASE STUDY

Medic 102 responds to the scene of what appears to be a minor fall down three steps at a local shopping mall. The patient, a 36-year-old male, is at the base of the stairs, complaining of pain and swelling of the right knee and right flank. He is difficult to get a clear history from and appears somewhat confused.

The initial assessment reveals a very thin patient who states his name is C.J. He is alert to name only and is confused as to how he came to be on the floor. He is tachypneic and tachycardic, with a weakly palpable radial pulse and obvious profuse diaphoresis. As C.J. appears shocky and complains of back pain, Christian and Victoria, the responding paramedics, immediately place him supine and logroll him on to a backboard. While they are logrolling C.J., Christian and Victoria note a large area of ecchymosis on his right flank. They initiate an IV of normal saline and administer a fluid bolus. They begin high-flow oxygen therapy with a nonrebreather face mask.

After they quickly place C.J. in the squad, Christian initiates rapid transport while Victoria performs a more complete assessment. Additional findings include a large joint effusion of the right knee and a medic alert tag on a wrist bracelet that reads "Hemophilia A." C.J. is responding to the

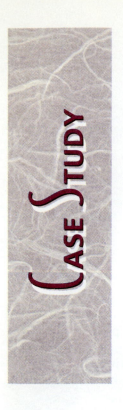

fluid bolus and oxygen and is becoming less confused. Vital signs reflect a blood pressure of 90/60, a pulse of 120, and respirations of 24. Victoria applies a splint to C.J.'s right knee and calls in to medical direction at Southside Medical Center. She alerts them that they are transporting a patient with hemophilia A and a probable hemarthrosis and retroperitoneal hematoma from a fall. In anticipation of the patient's arrival, the emergency physician alerts the hospital pharmacy to send Factor VIII to the department. In addition, he alerts the trauma team. The transport is uneventful and the paramedics of Medic 102 turn C.J. over to the emergency department team. It seems that C.J. is well known to the emergency department staff because of his illness. They quickly begin therapy with Factor VIII and administer intravenous fluids and packed red blood cells. The emergency physician performs an arthrocentesis of the right knee, primarily to help with pain. He removes 160 ml of blood from the knee. The patient is stabilized in the emergency department and then admitted to the medical floor for additional therapy.

INTRODUCTION

✱ **hematology** the study of blood and the blood-forming organs.

Hematology is the study of the blood and the blood-forming organs. It exemplifies the way that multiple organ systems interact to maintain homeostasis, the normal balance of body functions. Hematological disorders are common and include red blood cell disorders, white blood cell disorders, platelet disorders, and coagulation problems. Although these disorders are common, they rarely are the primary cause of a medical emergency. They usually accompany other ongoing disease processes. Some hematological diseases are genetic in origin. Hemophilia A is a classic example. It is a sex-linked disease that causes abnormally low levels of an essential blood clotting protein (Factor VIII). It affects approximately 1–2 persons per 10,000 in the United States. Some hematological diseases are more common in certain ethnic groups. For example, among the population as a whole, sickle cell anemia is relatively uncommon. However, among African-Americans specifically, 8 percent of the population has sickle cell trait. In addition to their primary effects, hematological disorders may predispose patients to infection and intolerance to exercise, hypoxia, acidosis, and blood loss.

Patients with hematological problems often complain of signs and symptoms that do not point directly to a specific disease process. Careful examination and history taking may be necessary to further clarify the diagnosis. Often, however, laboratory findings will be needed to confirm the diagnosis. Thus, the final diagnosis of patients for whom you provide prehospital care is often not immediately apparent. You must use your assessment skills to recognize and treat injuries, pain, and instabilities, while formulating a field impression that enables you to anticipate further complications and thus enhance patient outcome and survivability. Because of this, it is essential that you have a good understanding of the basic pathophysiological processes of your patients' disease, including hematological disorders.

ANATOMY, PHYSIOLOGY, AND PATHOPHYSIOLOGY

The hematopoietic system consists of blood (both cells and plasma), bone marrow, the liver, the spleen, and the kidneys. The cellular components of blood are formed by the differentiation of a **pluripotent stem cell** in a process termed **hematopoiesis.** In the fetus, hematopoiesis occurs first outside of the bone marrow *(extramedullary hematopoiesis)* in the liver, spleen, lymph nodes, and thymus. By the fourth month, the developing bone marrow begins to produce blood cells *(intramedullary hematopoiesis)*. After birth, the bone marrow is the primary site of blood cell production and extramedullary hematopoiesis greatly diminishes, occurring mostly in the liver and spleen. By adulthood, hematopoiesis occurs exclusively in the bone marrow unless a pathological state exists.

In hematopoiesis, the stem cell reproduces to maintain a constant population of cells. Some stem cells then further differentiate into myeloid *multipotent* stem cells that, in turn, differentiate into unipotent progenitors. These unipotent progenitors ultimately mature into basophils, eosinophils, neutrophils, monocytes (types of white blood cells), erythrocytes (red blood cells), and thrombocytes (platelets.) Pluripotent stem cells may also differentiate into common lymphoid stem cells that ultimately mature into lymphocytes (another type of white cell). The kidney, and to a lesser extent the liver, produce **erythropoietin,** the hormone responsible for red blood cell production. The liver also removes toxins from the blood and produces many of the clotting factors and proteins in plasma. The spleen, an important part of the immune system, has cells that scavenge abnormal blood cells and bacteria.

Blood volume normally remains relatively constant at about six percent of total body weight. With an average of 80–85 milliliters of blood per kilogram of body weight, a person who weighs 75 kilograms has approximately 6 liters of blood. The body can easily handle up to about one-half liter of lost blood or fluid. An example is routine blood donations where healthy donors tolerate the blood loss without complication.

The major determinants of the blood volume are red cell mass and plasma volume. Red blood cells remain confined to the intravascular compartment. If their destruction remains constant, then only changes in the rate of production can alter the size of the circulating red cell mass. The plasma volume on the other hand can rapidly change due to fluid shifts between the intravascular and extravascular space. These fluid shifts help to preserve circulating blood volume in the event of acute hemorrhage. Other compensatory mechanisms include vasoconstriction, tachycardia, and increased cardiac contractility to maintain adequate tissue perfusion until significant losses overwhelm these measures. When these compensatory measures fail, the patient enters decompensated shock. Fortunately, young healthy individuals' bodies can compensate for loss of as much as 25–30 percent of blood volume.

COMPONENTS OF BLOOD

Blood consists of liquid, or plasma, and of formed elements—red blood cells, white blood cells, and platelets.

Plasma

Plasma is a thick, pale yellow fluid that is 90–92 percent water and 6–7 percent proteins. Fats, carbohydrates, electrolytes, gases, and certain chemical messengers comprise the remaining 2–3 percent. Plasma transports the cellular components of blood and dissolved nutrients throughout the body and, at the same

Content Review

HEMATOPOIETIC SYSTEM COMPONENTS
- Blood
- Bone marrow
- Liver
- Spleen
- Kidneys

✱ **pluripotent stem cell** a cell from which the various types of blood cells can form.

✱ **hematopoiesis** the process through which pluripotent stem cells differentiate into various types of blood cells.

✱ **erythropoietin** the hormone responsible for red blood cell production.

Content Review

COMPONENTS OF BLOOD
- Plasma
- Formed elements
—Red blood cells
—White blood cells
—Platelets

✱ **plasma** thick, pale yellow fluid that makes up the liquid part of the blood.

time, transports waste products from cellular metabolism to the liver, kidneys, and lungs, where they can be removed from the body.

Most plasma components can move back and forth across the capillary membranes to the interstitial fluid. However, plasma proteins, such as albumin, are large molecules and have great difficulty diffusing across the membranes. This is fortunate, since they remain in the plasma to help retain water in the capillaries. This is known as *osmotic pull,* or *oncotic pressure.* Plasma proteins perform many other functions, including clotting of blood, dismantling of clots, buffering of the blood's acid/base balance, transporting hormones and regulating their effects, and providing a source of energy.

Electrolytes are also found in the plasma. These are chemical substances that dissociate into charged particles in water. They are essential for nerve conduction, muscle contraction, and water balance. They can easily diffuse across capillary membranes based on their concentration gradients. Carbohydrates in plasma are generally in the form of glucose, the primary energy source for all body tissues. Glucose is especially important to brain cells as they cannot obtain energy from fat metabolism. (As you learned in Chapter 4, glucose cannot diffuse across most cell membranes without assistance from the hormone insulin.) Plasma also performs a role in gas transport. In addition to being carried by red blood cells, carbon dioxide and oxygen are dissolved and transported in plasma.

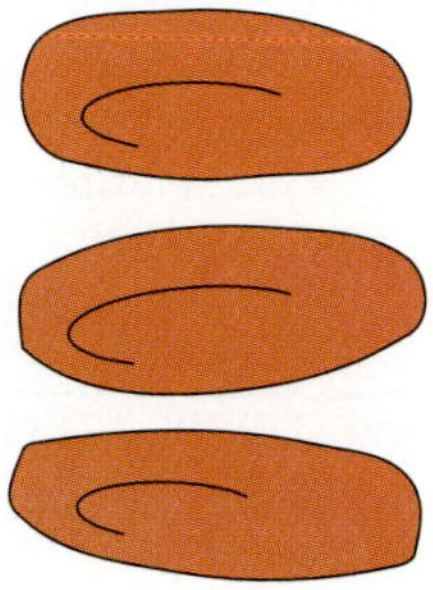

Red Blood Cells

The primary function of blood is to transport oxygen from the lungs to the tissues. At rest, the body consumes about 4 ml of oxygen per kilogram of body weight every minute. Because it stores little oxygen, the body would quickly succumb to anoxia without the continued transport provided by the blood.

The red blood cell (RBC), or **erythrocyte,** is a biconcave disc that does not have a nucleus when mature (Figure 9-1). It contains **hemoglobin** molecules that transport oxygen. Hemoglobin comprises four subunits of *globin,* each bonded to a *heme* (iron containing) molecule. Each globin subunit can bind with one oxygen molecule; thus, each complete hemoglobin molecule can carry up to four oxygen molecules. When all four subunits are carrying an oxygen molecule, the hemoglobin is 100 percent saturated. When fully saturated, each gram of hemoglobin can transport 1.34 milliliters of oxygen.

Oxygen Transport The effectiveness of oxygen transport depends on many factors. Red blood cell mass (the number of red blood cells present) is obviously a factor in oxygen transport. The greater the number of red blood cells, the greater will be the potential oxygen carrying capacity. The percentage of oxygen bound to hemoglobin increases as the pO_2 increases. This is illustrated in the oxygen-hemoglobin dissociation curve (Figure 9-2). Normal pO_2 is approximately 95 mmHg. Based on this, the oxygen-hemoglobin dissociation curve indicates that normal oxygen saturation is about 97 percent. Hemoglobin's affinity for oxygen is also a factor in oxygen transport. Several factors affect oxygen affinity, including pH, pCO_2, concentration of 2,3-DPG, and temperature.

The lower the pH (that is, the more acidic the blood), the more readily hemoglobin will release oxygen. This shifts the oxygen-hemoglobin dissociation curve to the right. In contrast, alkalosis makes hemoglobin bind to oxygen more tightly. This shifts the oxygen-hemoglobin dissociation curve to the left (Figure 9-3). The pCO_2 is directly related to the pH. Thus, in the lungs, as pCO_2 decreases with diffusion of CO_2 into the alveoli, the quantity of oxygen that binds with the hemoglobin increases. The opposite effect occurs when the blood reaches the tissues. There, waste CO_2 from the tissues diffuses into the blood, causing the hemoglobin to give up more oxygen to the tissues. This is called the **Bohr effect.**

Red blood cells

FIGURE 9-1   Red blood cells.

* **erythrocyte** red blood cell.

* **hemoglobin** oxygen-bearing molecule in the red blood cells. It is made up of iron-rich red pigment called *heme* and a protein called *globin.*

* **Bohr effect** phenomenon in which a decrease in pCO_2/acidity causes an increase in the quantity of oxygen that binds with the hemoglobin and, conversely, an increase in pCO_2/acidity causes the hemoglobin to give up a greater quantity of oxygen.

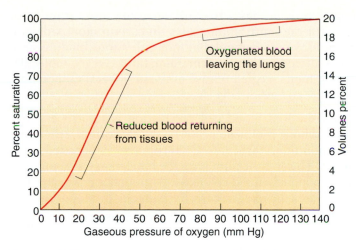

FIGURE 9-2   The oxygen-hemoglobin dissociation curve.

Except for hemoglobin, the most abundant chemical in red blood cells is **2,3-diphosphoglycerate (2,3-DPG)**. During prolonged periods of hypoxia, the level of 2,3-DPG increases. This shifts the oxygen-hemoglobin dissociation curve to the right and can increase the pO_2 in the plasma as much as 10 percent more than it otherwise would have been. However, the increased 2,3-DPG makes it more difficult for oxygen to combine with hemoglobin in the lungs. This effect casts doubt on whether 2,3-DPG's effect in hypoxia is as beneficial as was once thought.

An elevation in the body temperature causes a shift to the right of the oxygen-hemoglobin dissociation curve and a decrease in hemoglobin's affinity for blood. Conversely, a fall in body temperature causes hemoglobin to bind oxygen more tightly. During periods of hyperthermia and pyrexia (fever), hemoglobin's decreased affinity for oxygen enhances oxygenation of the peripheral tissues and end organs.

Exercise has several effects on oxygen affinity. First, exercise causes the production and release of carbon dioxide and other acids, especially from the large muscles. It also increases body temperature. Thus, both a decrease in pH and an increase in body temperature will cause hemoglobin to release oxygen more readily. This serves to enhance peripheral tissue oxygenation during strenuous exercise and work.

Importantly, other substances can compete with oxygen for hemoglobin's binding sites. The greater a substance's affinity for the binding sites, the more readily the substance will bind with hemoglobin. The classic example is carbon

✱ **2,3-diphosphoglycerate (2,3-DPG)** chemical in the red blood cells that affects hemoglobin's affinity for oxygen.

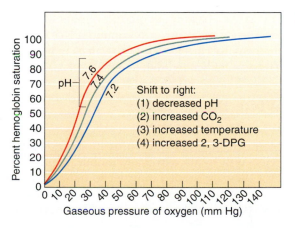

FIGURE 9-3   Effects of pH, increased carbon dioxide, temperature, and 2,3-DPG on the oxygen-hemoglobin dissociation curve.

monoxide (CO). Carbon monoxide has 210–250 times oxygen's affinity for hemoglobin and competes for the same binding sites. In carbon monoxide poisoning, when CO binds to one of the hemoglobin molecule's four binding sites, the hemoglobin molecule is altered so that the remaining three oxygen molecules are held more tightly. This inhibits oxygen release in the peripheral tissues, contributing to hypoxia, acidosis, and eventually shock.

Red Blood Cell Production Red blood cell production is termed **erythropoiesis.** Erythropoietin, a hormone produced primarily by the kidney, stimulates the bone marrow's production of erythrocytes. Erythropoietin is secreted when the renal cells sense hypoxia. This in turn stimulates the bone marrow to increase RBC production, resulting in increased red cell mass. Although a relatively slow process, this effectively increases the oxygen carrying capacity of blood, thereby increasing oxygen delivery to the tissues.

The red blood cell lives approximately 120 days. Hemorrhage, **hemolysis** (destruction of the RBC), or **sequestration** of the RBCs by the liver or spleen may significantly reduce its life span. Hemorrhage may occur outside the body or be hidden within a body cavity such as the peritoneum, retroperitoneum, or GI tract. Hemolysis may occur within the circulatory system in sickle cell disease and in rare autoimmune anemias. The spleen and liver contain specialized scavenger cells called macrophages (a type of white blood cell) that can remove damaged or abnormal red blood cells from the circulation.

Laboratory Evaluation of Red Blood Cells and Hemoglobin Red blood cells (RBCs) are quantified or measured and reported in two ways: red blood cell count and hematocrit. The red blood cell count is the total number of RBCs reported in millions per cubic millimeter (mm^3) of blood. Normal values vary with age and sex but in general run between 4.2 and 6.0 million/mm^3. The **hematocrit** is the packed cell volume of red blood cells per unit of blood (Figure 9-4). This measurement is obtained by placing a sample of blood in a centrifuge and spinning it at high speed so that the cellular elements separate from the plasma. The red blood cells are the heaviest blood component since they carry the iron-containing pigment hemoglobin. They are forced to the bottom of the tube. Above the red blood cells are the white blood cells. On the top of the specimen is the plasma, which consists primarily of water. The RBCs' column height is divided by the blood's total column height (cellular component plus plasma) and reported as a percentage. Normal values range between 40 and 52 percent, with females generally running a few percentage points below males.

Another way to determine the status of the red blood cell is to measure the concentration of hemoglobin present. This is typically expressed as the number of grams of hemoglobin present per deciliter of whole blood. The hemoglobin concentration will decrease in two ways. First, when the number of red blood cells present is below normal, the hemoglobin will also be below normal. In some cases, the red blood cell volume can be normal, but the amount of hemoglobin present may be decreased. In emergency medicine, it is commonplace to measure the hemoglobin in addition to the hematocrit (H&H). Both values indicate red blood cell volume and capability. The normal hemoglobin in a man is 12.0–15.0 g/dl; for females, it is 10.5–14.0 g/dl.

White Blood Cells

White blood cells, called **leukocytes** or white corpuscles, circulate through the bloodstream and tissues, providing protection from foreign invasion. White blood cells (WBCs) are extremely mobile, traveling through the blood stream to wherever they are needed in order to fight infection. A large population of leukocytes does not move freely within the blood stream but instead is attached to the blood vessels' walls. These *marginated* leukocytes may quickly return to the circulating

✱ erythropoiesis the process of producing red blood cells.

✱ hemolysis destruction of red blood cells.

✱ sequestration the trapping of red blood cells by an organ such as the spleen.

✱ hematocrit the packed cell volume of red blood cells per unit of blood.

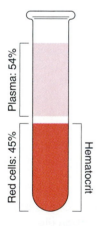

FIGURE 9-4 Hematocrit, including plasma.

✱ leukocyte white blood cell.

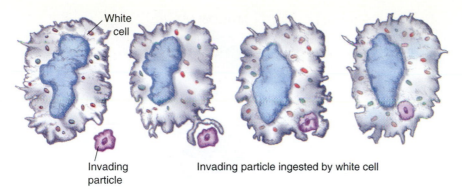

White cell

Invading particle

Invading particle ingested by white cell

FIGURE 9-5   White blood cells engulfing and destroying an invader in the process called phagocytosis.

pool in response to stress, corticosteroids, seizures, epinephrine, and exercise. This process is called *demargination*. Marginated leukocytes that attach more firmly to the vascular lining through *adhesion* may then leave the blood vessels by *diapedesis*. This enables the leukocytes to squeeze between the cells lining the blood vessels and to follow chemical signals (**chemotaxis**) to the infection site. There, they may engulf and destroy an invader by **phagocytosis** (Figure 9-5). Others stimulate either chemical or immune responses to fight infection.

Healthy people have from 5,000 to 9,000 white blood cells per microliter of blood. An infection can increase that number to more than 16,000. An increase in the white blood cell number is a classic sign of bacterial infection. White blood cells originate in the bone marrow from undifferentiated stem cells. Through a process termed **leukopoiesis,** these stem cells respond to specific growth factors that allow them to differentiate into three main -blasts (immature forms): *myeloblasts, monoblasts,* and *lymphoblasts.*

White blood cells are categorized as *granulocytes, monocytes,* or *lymphocytes* (Figure 9-6).

* **chemotaxis** the movement of white blood cells in response to chemical signals.

* **phagocytosis** process in which white blood cells engulf and destroy an invader.

* **leukopoiesis** the process through which stem cells differentiate into the white blood cells' immature forms.

Content Review

WHITE BLOOD CELL -BLASTS

- Myeloblasts
- Monoblasts
- Lymphoblasts

Content Review

WHITE BLOOD CELL CATEGORIES

- Granulocytes
- Monocytes
- Lymphocytes

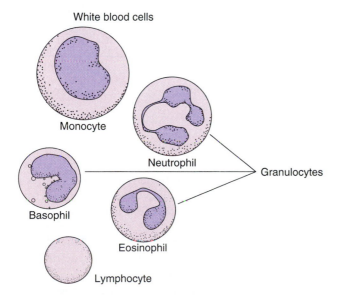

White blood cells

Monocyte

Neutrophil

Basophil

Eosinophil

Granulocytes

Lymphocyte

FIGURE 9-6   Types of white blood cells.

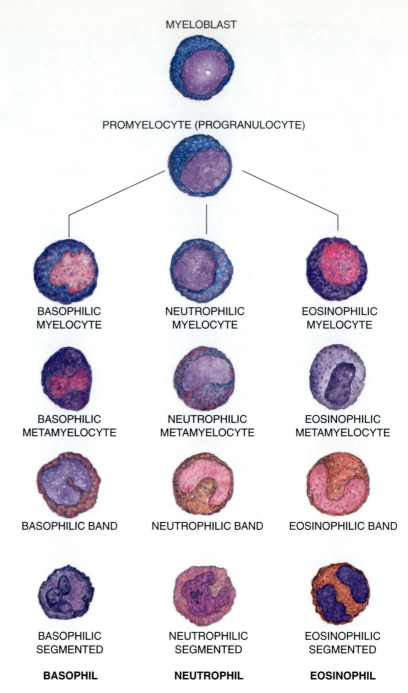

MYELOBLAST

PROMYELOCYTE (PROGRANULOCYTE)

BASOPHILIC MYELOCYTE	NEUTROPHILIC MYELOCYTE	EOSINOPHILIC MYELOCYTE
BASOPHILIC METAMYELOCYTE	NEUTROPHILIC METAMYELOCYTE	EOSINOPHILIC METAMYELOCYTE
BASOPHILIC BAND	NEUTROPHILIC BAND	EOSINOPHILIC BAND
BASOPHILIC SEGMENTED	NEUTROPHILIC SEGMENTED	EOSINOPHILIC SEGMENTED
BASOPHIL	**NEUTROPHIL**	**EOSINOPHIL**

FIGURE 9-7   Granulocyte maturation.

Granulocytes Granulocytic white blood cells, so named for the granules they contain, form from stem cells that differentiate in the bone marrow in response to hormonal stimulation. These cells mature through several stages from myeloblast to promyelocyte, myelocyte, metamyelocyte, band form, and mature form (Figure 9-7). Their mature forms are classified by the type of stain they absorb. *Basophils* absorb basic stains and have blue granules. *Eosinophils* absorb acidic stains and contain red granules. *Neutrophils* absorb neither acidic nor basic stains well and contain pale blue and pink granules.

Basophils   Basophils are granulocytes that primarily function in allergic reactions. Within their granules they store all of the histamine in the circulating blood. In response to an allergic stimulus, the cells degranulate, releasing histamines that cause vasodilation, bronchoconstriction, rhinorrhea, increased vascular permeability, and increased neutrophil and eosinophil chemotaxis. Basophils also contain heparin, which breaks down blood clots.

Eosinophils Eosinophils are highly specialized members of the granulocytic series. They can inactivate the chemical mediators of acute allergic reactions, thereby modulating the anaphylactic response. They also contain **major basic protein (MBP)**, which they release in conjunction with an antibody response shown to fight parasitic infections.

Neutrophils The neutrophils' primary function is to fight infection. They leave the blood stream by diapedesis and engulf and kill microorganisms that have invaded the body. Once they have phagocytized the microorganism, primary and secondary granules within the neutrophil fuse with the phagosome, and the organism is killed and digested. In severe infections the total neutrophil count may rise rapidly, with immature (band) forms apparent on the peripheral blood smear under microscopic examination. If the neutrophil count is low (**neutropenia**), the body cannot mount an appropriate response to infection, and the infection may overwhelm the body's defenses and kill the individual. Neutropenia may result from primary bone marrow disorders that decrease production, from overwhelming infection, viral syndrome, autoimmune disease, or drugs, and from nutritional deficiencies.

Monocytes Monocytes are unique in that after their initial phase of maturation they are released into the circulation and can remain there as circulating monocytes or migrate to distant sites to further mature into free or fixed tissue macrophages. Macrophages, the "garbage collectors" of the immune system, engulf both foreign invaders and dead neutrophils. They also can attack tumor cells and participate in tissue repair. Monocytes and macrophages also secrete growth factors to stimulate production of granulocytes and red blood cells. Some macrophages are fixed within tissues, residing in the liver, spleen, lungs, and lymphatic system. These cells are part of the reticuloendothelial system. They remove foreign matter, cellular debris, and proteins from the blood. After engulfing foreign proteins or infectious agents, these fixed macrophages of the reticuloendothelial system can stimulate lymphocyte production in an immune response against these agents.

Lymphocytes Lymphocytes are the primary cells involved in the body's immune response. They are located throughout the body in the circulating blood as well as in other tissues such as lymph nodes, circulating in lymph fluid, bone marrow, spleen, liver, lungs, intestine, and skin. Lymphocytes are characteristically small, round, white blood cells containing no granules on staining. However similar they may appear, these cells are highly specialized. They contain surface receptor sites specific to a single antigen (foreign protein) and stand ready to initiate the immune response to rid the body of that particular substance or infectious agent.

Immunity The two basic subpopulations of lymphocytes are T cells and B cells. T cells mature in the thymus gland, located in the mediastinum, and then migrate throughout the body. They are responsible for developing *cell-mediated*, or *cellular, immunity*. Once an antigen activates them, they generate other cells called effector cells that are responsible for delayed-type hypersensitivity reactions, tumor suppression, graft rejection (organ transplant rejections), and defense against intracellular organisms. B cells produce antibodies to combat infection, which is termed *humoral immunity*. They originate in the bone marrow and then migrate to peripheral lymphatic tissues. There they can be exposed to antigens from invading organisms and respond by producing the specific antibodies necessary to defend against them. Some

* **major basic protein (MBP)** a larvacidal peptide.

* **neutropenia** a low neutrophil count.

of these B cells' lines are maintained and give the body a "memory" of the previous infection. When the body is subsequently exposed to the same antigen or infection, it generates a rapid response to quickly overwhelm the infection (Volume 3, Chapter 11).

Autoimmune Disease Autoimmune disease occurs when the body makes antibodies against its own tissues. These antibodies may be limited to specific organs, such as the thyroid, as occurs in *Hashimoto's thyroiditis*. Or, they may involve virtually every tissue type as in the antinuclear antibodies of *systemic lupus erythematosis (SLE)* that attack the body's cell nuclei. Several anemias result from autoimmunity and will be discussed later in this chapter. Mechanisms for the development of autoimmune disease include genetic factors and viral infections.

Alterations in Immune Response Several factors can alter the body's immune response. For example, patients who receive an organ transplant must take drugs that inhibit cellular immunity and prevent graft rejection. If they do not, the T cells will recognize the new organ as "not self" and begin the process of attacking it. This is called rejection. Unfortunately, organ recipient immunosuppressed patients are at risk for infections from many different organisms including bacteria, viruses, fungi, and protozoa. Human immunodeficiency virus (HIV) effectively destroys cell-mediated immunity by selectively attacking and ultimately killing T cells. This also leaves the patient at risk for opportunistic infections against which the body cannot defend itself, ultimately killing him. Patients who have cancer are often immunocompromised by the disease itself or by chemotherapy agents that also attack the bone marrow. These agents decrease leukocyte production to extremely low levels, leaving the body defenseless against infection. As a paramedic, you must protect your immunosuppressed patients from undue exposure to infection by good hand-washing technique, correct IV technique, and proper wound care. If you have an infection, you must take precautions not to transmit it to your patients. If the infection is highly contagious, as in influenza or chicken pox, you may have to work in a non-patient-care setting.

Inflammatory Process The **inflammatory process** is a nonspecific defense mechanism that wards off damage from microorganisms or trauma. It attempts to localize the damage while destroying the source, at the same time facilitating repair of the tissues. Causes of the inflammatory process may be an infectious agent, trauma, chemical, or immunologic. After local tissue injury occurs, the damaged tissues release chemical messengers that attract white blood cells (chemotaxis), increase capillary permeability, and cause vasodilation. If bacteria are present, responding neutrophils or macrophages will phagocytize them and tissue repair begins. The greater capillary permeability and vasodilation allows increased blood flow to the area and enables fluid to leak out of the capillaries. The process of local inflammation results in redness, warmth, swelling, and usually pain. The pain serves as a reminder against overuse, allowing time for rest and repair. Systemic inflammation is an inflammatory reaction, often in response to a bacterial infection. Fever is a common symptom and likely occurs in response to chemical mediators that macrophages release in response to the infectious agent. These chemical mediators act on the brain and lead to stimulation of the sympathetic nervous system, which causes vasoconstriction, heat conservation, and fever. The macrophages also release factors that stimulate the release of leukocytes from the bone marrow, leading to an elevated white blood cell count.

Platelets

Platelets, or **thrombocytes**, are small fragments of large cells called *megakary-ocytes*. Like the other blood cells described so far, megakaryocytes come from an undifferentiated stem cell in the bone marrow. The hormone *thrombopoi-etin* stimulates these stem cells to differentiate through several stages into megakaryocytes, which then mature and break up into platelets, small frag-ments without nuclei. The normal number of platelets ranges from 150,000 to 450,000 per microliter of blood. As they function to form a plug at an initial bleeding site and also secrete factors important in clot formation, too few platelets, a condition called *thrombocytopenia*, can lead to bleeding problems and blood loss. Too many platelets, *thrombocytosis*, may cause abnormal clot-ting, plugs in vessels, and emboli that may travel to the extremities, heart, lungs, or brain. Platelets survive from seven to ten days and are removed from circulation by the spleen.

Platelets are activated when they contact injured tissue. This contact stimu-lates an enzyme within the platelet, causing the surface to become "sticky," which in turn leads the platelets to aggregate and form a plug. Platelets also ad-here to the damaged tissue to keep the plug in place. As the platelets aggregate, they release chemical messengers that also activate the blood clotting system.

HEMOSTASIS

Hemostasis—from *hemo* (blood) and *stasis* (standing still)—is the term used to describe the combined three mechanisms that work to prevent or control blood loss. These mechanisms include:

- Vascular spasms
- Platelet plugs
- Stable fibrin blood clots (coagulation)

When a blood vessel tears, the smooth muscle fibers (*tunica media*) in the ves-sel walls contract. This causes vasoconstriction and reduces the size of the tear. Less blood flows through the constricted area, effectively limiting blood loss, and the smaller tear makes it easier for a platelet plug to develop and stop blood loss. At any tear in a blood vessel, platelets aggregate and adhere to collagen, a connective tissue that supports the blood vessels. This forms a platelet plug, which acts much like bubble gum stuck into a hole. The plug is unstable, how-ever, and would permit the vessel to bleed again if not for the formation of a sta-ble fibrin clot. This process, blood coagulation, is initiated in part by the platelet plug (Figure 9-8).

Due to the smoothness of the *tunica intima*, the blood vessels' innermost lining, blood normally flows through the vessels without frictional damage to cells or platelets. Damage to cells or to the vessel lining, however, starts the coagulation cascade. This cascade, or sequence of events, can be activated ei-ther by damage to vessels (extrinsic pathway) or by trauma to blood from tur-bulence (intrinsic pathway). Either results in the cascade's progression to a clot. Most clotting proteins are produced in the liver and circulate in an inac-tive state. The best known of these are *prothrombin* and *fibrinogen*. The dam-aged cells send out a chemical message that activates a specific clotting factor. This activates each protein in turn, until a stable fibrin clot forms. To com-pletely stop the bleeding, the coagulation cascade relies on the platelet plug

✴ thrombocyte blood platelet.

✴ hemostasis the combined three mechanisms that work to pre-vent or control blood loss.

FIGURE 9-8   Clot formation.

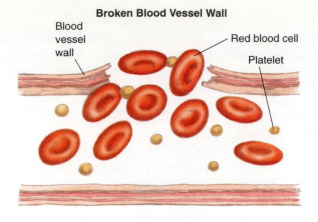

Broken Blood Vessel Wall

Blood
vessel
wall

Red blood cell

Platelet

Clot Formation

Fibrin

Activated platelet

and the clotting factors to interact. Once the bleeding stops, the inflammatory and healing processes can begin. The coagulation cascade can be summarized thus (See Figure 9-9):

1. a. *Intrinsic pathway.* Platelets release substances that lead to the formation of prothrombin activator

or

   b. *Extrinsic pathway.* Tissue damage causes platelet aggregation and the formation of prothrombin activator.
2. *Common pathway.* The prothrombin activator, in the presence of calcium, converts prothrombin to thrombin.
3. *Thrombin.* In the presence of calcium, thrombin converts fibrinogen to stable fibrin, which then traps blood cells and more platelets to form a clot.

The development of a clot does not end the coagulation cascade. What the body can do it usually can undo, given sufficient time. Once a fibrin clot is formed, it releases a chemical called *plasminogen*. Plasminogen is converted to *plasmin* and is then capable of dismantling, or lysing, a clot through the process of **fibrinolysis.** A clot's dismantling generally takes from hours to days. By that time, scarring has begun.

✱ **fibrinolysis** the process through which plasmin dismantles a blood clot.

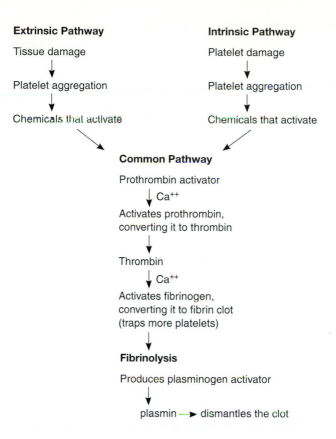

Extrinsic Pathway

Tissue damage
↓
Platelet aggregation
↓
Chemicals that activate

Intrinsic Pathway

Platelet damage
↓
Platelet aggregation
↓
Chemicals that activate

Common Pathway

Prothrombin activator
↓ Ca^{++}
Activates prothrombin, converting it to thrombin
↓
Thrombin
↓ Ca^{++}
Activates fibrinogen, converting it to fibrin clot (traps more platelets)
↓
Fibrinolysis

Produces plasminogen activator
↓
plasmin ⟶ dismantles the clot

FIGURE 9-9 The coagulation cascade.

Thrombosis (clot formation), when it occurs in coronary arteries or cerebral vasculature, may lead to heart attack and stroke. To stimulate or speed fibrinolysis and thus breakdown clots, medical researchers have developed several thrombolytic agents. These agents may help reestablish blood flow to these vital organs, limiting or preventing tissue death, and thus helping to prevent the patient's disability or death. Thrombolytics are effective only against blockages whose components include a fibrin clot.

Patients who lack certain clotting factors can have bleeding disorders that may complicate their assessment and treatment. Other patients take medications that decrease the effectiveness of platelets or the coagulation cascade. Recall that an enzyme on a platelet membrane makes the membrane sticky. Certain medications such as aspirin, dipyridamole (Persantine), and ticlopidine (Ticlid) irreversibly alter the enzyme, thus decreasing the platelets' ability to aggregate and initiate the coagulation cascade. Other medications such as heparin and warfarin (Coumadin) cause changes within the clotting cascade that prevent clot formation. Heparin, in conjunction with antithrombin III (a naturally occurring thrombin inactivator), rapidly inactivates thrombin, which then prevents formation of the fibrin clot. Warfarin (Coumadin) blocks vitamin K activity necessary to generate the activated forms of clotting factors II, VII, IX, and X, effectively interrupting the clotting cascade.

Vitamin K (AquaMEPHYTON) enhances clotting. Certain byproducts of tobacco smoking (especially in females on birth control pills) also enhance clotting. Relative or complete immobility, trauma, polycythemia (high red blood cell count), and cancer may also lead to increased clotting as blood becomes relatively stagnant. This allows platelet activation to begin, which leads to clotting. To counteract the effects of decreased activity, many patients take aspirin or other antiplatelet inhibitors and wear compressive stockings to facilitate venous drainage from the lower extremities.

✱ **thrombosis** clot formation, which is extremely dangerous when it occurs in coronary arteries or cerebral vasculature.

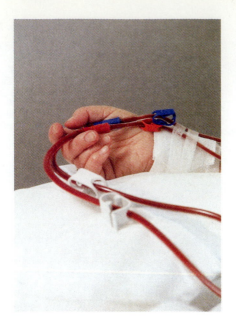

FIGURE 9-10   Blood
transfusion.

BLOOD PRODUCTS AND BLOOD TYPING

A blood transfusion is the transplantation of blood or a component of blood from one person to another. It is accomplished by IV infusion (Figure 9-10). Various types of transfusions are given for various purposes (Table 9-1).

In the 1800s when patients received blood from others, some had a reaction that led to multiple organ failure and death. Karl Landsteiner discovered the reason for this was reaction **antigens,** proteins on the surface of the donor's red blood cells that the patient's body recognized as "not self." Following transfusion, antibodies in the patient's own blood attacked the foreign antigens present in the transfused blood. Landsteiner named the antigens A and B and the opposing antibodies anti-A and anti-B. Someone with A antigen on his red blood cells would have anti-B antibodies. His blood type would be A. Someone with B antigens on the red blood cell surface would have anti-A antibodies; his type would be B. Some people's red blood cells have both antigens on their surface but neither antibody. Their blood type is AB. Others have neither antigen but both antibodies; their blood type is O (for zero antigens, but pronounced "Oh"). Blood type is an inherited trait. Approximately 45 percent of the United States population has type O, 39 percent type A, 11 percent type B, and 5 percent type AB.

Since only the antibodies recognize and attack foreign tissue, a person with no antibodies (type AB) can receive any blood type in an emergency, and the body will not attack the cells. So a person with type AB blood is called a *universal recipient.* Conversely, blood with no antigens to any other blood group type (type O) would not trigger a reaction, as the recipient's blood recognizes nothing "foreign." So people with type O blood are called *universal donors.*

Crossmatching blood involves checking samples from both donor and recipient to ensure the greatest compatibility. If a donor's blood does not clump together, or agglutinate, when mixed with the recipient's blood, they are compatible. Reliance on the universal donor and recipient concept is useful only in an emergency, when there is no time to check samples.

✱ **antigen** protein on the surface of a donor's red blood cells that the patient's body recognizes as "not self."

Content Review

BLOOD TYPES

- A
- B
- AB
- O

Table 9-1 TYPES OF TRANSFUSIONS

Type of Transfusion	Contents	Use
Whole blood	All cells, platelets, clotting factors, and plasma	Replace blood loss from hemorrhage
Packed red blood cells (PRBCs)	Red blood cells and some plasma	Replace red blood cells in anemic patients
Platelets	Thrombocytes and some plasma	Replace platelets in a patient with thrombocytopenia
Fresh frozen plasma (FFP)	Plasma, a combination of fluids, clotting factors, and proteins	Replace volume in a burn patient or in hypovolemia secondary to low oncotic pressure
Clotting factors	Specific clotting factors needed for coagulation	Replace factors missing due to inadequate production as in hemophilia

Blood transfusion is not as simple as that, however. Approximately 40 years after the discovery of A and B antigens, Landsteiner and A.S. Weiner observed another antigen present on red blood cells. Research leading to this antigen's discovery used rhesus monkey blood, so the antigen was called the Rh factor. If a person has the Rh factor, he is Rh positive; if not, he is Rh negative. As many as 500 other lesser antigens have since been identified but they usually do not cause the severe hemolytic reaction seen in the patients sensitized to the Rh factor. *Erythroblastosis fetalis,* more commonly called hemolytic disease of the newborn, can lead to a fatal hemolytic reaction in neonates. In this disease, the mother who is Rh⁻ is sensitized by previous exposure to the Rh antigen during a previous pregnancy with an Rh⁺ child or from a previous blood transfusion. Therefore, if she subsequently becomes pregnant with an Rh⁺ child, the mother produces antibodies that attack the fetus's red blood cells, leading to a severe and often fatal hemolytic reaction. Fortunately, the incidence of hemolytic disease of newborns has been declining due to the administration of Rh immune globulin (RhoGAM) to mothers. This inhibits formation of anti-Rh antibodies. Additionally, transfusions in *utero* or fetal exchange transfusions immediately after birth can diminish or eliminate the likelihood of infant death.

TRANSFUSION REACTIONS

There are many types of transfusion reactions. One, hemolytic transfusion reaction, occurs when a donor's and recipient's blood are not compatible. Antigens on the donor's red blood cells trigger a response from the antibodies in the recipient's blood. The antibodies attach to the red blood cells, which are then *hemolyzed,* or taken up by the fixed macrophages of the spleen's reticuloendothelial system.

Signs and symptoms of a hemolytic transfusion reaction may include facial flushing, hyperventilation, tachycardia, and a sense of dread. Hives may appear on the skin, and the patient may develop chest pain, wheezing, fever, chills, and cyanosis. Flank pain may occur as small clots begin to clog the microvasculature of the kidneys, which can lead to kidney failure requiring dialysis. The damage can be permanent.

If you are caring for a patient receiving a blood transfusion and he develops what you believe to be a hemolytic reaction, stop the transfusion immediately.

If a patient receiving a blood transfusion develops what you believe to be a hemolytic reaction, stop the transfusion immediately.

Change all associated IV tubing and initiate IV therapy with normal saline or lactated Ringer's solution. Administer a bolus as necessary to maintain good perfusion and blood pressure. Furosemide (Lasix) is often administered to promote diuresis. Low dose dopamine (2–5 mcg/kg/minute) should be considered along with the IV fluid to help maintain adequate renal perfusion. If you observe evidence of an allergic reaction, you can give diphenhydramine (Benadryl) 25–50 mg IV to help with some of the histamine-mediated effects such as itching or hives. In extreme cases of anaphylactic reaction, you may need to administer IV epinephrine if the patient is hypotensive or demonstrates severe bronchospasm.

The most common transfusion reaction is the febrile nonhemolytic reaction. It is caused by sensitization to antigens on the white blood cells, platelets, or plasma proteins. Signs and symptoms include headache, fever, and chills. As with any other transfusion reaction, always stop the transfusion before attempting to treat it. After stopping the blood product, change all tubing, and initiate normal saline IV. Patients are often given diphenhydramine (Benadryl) and an antipyretic (ibuprofen, acetaminophen) for the fever. No further treatment may be necessary, as this reaction rarely progresses to more serious complications. However, close observation is required to exclude development of a hemolytic reaction. In the event of any transfusion reaction, return all blood bags, tubing, and filters to the blood bank for analysis. Medical direction may order you to take blood and urine samples.

Because blood transfusion adds fluid to the system, a patient may experience signs and symptoms of circulatory overload. In fact, signs and symptoms are the same as those for left ventricular failure and may include pulmonary edema, dyspnea, and chest pain. Hypotension is not usually a problem, and you may treat the patient successfully by slowing the heart rate and administering diuretics.

GENERAL ASSESSMENT AND MANAGEMENT

In general, patients with disorders of the hematopoietic system may present with a variety of complaints and physical findings. Patients with infection, white blood cell abnormalities (immunocompromised and prone to infection), or transfusion reactions may present with febrile symptoms. Subsequently, these patients may develop hemodynamic instability as infection progresses to sepsis or as the transfusion reaction leads to a hemolytic reaction, renal failure, and disseminated intravascular coagulation (DIC). Acute hemodynamic compromise can also be found in patients with anemia secondary to acute blood loss, coagulation defects, or autoimmune disease. These disease processes may not be easily differentiated in the field and often require significant laboratory testing to confirm the diagnosis. In most cases, however, if you obtain a careful history, you will have a good working diagnosis.

Most hematopoietic disorders are chronic conditions that present with acute exacerbation when the patient is exposed to an additional stress such as infection or trauma. Treatment of patients with disorders of the hematopoietic system, in most cases, is supportive. Some patients may have hemodynamic instability from blood or fluid loss. These patients may require intravenous fluids to support end-organ perfusion and prevent shock. In addition, they should receive oxygen therapy to prevent hypoxia from poor perfusion and diminished oxygen carrying capacity of the blood. It is important to recognize the need for rapid transport in patients with hemodynamic instability who may require transfusion or other definitive care measures. Always contact medical direction for questions or problems.

SCENE SIZE-UP

Assessment of the patient with a possible hematopoietic abnormality begins the same as for any other patient. Perform a scene size-up and take BSI precautions. During your approach, form a general impression of the patient. Is the patient a trauma or medical patient? In how much distress is the patient?

INITIAL ASSESSMENT

Complete an initial assessment for life threats. Determine responsiveness and assess the airway, breathing, and circulation. Alterations in the hematopoietic system may present as life-threatening bleeds or overwhelming infections with septic shock. Do not spend time obtaining a complete set of vital signs during the initial assessment. Check the ABCs and quickly determine your priority for transport. Critical or unstable patients should be considered candidates for expeditious transport.

FOCUSED HISTORY AND PHYSICAL EXAM

Next, complete a focused history and physical exam. Use your general impression to choose a format for a responsive or unresponsive medical patient or trauma patient with significant or nonsignificant mechanism of injury. Each format follows a sequence of history gathering and examination designed to meet the needs of that particular patient. Trauma patients and unresponsive medical patients often present life-threatening problems that are noted in your initial assessment.

SAMPLE History

For a responsive medical patient, obtain a SAMPLE history and perform a physical exam. Obtain a set of vital signs and place the pulse oximeter. Keep in mind that an anemic patient will have increased heart and respiratory rates as his body attempts to compensate for less oxygen reaching the tissues. Ask for the chief complaint—why did the patient call for assistance? What signs or symptoms (SAMPLE) accompanied or preceded the complaint? Pay attention to generalized complaints such as fatigue, lethargy, malaise, apprehension, or confusion. These may indicate inadequate oxygen delivery to the tissues. Have there been any unusual skin changes such as coloring or bruising? Does the patient complain of itching? Inquire about lymph node enlargement (swollen glands), sore throat, or pain upon swallowing. These may indicate infection.

Any change in the blood's ability to deliver oxygen to the body will appear in the cardiovascular and respiratory systems. Note dyspnea, palpitations, and dizziness with changes in the patient's position. Patients with hematological problems may suffer syncope. Did the patient have a syncopal episode or is he just weak? Syncope can be due to several factors but is often related to a sudden change in position in a patient who has a marked anemia. Bleeding abnormalities may be disguised as gastrointestinal upset. Ask about overt bleeding with vomiting or diarrhea, but do not overlook complaints of nausea or anorexia, vomiting of "coffee ground" material, or having black tarry or cranberry, sticky, odoriferous stools. Many patients will notice bleeding of the gums when they brush their teeth. This can, on occasion, be hard to control. Atraumatic bleeding of the gums almost always points to an underlying hematologic abnormality. Ask about changes in urination, hematuria (blood in the urine), and alterations in the usual menstrual pattern in females. Keep in mind that hematological disorders are often diagnosed when the patient seeks assistance for another medical condition.

Keep in mind that hematological disorders are often diagnosed when the patient seeks assistance for another medical condition.

Determine any allergies (SAMPLE). Be sure to ask about use of prescription or over-the-counter medications (SAMPLE). Make note of the patient's medication, dose, and the condition for which he takes the medication. Also, if time allows, note the dosing schedule of the medications. Ask about compliance. Does the patient take medication as prescribed? When was the last dose taken? Medications that may indicate an alteration in the hematologic system, or that might make the patient more susceptible to an alteration in the system, include pain relievers, antibiotics, anticoagulants, hormones, and medications for heart disease, arthritis, and seizures.

When asking about past medical history (SAMPLE), make note of surgeries such as a splenectomy, heart-valve replacement, or placement of long-term venous-access devices. Ask about bloodborne infections such as HIV or hepatitis B or C. Make note of liver or bone marrow disease or cancers. Include questions about family history such as hemophilia, sickle cell disease, cancer, or death at an early age that was not trauma related. Inquire also about social habits such as smoking, alcohol consumption, IV drug use, or long-term exposure to chemicals or radiation.

If you find a significant history, ask about the last episode of an incident or last use of a medication. Remember to include the usual questions about last oral intake (SAMPLE). Also, inquire about any unusual events (SAMPLE) that preceded the onset of the complaint such, as the start of a new medication, recent transfusion, fall, or injury.

Physical Exam

When performing the physical exam, evaluate each system methodically as you would in any other patient. If the history suggests a hematopoietic problem, look for potential pathology during the physical exam that may confirm your working diagnosis and be a clue to developing complications.

- *Nervous system* Always evaluate the nervous system in any patient with a suspected hematological problem. First, note the patient's level of consciousness using the AVPU system. Be alert for other nervous system disorders. Many patients with hematological problems will complain of being "weak and dizzy." Try to clarify this further. Is the patient fatigued, weak all over, or does he have focal weakness? Is he dizzy or is he suffering true vertigo? Both can be associated with hematological problems such as anemia. Ask if the patient has any numbness or motor deficits. Pernicious anemia can cause sensory deficits that are often unilateral. Try to determine whether the patient had a syncopal episode. What were the patient's condition and position immediately prior to the syncopal episode? Many of the hematological diseases, especially the autoimmune diseases, will affect the eye. Always examine the eyes for abnormalities. Question the patient about any visual disturbances or visual loss. In addition to the autoimmune diseases, sickle cell anemia is notorious for causing eye problems.
- *Skin* Note the patient's skin color (Figure 9-11). Jaundice (yellow skin) may indicate liver disease or hemolysis of red blood cells, while a florid (reddish) appearance is often associated with polycythemia. Patients with anemia typically exhibit pallor. Observe for petechiae (tiny red dots in the skin), purpura (large purplish blotches related to multiple hemorrhages into the skin), and bruising. Inquire about pruritus (itching). Patients with hematological disorders often develop pruritus. Some hematological problems, such as sickle cell

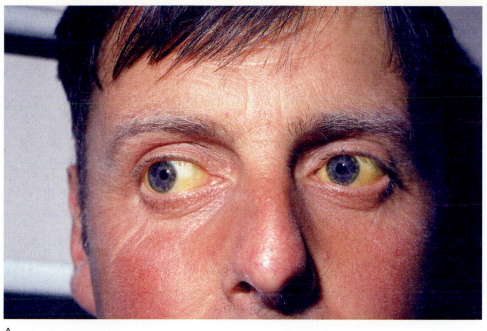

A

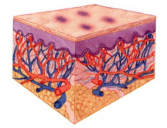

Petechiae – Reddish-purple spots, diameter less than 0.5 cm

B

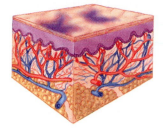

Purpura – Reddish-purple blotches, diameter more than 0.5 cm

C

FIGURE 9-11   Abnormal skin colors: A) jaundice, B) petechiae, C) purpura.

anemia, cause the destruction of red blood cells. This results in hemoglobin's spilling into the circulatory system. Macrophages then break down the hemoglobin. The iron is removed and transported to the bones or liver. The porphyrin portion of the hemoglobin is subsequently converted into bilirubin, which is taken up by the liver. An excess of bilirubin, either from liver disease or from the breakdown of hemoglobin associated with the hemolytic anemias, can cause pruritis. Often, patients will develop itching over a bruise. As the hemoglobin breaks down within the bruise, the localized accumulation of bilirubin causes the itching. This is most common 1–2 weeks after the bruise occurs. When examining the skin, be alert for any evidence of prolonged bleeding. The patient may have several bandages over relatively minor wounds where he could not stop the bleeding.

- *Lymphatic* The lymphatic system is affected early in hematopoietic diseases, especially those of the immune system. During your physical exam, pay particular attention to the lymph nodes. Palpate the lymph nodes of the neck, clavicle, axilla, and groin. Note any enlargement. Compare sides. Splenomegaly (an enlarged spleen) is also often present, but this can be hard to examine in the field.

- *Gastrointestinal* The gastrointestinal effects of hematological problems can be quite varied. Epistaxis (nosebleed) is common. The nasal mucosa is quite vascular as it warms and humidifies the inhaled air. A slight crack in the nasal mucosa can result in brisk bleeding. This is a particular problem in people with blood clotting abnormalities, as stopping the bleeding is very difficult for them. These patients may swallow a great deal of blood and may become nauseated. Also, blood acts as a cathartic (laxative). Patients who swallow even moderate amounts of blood will often report loose bowel movements. These are often dark (melena). Blood present in emesis may be bright red or appear like coffee grounds.

Bleeding gums are often associated with a decreased platelet count.

Bleeding of the gums is one of the earliest findings of hematological problems. Patients with blood clotting abnormalities and low platelet levels will often develop atraumatic bleeding of the gums. Any patient with bleeding gums requires a detailed investigation for a possible hematological disorder. Gingivitis (infection of the gums) can be due to poor hygiene, disease, or both. However, chronic gingivitis should cause increased suspicion of a hematological disorder, especially involving the immune system. Also, gingivitis increases a patient's risk of developing sepsis. Slight trauma, such as brushing the teeth, can cause the bacteria to enter the circulatory system, resulting in generalized sepsis. Always note the presence of gingivitis when examining for bleeding gums. Ulcerations of the gums and oral mucosa are typically due to viral diseases. These infections are more common in immunosuppressed patients. Thrush (yeast infection in the mouth) in adults is almost always associated with AIDS. (Thrush in children is common and not a reason for concern.)

An oral yeast infection in an adult is commonly associated with AIDS.

The liver plays a major role in manufacturing many of the substances required for blood clotting. Liver disease can slow blood clotting. This is most evident in a prolonged prothrombin (PT) time. Also, as the liver fails, the bilirubin level will increase, resulting in jaundice. Thus, any patient with jaundice should be evaluated for liver disease.

Abdominal pain is not uncommon in persons with hematological disease. Two of the major organs associated with the hematopoeitic system, the liver and spleen, are in the abdomen. Problems with the spleen, liver, or both can lead to abdominal pain. Splenomagaly is common in hematological problems, as the spleen is active in the removal of abnormal or aged red cells. In some of the anemias, especially the hemolytic anemias, the spleen can become markedly enlarged. Patients with sickle cell anemia will often develop splenic infarcts as sickled cells accumulate and block blood supply to parts of the spleen. By the time children with sickle cell disease are 5 years of age, they are virtually asplenic (without a spleen), as the disease has completely infarcted their spleen. Because the spleen is not functional, these patients are placed at increased risk of infection, especially by encapsulated bacteria.

- *Musculoskeletal* Many hematopoietic problems are autoimmune in nature. That is, a problem develops in which the immune system has trouble determining which tissues are self and which are nonself. Autoimmune diseases such as rheumatoid arthritis result from the body's immune system attacking various tissues in the joints. This can cause arthralgia (pain and swelling of the joints). Autoimmune diseases tend to affect more than one joint, whereas infectious processes tend to affect only a single joint. Patients with blood clotting disorders such as hemophilia will often develop hemarthrosis (bleeding into a joint) with only minor trauma. This can result in an extremely swollen, discolored, and painful joint. Always inquire about joint pain and examine the major joints in any patient suspected of having hematopoietic disease.

- *Cardiorespiratory* The effects of hematopoietic problems on the cardiorespiratory system are varied. Patients with anemia will often develop dyspnea, tachycardia, and chest pain from the increased cardiac work caused by the anemia. In severe cases, patients can develop high-output heart failure, where the heart works excessively hard to compensate for a profound anemia. If untreated, heart failure and pulmonary edema can result. Patients with bleeding disorders may report expectorating blood with coughing. This can be due to small tears in the respiratory mucosa from the coughing. Normally, these heal quickly. Patients with bleeding disorders, however, will continue to bleed, resulting in potential airway obstruction and, in severe cases, shock. Always auscultate for breath sounds. Note crackles or rhonchi indicative of heart problems or infection.

Be alert for high-output heart failure in patients with severe anemia.

- *Genitourinary* The genitourinary effects of hematopoietic problems are typically due to bleeding disorders or infection. Bleeding disorders can cause hematuria (blood in the urine) and blood in the scrotal sac in males. A woman who still has her uterus may develop menorrhagia (heavy menstrual bleeding) or frank vaginal bleeding (dysfunctional uterine bleeding). Immunocompromised patients are at increased risk for developing genitourinary infections. These can range from recurrent urinary tract infections to severe sexually transmitted diseases. Sickle cell anemia, especially in the later stages, can cause priapism. This is a prolonged, painful erection due to obstruction of the blood vessels that drain the penis and allow for detumescence. Sickle cell disease is the most common cause of priapism in the emergency setting. All of these require additional evaluation in the emergency department. Detailed evaluation of the genitourinary system is not appropriate for field settings.

Sickle cell disease is a common cause of priapism in the emergency setting.

GENERAL MANAGEMENT OF HEMATOPOIETIC EMERGENCIES

Pay close attention to the airway and ventilation status of patients experiencing any alteration in the hematopoietic system. Place the patient on high-concentration supplemental oxygen and monitor breathing for difficulty or fatigue. Be ready to assist ventilations with a bag-valve mask.

Assess the circulatory system. Consider fluid volume replacement, but remember that crystalloid solutions cannot carry oxygen. Too much fluid can "dilute" the blood and reduce its capacity per unit volume to carry oxygen. Be alert for dysrhythmias and treat accordingly. Based on your assessment and evaluation, create the optimum environment for the blood to perform its tasks of oxygen delivery and waste product removal. Creating such an environment may

Pay close attention to the airway and ventilation status of patients experiencing any alteration in the hematopoietic system.

include giving the patient aspirin to inhibit platelet aggregation or ventilating the patient to compensate for acidosis and to allow oxygen to unload from hemoglobin at the tissues.

Transport the patient to the appropriate facility, provide comfort measures including analgesia, and provide psychological support to both the patient and his family.

MANAGING SPECIFIC PATIENT PROBLEMS

Remember that many hematological problems occur in conjunction with other illnesses.
🗝

The rest of this chapter will detail the more common hematopoietic diseases that you might encounter in prehospital care. Again, it is important to remember that many hematological problems occur in conjunction with other illnesses. For example, someone with a cancer or significant renal disease quite commonly will have a coexisting anemia. In the following sections we will first examine diseases of the red blood cells. These are the most common hematological problems encountered. Second, we will look at the white blood cell diseases. These include the leukemias, lymphomas, and similar illnesses. Finally, we will present diseases of the platelets and blood coagulation disorders.

DISEASES OF THE RED BLOOD CELLS

* **polycythemia** an excess of red blood cells.

* **anemia** an inadequate number of red blood cells or inadequate hemoglobin within the red blood cells.

Red blood cell diseases result in too many red blood cells, too few red blood cells, or improperly functioning red blood cells. An excess of red blood cells is called **polycythemia.** Although uncommon, several conditions can cause polycythemia. An inadequate number of red blood cells or inadequate hemoglobin within the red blood cells is called **anemia.** Anemia is common, and several types are frequently encountered. Finally, red blood cell function can be impaired. Most commonly, this is due to problems with either hemoglobin structure and function or with the red blood cell membrane. Problems with red blood cell function include the thallasemias and sickle cell anemia.

Anemias

Content Review

DISEASES OF THE RED BLOOD CELLS
* Anemia
* Sickle cell disease
* Polycythemia

The most common diseases of the red blood cells are the anemias. Anemia is typically classified as a hematocrit of less than 37 percent in women or less than 40 percent in men. Most patients with anemia will remain asymptomatic until the hematocrit drops below 30 percent. The decreased hematocrit in anemia is due to a reduction in the number of red blood cells or in the amount or quality of hemoglobin in the red blood cells. Anemia is actually a sign of an underlying disease process that is either destroying red blood cells and hemoglobin or decreasing the production of red blood cells and hemoglobin. Blood loss, either acute or chronic, also can cause anemia. Anemia can be a self-limited disease or it can be a lifelong illness requiring periodic transfusions. Anemias that result from the destruction of red blood cells are called hemolytic anemias. These can be hereditary or acquired. Examples of hereditary hemolytic anemias include sickle cell anemia, thalassemia, and glucose-6-phosphate dehydrogenase deficiency (G6PD). Acquired hemolytic anemias can result from immune system disorders, drug effects, or environmental effects. Anemias caused by inadequate red blood cell production include such problems as iron deficiency anemia, pernicious anemia, and anemia of chronic disease. Table 9-2 shows the numerous types of anemia, all of which must be confirmed by laboratory diagnosis.

Anemia is a sign, not a disease process in itself. Since the red blood cells' primary purpose is to transport oxygen, anemia results in hypoxia. The signs and symptoms of anemia vary, depending upon the rapidity of its onset and

Table 9-2	TYPES OF ANEMIA	
Cause	**Type**	**Pathophysiology**
Inadequate production of red blood cells	Aplastic	Failure to produce red blood cells
	Iron deficiency	Iron is primary component of hemoglobin
	Pernicious	Vitamin B_{12} is necessary for correct red blood cell division during its development
	Sickle cell	Genetic alteration causes production of a hemoglobin that changes shape of red blood cell to a *C*, or sickle, in low oxygen states
Increased red blood cell destruction	Hemolytic	Body destroys red blood cells at greater rate than production; red blood cell parts interfere with blood flow
Blood cell loss or dilution	Chronic disease	Hemorrhage leads to cell loss while excessive fluid leads to a dilution of red blood cell concentration

upon the patient's age and underlying general health. A mild anemia may not exhibit signs or symptoms until the body is stressed, as during exercise. Then a mild dyspnea, fatigue, palpitations, and syncope may be present. Chronic anemias may present signs or symptoms of pica (the craving of unusual substances such as clay or ice), headache, dizziness, ringing in the ears, irritability or difficulty concentrating, pallor, and tachycardia. Angina pectoris can be an important indicator.

If anemia develops rapidly, the body does not have time to compensate for the change. Signs and symptoms of shock may be present, including postural hypotension and decreased cardiac output, resulting in a shunting of blood away from the periphery to the heart, lungs, and brain. Compensatory mechanisms can cause diaphoresis, pallor, cool skin, anxiety, thirst, and air hunger. If the anemia's onset is slower, the body can adjust to oxygen's reduced availability with a right shift of the oxyhemoglobin dissociation curve and an increase in plasma volume.

Prehospital treatment of anemia is primarily symptomatic. Direct your attention at maximizing oxygenation, stemming blood loss, and transporting to a medical facility for treatment of the cause. Start volume replacement if there is evidence of dehydration.

Sickle Cell Disease

Sickle cell anemia, often termed "sickle cell disease," is a disorder of red blood cell production. Normal hemoglobin is very flexible, and the red blood cell can pass easily through the tiny capillaries. Sickle hemoglobin has an abnormal chemical sequence that gives red blood cells a *C*, or sickle, shape when oxygen levels are low (Figure 9-12). Patients with sickle cell disease will have a chronic anemia that results from destruction of abnormal red blood cells (hemolytic anemia). The average

✴ **sickle cell anemia** an inherited disorder of red blood cell production, so named because the red blood cells become sickle-shaped when oxygen levels are low.

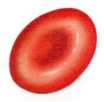
Normal red blood cell

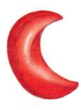
Sickle cell

FIGURE 9-12 A normal red blood cell contrasted with a sickle cell.

life span of sickled red blood cells is 10–20 days compared to 120 days for normal red blood cells. In addition, sickled red blood cells increase the blood's viscosity, leading to sludging and obstruction of the capillaries and small blood vessels. Blockage of blood flow to various tissues and organs is common and usually occurs following a period of stress. This process, called a vasoocclusive crisis, is characteristic of sickle cell anemia. Because of the vasoocclusive crisis, tissues and organs are eventually damaged. Adult sickle cell patients often have multiple organ problems, including cardiopulmonary disease, renal disease, and neurological disorders.

Sickle cell disease is inherited. It primarily affects African-Americans although other ethnic groups can be affected. These include Puerto Ricans and people of Spanish, French, Italian, Greek, and Turkish heritage. If both parents carry a gene for sickle cell anemia, the chances are one in four that the child will have normal hemoglobin. The chances are two in four that he will have both normal hemoglobin and sickle hemoglobin, which is referred to as *sickle cell trait*. The chances are one in four that he will have only sickle hemoglobin (no normal hemoglobin.) This condition is referred to as *sickle cell disease.*

Patients with sickle cell disease will develop three types of problems. *Vasoocclusive crises* cause musculoskeletal pain, abdominal pain, priapisms, pulmonary problems, renal crises (renal infarctions), and central nervous system crises (cerebral infarctions). In addition, they will develop *hematological crises* that consist of a fall in the hemoglobin level, sequestration of red blood cells in the spleen, and problems with bone marrow function. In severe cases, the bone marrow can shut down, causing an aplastic crisis. These are usually self-limited. Finally, sickle cell patients often develop *infectious crises*. They are functionally immunosuppressed, and the loss of splenic function makes them particularly vulnerable to encapsulated bacteria. Infections become common and are often the cause of death in sickle cell anemia.

Prehospital care for patients in sickle cell crisis is primarily supportive. Begin high-flow oxygen to saturate as much hemoglobin as possible. Initiate IV therapy with an isotonic crystalloid solution. These patients are often dehydrated and hydration will sometimes help with the vasoocclusive process. Venous access is sometimes difficult in older patients with sickle cell disease due to the large number of IV starts they have required in their lifetime. Placing a central line is occasionally necessary. Vasoocclusive crises can be extremely painful. Start analgesic therapy in the field, if possible. Often these patients will require large amounts of narcotics for pain control. Always consult medical direction if there is a question regarding management. Transport is indicated.

Polycythemia

Polycythemia is an abnormally high hematocrit. It is due to excess production of red blood cells. Polycythemia is a relatively rare disorder and typically occurs in patients 50 years of age or older. It can occur secondarily to dehydration. The increased red blood cell load increases the patient's risk of thrombosis. Most deaths from polycythemia are due to thrombosis.

Polycythemia's signs and symptoms vary. The principal finding is a hematocrit of 50 percent or greater. The patient will usually have an increased number of white blood cells and platelets. However, the large number of red blood cells may cause a platelet dysfunction. This can result in bleeding abnormalities such as epistaxis, spontaneous bruising, and gastrointestinal bleeding. Patients with polycythemia may complain of headache, dizziness, blurred vision, itching, and gastrointestinal disease. Severe cases can result in congestive heart failure.

The prehospital treatment of polycythemia is supportive. Assure that the airway and breathing are adequate. Administer supplemental oxygen as required. Initiate an IV with an isotonic crystalloid solution. The principal treatment is phlebotomy, which removes excess red blood cells.

Content Review

SICKLE CELL CRISES
• Vasoocclusive
• Hematological
• Infectious

* **polycythemia** an abnormally high hematocrit.

DISEASES OF THE WHITE BLOOD CELLS

The white blood cells are the body's principal defense system. Problems with white blood cells typically result from too few white blood cells (**leukopenia**), too many white blood cells (**leukocytosis**), or improper white blood cell function. The neutrophil is the main blood component protecting against a bacterial or fungal reaction. A reduction in the number of neutrophils (**neutropenia**) predisposes the patient to bacterial and fungal infections.

Leukopenia/Neutropenia

The status of the white blood cells is easily determined by obtaining a complete blood count. A normal white blood cell count ranges from 5,000 to 9,000 per cubic millimeter of blood. A decrease in the number of white blood cells indicates a problem with white-blood-cell production in the marrow or destruction of white blood cells. Because bacterial infections pose a major risk to humans, an absolute neutrophil count is a better indicator of the immune system's status. The prehospital treatment of leukopenia/neutropenia is supportive. Pay special attention to preventing infection in the patient, as his immune system is overstressed or may be functioning inadequately.

Leukocytosis

Leukocytosis is an increase in the number of circulating white blood cells. This occurs when the body is exposed to an infectious agent or is particularly stressed. Following exposure, the immune system is stimulated and the marrow and spleen start releasing white blood cells to help the body fight infection. A white blood cell count between 10,800 and 23,000 per cubic millimeter of blood is characteristic of a bacterial infection. During periods of stress, immature neutrophils may be released into the circulation. These differ from mature neutrophils in that they have a segmented nucleus. These cells are referred to as "bands" or "segs." An increase in the number of bands is indicative of a significant bacterial infection. Causes of leukocytosis include bacterial infection, rheumatoid arthritis, DKA, leukemia, pain, and exercise. Viral infections tend to have little effect on the white blood cell count or, in some cases, actually cause a decrease in the white blood cell count. A white blood cell count greater than 30,000 per cubic millimeter is called a *leukemoid reaction*. A white blood cell count this high indicates a problem with excess white blood cell production. Any patient with a significantly elevated white blood cell count should be evaluated for possible leukemia.

Leukemia

Leukemias are cancers of hematopoietic cells. Precursors of white blood cells in the bone marrow begin to replicate abnormally. The cells proliferate initially in the bone marrow and then spread to the peripheral blood. Leukemias affect approximately 13 in 100,000 persons. They are classified by the type of cell or cells involved. The most common types of leukemia are:

- Acute lymphocytic leukemia (ALL)
- Acute myelogenous leukemia (AML)
- Chronic lymphocytic leukemia (CLL)
- Chronic myelogenous leukemia (CML)
- Hairy cell leukemia

* **leukopenia** too few white blood cells.

* **leukocytosis** too many white blood cells.

Content Review

DISEASES OF THE WHITE BLOOD CELLS
- Leukopenia/Neutropenia
- Leukocytosis
- Leukemia
- Lymphoma

* **neutropenia** a reduction in the number of neutrophils.

* **leukemia** a cancer of the hematopoietic cells.

Discussion of the pathology of the various leukemias is not within the scope of this text. ALL is primarily a disease of children and young adults. CML occurs in both children and adults. AML, CLL, and hairy cell leukemia tend to occur in the sixth and seventh decades of life. Medicine has made significant advances in the treatment of leukemia. Treatments such as chemotherapy, radiation therapy, and bone marrow transplantation have resulted in cures of certain types of leukemias. The treatment of pediatric leukemia is one of the great successes of modern medicine. More than 50 percent of pediatric patients with ALL live a normal life with the disease in remission or cured. Infections are a common complication of leukemia, primarily due to the low number of circulating neutrophils. Deaths from leukemias are typically secondary to infection or bleeding.

The signs and symptoms of leukemia vary. Most patients will have a moderate to severe anemia as the cancerous cell production overwhelms the bone marrow. Thrombocytopenia (an abnormal decrease in platelets) is common for the same reason. Many leukemia patients will present with bleeding, usually due to the thrombocytopenia. With the initial presentation, leukemia patients will appear acutely ill. They will be febrile and weak, usually due to a secondary infection. Various lymph nodes may be enlarged. Patients often have a history of weight loss and anorexia. In addition, liver and spleen enlargement are typical, resulting in a sensation of abdominal fullness or abdominal pain. The sternum may be tender, secondary to the increased bone marrow activity. Fatigue is a common complaint.

The prehospital treatment of the patient with leukemia is primarily supportive. Place the patient in a position of comfort. Administer supplemental oxygen via a nonrebreather mask. Initiate an IV with an isotonic crystalloid solution such as lactated Ringer's or normal saline. Consider a fluid bolus if the patient is dehydrated. If the patient is having pain secondary to the leukemia, consider administration of an analgesic. Remember, leukemia patients are at increased risk of developing infection. Employ proper isolation techniques.

Employ proper isolation techniques for leukemia patients, who are at increased risk of developing infection.

Lymphomas

Lymphomas are cancers of the lymphatic system. Malignant lymphoma is typically classified as follows:

* Hodgkin's lymphoma
* Non-Hodgkin's lymphoma

Malignant lymphoma is classified by the cell type involved, which indicates the stem cell from which the malignancy arises. In the United States, each year approximately 40,000 persons are diagnosed with non-Hodgkin's lymphoma, and 7,500 are diagnosed with Hodgkin's lymphoma. The long-term survival rate is much better with Hodgkin's lymphoma. In fact, many patients with Hodgkin's lymphoma who have been treated with radiation, chemotherapy, or both are considered cured.

The most common presenting sign of non-Hodgkin's lymphoma is painless swelling of the lymph nodes. The majority of patients with Hodgkin's lymphoma typically have no related symptoms. Patients with lymphoma may report fever, night sweats, anorexia, weight loss, fatigue, and pruritis. Treat patients with lymphomas symptomatically. Place the patient in a position of comfort. Administer supplemental oxygen via a nonrebreather mask. Initiate an IV with an isotonic crystalloid solution such as lactated Ringer's or normal saline. Consider a fluid bolus if the patient is dehydrated. If the patient is having pain secondary to the lymphoma, consider administration of an analgesic. As with leukemia patients, lymphoma patients are at increased risk of developing infection. Employ proper isolation techniques.

* **lymphoma** a cancer of the lymphatic system.

Lymphoma patients are at increased risk of developing infection. Use proper isolation techniques.

Diseases of the Platelets/ Blood Clotting Abnormalities

Various disorders can affect the platelets or the body's blood clotting system. Some of these are hereditary, while others may be acquired. Examples of platelet abnormalities include thrombocytosis (increased platelets) and thrombocytopenia (reduced platelets). Various disorders can affect the coagulation system. These include hemophilia A, hemophilia B (Christmas disease), and others.

Thrombocytosis

Thrombocytosis is an increase in the number of platelets, usually due to increased platelet production (essential thrombocytosis). It is also seen in polycythemia vera where both red blood cells and platelets are increased. Thrombocytosis often complicates chronic myelogenous leukemia. Thrombcytosis can be secondary to other disorders such as malignant diseases, hemolytic anemias, acute hemorrhage, and autoinflammatory diseases. Most patients with thrombocytosis are asymptomatic. Prehospital treatment is supportive.

✷ **thrombocytosis** an abnormal increase in the number of platelets.

Thrombocytopenia

Thrombocytopenia is an abnormal decrease in the number of platelets. It is due to decreased platelet production, sequestration of platelets in the spleen, destruction of platelets, or any combination of the three. Many drugs can induce thrombocytopenia. *Acute idiopathic thrombocytopenia purpura (ITP)* results from destruction of platelets by the immune system. It is most commonly seen in children following a viral infection. ITP is characterized by easy bruising, bleeding, and a falling platelet count. Chronic ITP usually occurs in adult women and is often associated with autoimmune disease. Prehospital treatment is supportive.

✷ **thrombocytopenia** an abnormal decrease in the number of platelets.

Hemophilia

Hemophilia is a blood disorder in which one of the proteins necessary for blood clotting is missing or defective. A deficiency of factor VIII is called hemophilia A. A deficiency of factor IX is known as hemophilia B (Christmas disease). Hemophilia A is the most common inherited disorder of hemostasis. The severity of the disease is directly related to the amount of circulating factor VIII available. Patients are classified as mild, moderate, or severe, based upon the amount of circulating factor VIII. Hemophilia B is more rare, but also more severe, than hemophilia A.

When a person with hemophilia is injured, the bleeding will take longer to stop because the body cannot form stable fibrin clots. Simple trauma such as nosebleeds or tooth extractions can lead to prolonged, occasionally life-threatening bleeds. In extensive trauma such as pelvic fractures blood loss can be overwhelming. A common problem with hemophilia is hemarthrosis (bleeding into the joint space). This can result from even the most minor trauma. Eventually, repeated bleeding episodes will lead to permanent joint damage.

Hemophilia is a sex-linked, inherited bleeding disorder (Figure 9-13). The gene with the defective information is carried on the X chromosome. Females have two X chromosomes, one from their mother and one from their father. If one chromosome has the defective gene and the other does not, the disease is not expressed. Females who have one X chromosome containing the defective gene are referred to as carriers. Males, however, have an X chromosome from their mother and a Y chromosome from their father. If that

✷ **hemophilia** a blood disorder in which one of the proteins necessary for blood clotting is missing or defective.

MOTHER		FATHER	
X (healthy)	x (hemophilia gene-carrier)	X (healthy)	Y (healthy)
DAUGHTER XX (both healthy)	DAUGHTER Xx (carrier of trait-no disease)	SON XY no disease	SON xY hemophilia

FIGURE 9-13 Familial (sex-linked) characteristics of hemophilia.

X chromosome carries the defective gene, males will express the disease. Hemophilia A affects approximately 1 in 10,000 males. A female, on the other hand, can inherit hemophilia only if she receives two X chromosomes that express the disease. That is, she must be the offspring of a carrier mother and a father with hemophilia.

The signs and symptoms of hemophilia include numerous bruises, deep muscle bleeding characterized as pain or a "pulled muscle," and the joint bleeding called hemarthrosis. Most patients will be aware of their diagnosis and will tell you. Some may wear Medic-Alert bracelets or similar devices.

Hemophiliacs can be treated in the hospital with infusions of factor VIII. In addition to factor VIII, some hemophiliacs will require blood transfusions due to bleeding from trauma. Unfortunately, before blood and blood products were routinely tested, transfusions infected many hemophiliacs with the human immunodeficiency virus, hepatitis B, and/or hepatitis C.

Prehospital treatment of the patient with hemophilia should be comprehensive. The normal hemostatic mechanisms of vasoconstriction and platelet aggregation will still occur, but the platelet plug will not be stable, due to the deficiency of factor VIII. Thus, you should be attentive to prolonged bleeding or possible rebleeds. The hemophiliac is at risk of both. Administer supplemental oxygen via a nonrebreather mask and initiate IV therapy with an isotonic crystalloid such as normal saline. Be careful to help prevent additional trauma, which can result in further hemorrhage. If the patient sustained a joint injury with resultant hemarthrosis, splinting the extremity will sometimes help control pain. Occasionally, analgesics will be required.

If your patient has hemophilia, be especially careful to help prevent additional trauma, which can result in further hemorrhage.

* von Willebrand's disease condition in which the vWF component of factor VIII is deficient.

Von Willebrand's Disease

Factor VIII actually consists of several components. One of these components is factor VIII:vWF, also called von Willebrand's factor. In **von Willebrand's disease,** this component of factor VIII is deficient. It is produced by the endothelial cells and is necessary for normal platelet adhesion. Thus, in addition to the clotting problem, platelet function is abnormal in patients with von Willebrand's disease. While the disease is inherited, it is not sex linked, equally affecting both females and males. A sign of this disease is excessive bleeding, primarily after surgery or injury. It is not associated with the deep muscle or joint bleeding of hemophilia, nor is it usually as serious, although nosebleeds, excessive menstruation, and gastrointestinal bleeds can occur. Prehospital treatment is supportive. Aspirin is generally contraindicated as it further inhibits platelet aggregation, thus exacerbating the disease. Definitive treatment is the administration of von Willebrand factor.

OTHER HEMATOPOIETIC DISORDERS

Other hematopoietic disorders that you may encounter in the prehospital setting include disseminated intravascular coagulation and multiple myeloma.

Disseminated Intravascular Coagulation

Disseminated intravascular coagulation (DIC), also called consumption coagulopathy, is a disorder of coagulation caused by systemic activation of the coagulation cascade. Normally, inhibitory mechanisms localize coagulation to the affected area. A combination of protein inhibitors, rapid blood flow, and absorption of the fibrin clot restricts circulating free thrombin to the site of coagulation. In DIC, circulating thrombin cleaves fibrinogen to form fibrin clots throughout the circulation. This can cause widespread thrombosis and, occasionally, end-organ ischemia. Bleeding is the most frequent sign of DIC and is due to the reduced fibrinogen level, consumption of coagulation factors, and thrombocytopenia. DIC most commonly results from sepsis, hypotension, obstetric complications, severe tissue injury, brain injury, cancer, and major hemolytic transfusion reactions. The disease is quite grave. Its signs include oozing blood at venipuncture and wound sites. The patient may exhibit a purpuric rash, often over the chest and abdomen. Minute hemorrhages may be noted just under the skin. Prehospital care is symptomatic. The patient with DIC may be hemodynamically unstable and may require intravenous fluids. Definitive treatment includes the administration of fresh frozen plasma and platelets.

✱ **disseminated intravascular coagulation (DIC)** a disorder of coagulation caused by systemic activation of the coagulation cascade.

Multiple Myeloma

Multiple myeloma is a cancerous disorder of plasma cells. Plasma cells are a type of B cell responsible for producing immunoglobulins (antibodies). The disease is rarely found in persons under the age of 40. Approximately 14,000 new cases are diagnosed each year. Usually, multiple myeloma begins with a change or mutation in a plasma cell in the bone marrow. These cancerous plasma cells crowd out healthy cells and lead to a reduction in blood cell production. The patient then becomes anemic and prone to infection.

✱ **multiple myeloma** a cancerous disorder of plasma cells.

The first sign of multiple myeloma often is pain in the back or ribs. The diseased marrow weakens the bones and *pathological fractures* (those occurring with minimal or no trauma) may occur. The resulting anemia leads to fatigue, and reduced platelet production places the patient at risk for bleeding. Laboratory evaluation will reveal an elevation in the level of a circulating antibody or part of an antibody (light chain). This is due to the proliferation of plasma cells. Despite this, the patient is at increased risk of infection, as the plasma cells do not secrete specific antibodies in response to infection. In addition, the calcium level is often elevated in multiple myeloma due to bone destruction. This can lead to renal failure.

Treatment of multiple myeloma includes chemotherapy, radiation, and bone marrow transplants. Prehospital care is supportive. Establish an IV of isotonic crystalloid solution. Consider a fluid bolus if there are symptoms of dehydration. Multiple myeloma can be very painful due to the proliferation of the plasma cells and destruction of the marrow. Consider analgesics if pain is severe. It is not uncommon for EMS to be summoned following a pathological fracture in a patient with multiple myeloma. Again, these are very painful, and you should start analgesic therapy if so indicated.

SUMMARY

Hematology is the study of blood and blood-forming organs. Blood consists of a liquid portion, or plasma, and the formed elements—red blood cells, white blood cells, and platelets. Each component of blood has various functions. Plasma draws water into the capillaries, and it assists in clotting blood, dismantling clots, buffering the blood's acid/base balance, transporting hormones and regulating their effects, and providing a source of energy. Red blood cells, composed of hemoglobin, transport oxygen to the body tissues and remove wastes such as carbon dioxide. White blood cells protect the body from foreign invasion through the processes of chemotaxis and phagocytosis. Platelets travel to the site of damaged tissue and help to prevent blood loss.

Hemostasis is the body's way of preventing or controlling blood loss. The three phases of hemostasis include vascular spasm, development of the platelet plug, and formation of a stable fibrin clot (blood coagulation).

Numerous conditions and diseases affect the hematic system, with varying and sometimes disastrous outcomes. As a paramedic, you must understand hematology because breakdowns in the hematological system can complicate patient assessment and care.

YOU MAKE THE CALL

Your crew is just starting a Sunday afternoon barbecue lunch when the call comes in to respond to a patient who is hemorrhaging due to a lawn mower accident. The accident occurred at 2424 Eighth Avenue, which is just around the corner from your location, and you arrive within minutes. As you approach the scene, you see that the lawn mower has been turned off and a middle-aged man is calling for you to come quickly. The man's 17-year-old son, Jim, was walking through the yard when a sharp stone was kicked out from the blades and struck him in the arm. He has a nasty laceration to his left upper arm, which is spurting blood with each pulse beat. Jim is trying vainly to stem the bleeding.

While you administer oxygen and apply pressure during the initial assessment, your EMT partner, Tina, obtains a set of vital signs. The pulse is 110 and regular; the respiratory rate is 22 and nonlabored; the blood pressure is 112/84.

After you transport the patient to the hospital, the hospital staff closes the patient's wound, but they are concerned about a possible infection at the wound site.

1. What hemostatic responses will seek to control this blood loss?
2. Why are the heart rate and respiratory rate elevated?
3. What will the body do to replace red blood cells?
4. What body mechanisms will fight off an infection?

See Suggested Responses at the back of this book.

FURTHER READING

Hawley, Kelly. "Pernicious Anemia." *American Journal of Nursing,* 11 (November 1996): 52–53.

McCance, Kathryn L. and Sue E. Heuther. *Pathophysiology. The Biologic Basis for Disease in Adults and Children.* 3rd ed. St. Louis: Mosby, 1998.

Ross, Clare. "A Trauma Patient With Sickle Cell Disease." *Journal of Emergency Nursing* (June 1997): 211–213.

Snyder, Claudine L. et al. "Confronting a Tempest: Acute Leukemia." *Nursing* (February 1997): 32aa–32dd.

Warmkessel, Jeanne A. "Caring for a Patient with Non-Hodgkin's Lymphoma." *Nursing* (June 1997): 48–49.

ON THE WEB

Visit Brady's Paramedic Website at www.bradybooks.com/paramedic.

CHAPTER 10

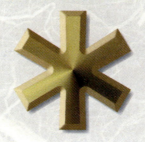

Environmental Emergencies

Objectives

After reading this chapter, you should be able to:

1. Define "environmental emergency." (p. 505)
2. Describe the incidence, morbidity, and mortality associated with environmental emergencies. (p. 525)
3. Identify risk factors most predisposing to environmental emergencies. (p. 505)
4. Identify environmental factors that may cause illness or exacerbate a preexisting illness or complicate treatment or transport decisions. (p. 505)
5. Define "homeostasis" and relate the concept to environmental influences. (p. 505–506)
6. Identify normal, critically high, and critically low body temperatures. (p. 509)
7. Describe several methods of temperature monitoring. (p. 508)
8. Describe human thermal regulation, including system components, substances used, and wastes generated. (pp. 506–510, 517)
9. List the common forms of heat and cold disorders. (pp. 510–516)

Continued

10. List the common predisposing factors and preventive measures associated with heat and cold disorders. (pp. 510–511, 517–518)

11. Define heat illness, hypothermia, frostbite, near-drowning, decompression illness, and altitude illness. (pp. 510, 517, 523, 525, 531, 536)

12. Describe the pathophysiology, signs and symptoms, and predisposing factors, preventive actions, and treatment for heat cramps, heat exhaustion, heatstroke, and fever. (pp. 511–516)

13. Describe the contribution of dehydration to the development of heat disorders. (p. 515)

14. Describe the differences between classical and exertional heatstroke. (p. 514)

15. Identify the fundamental thermoregulatory difference between fever and heatstroke. (p. 516)

16. Discuss the role of fluid therapy in the treatment of heat disorders. (p. 515)

17. Describe the pathophysiology, predisposing factors, signs, symptoms, and management of the following:
    a. hypothermia (pp. 517–523)
    b. superficial and deep frostbite (pp. 523–524)
    c. near-drowning (pp. 525–528)
    d. decompression illness (pp. 531, 532–534)
    e. diving emergency (pp. 530–536)
    f. altitude illness (pp. 536–539)

18. Identify differences between mild, severe, chronic and acute hypothermia. (p. 518)

19. Discuss the impact of severe hypothermia on standard BCLS and ACLS algorithms and transport considerations. (pp. 520–523)

20. Differentiate between fresh-water and saltwater immersion as they relate to near-drowning. (pp. 526–527)

21. Discuss the incidence of "wet" versus "dry" drownings and the differences in their management. (pp. 525–526)

22. Discuss the complications and protective role of hypothermia in the context of near-drowning. (pp. 525, 527–528)

23. Define self contained underwater breathing apparatus (scuba). (p. 528)

24. Describe the laws of gases and relate them to diving emergencies and altitude illness. (pp. 528–529)

25. Differentiate between the various diving emergencies. (pp. 530–531)

26. Identify the various conditions that may result from pulmonary over-pressure accidents. (pp. 531, 534)

27. Describe the function of the Divers Alert Network (DAN) and how its members may aid in the management of diving related illnesses. (pp. 535–536)

28. Describe the specific function and benefit of hyperbaric oxygen therapy for the management of diving accidents. (p. 533)

29. Define acute mountain sickness (AMS), high altitude pulmonary edema (HAPE), and high altitude cerebral edema (HACE). (pp. 538–539)

30. Discuss the symptomatic variations presented in progressive altitude illnesses. (pp. 538–539)

31. Discuss the pharmacology appropriate for the treatment of altitude illnesses. (pp. 537–539)

32. Given several pre-programmed simulated environmental emergency patients, provide the appropriate assessment, management, and transportation. (pp. 505–544)

CASE STUDY

Today is Sunday and you and your partner are staffing Medic 7. Because of the bad weather, you pick up your partner from his home in your four-wheel-drive sport utility vehicle and ride together to work at the Thunder Bay station. It is another bitterly cold January day, so you warm up with a mug of hot chocolate, awaiting what the day will bring. Suddenly, central dispatch calls in a "priority A" situation at 1050 Ventura Road, a downtown office building in the bar and nightclub district. Apparently, someone on the way to work found an unconscious man lying in the snow. You and you partner depart immediately.

Upon arrival you find an approximately 20-year-old male huddled and shivering on the ice-covered ground. His breathing is shallow and irregular. He is quite stuporous and confused but manages to tell you that he had been out celebrating his twenty-first birthday last night and early this morning. He thinks he passed out here a couple of hours ago but really is not sure.

Your assessment reveals that the patient is bradycardic and mildly hypotensive. His core temperature is 86° F (30° C). While you are speaking with the patient, he stops shivering and his speech becomes unintelligible. You and your partner gently and slowly put him in the ambulance, remove his wet clothing, apply cardiac and core temperature monitors, and then place warm water bottles at his head, neck, chest, and groin. Your partner notes his core temperature has dropped to 85° F (29.4° C).

En route to Foothills General Hospital, your vehicle passes through a bumpy area of road construction, jostling your patient considerably. The alarms go off, and ventricular fibrillation appears on the monitor. Vitals are absent after checking for two minutes. Your partner administers 200J, 300J, and 360J shocks without success. You intubate the patient, ventilate with warmed oxygen, and begin chest compressions. You give no medications through the IV.

In the emergency department, the patient is gradually rewarmed, using active techniques. Once the core temperature is above 86° F (30°C), the usual ACLS protocols are initiated. The patient is converted from ventricular fibrillation and slowly regains vital signs and is eventually admitted to the ICU. Following admission, he does well and is discharged five days later. The day before his discharge you and your partner stop by to check his progress. He reports that he is doing very well but does not remember the prehospital care or the ambulance ride. The patient is adamant about one thing, however. He vows never to drink alcohol again.

INTRODUCTION

The *environment* can be defined as all of the surrounding external factors that affect the development and functioning of a living organism. Human beings obviously depend on the environment for life. But they also must be protected from its extremes. When factors such as temperature, weather, terrain, and atmospheric pressure act on the body, they can create stresses that the body is unable to compensate for. A medical condition caused or exacerbated by such environmental factors is known as an **environmental emergency.**

Environmental emergencies include a variety of conditions such as heatstroke, hypothermia, drowning or near-drowning, altitude sickness, nuclear radiation, and diving accidents or barotraumas, among others. Such emergencies often call for special rescue resources.

Although environmental emergencies can affect anyone, several risk factors predispose certain individuals to developing environmental illnesses. These factors include:

- Age—Very young children and older adults do not tolerate environmental extremes very well.
- Poor general health
- Fatigue
- Predisposing medical conditions
- Certain medications—either prescription or over-the-counter

Environmental factors must also be considered when determining the risk for environmental emergencies. For example, climate in a particular place may vary greatly from moment to moment. Areas where change in temperature can be drastic over the course of the day may catch unwary individuals off guard. For example, desert areas can have temperatures of 105° F during the day but drop below freezing at night, placing unprepared travelers in a difficult situation. Temperatures in parts of southern Alberta can change drastically when the Chinook winds kick up. Other considerations include the current season, local weather patterns, atmospheric pressures (high altitude or underwater), and the type of terrain, which can cause injury or hinder rescue efforts.

As a paramedic, you will frequently be called upon to treat medical emergencies related to environmental conditions. It is critical that you understand the particular conditions that prevail in your region. If you live in a mountain area, near large caves, in an area with swift moving water, or in a resort area where diving is prominent, you need to be familiar with the specialized rescue resources these situations may require and the particular environmental emergencies they may cause. Understanding their causes and underlying pathophysiologies can help you recognize these emergencies promptly and manage them effectively.

Although many environmental factors can result in medical emergencies, this chapter will focus primarily on problems related to temperature extremes, drowning or near-drowning, diving emergencies, high altitude illness, and nuclear radiation.

＊ environmental emergency a medical condition caused or exacerbated by the weather, terrain, atmospheric pressure, or other local factors.

HOMEOSTASIS

In order for the human body to function properly, it must interact with the environment to obtain oxygen, nutrients, and other necessities, but it must also avoid being damaged by extreme external environmental conditions. The process of maintaining constant suitable conditions within the body is called **homeostasis.** Various body systems respond in an effort to maintain the correct core and peripheral temperature, oxygen level, and energy supply to maintain life.

＊ homeostasis the natural tendency of the body to maintain a steady and normal internal environment.

The following sections address how the body attempts to maintain these normal settings and what happens when certain environmental conditions exceed the ability of the body to compensate.

PATHOPHYSIOLOGY OF HEAT AND COLD DISORDERS

MECHANISMS OF HEAT GAIN AND LOSS

The body gains and loses heat in two ways, from within the body itself and by contact with the external environment.

The body receives heat from or loses it to the environment via the thermal gradient. The **thermal gradient** is the difference in temperature between the environment (the ambient temperature) and the body. The ambient temperature is usually different from body temperature. If the environment is warmer than the body, heat flows from the environment to the body. If the body is warmer than the environment, heat flows from the body to the environment. Other environmental factors, including wind and relative humidity (the percentage of water vapor in the air), also affect heat gain and loss.

The mechanisms by which heat is generated within the body and by which heat is gained or lost to the environment are discussed in more detail in the following sections.

* **thermal gradient** the difference in temperature between the environment and the body.

THERMOGENESIS (HEAT GENERATION)

The amount of heat in the body continually fluctuates as a result of the heat generated or gained and the heat lost. The body gains heat from both external and internal sources. In addition to the heat the body absorbs from the environment, the body also generates heat through energy-producing chemical reactions (metabolism).

The creation of heat is called **thermogenesis.** There are several types of thermogenesis. One is *work-induced thermogenesis* that results from exercise. Our muscles need to create heat because warm muscles work more effectively than cold ones. One way muscles can produce heat is by shivering. Another type, *thermoregulatory thermogenesis,* is controlled by the endocrine system. The hormones norepinephrine and epinephrine can cause an immediate increase in the rate of cellular metabolism, which in turn increases heat production. The last type, metabolic thermogenesis, or *diet-induced thermogenesis,* is caused by the processing of food and nutrients. When a meal is eaten, digested, absorbed, and metabolized, heat is produced as a by-product of these activities.

* **thermogenesis** the production of heat, especially within the body.

THERMOLYSIS (HEAT LOSS)

The heat generated by the body is constantly lost to the environment. This occurs because the body is usually warmer than the surrounding environment. The transfer of heat into the environment occurs through the following mechanisms (Figure 10-1):

* **Conduction.** Direct contact of the body's surface to another, cooler object causes the body to lose heat by conduction. Heat flows from higher temperature matter to lower temperature matter.
* **Convection.** Heat loss to air currents passing over the body is called convection. Heat, however, must first be conducted to the air before being carried away by convection currents.
* **Radiation.** An unclothed person will lose approximately 60 percent of total body heat by radiation at normal room temperature. This

* **conduction** moving electrons, ions, heat, or sound waves through a conductor or conducting medium.

* **convection** transfer of heat via currents in liquids or gases.

* **radiation** transfer of energy through space or matter.

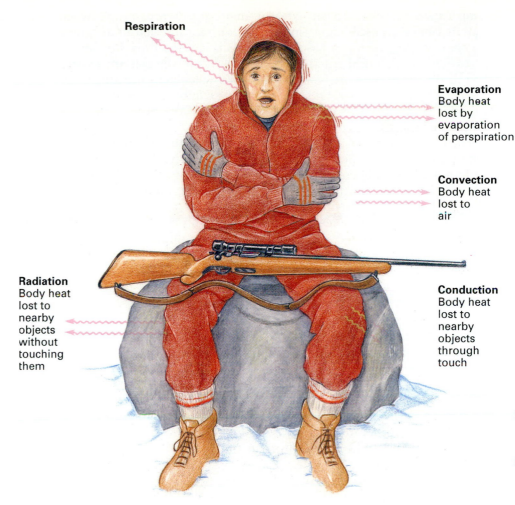

Respiration

Evaporation
Body heat
lost by
evaporation
of perspiration

Convection
Body heat
lost to
air

Radiation
Body heat
lost to
nearby
objects
without
touching
them

Conduction
Body heat
lost to
nearby
objects
through
touch

FIGURE 10-1   Heat loss by the body.

heat loss is in the form of infrared rays. All objects not at absolute zero temperature will radiate heat into the atmosphere.

- **Evaporation.** Evaporation is the change of a liquid to vapor. Evaporative heat loss occurs as water evaporates from the skin. Additionally, a great deal of heat loss occurs through evaporation of fluids in the lungs. Water evaporates from the skin and lungs at approximately 600 mL/day.

- **Respiration.** Respiration combines the mechanisms of convection, radiation, and evaporation. It accounts for a large proportion of the body's heat loss. Heat is transferred from the lungs to inspired air by convection and radiation. Evaporation in the lungs humidifies the inspired air (adds water vapor to it). During expiration this warm, humidified air is released into the environment, creating heat loss.

THERMOREGULATION

Thermoregulation is the maintenance or regulation of temperature. The body temperature of the deep tissues, commonly called the **core temperature,** usually does not vary more than a degree or so from its normal 98.6° (37° C). A naked

✳ **evaporation** change from liquid to a gaseous state.

✳ **respiration** the exchange of gases between a living organism and its environment.

✳ **thermoregulation** the maintenance or regulation of a particular temperature of the body.

✳ **core temperature** the body temperature of the deep tissues, which usually does not vary more than a degree or so from its normal 37° C (98.6° F).

Content Review

COMPARATIVE BODY TEMPERATURES

Celsius	Fahrenheit
40.6°	105°
37.8°	100°
37°	98.6°
35°	95°
32°	89.6°
30°	86°
20°	68°

* **hypothalamus** portion of the diencephalon producing neurosecretions important in the control of certain metabolic activities, including body temperature regulation.

* **negative feedback** a mechanism of response that serves to maintain a state of internal constancy, or homeostasis. Changes in the internal environment trigger mechanisms that reverse or negate the change, hence the term "negative feedback."

* **basal metabolic rate (BMR)** rate at which the body consumes energy just to maintain stability; the basic metabolic rate (measured by the rate of oxygen consumption) of an awake, relaxed person 12 to 14 hours after eating and at a comfortable temperature.

* **exertional metabolic rate** rate at which the body consumes energy during activity. It is faster than the basic metabolic rate.

person can be exposed to an external environment ranging anywhere from 55° F to 144° F and still maintain a fairly constant internal body temperature. This characteristic of warm-blooded animals is called *steady-state metabolism*. The various biochemical reactions occurring within the cell are most efficient when the body temperature is within this narrow temperature range.

Evaluation of peripheral body temperature can be measured by touch or by taking the temperature by oral or axillary means. Core body temperatures can be measured using tympanic or rectal thermometers.

The body maintains a balance between the production and loss of heat almost entirely through the nervous system and negative feedback mechanisms. The **hypothalamus,** located at the base of the brain, is responsible for temperature regulation. It functions as a thermostat, controlling temperature through the release of neurosecretions (secretions produced by nerve cells). When the hypothalamus senses an increased body temperature, it shuts off the mechanisms designed to create heat, for example, shivering. When it senses a decrease in body temperature, the hypothalamus shuts off mechanisms designed to cool the body, for example, sweating. Because the action involved requires stopping, or negating, a process, it is called a **negative feedback** system.

When the heat regulating function of the hypothalamus is disrupted, the result can be an abnormally high or low body temperature. At the extremes, such abnormal temperatures can result in death (Figure 10-2).

Thermoreceptors

Although the hypothalamus plays a key role in body temperature regulation, temperature receptors in other parts of the body also help to moderate temperatures. There are thermoreceptors in the skin and certain mucous membranes (peripheral thermoreceptors) as well as in certain deep tissues of the body (central thermoreceptors). The skin has both cold and warm receptors. Because cold receptors outnumber warm receptors, peripheral detection of temperature consists mainly of detecting cold rather than warmth. Deep body temperature receptors lie mostly in the spinal cord, abdominal viscera, and in or around the great veins. These receptors are exposed to the body's core temperature rather than the peripheral temperature. They also respond mainly to cold rather than warmth. Both peripheral and central thermoreceptors act to prevent lowering of the body temperature.

Metabolic Rate

The **basal metabolic rate (BMR)** is the metabolism that occurs when the body is completely at rest. It is the rate at which the body consumes energy just to maintain itself—the rate of metabolism that maintains brain function, circulation, and cell stability. Any additional activity that the body performs demands energy consumption beyond that supported by the basal rate, metabolizing more nutrients and releasing more calories (units of heat). The rate of metabolism that supports this additional activity is called an **exertional metabolic rate.**

The body continually adjusts the metabolic rate in order to maintain the temperature of the core (where the crucial structures like the heart and brain are located). The body also achieves temperature maintenance by dilating some blood vessels and constricting others so that the blood carries the excess heat from the core to the periphery where it is close to the skin. This allows heat to dissipate through the skin into the environment.

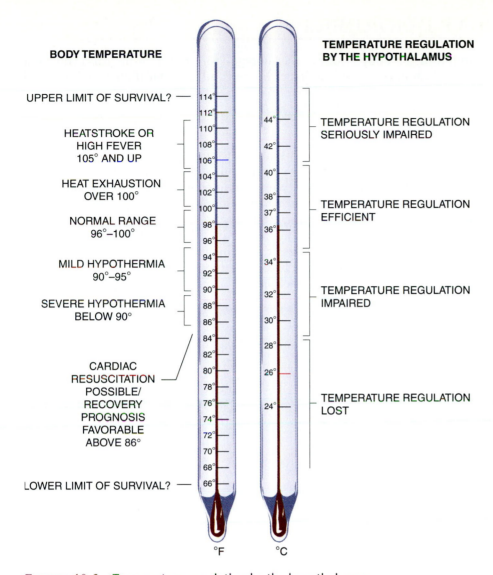

BODY TEMPERATURE

UPPER LIMIT OF SURVIVAL? — 114°

112°

HEATSTROKE OR
HIGH FEVER
105° AND UP

HEAT EXHAUSTION
OVER 100°

NORMAL RANGE
96°–100°

MILD HYPOTHERMIA
90°–95°

SEVERE HYPOTHERMIA
BELOW 90°

CARDIAC
RESUSCITATION
POSSIBLE/
RECOVERY
PROGNOSIS
FAVORABLE
ABOVE 86°

LOWER LIMIT OF SURVIVAL? — 66°

°F   °C

**TEMPERATURE REGULATION
BY THE HYPOTHALAMUS**

TEMPERATURE REGULATION
SERIOUSLY IMPAIRED

TEMPERATURE REGULATION
EFFICIENT

TEMPERATURE REGULATION
IMPAIRED

TEMPERATURE REGULATION
LOST

FIGURE 10-2 Temperature regulation by the hypothalamus.

Conversely, when the environment is too cold, *counter-current heat exchange* is used to shunt warm blood away from the superficial veins near the skin and back into the deep veins near the core to keep vital structures warm. Another body response that counters a cold environment is shivering, a physical activity that increases metabolism and generates heat.

It is important to note that these various mechanisms can create a difference between the core body temperature and the peripheral body temperature. Core temperature is the crucial measurement since, as noted, the core is where the major organs are located. Therefore, it is important in any heat-related or cold-related emergency to obtain a core temperature reading such as from the rectum. Oral and axillary temperatures may provide convenient approximations in some situations but may lead to incorrect interventions if relied upon for treatment of the patient with an environmental illness.

HEAT DISORDERS

Disruption of the body's normal thermoregulatory mechanisms can produce a number of heat illnesses, such as hyperthermia and fever. **Heat illness** is increased *core body temperature (CBT)* due to inadequate thermolysis.

HYPERTHERMIA

Hyperthermia is a state of unusually high body temperature, specifically the core body temperature. Hyperthermia is usually caused by heat transfer from the external environment that the body cannot compensate for. Occasionally it is caused by excessive generation of heat within the body.

As the body attempts to eliminate this excessive heat, you will see the general signs of thermolysis (heat loss). These signs are caused by the body's two chief methods of heat dissipation, sweating (which leads to evaporative heat loss) and vasodilation (which allows the blood to carry heat to the periphery for dissipation through the skin). These include:

- Diaphoresis (sweating)
- Increased skin temperature
- Flushing

As heat illness progresses, you will also note signs of thermolytic inadequacy (the failure of the body's thermoregulatory mechanisms to compensate adequately):

- Altered mentation
- Altered level of consciousness

Hyperthermia can manifest as heat cramps, heat exhaustion, or heatstroke, which will be discussed in following sections.

PREDISPOSING FACTORS

Age, general health, and medications are predisposing factors in hyperthermia. Factors that may contribute to a susceptibility to hyperthermia include:

- *Age of the patient*—Pediatric and geriatric populations can tolerate less variation in temperature and their heat regulating mechanisms are not as responsive as those of young adult and adult populations.
- *Health of the patient*—Diabetics can become hyperthermic more easily because they develop **autonomic neuropathy.** This condition damages the autonomic nervous system, which may interfere with thermoregulatory input and with vasodilation and perspiration, which normally dissipate heat.
- *Medications*—Various medications can affect body temperature in the following ways:
  - *Diuretics* predispose to dehydration, which worsens hyperthermia.
  - *Beta blockers* interfere with vasodilation and reduce the capacity to increase heart rate in response to volume loss and may also interfere with thermoregulatory input.
  - *Psychotropics and antihistamines,* such as antipsychotics and phenothiazines, interfere with central thermoregulation.

- *Level of acclimatization*—**Acclimatization** is the process of becoming adjusted to a change in environment. In response to an environmental change, reversible changes in body structure and function take place that help to maintain homeostasis.
- *Length of exposure*
- *Intensity of exposure*
- *Environmental factors* such as humidity and wind

PREVENTIVE MEASURES

Ideally, prevention of heat disorders is preferable to treating an illness already in progress. Measures to prevent hyperthermia include the following:

- Maintain adequate fluid intake, remembering that thirst is an inadequate indicator of dehydration.
- Allow time for gradual acclimatization to being out in the heat. Acclimatization results in more perspiration with lower salt concentration and increases body-fluid volume.
- Limit exposure to hot environments.

SPECIFIC HEAT DISORDERS

Inevitably, you will be required to respond to heat-related emergencies: heat cramps, heat exhaustion, or heatstroke. Heat cramps and heat exhaustion result from dehydration and depletion of sodium and other electrolytes. Heatstroke, a far more serious and potentially life-threatening condition, results from the failure of the body's thermoregulatory mechanisms.

Signs and symptoms and emergency care procedures for heat cramps, heat exhaustion, and heatstroke are discussed in the following sections and summarized in Procedure 10–1.

Heat (Muscle) Cramps

Heat cramps are muscle cramps caused by overexertion and dehydration in the presence of high atmospheric temperatures. Sweating occurs as sodium (salt) is transported to the skin. Because "water follows sodium," water is deposited on the skin surface where evaporation occurs, aiding in the cooling process. Since sweating involves not only the loss of water but also the loss of electrolytes (such as sodium), intermittent cramping of skeletal muscles may occur. Heat cramps are painful but are not considered to be an actual heat illness.

Signs and Symptoms The patient with heat cramps will present with cramps in the fingers, arms, legs, or abdominal muscles. He will generally be mentally alert with a feeling of weakness. He may feel dizzy or faint. Vital signs will be stable. Body temperature may be normal or slightly elevated. The skin is likely to be moist and warm.

Treatment Treatment of the patient with heat cramps is usually easily accomplished:

1. *Remove the patient from the environment.* Place the patient in a cool environment such as a shaded area or the air conditioned back of the ambulance.

Procedure 10-1   Heat Disorders.

Condition	Muscle Cramps	Mental Status	Respirations	Pulse	Blood pressure	Body temperature	Other possible
Heat cramps	Yes	Alert	Normal	Normal	Normal	Normal	Weakness, dizziness, faintness
Heat exhaustion	Sometimes	Anxiety to possible loss of consciousness	Rapid, shallow	Weak	Normal	Somewhat elevated	Headache, paresthesia, diarrhea
Heatstroke	No	Confusion, disorientation, or loss of consciousness	Deep, rapid; later shallow, slowing	Rapid, full; later slowing	Low	Very high	Seizures

10-1a   Heat Cramps.

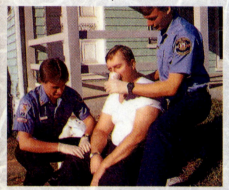

EMERGENCY CARE
- Remove patient from hot environment. Place in a cool, shaded, or air-conditioned area.
- Administer oral fluids if patient is alert and able to swallow or an IV of normal saline.

10-1b   Heat Exhaustion.

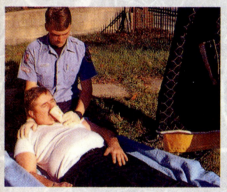

EMERGENCY CARE
- Remove patient from hot environment. Place in a cool, shaded, or air-conditioned area.
- Administer oral fluids if patient is alert and able to swallow or an IV of normal saline.
- Place patient in a supine position.
- Remove some clothing and fan the patient. Be careful not to cool to the point of chilling or causing shivering.
- Treat for shock if shock is suspected. However, do not cover the patient to the point of overheating.

10-1c   Heatstroke.

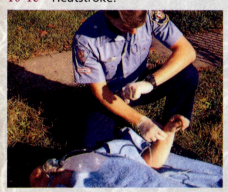

EMERGENCY CARE
- Remove patient from hot environment. Place in a cool, shaded, or air-conditioned area.
- Initiate rapid active cooling en route to the hospital. Remove clothing and cover patient with sheets soaked in tepid water. Lower body temperature to 102° F/30° C. Avoid cooling to a lower temperature.
- Administer high-flow oxygen by nonrebreather mask.
- If patient is alert and able to swallow, administer oral fluids. Begin one or two IVs of normal saline, wide open.
- Monitor the ECG.
- Avoid vasopressors and anticholinergic drugs.
- Monitor the body temperature.

In the case of severe cramps:

2. *Administer an oral saline solution* (approximately 4 teaspoons of salt to a gallon of water) or a sports drink. Do NOT administer salt tablets, which are not absorbed as readily and may cause stomach irritation and ulceration or hypernatremia. *If the patient is unable to take fluids orally, an IV of normal saline may be needed.*

Some EMS systems recommend massaging the painful muscles. Application of moist towels to the patient's forehead and over the cramped muscles may also be helpful.

Heat Exhaustion

Heat exhaustion, which is considered to be a mild heat illness, is an acute reaction to heat exposure. It is the most common heat-related illness seen by prehospital personnel. An individual performing work in a hot environment will lose 1 to 2 liters of water an hour. Each liter lost contains 20 to 50 milliequivalents of sodium. The resulting loss of water and sodium, combined with general vasodilation, leads to a decreased circulating blood volume, venous pooling, and reduced cardiac output.

Dehydration and sodium loss due to sweating account for the presenting symptoms. However, these signs and symptoms are not exclusive to heat exhaustion. Instead, they mimic those of an individual suffering from fluid and sodium loss from any of a number of other causes. A history of exposure to high environmental temperatures is needed to obtain an accurate assessment.

If not treated, heat exhaustion may progress to heatstroke.

Signs and Symptoms Signs and symptoms that you may encounter include increased body temperature (over 100° F or 37.8° C), skin that is cool and clammy with heavy perspiration, breathing that is rapid and shallow, and a weak pulse. There may be signs of active thermolysis such as diarrhea and muscle cramps. The patient will feel weak and, in some cases, may lose consciousness. There may be central nervous system (CNS) symptoms such as headache, anxiety, paresthesia, and impaired judgment or even psychosis.

Treatment Prehospital management of the patient with heat exhaustion is aimed at immediate cooling and fluid replacement. Steps include:

1. *Remove the patient from the environment.* Place the patient in a cool environment such as a shaded area or the air-conditioned ambulance.
2. *Place the patient in a supine position.*
3. *Administer an oral saline solution* (approximately 4 teaspoons of salt to a gallon of water) or a sports drink. Do NOT administer salt tablets, which are not absorbed as readily and may cause stomach irritation and ulceration or hypernatremia. *If the patient is unable to take fluids orally, an IV of normal saline may be needed.*
4. *Remove some clothing and fan the patient.* Remove enough clothing to cool the patient without chilling him. Fanning increases evaporation and cooling. Again, be careful not to cool the patient to the point of chilling. If the patient begins to shiver, stop fanning and perhaps cover the patient lightly.
5. *Treat for shock, if shock is suspected.* However, be careful not to cover the patient to the point of overheating him.

* **heat exhaustion** a mild heat illness; an acute reaction to heat exposure.

Symptoms should resolve with fluids, rest, and supine posturing with knees elevated. If they do not, consider that the symptoms may be due to an increased core body temperature, which is predictive of impending heatstroke and should be treated aggressively, as outlined in the following section.

Heatstroke

Heatstroke is a true environmental emergency.

Heatstroke is a true environmental emergency that occurs when the body's hypothalamic temperature regulation is lost, causing uncompensated hyperthermia. This in turn causes cell death and damage to the brain, liver, and kidneys. There is no arbitrary core temperature at which heatstroke begins. However, heatstroke is generally characterized by a body temperature of at least 105° F (40.6° C), central nervous system disturbances, and usually the cessation of sweating.

Signs and Symptoms Sweating is thought to stop due to destruction of the sweat glands or when sensory overload causes them to temporarily dysfunction. However, the patient's skin may be either dry or covered with sweat that is still present on the skin from earlier exertion. In either case, the skin will be hot.

The patient may present with the following signs and symptoms:

- Cessation of sweating
- Hot skin that is dry or moist
- Very high core temperature
- Deep respirations that become shallow, rapid at first but may later slow
- Rapid, full pulse, may slow later
- Hypotension with low or absent diastolic reading
- Confusion or disorientation or unconsciousness
- Possible seizures

Classic heatstroke commonly presents in those with chronic illnesses, with the increased core body temperature due to deficient thermoregulatory function. Predisposing conditions include age, diabetes, and other medical conditions. In this type of heatstroke hot, red, dry skin is common.

Exertional heatstroke commonly presents in those who are in good general health, with the increased core body temperature due to overwhelming heat stress. There is excessive ambient temperature as well as excessive exertion with prolonged exposure and poor acclimatization. In this type of heatstroke you will find that, although sweating has ceased and the skin is hot, moisture from prior sweating may still be present.

If the patient develops heatstroke due to exertion, he may go into severe metabolic acidosis caused by lactic acid accumulation. Hyperkalemia (excessive potassium in blood) may also develop because of the release of potassium from injured muscle cells, renal failure, or metabolic acidosis.

The heatstroke patient should be cooled immediately and given fluids.

Treatment Prehospital management of the heatstroke patient is aimed at immediate cooling and replacement of fluids. Steps include:

1. *Remove the patient from the environment.* This first step is essential. If you do not remove the patient from the hot environment, any other measures will be only minimally useful. Move the patient to a cool environment, such as the air-conditioned ambulance.

2. *Initiate rapid active cooling.* Body temperature must be lowered to 102° F (39° C). A target of 102° F (39° C) is used to avoid an overshoot. This can be accomplished en route to the hospital.

Remove the patient's clothing and cover the patient with sheets soaked in tepid water. Fanning and misting may also be used if necessary. Refrain from over-cooling, as this may cause reflex hypothermia (low body temperature). This results in shivering, which can raise the core temperature again. Tepid water is used because ice packs and cold-water immersion may affect peripheral thermoreceptors, producing reflex vasoconstriction and shivering.

3. *Administer oxygen.* Administer high-flow oxygen by nonrebreather mask. If respirations are shallow, assist with a bag-valve-mask unit supplied with 100 percent oxygen. Utilize pulse oximetry, if available.

4. *Administer fluid therapy if the patient is alert and able to swallow.*
   – *Oral fluids.* In many cases oral fluid therapy will be all that is needed. Some salt additive is beneficial, but salt tablets should be avoided as they may cause gastrointestinal irritation and ulceration or hypernatremia. There is a very limited need for other electrolytes in oral rehydration.
   – *Intravenous fluids.* Begin 1 to 2 IVs, using normal saline. Initially infuse them wide open.

5. *Monitor the ECG.* Cardiac dysrhythmias may occur at any time. S-T segment depression, non-specific T-wave changes with occasional PVCs, and supraventricular tachycardias are common.

6. *Avoid vasopressors and anticholinergic drugs.* These agents may potentiate heatstroke by inhibiting sweating. They can also produce a hypermetabolic state in the presence of high environmental temperatures and relatively high humidity.

7. *Monitor body temperature.* EMS systems operating in extremely warm climates should carry some device to record the body temperature, whether a simple rectal thermometer or a sophisticated electronic device. Simple glass thermometers generally do not measure above 106° F (41° C) or below 95° F (35° C). This may become significant during long transport when it is essential to detect changes in the patient's condition.

ROLE OF DEHYDRATION IN HEAT DISORDERS

Dehydration often goes hand in hand with heat disorders because it inhibits vasodilation and therefore thermolysis. Dehydration leads to orthostatic hypotension (increased pulse and decreased blood pressure on rising from a supine position) and the following symptoms which may occur along with the signs and symptoms of heatstroke:

- Nausea, vomiting, and abdominal distress
- Vision disturbances
- Decreased urine output
- Poor skin turgor
- Signs of hypovolemic shock

When these signs and symptoms are present, rehydration of the patient is critical. Oral fluids may be administered if the patient is alert and not nauseated. Administration of IV fluids may be necessary, especially if the patient has an altered mental status or is nauseated. It is not uncommon for the adult patient with moderate to severe dehydration to require 2–3 liters of IV fluids (occasionally more!).

Dehydration often goes hand in hand with heat disorders.

Thirst is a poor indication of the degree of dehydration present.

FEVER (PYREXIA)

✻ **pyrexia** fever, or above-normal body temperature.

✻ **pyrogen** any substance causing a fever, such as viruses and bacteria or substances produced within the body in response to infection or inflammation.

A fever (**pyrexia**) is the elevation of the body temperature above the normal temperature for that person. (An individual person's normal temperature may be one or two degrees above or below 98.6° F or 37° C.) The body develops a fever when pathogens enter and cause infection, which in turn stimulates the production of pyrogens.

Pyrogens are any substances that cause fever, such as viruses and bacteria or substances produced within the body in response to infection or inflammation. They reset the hypothalamic thermostat to a higher level. Metabolism is increased, which produces the elevation of temperature. The increased body temperature fights infection by making the body a less hospitable environment for the invading organism. The hypothalamic thermostat will reset to normal when pyrogen production stops or when pathogens end their attack on the body.

Fever is sometimes difficult to differentiate from heatstroke, and neurological symptoms may present with either, but there is usually a history of infection or illness with a fever. While the heatstroke patient usually has a history of exertion and exposure to high ambient temperatures, this is not always the case. In some cases, heatstroke can be caused by impaired functioning of the hypothalamus without exertion or exposure to ambient heat. Treat for heatstroke if you are unsure which it is.

When unsure if the problem is heatstroke or fever, treat for heatstroke.

Although fever may be beneficial, it can be disconcerting to the parents of children with fever. In addition, fever can be uncomfortable for the patient. If the patient is uncomfortable, measures should be taken to treat the fever. Also, if a child has a history of febrile seizures, the fever should be treated. Parents will often have their febrile children wrapped in several layers of clothing or blankets because the child is "cold." These should be removed, leaving only the diaper or underclothes, exposing the child to the ambient air. This will allow a controlled cooling.

Do not use sponge baths to cool febrile children.

Consider administering an antipyretic, primarily for patient comfort. This is especially important in services with long transportation times.

Sponge baths and cool-water immersion should not be used. These cause a rapid drop in the body core temperature and result in shivering. This again elevates the core temperature, which complicates the process. Several medications are good antipyretics (that is, they lower body temperature in fever). These include acetaminophen (Tylenol) and ibuprofen (Motrin). Many EMS systems will utilize an antipyretic in the treatment of fever, particularly in pediatric patients. Liquid acetaminophen and ibuprofen are easy to administer and effective. Acetaminophen is also available in a suppository form for patients with active vomiting. These antipyretics are typically dosed based on the patient's weight:

- *Acetaminophen*—15 mg/kg for pediatric patients; adult dose is typically 650 mg
- *Ibuprofen*—10 mg/kg for pediatric patients; adult dose is typically 600–800 mg

These liquid medications should be dosed with syringes as teaspoons are inaccurate measuring devices. EMS services with prolonged transport times should consider the use of antipyretics for patient comfort as well as for the prevention of febrile seizures.

COLD DISORDERS

Disruption of the body's normal thermoregulation may produce cold-related disorders such as hypothermia, frostbite, and trench foot.

Content Review

COLD DISORDERS
Hypothermia
Frostbite
Trench foot

HYPOTHERMIA

Hypothermia is a state of low body temperature, specifically low core temperature. When the core temperature of the body drops below 95° F (35° C), an individual is considered to be hypothermic. Hypothermia can be attributed to inadequate thermogenesis, excessive cold stress, or a combination of both.

MECHANISMS OF HEAT CONSERVATION AND LOSS

Exposure to cold normally triggers compensatory mechanisms designed to conserve and generate heat in order to maintain a normal body temperature. One such mechanism is piloerection (hair standing on end, "goose bumps") to impede air flow across the skin. Shivering and increased muscle tone occur, resulting in increased metabolism. There is peripheral vasoconstriction with an increase in cardiac output and respiratory rate. When these mechanisms can no longer adequately compensate for heat lost from the body surface, the body temperature falls. As the body temperature falls, so do the metabolic rate and cardiac output.

As discussed, major mechanisms of body heat loss are conduction, convection, radiation, evaporation, and respiration. Heat loss can be increased by the removal of clothing (decreased insulation, increased radiation), the wetting of clothing by rain or snow (increased conduction and evaporation), air movement around the body (increased convection), or contact with a cold surface or cold-water immersion (increased conduction).

PREDISPOSING FACTORS

Several factors can contribute to the risk of developing hypothermia. They also contribute to the severity of damage if cold injury occurs. Risk factors that increase the danger of developing hypothermia include:

- *Age of the patient*—Pediatric or geriatric patients cannot tolerate cold environments and have less responsive heat generating mechanisms to combat cold exposure. Elderly persons often become hypothermic in environments that seem only mildly cool to others.

- *Health of the patient*—Hypothyroidism suppresses metabolism, preventing patients from responding appropriately to cold stress. Malnutrition, hypoglycemia, Parkinson's disease, fatigue, and other medical conditions can interfere with the body's ability to combat cold exposure.

- *Medications*—Some drugs interfere with proper heat generating mechanisms. These include narcotics, alcohol, phenothiazines, barbiturates, antiseizure medications, antihistamines and other allergy medications, antipsychotics, sedatives, antidepressants, and various pain medications such as aspirin, acetaminophen, and NSAIDs.

- *Prolonged or intense exposure*—The length and severity of cold exposure have a direct effect on morbidity and mortality.

- *Coexisting weather conditions*—High humidity, brisk winds, or accompanying rain can all magnify the effect of cold exposure on the human body by accelerating the loss of heat from skin surfaces.

PREVENTIVE MEASURES

Certain precautions can decrease the risk of morbidity related to cold injury.

- Dress warmly.
- Get plenty of rest to maximize the ability of heat generating mechanisms to replenish energy supplies.
- Eat appropriately and at regular intervals to support metabolism.
- Limit exposure to cold environments.

DEGREES OF HYPOTHERMIA

Hypothermia can be classified as mild or severe, as follows:

- *Mild*—a core temperature greater than 90° F (32° C) with signs and symptoms of hypothermia
- *Severe*—a core temperature less than 90° F (32° C) with signs and symptoms of hypothermia

Initially some patients may exhibit *compensated* hypothermia. In this case signs and symptoms of hypothermia will be present but with a normal core body temperature, temporarily maintained by thermogenesis. As energy stores from the liver and muscle glycogen are exhausted, the core body temperature will drop.

The onset of symptoms may be *acute,* as occurs when a person suddenly falls through ice into a frigid lake. *Subacute* exposure can occur in situations such as when mountain climbers are trapped in a snowy, cold environment. Finally, *chronic* exposure to cold is a growing problem in our inner cities where homeless people endure frequent and prolonged cold stress without shelter.

In some cases cold exposure is the primary cause of hypothermia, but in others, hypothermia may develop secondary to other problems, such as medical problems. For example, hypothyroidism depresses the body's heat-producing mechanisms. Brain tumors or head trauma can depress the hypothalamic temperature control center, causing hypothermia. Other conditions such as myocardial infarction, diabetes, hypoglycemia, drugs, poor nutrition, sepsis, or old age can also contribute to metabolic and circulatory disorders that predispose to hypothermia. Any patient thought to have hypothermia, but with no history of exposure to a cold environment, should be assessed for any predisposing factors. Evaluate the patient for level of consciousness, cool skin, and shivering. Also, evaluate the rectal temperature. A rectal temperature of less than 95° F (35° C) indicates hypothermia. Key findings at different degrees of hypothermia are summarized in Table 10-1.

Patients who experience body temperatures above 86° F (30° C) will usually have a favorable prognosis. Those with temperatures below 86° F (30° C) show a significant increase in mortality rate. Remember that most thermometers used in medicine do not register below 95° F (35° C). EMS systems in colder areas should carry special thermometers for recording subnormal temperature readings as there is no reliable correlation between signs and symptoms and actual core body temperature.

Services operating in colder environments should carry specialized hypothermia thermometers for cold exposure victims.

Signs and Symptoms

Signs and symptoms of hypothermia are summarized in Table 10-2. Patients experiencing mild hypothermia (core temperature >90° F or 32° C) will generally exhibit shivering. The patient may be lethargic and somewhat dulled

Table 10-1		KEY FINDINGS AT DIFFERENT DEGREES OF HYPOTHERMIA
C°	**F°**	**Clinical Findings**
37.6	99.6	Normal rectal temperature
37	98.6	Normal oral temperature
36	96.8	Metabolic rate increased
35	95	Maximum shivering seen
		Impaired judgment
34	93.2	Amnesia
		Slurred speech
33	91.4	Severe clouding of consciousness/apathy
		Uncoordinated movement
32	89.6	Most shivering ceases
		Pupils dilate
31	87.8	Blood pressure may no longer be obtainable
30	86	Atrial fibrillation/other dysrhythmias develop
		Pulse and cardiac output decreased by 33%
29	84.2	Progressive decrease in pulse and breathing
		Progressive decrease in level of consciousness
28	82.4	Pulse and oxygen consumption decreased by 50%
		Severe slowing of respiration
		Increased muscle rigidity
		Loss of consciousness
		High risk of ventricular fibrillation
27	80.6	Loss of reflexes and voluntary movement
		Patients appear clinically dead
26	78.8	No reflexes or response to painful stimuli
25	77	Cerebral blood flow decreased by 66%
24	75.2	Marked hypotension
22	71.6	Maximum risk for ventricular fibrillation
19	66.2	Flat electroencephalogram (EEG)
18	64.4	Asystole
16	60.8	Lowest reported adult survival from accidental exposure
15.2	59.2	Lowest reported infant survival from accidental exposure
10	50	Oxygen consumption 8% of normal
9	48.2	Lowest reported survivor from therapeutic exposure

mentally. (In some cases, however, they may be fully oriented.) Muscles may be stiff and uncoordinated, causing the patient to walk with a stumbling, staggering gait.

Patients experiencing severe hypothermia (core temperature <90° F or 32° C) may be disoriented and confused. As their temperatures continue to fall, they will proceed into stupor and complete coma. Shivering will usually stop, and physical activity will become uncoordinated. Muscles may be stiff and rigid. Continuous cardiac monitoring is indicated for anyone experiencing hypothermia. The ECG

Table 10-2	HYPOTHERMIA: SIGNS AND SYMPTOMS	
Mild		**Severe**
Lethargy		No shivering
Shivering		Dysrhythmias, asystole
Lack of coordination		Loss of voluntary muscle control
Pale, cold, dry skin		Hypotension
Early rise in blood pressure, heart, and respiratory rates		Undetectable pulse and respirations

✱ **J wave** ECG deflection found at the junction of the QRS complex and the ST segment. It is associated with hypothermia and seen at core temperatures below 32° C, most commonly in leads II and V₆; also called an *Osborn wave*.

will frequently show pathognomonic (indicative of a disease) **J waves**, also called Osborn waves, associated with the QRS complexes (Figure 10-3), but these are not useful diagnostically. Atrial fibrillation is the most common presenting dysrhythmia seen in hypothermia. As the body cools, however, the myocardium becomes progressively more irritable and may develop a variety of dysrhythmias. In severe hypothermia, bradycardia is inevitable.

Ventricular fibrillation becomes more probable as the body's core temperature falls below 86° F (30° C). The severely hypothermic patient requires assessment of pulse and respirations for at least 30 seconds every 1 to 2 minutes.

Treatment for Hypothermia

All victims of hypothermia should have the following care (see also Figure 10-4):

1. *Remove wet garments.*
2. *Protect against further heat loss and wind chill.* Use *passive external warming* methods such as application of blankets, insulating materials, and moisture barriers.
3. *Maintain the patient in a horizontal position.*
4. *Avoid rough handling,* which can trigger dysrhythmias.
5. *Monitor the core temperature.*
6. *Monitor the cardiac rhythm.*

Rewarming is not the mirror image of the cooling process.
⚷

Active Rewarming Victims of mild hypothermia may also be rewarmed, using *active external methods*. This includes the use of warmed blankets and/or heat packs placed over areas of high heat transfer with the core: the base of the neck, the axilla,

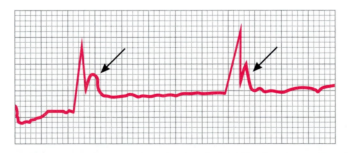

FIGURE 10-3 ECG tracing showing J wave following the QRS complex as seen in hypothermia.

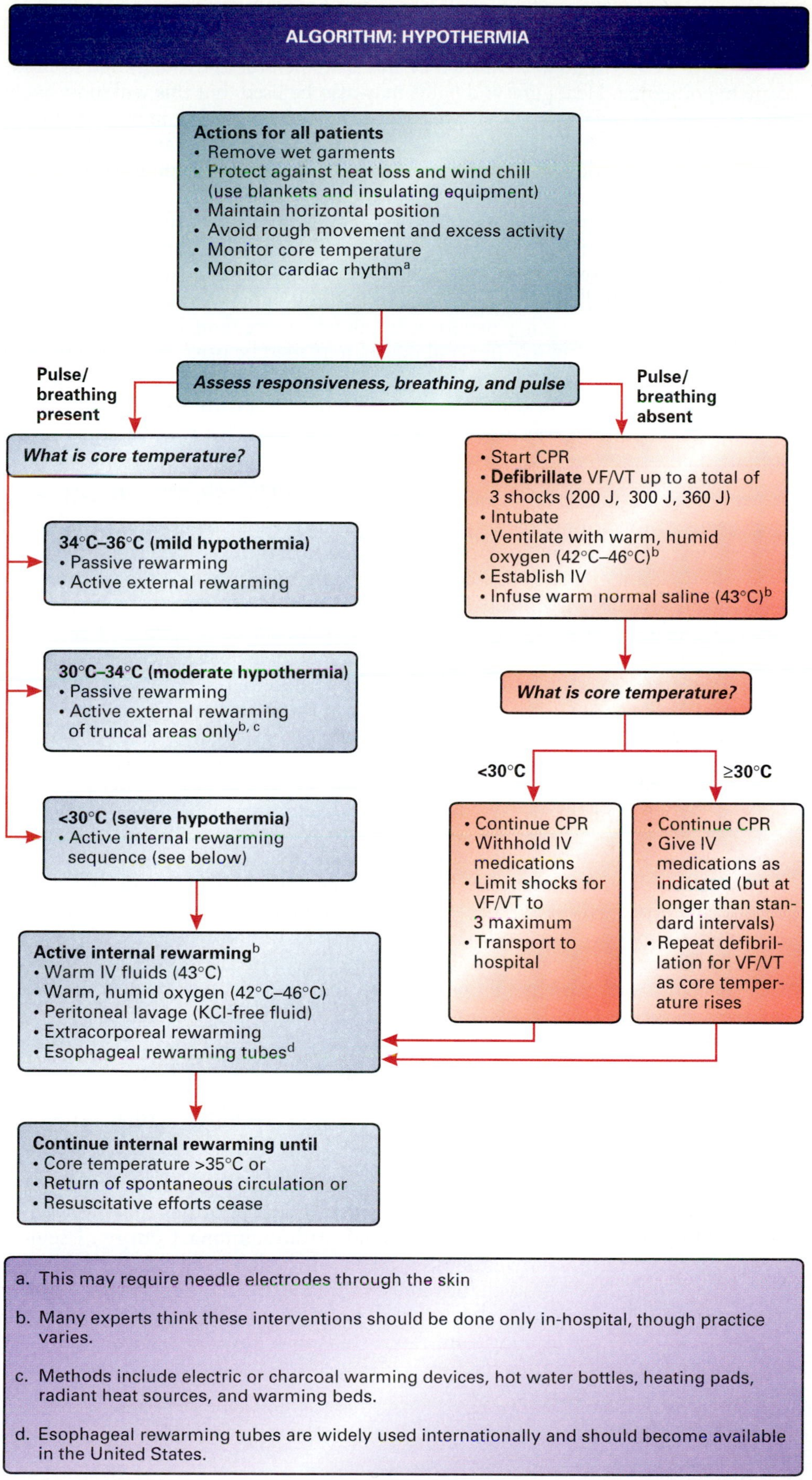

FIGURE 10-4 Algorithm for treatment of hypothermia. Adapted with permission. Journal of the American Medical Association, October 28, 1992, Volume 268, No. 16, *Guidelines for Cardiopulmonary Resuscitation and Emergency Cardiac Care*, p. 2245. © 1992 American Medical Association.

ALGORITHM: HYPOTHERMIA

Actions for all patients
- Remove wet garments
- Protect against heat loss and wind chill (use blankets and insulating equipment)
- Maintain horizontal position
- Avoid rough movement and excess activity
- Monitor core temperature
- Monitor cardiac rhythm[a]

Assess responsiveness, breathing, and pulse

Pulse/breathing present

What is core temperature?

34°C–36°C (mild hypothermia)
- Passive rewarming
- Active external rewarming

30°C–34°C (moderate hypothermia)
- Passive rewarming
- Active external rewarming of truncal areas only[b, c]

<30°C (severe hypothermia)
- Active internal rewarming sequence (see below)

Pulse/breathing absent
- Start CPR
- **Defibrillate** VF/VT up to a total of 3 shocks (200 J, 300 J, 360 J)
- Intubate
- Ventilate with warm, humid oxygen (42°C–46°C)[b]
- Establish IV
- Infuse warm normal saline (43°C)[b]

What is core temperature?

<30°C
- Continue CPR
- Withhold IV medications
- Limit shocks for VF/VT to 3 maximum
- Transport to hospital

≥30°C
- Continue CPR
- Give IV medications as indicated (but at longer than standard intervals)
- Repeat defibrillation for VF/VT as core temperature rises

Active internal rewarming[b]
- Warm IV fluids (43°C)
- Warm, humid oxygen (42°C–46°C)
- Peritoneal lavage (KCl-free fluid)
- Extracorporeal rewarming
- Esophageal rewarming tubes[d]

Continue internal rewarming until
- Core temperature >35°C or
- Return of spontaneous circulation or
- Resuscitative efforts cease

a. This may require needle electrodes through the skin

b. Many experts think these interventions should be done only in-hospital, though practice varies.

c. Methods include electric or charcoal warming devices, hot water bottles, heating pads, radiant heat sources, and warming beds.

d. Esophageal rewarming tubes are widely used internationally and should become available in the United States.

Cold Disorders **521**

and the groin. Be sure to insulate between the heat packs and the skin to prevent burning. Intravenous fluid heaters (i.e. Hot I.V.) can be used to warm the IV fluid to 95° to 100° F/ 35° to 38° C. Warmed IV fluids are helpful in treating mild to moderate hypothermia. Heat guns and lights may also be used, but this will most likely take place in the emergency department. Warm water immersion in water between 102° and 104° F (39° to 40° C) may be used but can induce rewarming shock (see below), so this method also has little application in an out-of-hospital setting.

Active rewarming of the severely hypothermic patient is best carried out in the hospital using a prearranged protocol. Most patients who die during rewarming die from ventricular fibrillation, the risk of which is related to both the depth and the duration of hypothermia. Rough handling of the hypothermic patient may also induce ventricular fibrillation. Active rewarming should not be attempted in the field unless travel to the emergency department will take more than 15 minutes.

If such is the case, active internal means may also be used, including the use of warmed (102° to 104° F/38° to 40° C) humidified oxygen, and administration of warmed IV fluids (also warmed to 102° to 104° F/38° to 40° C). This is crucial to prevent further heat loss, but actual heat transferred is minimal, so there is limited contribution to the rewarming effort.

Rewarming Shock While application of warmed blankets is a safe and effective means of rewarming the hypothermic patient, application of external heat, as with heat packs, is usually not recommended in the prehospital setting. For effective rewarming, more heat transference is generally required than is possible with out-of-hospital methods. Additionally, application of external heat may result in *rewarming shock* by causing reflex peripheral vasodilatation. This reflex vasodilation causes the return of cool blood and acids from the extremities to the core. This may cause a paradoxical "afterdrop" core temperature decrease and further worsen core hypothermia. This, in turn, may cause the blood pressure to fall, especially when there is also volume depletion.

If active rewarming is necessary in the prehospital setting, for example when transport is delayed, administration of warmed IV fluids during rewarming can prevent the onset of rewarming shock.

Cold Diuresis Volume depletion can occur as a result of *cold diuresis*. Core vasoconstriction causes increased blood volume and blood pressure, so the kidneys remove excess fluid to reduce the pressure, thus causing diuresis. A warmed IV volume expander (e.g., normal saline) should be used both to prevent rewarming shock and to replace fluid lost from cold diuresis.

The conscious patient who is able to manage his airway may be given warmed, sweetened fluids. Alcohol and caffeine should be avoided.

Resuscitation

There are certain resuscitation considerations when handling cardiac arrest victims with core temperatures below 86° F (30° C).

Basic Cardiac Life Support BLS providers should start cardiopulmonary resuscitation (CPR) immediately, although pulse and respirations may need to be checked for longer periods to detect minimal cardiopulmonary efforts. Use normal chest compression and ventilation rates and ventilate with warmed, humidified oxygen. If an AED is available and ventricular fibrillation is detected, three shocks may be given. Further shocks should be avoided until after rewarming to above 86° F. CPR, rewarming, and rapid transport should immediately follow the three defibrillation attempts.

Advanced Cardiac Life Support Since there is no increased risk of inducing ventricular fibrillation from orotracheal or nasotracheal intubation, ALS

Active rewarming of the severely hypothermic patient should be deferred until the patient is at the hospital unless transport time is long and rewarming is ordered by medical direction.

providers may intubate the patient and ventilate with warmed, humidified oxygen. Drug metabolism is reduced however, so administered medications, such as epinephrine, lidocaine and procainamide may accumulate to toxic levels if used repeatedly in the severely hypothermic victim. In addition, administered drugs may remain in the peripheral circulation. When the patient is rewarmed and perfusion resumes, large, toxic boluses of these medications may be delivered to the central circulation and target tissues. Lidocaine and procainamide may also paradoxically lower the fibrillatory threshold in a hypothermic heart and increase resistance to defibrillation. Bretylium and magnesium sulfate however, may be effective even in hypothermic hearts.

The American Heart Association recommends that, if the patient fails to respond to initial defibrillation attempts or initial drug therapy, subsequent defibrillations or boluses of medication should be avoided until the core temperature is about 86° F (30° C). This is because it is generally impossible to electrically defibrillate a heart that is colder than 86° F. Active core rewarming techniques are the primary modality in hypothermia victims who are either in cardiac arrest or unconscious with a slow heart rate.

If the hypothermic cardiac arrest patient fails to respond to initial defibrillation attempts or drug therapy, avoid subsequent defibrillations or medication until the core temperature is about 86° F (30° C). It is generally impossible to defibrillate a heart that is colder than 86° F.

Techniques that may be used include the administration of heated, humidified oxygen and warmed intravenous fluids, preferably normal saline, infused centrally at rates of 150 to 200 mL an hour to avoid overhydration. Peritoneal lavage with warmed potassium-free fluid administered 2 L at a time may be used, as may extracorporeal blood warming with partial cardiac bypass. Obviously some of these techniques may only be carried out in a hospital setting.

Transportation

When transporting a hypovolemic patient, remember that gentle transportation is necessary due to myocardial irritability and that the patient should be kept level or slightly inclined with head down. Contact the receiving hospital for general rewarming options. When determining your destination, consider the availability of cardiac bypass rewarming.

FROSTBITE

Frostbite is environmentally induced freezing of body tissues (Figure 10-5). As the tissues freeze, ice crystals form within and water is drawn out of the cells into the extracellular space. These ice crystals expand, causing the destruction of cells.

✱ **frostbite** environmentally induced freezing of body tissues causing destruction of cells.

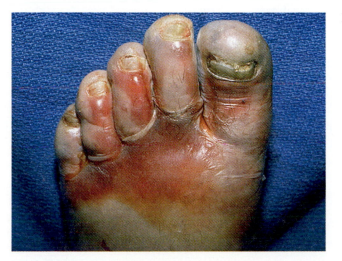

FIGURE 10-5 Frostbite.

During this process, intracellular electrolyte concentrations increase, further destroying cells. Damage to blood vessels from ice crystal formation causes loss of vascular integrity, resulting in tissue swelling and loss of distal nutritional flow.

Superficial and Deep Frostbite

Generally, there are two types of frostbite: superficial and deep. **Superficial frostbite** (frostnip) exhibits some freezing of epidermal tissue, resulting in initial redness, followed by blanching. There will also be diminished sensation. **Deep frostbite** affects the epidermal and subcutaneous layers. There is a white appearance and the area feels hard (frozen) to palpation. There is also loss of sensation in deep frostbite.

Frostbite mainly occurs in the extremities and in areas of the head and face exposed to the environment. Subfreezing temperatures are required for frostbite to occur, although they are not necessary to produce hypothermia. Many patients who have frostbite will also have hypothermia.

There can be tremendous variation in how an individual can present with frostbite. For example, some patients feel little pain at onset. Others will report severe pain. A certain degree of compliance may be felt beneath the frozen layer in superficial frostbite, but in deep frostbite, the frozen part will be hard and noncompliant.

Treatment for Frostbite

In treating frostbite, take the following recommended steps:

Do not thaw frozen flesh if there is any possibility of refreezing. Do not massage the frozen area or rub it with snow.

- Do not thaw the affected area if there is any possibility of refreezing.
- Do not massage the frozen area or rub with snow. Rubbing the affected area may cause ice crystals within the tissues to damage the already injured tissues more seriously.
- Administer analgesia prior to thawing.
- Transport to the hospital for rewarming by immersion. If transport will be delayed, thaw the frozen part by immersion in a 102–104° F (39°–40° C) water bath. Water temperature will fall rapidly, requiring additions of warm water throughout the process.
- Cover the thawed part with loosely applied dry, sterile dressings.
- Elevate and immobilize the thawed part.
- Do not puncture or drain blisters.
- Do not rewarm frozen feet if they are required for walking out of a hazardous situation.

TRENCH FOOT

Trench foot (immersion foot) is similar to frostbite, but it occurs at temperatures above freezing. It is rarely seen in the civilian population. It received its name in World War I, when troops confined to trenches with standing cold water developed progressive symptoms over days. Symptoms are similar to frostbite, but there may be pain. Blisters may form upon spontaneous rewarming.

Treatment of Trench Foot

Treatment of trench foot requires early recognition of developing symptoms and immediate steps to warm, dry, aerate, and elevate the feet. Measures to prevent trench foot are most effective, such as avoiding prolonged exposure to standing water, changing wet socks frequently, and never sleeping in wet boots or socks.

NEAR-DROWNING AND DROWNING

Drowning is asphyxiation resulting from submersion in liquid. There has been an attempt made to differentiate between the terms drowning and near-drowning. The term *drowning* means that death occurred within 24 hours of submersion, while the term **near-drowning** indicates that death either did not occur or occurred more than 24 hours after submersion.

It is estimated that in the United States, approximately 4,500 persons die annually due to drowning. Many more sustain serious injury due to near-drowning. This makes drowning the third most common cause of accidental death in the United States. Approximately 40 percent of these deaths are in children under 5 years of age. There is a second peak incidence in teenagers and a final third peak in the elderly as a result of accidental bathtub drownings. Approximately 85 percent of near-drowning victims are male, and two-thirds of these do not know how to swim. Most commonly, these situations are due to fresh-water submersion, especially in swimming pools. Unfortunately, alcohol use by the victim or the supervising adult is frequently associated with this type of accident.

It is important to note that other emergency conditions are often associated with near-drowning. If the cause of the submersion is unknown, you must consider the possibility of trauma and treat the patient accordingly.

Frequently the submersion occurs in cold water, causing hypothermia. Hypothermia slows the body's metabolic processes thereby decreasing the need for oxygen. This can have a protective effect on organs and tissues which become hypoxic (low in oxygen) in submersion situations. However, it is important to treat the hypoxia first, once you have initiated rescue.

Pathophysiology of Drowning and Near-Drowning

As a paramedic, you need to understand the sequence of events in drowning or near-drowning. Following submersion, if the victim is conscious, he will undergo a period of complete apnea for up to three minutes. This apnea is an involuntary reflex as the victim strives to keep his head above water. During this time, blood is shunted to the heart and brain because of the mammalian diving reflex, which is described later in this chapter.

When the victim is apneic, the $PaCO_2$ in the blood rises to greater than 50 mmHg. Meanwhile, the PaO_2 of the blood falls below 50 mmHg. The stimulus from the hypoxia ultimately overrides the sedative effects of the hypercarbia, resulting in central nervous system stimulation.

Dry Versus Wet Drowning

Until unconscious, the victim experiences a great deal of panic. During this stage the victim makes violent inspiratory and swallowing efforts. At this point, copious amounts of water enter the mouth, posterior oropharynx, and stomach, stimulating severe laryngospasm (airway obstruction due to aspirated water) and bronchospasm. In approximately 10 percent of drowning victims, and in a much greater percentage of near-drowning victims, this laryngospasm prevents the influx of water into the lungs. If a significant amount of water does not enter the lungs, it is referred to as a *dry drowning*. Conversely, if a laryngospasm does not occur, and a significant quantity of water does enter the lungs, it is referred to as a *wet drowning*.

The laryngospasm further aggravates the hypoxia, with coma ultimately ensuing. Persistent anoxia (absence of oxygen) results in a deeper coma. Following

* **drowning** asphyxiation resulting from submersion in liquid with death occurring within 24 hours of submersion.

* **near-drowning** an incident of potentially fatal submersion in liquid which did not result in death or in which death occurred more than 24 hours after submersion.

unconsciousness, reflex swallowing continues, resulting in gastric distention and increased risk of vomiting and aspiration. If untreated, hypotension, bradycardia, and death result in a short period.

Drowning and near-drowning are primarily due to asphyxia from airway obstruction in the lung secondary to the aspirated water or the laryngospasm. If, in a near-drowning episode, this process does not end in death, any fluid that has entered the lungs may cause lower-airway disease.

Fresh–Water Versus Saltwater Drowning

You should expect different physiological reactions in cases of fresh-water and saltwater drownings or near-drownings. However, these mechanistic differences do not make any difference in the end metabolic result or in the prehospital management.

Fresh–Water Drowning In fresh-water drowning or near-drowning, the large surface area of the alveoli and small airways allow a massive amount of hypotonic water to diffuse across the alveolar/capillary membrane and into the vascular space. This results in hemodilution, an expansion in blood plasma volume and relative reduction in red blood cell concentration. *Hemodilution* produces a thickening of the alveolar walls with inflammatory cells, hemorrhagic pneumonitis (bleeding lung inflammation), and destruction of surfactant.

Surfactant is a substance in the alveoli responsible for keeping the alveoli open. In drowning, some surfactant is lost when the capillaries of the alveoli are damaged. Plasma proteins then leak back into the alveoli, resulting in the accumulation of fluid in the small airways. This in turn leads to multiple areas of atelectasis—areas of alveolar collapse. Atelectasis causes shunting, which is the return of unoxygenated blood from the damaged alveoli to the bloodstream. In other words, blood is traveling through the lungs without being oxygenated. The result is hypoxemia (inadequate oxygenation of the blood) (Figure 10-6).

Saltwater Drowning In saltwater drowning or near-drowning, the hypertonic nature of sea water, which is 3 to 4 times more hypertonic than plasma, draws water from the bloodstream into the alveoli (Figure 10-6). This produces pul-

---

Although the physiology of fresh-water and saltwater drownings differ, there is no difference in the end result or in prehospital management.

✳ **surfactant** a compound secreted by cells in the lungs that regulates the surface tension of the fluid that lines the alveoli, important in keeping the alveoli open for gas exchange.

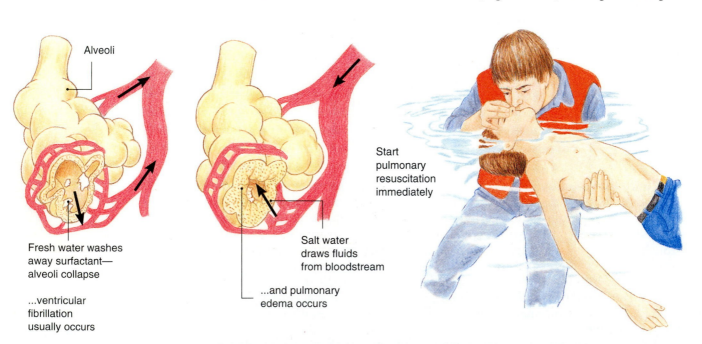

Alveoli

Fresh water washes away surfactant— alveoli collapse

...ventricular fibrillation usually occurs

Salt water draws fluids from bloodstream

...and pulmonary edema occurs

Start pulmonary resuscitation immediately

FIGURE 10-6 Pathophysiological effects of drowning.

monary edema, leading to profound shunting. The result is failure of oxygenation, producing hypoxemia. Additionally, respiratory and metabolic acidosis develop due to the retention of CO_2 and developing anaerobic (without-oxygen) metabolism.

Factors Affecting Survival

A number of factors have an impact on drowning and near-drowning survival rates. These include the cleanliness of the water, the length of time submerged, and the age and general health of the victim. Children have a longer survival time and a greater probability of a successful resuscitation. Even more significant is the water temperature. The concept of developing brain death after four to six minutes without oxygen is not applicable in cases of near-drowning in cold water. Some patients in cold water (below 68° F) can be resuscitated after 30 minutes or more in cardiac arrest. However, persons under water 60 minutes or longer usually cannot be resuscitated.

A possible contribution to survival may be the **mammalian diving reflex**. When a person dives into cold water, he reacts to the submersion of the face. Breathing is inhibited, the heart rate becomes bradycardic, and vasoconstriction develops in tissues relatively resistant to asphyxia. Meanwhile cerebral and cardiac blood flow is maintained. In this way, oxygen is sent and used only where it is immediately needed to sustain life. The colder the water, the more oxygen is diverted to the heart and brain. A common saying in emergency medicine states: "The cold-water drowning victim is not dead until he is warm and dead." In other words, a person who has been submerged in cold water may only seem to be dead, but due to the continued supply of oxygen to the heart and brain may indeed still be alive.

* **mammalian diving reflex** a complex cardiovascular reflex, resulting from submersion of the face and nose in water, that constricts blood flow everywhere except to the brain.

The cold-water drowning victim is not dead until he is warm and dead.

TREATMENT FOR NEAR-DROWNING

Since fresh-water and saltwater near-drownings both involve factors that disrupt normal pulmonary function, initial field treatment must be directed toward correcting the profound hypoxia. Take the following steps:

Never attempt to rescue a drowning victim unless you have been trained and have the necessary safety equipment.

- Remove the patient from the water as soon as possible. This should be done by a trained rescue swimmer.
- Initiate ventilation while the patient is still in the water. Rescue personnel should wear protective clothing if water temperature is less than 70° F. In addition, attach a safety line to the rescue swimmer. In fast water, it is essential to use personnel specifically trained for this type of rescue.
- Suspect head and neck injury if the patient experienced a fall or was diving. Rapidly place the victim on a long backboard and remove him from the water. Use C-spine precautions throughout care.
- Protect the patient from heat loss. Avoid laying the patient on a cold surface. Remove wet clothing and cover the body to the extent possible.
- Examine the patient for airway patency, breathing, and pulse. If indicated, begin CPR and defibrillation.
- Manage the airway using proper suctioning and airway adjuncts.
- Administer oxygen at a 100 percent concentration.
- Use respiratory rewarming, if available, and if transport time is longer than 15 minutes. (In the past, prophylactic abdominal thrusts

were used to clear the airway, but there are conflicting recommendations regarding the practice as there is no definitive scientific data to support this maneuver.)

- Establish an IV of lactated Ringer's or normal saline for venous access and run at 75 mL/hr. If indicated, carry out defibrillation.
- Follow ACLS protocols if the patient is normothermic. If the patient is hypothermic, treat him according to the hypothermia protocol presented earlier in the chapter.

Resuscitation is not indicated if immersion has been extremely prolonged (unless hypothermia is present) or if there is evidence of putrefaction (decomposition).

Adult Respiratory Distress Syndrome

More than 90 percent of near-drowning patients survive without *sequelae* (after effects). However, all near-drowning patients should be admitted to the hospital for observation since complications may not appear for 24 hours.

Adult respiratory distress syndrome (ARDS) is one of the more severe post-resuscitation complications, with a high rate of mortality. The physiologic stress of near-drowning causes the lungs to leak fluid into the alveoli. This fluid is loaded with various chemical factors that cause severe inflammation of the tissues and failure of the respiratory system. In addition, some of these patients have problems with pulmonary parenchymal injury, destruction of surfactant, aspiration pneumonitis, or pneumothorax. A number require an extended hospital stay due to renal failure, hypoxia, hypercarbia, and mixed metabolic and respiratory acidosis. The effects of cerebral hypoxia occasionally require treatment throughout hospitalization and beyond.

All near-drowning patients should be admitted to the hospital for observation since complications may not appear for 24 hours.

DIVING EMERGENCIES

Scuba diving has become an extremely popular recreational sport. Divers wear portable equipment containing compressed air, which allows the diver to breathe underwater. Although scuba diving accidents are fairly uncommon, inexperienced divers have a higher rate of injury. Scuba diving emergencies can occur on the surface, in three feet of water, or at any depth. The more serious emergencies usually occur following a dive. To better assess and care for diving injuries, you need to understand a few principles of pressure.

scuba abbreviation for *self-contained underwater breathing apparatus.* Portable apparatus that contains compressed air which allows the diver to breathe underwater.

THE EFFECTS OF AIR PRESSURE ON GASES

Water is an incompressible liquid. Fresh water has a density, or weight per unit of volume, of 62.4 pounds per cubic foot. Saltwater has a density of 64.0 pounds per cubic foot. This density can be equated to pressure, which is defined as the weight or force acting upon a unit area. Thus, a cubic foot of fresh water exerts a pressure ("weight") of 62.4 pounds over an area of one square foot. This measurement is typically stated in pounds per square inch (psi).

Humans at sea level live in an atmosphere of air, which is a mixture of gases. These gases weigh and exert a pressure of 14.7 pounds per square inch (760 mmHg). This pressure, however, may vary within the environment. For example, ascending to an altitude of one mile will decrease the atmospheric pressure by 17 percent to approximately 12.2 pounds.

To understand how air pressure affects diving accidents, you need to look at three physical laws: Boyle's Law, Dalton's Law, and Henry's Law.

Boyle's Law

Boyle's Law states that the volume of a gas is inversely proportional to its pressure if the temperature is kept constant. As you increase pressure, the gas is compressed into a smaller space. For example, doubling the pressure of a gas mixture will decrease its volume by one-half. The pressure of air at sea level is 14.7 lb./sq.in. or 760 mmHg. This pressure is called one "atmosphere absolute" or one "ata." Two ata occur at a depth of 33 feet of water, three ata occur at a depth of 66 feet of water, and so on. Therefore, one liter of air at the surface is compressed to 500 mL at 33 feet. At 66 feet, one liter of air would be compressed to 250 mL.

Dalton's Law

Dalton's Law states that the total pressure of a mixture of gases is equal to the sum of the partial pressures of the individual gases. The air we breathe is a mixture of nitrogen (about 78%), oxygen (about 21%), and carbon dioxide plus traces of argon, helium, and other rare gases (about 1%). Since the pressure of air at sea level is 760 mmHg, the pressure of nitrogen is about 593 mmHg, the pressure of oxygen is about 160 mmHg, and the pressure of carbon dioxide is somewhat less than 4 mmHg—each gas exerting its proportion of the total pressure of the mixture.

At different altitudes above sea level or depths below sea level, the pressure of air will change (less at higher altitudes, more at greater depths), but the component gases will still account for the same proportion of whatever the total pressure is at that level: nitrogen 78%, oxygen 21%, and carbon dioxide less than 1%.

Henry's Law

Henry's Law states that the amount of gas dissolved in a given volume of fluid is proportional to the pressure of the gas above it. When we descend below sea level, and the pressure bearing down on us increases, the gases that make up the air we breathe tend to dissolve in the liquids (mainly blood plasma) and tissues of the body.

Let us compare what happens to the two chief components of the air we breathe—oxygen and nitrogen—when a person descends to greater and greater depths below sea level. Much of the oxygen is used up in the normal metabolism of the cells, leaving only a small amount to be dissolved in the blood and tissues. Nitrogen, however, is an inert gas and, as such, is not used by the body. Therefore, a far greater quantity of nitrogen is available to dissolve in the blood and tissues as a person descends below sea level. In brief, at depths below sea level, oxygen metabolizes but nitrogen dissolves.

When the person ascends toward sea level again, the gases that are dissolved in the blood and tissues, being under less and less pressure, come out of the blood and tissues and, if the ascent is too rapid, form bubbles. To understand this phenomenon, compare the human body to a bottled carbonated soft drink—that is, a liquid in which carbon dioxide gas is dissolved. The gas is kept dissolved in the liquid by the cap on the bottle and a high-pressure gas under the cap, on top of the liquid. When the cap is removed and the pressure is released, the gas bubbles out of the liquid, causing a fizz that will sometimes rise completely out of the bottle.

In the following sections, we will discuss how the phenomena of gases and pressure can cause serious problems for divers.

PATHOPHYSIOLOGY OF DIVING EMERGENCIES

As noted above, gases are dissolved in the diver's blood and tissues under pressure. As the diver goes deeper into the water, pressure increases, causing more gas to dissolve in the blood (Henry's Law). According to Boyle's Law, these gases will have a smaller volume due to the increased ambient pressure. During *controlled* ascent, with decreasing pressure, dissolved gases come out of the blood and tissues slowly, escaping gradually through respiration.

If ascent is *too rapid*, however, the dissolved gases, mostly nitrogen, come out of solution and expand quickly, forming bubbles in the blood, brain, spinal cord, skin, inner ear, muscles, and joints. Once bubbles of nitrogen have formed in various tissues, it is difficult for the body to remove them. The ascending diver who comes to the surface too rapidly, not adhering to safety measures, is at risk of becoming a veritable living bottle of soda.

CLASSIFICATION OF DIVING INJURIES

Scuba diving injuries are due to barotrauma, pulmonary over-pressure, arterial gas embolism, decompression illness, cold, panic, or a combination of these. Accidents generally occur at one of the following four stages of a dive:

- On the surface
- During descent
- On the bottom
- During ascent

Injuries on the Surface

Surface injuries can involve any of several factors. One such factor can be entanglement of lines or entanglement in kelp fields while swimming to the area of the dive. Divers in these situations may panic, become fatigued, even drown. Another factor may be cold water that produces shivering and blackout. Boats in the area are another potential source of injury to the diver. To prevent such accidents, divers will usually mark the area of their dive with a flag. Maritime rules require boat operators to stay clear of a flagged area.

Injuries during Descent

* barotrauma injuries caused by changes in pressure. Barotrauma that occurs from increasing pressure during a diving descent is commonly called "the squeeze."

Barotrauma means injuries caused by changes in pressure. Barotrauma during descent is commonly called "the squeeze." It can occur if the diver cannot equilibrate the pressure between the nasopharynx and the middle ear through the eustachian tube. The diver can experience middle ear pain, ringing in the ears, dizziness, and hearing loss. In severe cases, rupture of the eardrum can occur. A diver who has an upper respiratory infection, and who therefore cannot clear the middle ear through the eustachian tube, should not dive. A similar lack of equilibration can occur in the sinuses, producing severe frontal headaches or pain beneath the eye in the maxillary sinuses.

Injuries on the Bottom

* nitrogen narcosis a state of stupor that develops during deep dives due to nitrogen's effect on cerebral function; also called "raptures of the deep."

Major diving emergencies while at the bottom of the dive often involve **nitrogen narcosis** (a state of stupor), commonly called "raptures of the deep." This is due to nitrogen's effect on cerebral function. The diver may appear to be intoxicated and may take unnecessary risks. Other emergencies occur when a diver runs low on or out of air. The diver who panics will exacerbate this situation by consuming even more oxygen and producing even more carbon dioxide.

Injuries during Ascent

Serious and life-threatening emergencies, many involving barotrauma, can occur during the ascent. For example, as during descent, an ascending diver may be unable to equilibrate inner ear and nasopharyngeal pressure.

Dives below 40 feet require staged ascent to prevent **decompression illness,** also called "the bends." This condition develops in divers subjected to rapid reduction of air pressure while ascending to the surface following exposure to compressed air, with formation of nitrogen bubbles causing severe pain, especially in the abdomen and the joints.

The most serious barotrauma that occurs during ascent is injury to the lung from **pulmonary over-pressure.** This can occur with a deep dive, or it can occur with a dive of as little as three feet below the surface. The injury results from the diver holding his breath during the ascent. As the diver ascends, the air in the lung, which has been compressed, expands. If it is not exhaled, the alveoli may rupture. If this occurs, the result will be structural damage to the lung and, possibly, **arterial gas embolism (AGE),** an air bubble, or air embolism, that enters the circulatory system from the damaged lung. Another result may be **pneumomediastinum,** the release of gas (air) through the visceral pleura into the mediastinum and pericardial sac around the heart as well as into the tissues of the neck. **Pneumothorax** is possible if the alveoli rupture into the pleural cavity. Air embolism can occur if the air ruptures into the pulmonary veins or arteries and returns to the left atrium and finally into the left ventricle and out into the systemic circulation.

GENERAL ASSESSMENT OF DIVING EMERGENCIES

In the early assessment of diving accidents, all symptoms of air embolism and decompression illness are considered together. Early assessment and treatment of a diving injury is of more importance than trying to distinguish the exact problem. One of your most important tasks in a diving-related injury is elicitation of a diving history or profile. There are several essential factors to consider. These include:

- Time at which the signs and symptoms occurred
- Type of breathing apparatus utilized
- Type of hypothermia protective garment worn
- Parameters of the dive:
  - Depth of dive(s)
  - Number of dives(s)
  - Duration of dive(s)
- Aircraft travel following a dive (in a pressurized cabin?)
- Rate of ascent
- Associated panic forcing rapid ascent
- Experience of the diver, for example, student, inexperienced, or "pro"
- Properly functioning depth gauge
- Previous medical diseases
- Old injuries
- Previous episodes of decompression illness
- Use of medications
- Use of alcohol

* **decompression illness** development of nitrogen bubbles within the tissues due to a rapid reduction of air pressure when a diver returns to the surface; also called "the bends."

* **pulmonary over-pressure** expansion of air held in the lungs during ascent. If not exhaled, the expanded air may cause injury to the lungs and surrounding structures.

* **arterial gas embolism (AGE)** an air bubble, or air embolism, that enters the circulatory system from a damaged lung.

* **pneumomediastinum** the presence of air in the mediastinum.

* **pneumothorax** a collection of air in the pleural space. Air may enter the pleural space from through an injury to the chest wall or through an injury to the lungs. In a *tension pneumothorax,* pressure builds because there is no way for the air to escape, causing lung collapse.

In a diving emergency, consider all symptoms of air embolism and decompression illness together. Early assessment and treatment are more important than identifying the exact problem.

Table 10-3	FACTORS RELATED TO THE DEVELOPMENT OF DECOMPRESSION ILLNESS
General Factors	**Individual Factors**
Cold water dives	Age—older individuals
Diving in rough water	Obesity
Strenuous diving conditions	Fatigue—lack of sleep prior to dive
History of previous decompression dive incident	Alcohol—consumption before or after dive
Overstaying time at given dive depth	History of medical problems
Dive at 80 feet or greater	
Rapid ascent—panic, inexperience, unfamiliarity with equipment	
Heavy exercise before or after dive to the point of muscle soreness	
Flying after diving (24 hour wait is recommended)	
Driving to high altitude after dive	

From a quick assessment of the patient's diving profile, you can rapidly determine if the diver is a likely candidate for a pressure disorder.

PRESSURE DISORDERS

Injuries caused by pressure, as noted earlier, are known as *barotrauma*. In the case of diving accidents, most barotrauma results from a pressure imbalance between the external environment and gases within the body. The following sections describe some of the most common forms of barotrauma involved in diving accidents.

Decompression Illness

Decompression illness develops in divers subjected to rapid reduction of air pressure after ascending to the surface following exposure to compressed air. A number of general and individual factors can contribute to the development of decompression illness, or the bends (Table 10-3). Decompression illness results as nitrogen bubbles come out of solution in the blood and tissues, causing increased pressure in various body structures and occluding circulation in the small blood vessels. This occurs in joints, tendons, the spinal cord, skin, brain, and inner ear. Symptoms develop when a diver rapidly ascends after being exposed to a depth of 33 feet or more for a time sufficient to allow the body's tissues to be saturated with nitrogen.

Signs and Symptoms The principal signs and symptoms of decompression illnesses are joint and abdominal pain, fatigue, paresthesias, and CNS disturbances. The nitrogen bubbles produced by rapid decompression are thought to produce obstruction of blood flow and lead to local ischemia, subjecting tissues to anoxic stress. In some cases, this stress may lead to tissue damage.

Treatment Patients with decompression illness usually seek medical treatment within 12 hours of ascent from a dive. Some patients may not seek treatment for as long as 24 hours after the last dive. It is generally safe to assume that signs or symptoms developing more than 36 hours after a dive cannot reasonably be attributed to decompression illness.

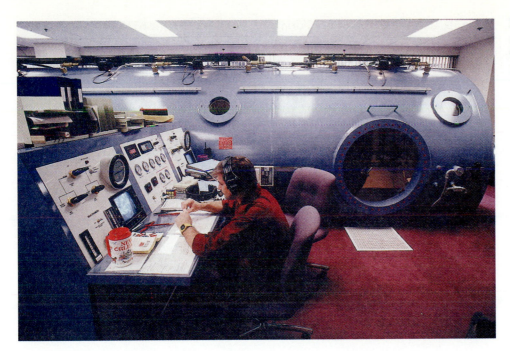

FIGURE 10-7 Hyperbaric oxygen chamber used in the treatment of decompression illness.

Decompression illness may require urgent definitive care through **recompression.** This can be accomplished by placing the patient in a **hyperbaric oxygen chamber** (Figure 10-7). There the patient is subjected to oxygen under greater-than-atmospheric pressure to force the nitrogen in the body to re-dissolve, then gradually decompressed to allow the nitrogen to escape without forming bubbles. However, prompt stabilization at the nearest emergency department should be accomplished before transportation to a recompression chamber.

Early oxygen therapy may reduce symptoms of decompression illness substantially. Divers who are administered high concentrations of oxygen have a considerably better treatment outcome. The following list outlines some of the steps in the prehospital management of decompression illnesses.

* Assess the ABCs.
* Administer CPR, if required.
* Administer oxygen at 100 percent concentration with a nonrebreather mask. An unconscious diver should be intubated.
* Keep the patient in the supine position.
* Protect the patient from excessive heat, cold, wetness, or noxious fumes.
* Give the conscious, alert patient nonalcoholic liquids such as fruit juices or oral balanced salt solutions.
* Evaluate and stabilize the patient at the nearest emergency department prior to transport to a recompression chamber. Begin IV fluid replacement with electrolyte solutions for unconscious or seriously injured patients. You may use lactated Ringer's or normal saline. Do not use 5 percent dextrose in water.
* If there is evidence of CNS involvement, administer dexamethasone, heparin, or Valium as ordered by medical direction.

✱ recompression resubmission of a person to a greater pressure so that gradual decompression can be achieved; often used in the treatment of diving emergencies.

✱ hyperbaric oxygen chamber recompression chamber used to treat patients suffering from barotrauma.

Recompression in a hyperbaric oxygen chamber may be required for the patient suspected of suffering decompression illness or an air embolism.

- If air evacuation is used, do not expose the patient to decreased barometric pressure. Cabin pressure must be maintained at sea level, or fly at the lowest possible safe altitude.
- Send the patient's diving equipment with the patient for examination. If that is impossible, arrange for local examination and gas analysis.

Pulmonary Over-Pressure Accidents

Lung overinflation due to rapid ascent is the common cause of a number of emergencies, particularly at shallow depths of less than 6 feet. Air can become trapped in the lungs by mucous plugs, bronchospasm, or simple breath holding. With rapid ascent, ambient pressure drops quickly, causing the trapped air to expand. Air expansion can rupture the alveolar membranes. This can result in hemorrhage, reduced oxygen and carbon dioxide transport, and capillary and alveolar inflammation. Air can also escape from the lung into other nearby tissues and cause pneumothorax and tension pneumothorax, subcutaneous emphysema, or pneumomediastinum.

Signs and Symptoms Divers with this type of condition will complain of substernal chest pain. Respiratory distress and diminished breath sounds are common findings on examination.

Treatment Treatment for this condition is the same as for pneumothorax caused by any other mechanism (see Chapter 1). Rest and supplemental oxygen are important but hyperbaric oxygen is not usually necessary.

Arterial Gas Embolism (AGE)

As described above, a pressure buildup in the lung can damage and rupture alveoli. This can allow air in the form of a large bubble to escape into the circulation. This air embolism, or arterial gas embolism, can travel to the left atrium and ventricle of the heart and out into various parts of the body where it may lodge and obstruct blood flow, causing ischemia and possibly infarct. Such obstruction of blood flow can have devastating effects triggered by cardiac, pulmonary, and cerebral compromise.

Signs and Symptoms Signs and symptoms of air embolism include onset within 2 to 10 minutes of ascent, a rapid and dramatic onset of sharp, tearing pain, and other symptoms related to the organ system affected by blocked blood flow. The most common presentation mimics a stroke with confusion, vertigo, visual disturbances, and loss of consciousness. Although rare, you may also encounter paralysis on one side of the body (hemiplegia), as well as cardiac and pulmonary collapse. If any person using SCUBA equipment presents with neurologic deficits during or immediately after ascent, an air embolism should be suspected. As death or serious disability can result, prompt medical treatment is crucial.

Treatment Management of air embolism includes the following steps:

- Assess ABCs.
- Administer oxygen by nonrebreather mask at 100 percent.
- Place the patient in a supine position.
- Monitor vital signs frequently.
- Administer IV fluids at a TKO rate.
- Administer a corticosteroid agent, if ordered by medical direction.
- Transport to a recompression chamber as rapidly as possible. If air transport is utilized, it is very important to use a pressurized aircraft or to fly at a low altitude.

Pneumomediastinum

As noted earlier, a pneumomediastinum is the release of gas (air) through the visceral pleura into the mediastinum and pericardial sac around the heart. It can result from a pulmonary over-pressure accident during rapid ascent from a dive.

Signs and Symptoms Signs and symptoms of a pneumomediastinum include substernal chest pain, irregular pulse, abnormal heart sounds, reduced blood pressure and narrow pulse pressure, and a change in voice. There may or may not be evidence of cyanosis.

Treatment The field management of pneumomediastinum includes:

- Administer high-concentration oxygen via nonrebreather mask.
- Start an IV lactated Ringer's or normal saline per medical direction.
- Transport to the emergency department.

Treatment generally ranges from observation to recompression for relief of acute symptoms. The patient should be observed for 24 hours for any other signs of lung overpressure. He should not be recompressed unless air embolism or decompression illness is also present.

Nitrogen Narcosis

Nitrogen narcosis develops during deep dives and contributes to major diving emergencies while the diver is at the bottom. With an elevated partial pressure, more nitrogen dissolves in the bloodstream. With higher concentrations of nitrogen in the body, including the brain, the result is intoxication and altered levels of consciousness very similar to the effects of alcohol or narcotic use. Between 70 and 100 feet these effects become apparent in most divers, but at 200 feet most divers become so impaired that they cannot do any useful work. At 300 to 350 feet unconsciousness occurs. The main concern with nitrogen narcosis is the same as with any person who is intoxicated while in a situation requiring alertness and common sense. Impaired judgment during a deep dive can cause accidents and unnecessary risk taking.

Signs and Symptoms Altered levels of consciousness and impaired judgment.

Treatment Treatment simply requires return to a shallow depth since this condition is self resolving on ascent. To avoid this problem altogether in deep dives, oxygen mixed with helium is used, since helium does not have the anesthetic effect of nitrogen.

OTHER DIVING-RELATED ILLNESSES

There are less frequent problems that can occur as a result of SCUBA diving. For example, oxygen toxicity caused by prolonged exposure to high partial pressures of oxygen can cause lung damage or even convulsions. Hyperventilation due to excitement or panic may lead to a decreased level of consciousness or muscle cramps and spasm. This will impair the diver's ability to function properly, possibly leading to injury. Inadequate breathing or faulty equipment may lead to increased CO_2 levels, or *hypercapnia*. This also may cause unconsciousness. Finally, poorly prepared air tanks may be contaminated with other gases, which can increase the risk of hypoxia, narcosis, and accidental injury.

DIVERS ALERT NETWORK (DAN)

Clearly, SCUBA diving has a unique set of potential problems. With the popularity of this activity rising so dramatically, it is important for EMS personnel in popular diving areas to become familiar with recognition and treatment of these problems. If assistance is needed, the Divers Alert Network (DAN) operates a non-profit consultation and referral service in affiliation with Duke University Medical Center. In an emergency, contact (919) 684-8111. For non-emergency situations call (919) 684-2948.

HIGH ALTITUDE ILLNESS

In contrast to illnesses related to diving and high atmospheric pressure, high altitude illnesses are caused by a decrease in ambient pressure. Essentially, high altitude is a low-oxygen environment. As noted in the discussion of Dalton's law, earlier, oxygen concentration in the atmosphere remains constant at 21 percent. Therefore, as you go higher and barometric pressure decreases, the partial pressure of oxygen also decreases (is 21 percent of a lower total pressure). Oxygen becomes less available, triggering a number of related illnesses as well as aggravating pre-existing conditions such as angina, congestive heart failure, chronic obstructive pulmonary disease, and hypertension.

Even in healthy individuals, ascent to high altitude, especially if it is very rapid, can cause illness. It is difficult to predict who will be affected and to what degree. The only predictor is the hypoxic ventilatory response.

Every year millions of visitors to mountains expose themselves to altitudes greater than 2,400 m (8,000 ft.) the altitude at which high altitude illnesses start to become manifest. For reference purposes, Denver, Colorado, is at 1,610 m where there is 17 percent less oxygen than at sea level. Aspen at 2,438 m has 26 percent less oxygen, and at the top of Mount Everest (8,848 m or 29,028 ft.) there is 66 percent less oxygen than at sea level. At *high altitude* (4,900 to 11,500 ft.) the hypoxic environment causes decreased exercise performance, although without major disruption of normal oxygen transport in the body. However, if ascent is very rapid, altitude illness will commonly occur at 8,000 feet and beyond. *Very high altitude* (11,500 to 18,000 ft.) will result in extreme hypoxia during exercise or sleep. It is important to ascend to these altitudes slowly allowing for acclimatization to the environment. *Extreme altitude* beyond 18,000 feet will cause severe illness in almost everyone.

Some of the signs and symptoms of altitude illness are malaise, anorexia, headache, sleep disturbances and respiratory distress that increases with exertion.

High altitude illnesses start to become manifest at altitudes greater than 8,000 ft.

PREVENTION

Acclimatization, exertion, sleep, diet, and medication are key considerations in preventing or limiting high altitude medical emergencies. A description of each follows.

Gradual Ascent

To avoid developing high altitude medical problems, it is important to allow a period of acclimatization. Slow, gradual ascent over days to weeks gives the body a chance to adjust to the hypoxic state caused by high altitudes. A person who would normally become short of breath, dizzy, and confused by a rapid drop in oxygen can function quite well if the oxygen level is decreased to the same level gradually over a long period of time. Acclimatization occurs through several mechanisms. They are:

- *Ventilatory Changes.* The *hypoxic ventilatory response (HVR)* is triggered by decreased oxygen. When oxygen is decreased, ventilation increases. This hyperventilation causes a decrease in CO_2, but the kidneys compensate by eliminating more bicarbonate from the body. In essence, the body resets its normal ventilation and operating level of CO_2. The process takes 4 to 7 days at a given altitude.

- *Cardiovascular Changes.* The heart rate increases at high altitude, allowing more oxygen to be delivered to the tissues. In addition, peripheral veins constrict, increasing the central blood volume. In response, the central receptors, which sense blood volume, induce a diuresis, which causes concentration of the blood. Unfortunately, pulmonary circulation also constricts in a hypoxic environment. This causes or exacerbates pre-existing hypertension and predisposes to developing high altitude pulmonary edema.

- *Blood Changes.* Within two hours of ascent to high altitude the body begins making more red blood cells to carry oxygen. Over time, this mechanism will significantly compensate for the hypoxic environment. It is this mechanism that fostered the idea of "blood-doping" during athletic competition, especially at high altitudes. Athletes donate their own blood long in advance of a competition at high altitude. This allows them time to rebuild their red blood cells. Just before the competition they receive a transfusion of their own blood to increase their oxygen carrying capacity. This practice is frowned upon by most athletic governing bodies.

Limited Exertion

Clearly, one of the easiest ways to avoid some effects of high altitude is to limit the amount of exertion. By limiting the body's need for oxygen, the effect of oxygen deprivation will be minimized.

Sleeping Altitude

Sleep is often disrupted by high altitude. Hypoxia causes abnormal breathing patterns and frequent awakenings in the middle of the night. Descending to a lower altitude for sleep improves rest and allows the body to recover from hypoxia. This practice will, however, interfere with the process of acclimatization.

High Carbohydrate Diet

Carbohydrates are converted by the body into glucose and rapidly released into the blood stream, providing quick energy. The theory that this is helpful in acclimatizing to high altitude is controversial.

Medications

Two medications will limit or prevent the development of medical conditions related to high altitude. They are:

- *Acetazolamide.* Acetazolamide (Diamox) acts as a diuretic. It forces bicarbonate out of the body, which greatly enhances the process of acclimatization as discussed above. The hypoxic ventilatory response reaches a new set point more quickly. This improves ventilation and oxygen transport with less alkalosis. In addition, the periodic breathing that occurs at high altitude is resolved, thereby preventing sudden drops in oxygen.

- *Nifedipine.* Nifedipine (Procardia, Adalat) is a medication usually used to treat high blood pressure. It causes blood vessels to dilate, preventing the increase in pulmonary pressure that often causes pulmonary edema.

Other treatments are currently under evaluation. Phenytoin (Dilantin), for example, is being studied because of its membrane stabilization effects. Steroids are commonly used but their efficacy is still controversial.

TYPES OF HIGH ALTITUDE ILLNESS

A variety of symptoms occur when the average person ascends rapidly to high altitude. These may range from fatigue and decreased exercise tolerance to headache, sleep disturbance, and respiratory distress. The following section will deal with some of the specific syndromes that will occur.

Acute Mountain Sickness (AMS)

Acute mountain sickness usually manifests in an unacclimatized person who ascends rapidly to an altitude of 2,000 m (6,600 ft.) or greater.

Signs and Symptoms The mild form of acute mountain sickness presents with the following symptoms:

- Lightheadedness
- Breathlessness
- Weakness
- Headache
- Nausea and vomiting

These symptoms can develop from 6 to 24 hours after ascent. More severe cases can develop especially if the person continues to ascend to higher altitudes. These symptoms include:

- Weakness (requiring assistance to eat and dress)
- Severe vomiting
- Decreased urine output
- Shortness of breath
- Altered level of consciousness

Mild AMS is self-limiting and will often improve within 1 to 2 days if no further ascent occurs.

Treatment Treatment of AMS consists of halting ascent, possibly lowering altitude, using acetazolamide (Diamox), and anti-nauseants such as prochlorperazine (Compazine) as necessary. It is not usually necessary to descend to sea level. Supplemental oxygen will relieve symptoms but is usually used only in severe cases. In severe cases oxygen, if available, will help. In addition, immediate descent is the definitive treatment. For very severe cases, hyperbaric oxygen may be necessary.

Definitive treatment of all high altitude illnesses is descent to a lower altitude. Administration of supplemental oxygen is also important.

High Altitude Pulmonary Edema (HAPE)

HAPE develops as a result of increased pulmonary pressure and hypertension caused by changes in blood flow at high altitude. Children are most susceptible, and men are more susceptible than women.

Signs and Symptoms Initially symptoms include dry cough, mild shortness of breath on exertion, and slight crackles in the lungs. As the condition progresses, so will the symptoms. Dyspnea can become quite severe and cause cyanosis. Coughing may be productive of frothy sputum, and weakness may progress to coma and death.

Treatment In the early stages, HAPE is completely and easily reversible with descent and the administration of oxygen. It is therefore critical to recognize the illness early and initiate appropriate treatment. If immediate descent is not possible, supplemental oxygen can completely reverse HAPE but requires 36 to 72 hours. Such a supply of oxygen is rarely available to mountain climbers. In this situation the portable hyperbaric bag can be very useful. This is a sealed bag that can be inflated to 2 psi, which simulates a descent of approximately 5,000 feet. Acetazolamide can be used to decrease symptoms. Medications such as morphine, nifedipine (Procardia), and furosemide (Lasix) have been used with some success, but they carry complications such as hypotension and dehydration and should be used with caution.

High Altitude Cerebral Edema (HACE)

The exact cause of high altitude cerebral edema is not known. It usually manifests as progressive neurological deterioration in a patient with AMS or HAPE. The increased fluid in the brain tissue causes a rise in intracranial pressure.

Signs and Symptoms The symptoms of high altitude cerebral edema include:

- Altered mental status
- Ataxia (poor coordination)
- Decreased level of consciousness
- Coma

Headache, nausea, and vomiting are less common. Occasionally actual focal neurological changes may occur.

Treatment As in all altitude illnesses, definitive treatment is descent to lower altitude. Oxygen and steroids may also help to improve recovery. If descent is not possible, the use of oxygen with steroids and a hyperbaric bag may be sufficient, although often unavailable. If coma develops, it may persist for days after descent to sea level but usually resolves, although sometimes leaving residual disability.

NUCLEAR RADIATION

Injury due to exposure to ionizing radiation occurs infrequently. However, the incidence of radiation emergencies has increased in recent years due to the expansion of nuclear medicine procedures and commercial nuclear facilities.

Keep in mind that radiation emergencies should be handled only by those with proper protective equipment and adequate training.

Radiation emergencies should be handled only by those with proper protective equipment and adequate training.

BASIC NUCLEAR PHYSICS

Radiation is a general term applied to the transmission of electromagnetic or particle energy. This energy can include nuclear energy, ultraviolet light, visible light, infrared, and x-ray. A radioactive substance emits ionizing radiation. Such a substance is referred to as a *radionuclide* or *radioisotope*.

To understand nuclear radiation, you might begin by taking a look at the structure of an atom and by becoming familiar with some of the basic terms associated with nuclear physics. The atom consists of various subatomic particles. These include:

- *Protons.* Positively charged particles that form the nucleus of hydrogen and that are present in the nuclei of all elements. The atomic number of the element indicates the number of protons present.
- *Neutrons.* Subatomic particles that are approximately equal in mass to a proton, but lack an electrical charge. As a free particle, a neutron has an average life of less than 17 minutes.
- *Electrons.* Minute particles with negative electrical charges that revolve around the nucleus of an atom. When emitted from radioactive substances, electrons are called beta particles.

You should also be familiar with the following two basic terms associated with nuclear medicine:

- *Isotopes (radioisotope).* Atoms in which the nuclear composition is unstable. That is, they give off **ionizing radiation.**
- *Half-life.* **Half-life** is the time required for half the nuclei of a radioactive substance to lose its activity due to radioactive decay.

A radioactive substance is one that emits ionizing radiation. There are four types of ionizing radiation. These include:

- *Alpha Particles.* Alpha particles are slow-moving, low-energy particles that usually can be stopped by such things as clothing and paper. When they contact the skin, they only penetrate a few cells deep. Because they can be absorbed (stopped) by a layer of clothing, a few inches of air, or the outer layer of skin, alpha particles usually constitute a minor hazard. However, they can produce serious effects if taken internally by ingestion or inhalation.
- *Beta Particles.* Smaller than alpha particles, beta particles are higher in energy. Although beta particles can penetrate air, they can be stopped by aluminum and similar materials. Beta particles generally cause less local damage than alpha particles, but they can be harmful if inhaled or ingested.
- *Gamma Rays.* Gamma rays are more highly energized and penetrating than alpha and beta particles. The origin of gamma rays is related to that of x-rays. Gamma radiation is extremely dangerous, carrying high levels of energy capable of penetrating thick shielding. Gamma rays easily pass through clothing and the entire body, inflicting extensive cell damage. They also create indirect damage by causing internal tissue to emit alpha and beta particles. Protection from gamma radiation can be provided by lead shielding.
- *Neutrons.* Neutrons are more penetrating than the other types of radiation. The penetrating power of neutrons is estimated to be 3 to 10 times greater than gamma rays, but less than the internal hazard associated with ingestion of alpha and beta particles. Exposure to neutrons causes direct tissue damage. However, in nuclear accidents, neutron exposure is not normally a problem for paramedics because neutrons tend to be present only near a reactor core.

---

* **ionizing radiation** electromagnetic radiation (e.g., x-ray) or particulate radiation (e.g., alpha particles, beta particles, and neutrons) that, by direct or secondary processes, ionizes materials that absorb the radiation. Ionizing radiation can penetrate the cells of living organisms, depositing an electrical charge within them. When sufficiently intense, this form of energy kills cells.

* **half-life** time required for half of the nuclei of a radioactive substance to lose activity by undergoing radioactive decay. In biology and pharmacology, the time required by the body to metabolize and inactivate half the amount of a substance taken in.

Table 10-4 DOSE-EFFECT RELATIONSHIPS TO IONIZING RADIATION

Whole Body Exposure

Dose (RAD)	Effect
5–25	Asymptomatic. Blood studies are normal.
50–75	Asymptomatic. Minor depressions of white blood cells and platelets in a few patients.
75–125	May produce anorexia, nausea, and vomiting, and fatigue in approximately 10–20% of patients within two days.
125–200	Possible nausea and vomiting. Diarrhea, anxiety, tachycardia. Fatal to less than 5% of patients.
200–600	Nausea and vomiting, diarrhea in the first several hours, weakness, fatigue. Fatal to approximately 50% of patients within six weeks without prompt medical attention.
600–1,000	Severe nausea and vomiting, diarrhea in the first several hours. Fatal to 100% of patients within two weeks without prompt medical attention.
1,000 or more	"Burning sensation" within minutes, nausea and vomiting within 10 minutes, confusion ataxia, and prostration within one hour, watery diarrhea within 1–2 hrs. Fatal to 100% within short time without prompt medical attention.

Localized Exposure

Dose (RAD)	Effect
50	Asymptomatic.
500	Asymptomatic (usually). May have risk of altered function of exposed area.
2,500	Atrophy, vascular lesion, and altered pigmentation.
5,000	Chronic ulcer, risk of carcinogenesis.
50,000	Permanent destruction of exposed tissue.

EFFECTS OF RADIATION ON THE BODY

Ionizing radiation cannot be seen, felt, or heard. Therefore, a detection instrument is required to measure the radiation given off by the radiation source. The most commonly used device is the *Geiger counter.* The rate of radiation is measured in roentgens per hour (R/hr) or milliroentgens per hour (mR/hr) (1,000 mR = 1R).

The unit of local tissue energy deposition is called *radiation absorbed dose (RAD). Roentgen equivalent in man (REM)* provides a gauge of the likely injury to the irradiated part of an organism. For all practical purposes, RAD and REM are equal in clinical value. When neutrons or other high-energy radiation sources are used, a *quality factor (QF)* is applied to determine the equivalent dose.

Simply stated, ionizing radiation causes alterations in the body's cell, primarily the genetic material (DNA). Depending upon the dosage received, the changes can be in cell division, cell structure, and cellular biochemical activities. Cell damage due to ionizing radiation is cumulative over a lifetime. If a person is exposed to ionizing radiation long enough, there will be a decreased number of white blood cells. Additionally, there may be defects in offspring, an increased incidence of cancer, and various degrees of bone marrow damage.

Detection of the first biological effects of exposure to ionizing radiation occurs at varying times (Table 10-4). Biological effects include:

- *Acute.* Effects appearing in a matter of minutes or weeks.
- *Long-term.* Effects appearing years or decades later.

FIGURE 10-8   Nuclear
radiation.

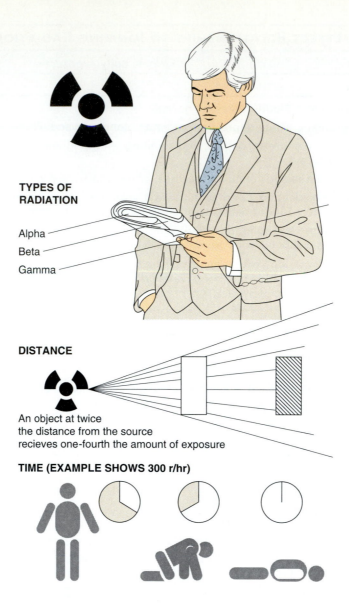

TYPES OF
RADIATION

Alpha

Beta

Gamma

DISTANCE

An object at twice
the distance from the source
recieves one-fourth the amount of exposure

TIME (EXAMPLE SHOWS 300 r/hr)

PRINCIPLES OF SAFETY

Limiting radiation exposure is based on three principles: time, distance, and shielding.

There are three basic principles that allow rescue personnel and patients to limit exposure to ionizing radiation. These are *time, distance,* and *shielding.* Determining exposure, absorption, and damage done by radiation requires specialized training. The amount of radiation received by a person depends upon the source of radiation, the length of time exposed, the distance from the source, and the shielding between the exposed person and the source (Figure 10-8). For example, the amount of radiation at the patient's initial location may be 300 R/hr. If exposure is for 20 minutes, this is the same radiation equivalent as working for one hour at a 100 R/hr scene.

The amount of radiation may drop off rapidly as the patient is decontaminated and moved away from the exposure. The distance from an ionizing radiation source is crucial since exposure is determined by the inverse square relationship. Doubling the distance away from a radiation source reduces the exposure by a factor of four. Conversely, halving the distance to a radiation source increases exposure by a factor of four.

There are basically two types of ionizing radiation accidents—clean and dirty. In a *clean accident,* the patient is exposed to radiation but is not contaminated by the radioactive substance, particles of radioactive dust, or radioactive liquids, gases, or smoke. If he is properly decontaminated before arrival of rescue personnel, there will be little danger, provided the source of the radiation is no longer exposed at the scene. After exposure to ionizing radiation, the patient is not radioactive. Therefore, he poses no hazard to rescue personnel.

In contrast, the *dirty* accident, often associated with fire at the scene of a radiation accident, exposes the patient to radiation and contaminates him with radioactive particles or liquids. The scene may be highly contaminated, although the primary source of radiation is shielded when rescue personnel arrive. Unless you are properly trained in dealing with this type of emergency, you may have to delay rescue procedures until properly trained technical assistance arrives.

MANAGEMENT

If you find yourself involved in a radioactive emergency, take the following precautionary steps:

- Park the rescue vehicle upwind to minimize contamination.
- Look for signs of radiation exposure. Radioactive packages are marked by clearly identifiable color-coded labels (Figure 10-9).
- Use portable instruments to measure the level of radioactivity. If dose estimates are significant, rotate rescue personnel.
- Normal principles of emergency care should be applied, for example, ABCs, shock management, and trauma care.
- Externally radiated patients pose little danger to rescue personnel. Initiate normal care procedures for injuries other than radiation.
- Internally contaminated patients (who have ingested or inhaled radioactive particles) pose little danger to rescue personnel. Normal care procedures should be undertaken. Collect body wastes. If assisted ventilation is required, use a bag-valve-mask unit or demand valve. If radioactive particles are inhaled, swab the nasal passages and save the swabs.

In a radiation accident, externally radiated and internally contaminated patients pose little danger to rescue personnel. Provide normal emergency care. Externally contaminated patients must be decontaminated before normal emergency care is initiated. Paramedic personnel and equipment must be decontaminated after the call.

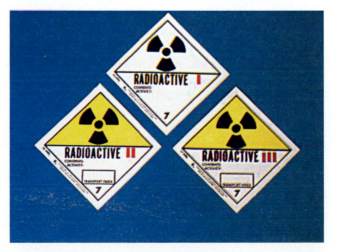

FIGURE 10-9   Radioactive warning labels.

- Externally contaminated patients (liquids, dirt, smoke) require decontamination. Following decontamination, initiate normal emergency care procedures. Decontamination of paramedic personnel and equipment is required after the call is completed.
- Patients with open, contaminated wounds require normal emergency care procedures. Avoid cross-contamination of wounds.

SUMMARY

Our environment provides us with all that we need to survive and prosper. The extremes of our environment, however, can have significant impact on human metabolism. Our bodies will, of course, compensate for these extremes, but sometimes it is not enough. Sometimes the heat gain or loss is too much. Sometimes the pressure change is too much. As a result, medical illnesses and emergencies arise. These can range from abnormal core body temperatures to decompensation, shock, and even death.

Basic knowledge of common environmental, recreational, and exposure emergencies is necessary in order for you to administer prompt and proper treatment in the prehospital setting. It is not easy to remember this type of information since these problems are not usually encountered on a daily basis. Remember the general principles involved. Remove the environmental influence causing the problem. Support the patient's own attempt to compensate. Finally, select a definitive care location and transport the patient as rapidly as possible.

In every case, remember that you must maintain your own safety. There are too many cases in which paramedics have lost their lives as a result of attempting a rescue for which they were not properly trained. Rapid action is always necessary when performing an environmental rescue. However, common sense must prevail.

YOU MAKE THE CALL

You and your partner, Christina, are paramedics stationed at Mike Leigh General Hospital in Lake Dulce, Colorado. You've enjoyed working at this beautiful mountain ski resort (elevation 8,815 ft.) even though you've only been doing it for a year. This morning you are expecting a busy day since this is the first day of Spring Break and hundreds of visitors have been arriving daily for their week-long romp in the snow.

Shortly after 10 a.m. a call comes in from the first-alert ski patrol. A skier on Mount Guilio is in unspecified distress. You and Christina hasten to your snowmobiles and proceed immediately to the slope. On arrival you find a 25-year-old man crouched in the snow, surrounded by curious onlookers. The ski patrol informs you that he is a scuba diving expert, Biff Western. Biff arrived yesterday with his wife Muffy to try skiing for the first time. Biff did not sleep well last night despite taking one sleeping pill he had brought with him. This morning he felt very tired, a condition that was aggravated by a dry cough he seemed to have developed. Now on his second run down the slope, the exertion has exhausted him. The ski patrol thinks he is becoming confused and disoriented. He is short of breath, weak, dizzy, and his cough has become productive of white frothy sputum.

On examination you find that Biff is breathing very rapidly. His heart is racing and his lips are tinged blue. Listening to the chest you note coarse diffuse crackles on inspiration. You and Christina share a momentary knowing glance then spring into action.

1. What illness are you probably dealing with?
2. What predisposing factors lead to this illness?
3. What is the definitive treatment for this condition?
4. If definitive treatment is not possible, what other measures can be used?

See Suggested Responses at the back of this book.

FURTHER READING

Auerbach, Paul S., ed. *Wilderness Medicine: Management of Wilderness and Environmental Emergencies.* 3rd ed. St. Louis: Mosby-Year Book, 1995.
Bledsoe, Bryan E., Dwayne E. Clayden, and Frank J. Papa. Prehospital Emergency Pharmacology. 4th ed. Upper Saddle River, N.J.: Brady, 1996.
"Environmental Injuries." In *Emergency Medicine: A Comprehensive Study Guide.* 4th ed, edited by Judith E. Tintinalli, et al. New York: McGraw-Hill, 1996.
Guyton, Arthur C. and John E. Hall. Textbook of Medical Physiology. 9th ed. Philadelphia: Saunders, 1995.

ON THE WEB

Visit Brady's Paramedic Website at www.bradybooks.com/paramedic.

CHAPTER 11

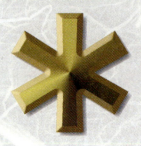

Infectious Disease

Objectives

After reading this chapter, you should be able to:

1. Describe the specific anatomy and physiology pertinent to infectious and communicable diseases. (pp. 557–560)

2. Define specific terminology identified with infectious/communicable diseases. (pp. 549–601)

3. Discuss public health principles relevant to infectious/communicable diseases. (pp. 549–550)

4. Identify public health agencies involved in the prevention and management of disease outbreaks. (p. 550)

5. List and describe the steps of an infectious process. (pp. 555–557)

6. Discuss the risks associated with infection. (pp. 549, 551, 555–557)

7. List and describe the stages of infectious diseases. (pp. 555–557)

8. List and describe infectious agents, including bacteria, viruses, fungi, protozoans, and helminths (worms). (pp. 550–554)

Continued

Objectives Continued

9. Describe characteristics of the immune system, including the categories of white blood cells, the reticuloendothelial system (RES), and the complement system. (pp. 557–560)

10. Describe the processes of the immune system defenses, including humoral and cell-mediated immunity. (pp. 557–560)

11. In specific diseases, identify and discuss the issues of personal isolation. (pp. 561–604)

12. Describe and discuss the rationale for the various types of personal protection equipment. (pp. 561–567)

13. Discuss what constitutes a significant exposure to an infectious agent. (pp. 567–568)

14. Describe the assessment of a patient suspected of, or identified as having, an infectious/communicable disease. (pp. 568–569)

15. Discuss the proper disposal of contaminated supplies such as sharps, gauze, sponges, and tourniquets. (pp. 561–565)

16. Discuss disinfection of patient care equipment and areas where patient care occurred. (pp. 566–567)

17. Discuss the seroconversion rate after direct significant HIV exposure. (pp. 560, 570–571)

18. Discuss the causative agent, body systems affected and potential secondary complications, routes of transmission, susceptibility and resistance, signs and symptoms, patient management and protective measures, and immunization for each of the following:
    - HIV (pp. 570–574)
    - Hepatitis A (pp. 574–575)
    - Hepatitis B (p. 575)
    - Hepatitis C (pp. 575–576)
    - Hepatitis D (p. 576)
    - Hepatitis E (p. 576)
    - Tuberculosis (pp. 576–579)
    - Meningococcal meningitis (pp. 582–583)
    - Pneumonia (pp. 579–580)
    - Tetanus (pp. 594–595)
    - Rabies (pp. 592–594)
    - Hantavirus (pp. 589–590)
    - Chicken pox (pp. 581–582)
    - Mumps (pp. 585–586)
    - Rubella (p. 586)
    - Measles (p. 585)
    - Pertussis (whooping cough) (p. 587)
    - Influenza (pp. 584–585)
    - Mononucleosis (pp. 587–588)
    - Herpes Simplex 1 and 2 (pp. 587–588, 598)
    - Syphilis (pp. 596–598)
    - Gonorrhea (p. 596)
    - Chlamydia (pp. 598–599)
    - Scabies (p. 601)
    - Lice (p. 600)
    - Lyme disease (pp. 595–596)
    - Gastroenteritis (pp. 590–591)

19. Discuss other infectious agents known to cause meningitis including streptococcus pneumonia, haemophilus influenza type B, and various varieties of viruses. (p. 582)

20. Identify common pediatric viral diseases. (pp. 581–582, 585–587)

21. Discuss the characteristics of and organisms associated with febrile and afebrile diseases including bronchiolitis, bronchitis, laryngitis, croup, epiglottitis, and the common cold. (pp. 584–590)

22. Articulate the pathophysiological principles of an infectious process given a case study of a patient with an infectious/communicable disease. (pp. 550–601)

23. Given several preprogrammed infectious disease patients, provide the appropriate body substance isolation procedure, assessment, management, and transport. (pp. 550–601)

Case Study

Elizabeth Fletcher and her partner, Stuart Pratt, are performing routine duties at the station one cool spring evening when the call comes in. They are dispatched to a local residence for a patient complaining of difficulty breathing.

Elizabeth and Stuart arrive to find a 52-year-old male sitting on the edge of his bed, complaining of shortness of breath. The patient's wife reports that his symptoms began as a cough and congestion. Over the last two weeks the symptoms have gradually worsened.

While Stuart gathers the history and records the patient's vital signs, Elizabeth begins the physical exam. The patient is an undernourished male who appears much older than his 52 years. His vital signs are blood pressure, 156/96; pulse, 118; respirations, 30 and slightly labored; temperature, 99.4°F via a tympanic thermometer. The patient's electrocardiogram shows a sinus tachycardia with occasional unifocal premature ventricular contractions. His skin is pale and dry. Oxygen saturation is 90 percent on room air and improves to 95 percent after several minutes of oxygen by simple plastic mask. Auscultation of the patient's chest reveals scattered dry crackles bilaterally. He coughs occasionally, but it is non-productive. He is a one-pack-per-day smoker with a 20 pack/year history. There is no history of obstructive lung disease. Before this episode, he has never experienced any difficulty breathing.

When Stuart questions him further, the patient admits to night sweats and loss of fifteen pounds of body weight over the past month. He has coughed up blood on at least three occasions during the past several days.

Elizabeth and Stuart place the patient on high-flow oxygen via a non-rebreather mask. They start an IV of normal saline at a to-keep-open rate. While they transport the patient to the emergency department, he remains stable and his shortness of breath improves. Upon arrival, the emergency physician diagnoses the patient with possible tuberculosis based upon the history and chest X-ray findings. The patient is admitted to an isolation room on a medical floor for treatment and subsequent evaluation by an infectious disease specialist.

The EMS system is notified about the possible exposure. Cultures for the bacterium that causes tuberculosis can take up to six weeks to complete. The paramedics involved in the call are informed about the possible exposure, and post-exposure protective measures are started. Cultures later confirm the diagnosis of tuberculosis. Fortunately, neither of the paramedics has been infected.

INTRODUCTION

Infectious diseases are illnesses caused by infestation of the body by biological organisms such as bacteria, viruses, fungi, protozoans, and helminths (worms). Most infectious disease states are not life-threatening and the patient recovers completely. Some types of infection, however, such as human immunodeficiency virus (HIV), hepatitis B virus (HBV), and acute bacterial meningitis, are particularly dangerous and may result in death or permanent disability.

All health care professionals must maintain a strong working knowledge of public health principles and infectious diseases. This is especially true for paramedics, who are often the first to encounter patients with communicable diseases. Early recognition and management of these patients may make a difference in how the patient is treated and may also ensure that care providers take necessary precautions to prevent the spread of the disease to others.

This chapter discusses infectious diseases, including the types of disease-causing organisms, functions of the immune system, and general pathophysiology of infectious diseases. It emphasizes the specific diseases, discussing those that you may encounter during interhospital transports or out-of-hospital care, especially those that you are most likely to encounter in the field.

* **infectious disease** illness caused by infestation of the body by biological organisms.

PUBLIC HEALTH PRINCIPLES

When dealing with infectious diseases, you must consider the impact of the disease process on the community as well as on the infected patient. An infectious agent is a "hazardous material" that can affect large numbers of people.

Epidemiologists, health professionals who study how infectious diseases affect populations, attempt to describe and predict how diseases move from individuals to populations. Through various clinically based studies and statistical techniques, they try to determine how effectively an infectious agent can travel through a population. Using the population of infected individuals as a standard, they attempt to predict those individuals in the larger population who may be most at risk for contracting the infectious agent. Recognizing that risk may be predictable, and not just random, is important. The characteristics of the host, the infectious agent, and the environment may yield clues as to how the infectious agent is transmitted and reveal individuals or populations susceptible to infection.

How a population is identified is important. It may be defined by such parameters as geographic boundary, workplace, school, correctional institution, age group, income level, or ethnic group. All of the characteristics of a certain population are known as its demographics. The population's tendency to expand, decline, or move is important as well. Besides stimulating social and economic progress, the movement of people and animals within and among other societies also provides a vehicle for infectious agents.

To track the progress of infection within a population, epidemiologists work backward through the chain of infection to determine the **index case,** that individual who first introduced the infectious agent to the population. From the index case, they then retrace the chain forward to verify their reconstruction of the infection's pattern.

To gauge a disease's potential impact on the community, paramedics must evaluate the host (patient), what they believe to be the infectious agent, and the environment. Based on that assessment, they may use more aggressive personal protective equipment. They must also consider the patient, those in the patient's

* **index case** the individual who first introduced an infectious agent to a population.

immediate environment, and those in the environment where the patient is being transported all to be at risk for infection. On a more personal level, paramedics must appreciate that they and their families could also be at risk.

PUBLIC HEALTH AGENCIES

Local agencies are the first line of defense in disease surveillance and outbreak.

Local agencies are the first line of defense in disease surveillance and outbreak. Municipal, city, and county agencies, including fire departments, ambulance services, and health departments, must cooperate to monitor and report the incidence and prevalence of disease.

At the state level, a designated agency (health department or board of health, for instance) generally monitors infectious diseases. These agencies may set policies requiring vaccinations and regulate or implement control programs in vector and animal control, food preparation, water, sewer, and other sanitation control programs. State and local laws sometimes require these agencies to meet or exceed federal guidelines and recommendations.

A number of federal agencies are involved in tracking the morbidity and mortality of infectious diseases. The U.S. Department of Health and Human Services (DHHS) Centers for Disease Control and Prevention (CDC) in Atlanta, Georgia, is the most visible federal agency. The CDC monitors national disease data and freely disseminates this information to all health care providers. It sends personnel nationally and internationally to assist with studying, characterizing, and managing serious disease outbreaks. The CDC is also involved in researching infectious diseases. The National Institute for Occupational Safety and Health (NIOSH), also under the aegis of DHHS, works with the U.S. Department of Labor's Occupational Safety and Health Administration (OSHA), in setting standards and guidelines for workplace and worker controls to prevent infectious diseases in the workplace. This level of federal government involvement would not be possible without the leadership of the U.S. Congress in establishing national health policies and in drafting the federal budget.

Other organizations and governmental agencies that might serve as resources to your organization include the Federal Emergency Management Agency (FEMA), the National Fire Protection Association (NFPA), the United States Fire Protection Administration (USFPA), and the International Association of Firefighters (IAFF). These groups develop helpful blueprints for incorporating OSHA, NIOSH, and other standards and guidelines into daily operations.

MICROORGANISMS

The vast majority of disease-causing organisms are microscopic (visible only under a microscope). These microorganisms surround us. They are on our skin and in the air we breathe, and they colonize virtually every orifice of our bodies. Some can even live in the highly acidic environment of our stomachs, which destroys other disease-producing microorganisms or deactivates their toxic products. Microorganisms that reside in our bodies without ordinarily causing disease are part of the *host defenses* known as **normal flora**. Normal flora help keep us disease-free by creating environmental conditions that are not conducive to disease-producing microorganisms, or **pathogens**. Competition between colonies of normal flora and pathogens also discourages the survival of pathogens. Common bacterial pathogens include *Staphylococci, Streptococci,* and *Enterobacteriaceae.* Certain viruses, rickettsiae, fungi, and protozoans are also pathogenic.

✳ normal flora organisms that live inside our bodies without ordinarily causing disease.

✳ pathogen organism capable of causing disease.

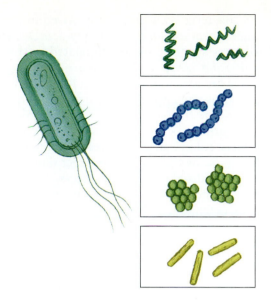

FIGURE 11-1 Bacteria are single-celled organisms that range in length from one to twenty micrometers.

Opportunistic pathogens are ordinarily nonharmful bacteria that cause disease only under unusual circumstances. Most opportunistic pathogens are normal flora. Patients who have a weakened immune system or who are under unusual stress become susceptible to diseases caused by opportunistic organisms. For example, the fungus *Pneumocystis carinii* is usually harmless but can cause a deadly form of pneumonia in patients with HIV. The fungus overwhelms the weakened immune system and begins to reproduce rapidly in the lungs. Left untreated, *Pneumocystis carinii* pneumonia may be fatal. Organ transplant recipients are also at increased risk for infectious diseases because they must take immunosuppressant medications to prevent organ rejection. A more common (and less harmful) opportunistic infection is thrush (oral candidiasis), often seen in patients who take broad spectrum antibiotics. As the antibiotic kills normal bacterial flora in the mouth, the fungus *Candida albicans* grows almost uninhibited on the tongue and in the pharynx, producing a white coating on the mucosa.

✳ **opportunistic pathogen** ordinarily nonharmful bacterium that causes disease only under unusual circumstances.

BACTERIA

Bacteria are microscopic single-celled organisms that range in length from one to twenty micrometers (Figure 11-1). They are living cells that are classified as *prokaryotes* because they do not have a distinct nuclear membrane and possess only one chromosome in the cytoplasm. Bacteria reproduce independently, but they require a host to supply food and a supportive environment. Some common diseases caused by pathogenic bacteria include sinusitis, otitis media, bacterial pneumonia, pharyngitis (strep throat), tuberculosis, and most urinary tract infections.

Most bacteria are easily identifiable with stains or by their appearance under a microscope. Similar colorfastness indicates similarities in cell wall structure and other anatomic features. The **Gram stain** is the most common method of differentiating bacteria. Bacteria this process turns purple are known as gram-positive bacteria; those it turns red are gram-negative. Because of the similarities in their cell walls, bacteria that stain alike may respond to similar treatments.

✳ **bacteria** microscopic single-celled organisms that range in length from one to twenty micrometers.

✳ **Gram stain** method of differentiating types of bacteria according to their reaction to a chemical stain process.

Bacteria are further categorized into groups based on their general appearance: cocci, or spheres, (staphylococcus, streptococcus) are round; rods (*Enterobacter* sp., *E. coli*) are elongated; and spirals (spirochetes, vibrio) are coiled. *Enterobacter* sp. and *E. coli* are gram-negative rods. *Staphylococci* and *streptococci* are gram-positive cocci. Regardless of how bacteria stain or appear under a microscope, it is the specific tissues and organs which are infected that chiefly determine the patient's signs and symptoms.

Pathogenic bacteria may harm their human hosts in a number of ways. Heavy colonization may result in direct damage to tissues as the bacteria feed. Bacteria may also cause indirect damage by releasing toxic chemicals that can have localized or systemic effects. The two general categories of toxins are exotoxins and endotoxins. This classification is no longer based primarily on where they originate, as their names imply, but by their chemical structures. **Exotoxins** are poisonous proteins shed by bacteria during bacterial growth. They stimulate the immune system to form antibodies to these proteins, and they may also be deactivated by chemicals, light, or heat. Exotoxins are more toxic than endotoxins. The infectious agent of toxic shock syndrome, *S. aureus,* releases an exotoxin, as does anthrax, which can be delivered as a biological weapon of mass destruction.

Endotoxins are composed of proteins, polysaccharides (large sugar molecules), and lipids. The immune system cannot form antibodies specific to a particular endotoxin unless both the protein and polysaccharide portions are present. Endotoxins come from the bacterial cell wall and are released when the bacterial cell is destroyed. They are more stable in heat than exotoxins. Only gram-negative bacteria make endotoxins. The skin lesions of meningococcemia and the signs of shock that sometimes accompany it are due to large amounts of endotoxin released by the infectious agent, *N. menningitidis.*

Most bacterial infections respond to treatment with antibiotics that are either **bactericidal** (kill bacteria) or **bacteriostatic** (inhibit bacterial growth or reproduction). Antibiotics are prescribed based on bacterial sensitivity; different antibiotics are required to treat different bacteria. Their administration usually decreases bacterial presence and reduces symptoms. Some types of bacterial infections respond quickly to antibiotics; others take longer. In recent years, a number of bacterial strains have developed resistance to antibiotic therapy, making treatment more difficult. The more a type of bacterium is exposed to an antibiotic, the greater the likelihood of its developing resistance. The overuse of antibiotics in both medical and veterinary settings has contributed to this serious problem. Resistant forms of tuberculosis (mycobacterium) are of particular concern. Antibiotics may now be ineffective against this disease, and its mortality rate is high. The willingness of some physicians to prescribe the newest antibiotics for relatively minor infections and the widespread addition of antibiotics to animal feed have only added to the problem.

Antimicrobial treatment alters the normal flora of the skin, mouth, mucosa, and gastrointestinal tract and often results in colonization of those areas by new microorganisms that resist antibiotics. In some cases, an antibiotic may kill normal flora and allow more virulent and dangerous opportunistic pathogens to multiply freely. This can lead to a secondary infection that is more severe than the original infection being treated. For all of these reasons, antibiotics should be prescribed cautiously.

VIRUSES

Viruses are much smaller than bacteria and can be seen only with an electron microscope (Figure 11-2). Viruses cannot reproduce and carry on metabolism by themselves. Therefore, they are considered to be neither prokaryotes nor eukaryotes.

✳ **exotoxin** toxic waste products released by living bacteria.

✳ **endotoxin** toxic products released when bacteria die and decompose.

✳ **bactericidal** capable of killing bacteria.

✳ **bacteriostatic** capable of inhibiting bacterial growth or reproduction.

✳ **virus** disease-causing organism that can be seen only with an electron microscope.

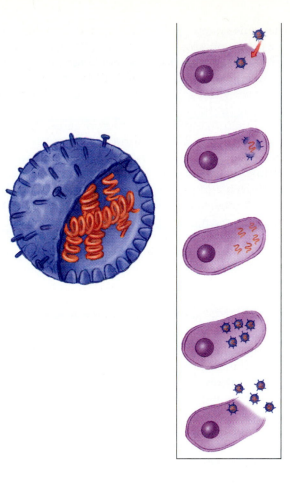

FIGURE 11-2 Viruses are much smaller than bacteria and can be seen only with an electron microscope. They grow and reproduce only within a host cell.

Instead, viruses are **obligate intracellular parasites**; that is, they can grow and reproduce only within a host cell. Once inside, the virus takes control of the host cell's protein synthesis mechanism and directs it to begin reproducing the virus. The cell then releases new virus particles, which infect nearby cells.

Since viruses "hide" inside the host's cells, they resist antibiotic treatment. Once a virus enters a host cell, it becomes part of that host cell, making selective eradication of the virus virtually impossible, as any treatment capable of killing the virus will generally kill the host cell as well. This is the major obstacle facing researchers as they work to find cures for HIV and other viruses.

Approximately 400 types of viruses have been identified. One frequently encountered viral disorder, the common cold, is caused by a number of different viruses (nearly 200) that all produce similar symptoms. Fortunately, most viral diseases are mild and self-limiting. They run their course until the patient's immune system eventually fights them off. A host is generally susceptible to any particular virus only once. Once a person's immune system develops active immunity against a particular type of virus, it becomes attuned to similar attacking viruses and will destroy them.

OTHER MICROORGANISMS

Prions are a new classification of disease-producing agents that microbiologists used to refer to as "slow viruses." They are neither prokaryotes nor eukaryotes but particles of protein, folded in such a way that proteases (enzymes that break down proteins) cannot act upon them. These protein particles accumulate in

✱ **obligate intracellular parasite** organism that can grow and reproduce only within a host cell.

✱ **prions** particles of protein, folded in such a way that protease enzymes cannot act upon them.

nervous system and brain tissue, destroying them and giving them a spongy appearance on gross examination. Prions are known to cause progressive, untreatable dementia in Kuru, Creutzfeldt-Jakob disease, mad cow disease, and fatal familial insomnia. Although EMS providers will rarely respond to patients with diseases caused by prions, a general discussion of infectious agents must acknowledge their existence.

Fungi are plant-like microorganisms, most of which are not pathogenic. Yeasts, molds, and mushrooms are types of fungi. Some fungi have a capsule around the cell wall that provides additional protection against phagocytes. While fungi compose a large part of the body's normal flora, they may become pathogenic in patients with compromised immune function, such as those with HIV. Fungi may also lead to disease states in patients taking broad-spectrum antibiotics. As the antibiotics kill off bacteria, the fungi are able to grow uninhibited. Fungi are a common cause of vaginal infections and often cause pneumonia in patients with weakened immune systems.

Protozoa are single-celled parasitic organisms with flexible membranes and the ability to move. Most protozoa live in the soil and ingest decaying organic matter. Although rarely a cause of disease in humans, they are considered opportunistic pathogens in patients with compromised immune function. These organisms may enter the body by the fecal-oral route or through a mosquito bite. Common diseases caused by protozoa include malaria and forms of gastroenteritis. Protozoa also cause vaginal infections (trichomoniasis) in women with normal immune function.

Parasites are common causes of disease where sanitation is poor (generally in developing countries). Occasional cases are seen in this country. Roundworms (ascarides) live in the intestinal mucosa and may reach 30–50 cm in length. Symptoms include abdominal cramping, fever, and cough. Diagnosis usually depends on finding eggs in the patient's stool.

Pinworms (*Enterobius vermicularis*) are common in the United States and in other civilized countries. It is estimated that 20 percent of children living in temperate climates harbor this disease. These tiny worms (3–10 mm long) live in the distal colon and crawl onto the anal mucosa to lay their eggs, usually when the host is asleep. Although the disease may remain asymptomatic, it is a common cause of anal pruritus (itching) and infection and is easily spread among children, especially in day-care centers. Children may carry the disease home and infect their entire family. This disease is often endemic among institutionalized children. Treatment involves a single dose of an antibiotic (mebendazole); all family members must be treated simultaneously to avoid reinfection.

Hookworms (*Ancylostoma duodenale, Necator americanus*) are found in warm, moist climates. This parasite infects an estimated 25 percent of the world's population, although it is relatively rare in the United States. The larvae are passed in the stool of infected animals. The disease is most commonly contracted when a barefoot child walks in a contaminated area. The larvae enter through the skin and migrate to the intestines, where they grip and irritate the intestinal wall and feed on blood. Epigastric pain and anemia are possible. Prevention involves wearing shoes; treatment is similar to that for pinworms.

Trichinosis (*Trichinella spiralis*) may be contracted by eating raw or inadequately cooked pork products, most commonly sausage. Females burrow into the intestinal wall and produce thousands of living larvae that migrate to skeletal muscle, where each forms a cyst and remains. Symptoms include gastrointestinal disturbances, edema (especially of the eyelids), fever, and a variety of other diffuse and secondary symptoms. If the worms invade the heart, lungs, or brain in large numbers, death may result. Diagnosis is made by finding encysted worms during examination of muscle biopsy. Mebendazole is the antibiotic of choice.

Other types of worms such as tapeworms and flukes are rarely encountered in the United States.

* fungus plant-like microorganism.

* protozoan single-celled parasitic organism with flexible membranes and the ability to move.

* parasite organism that lives in or on another organism.

* pinworm parasite that is 3–10 mm long and lives in the distal colon.

* hookworm parasite that attaches to the host's intestinal lining.

* trichinosis disease resulting from an infestation of *Trichinella spriralis.*

CONTRACTION, TRANSMISSION, AND STAGES OF DISEASE

As a paramedic you must understand the relationship between the pathophysiology and the assessment and management of patients with infections or diseases resulting from infections. This knowledge will prepare you for leadership in recognizing infectious diseases and curbing their transmission.

The interactions of host, infectious agent, and environment are the elements of disease transmission. Studying each of these factors individually and then looking for relationships among them often reveals how an infectious agent has been effectively transmitted. Infectious agents exist in all types of **reservoirs**—animals, humans, insects, and the environment. While inhabiting animal or insect reservoirs, they do not cause disease. Their presence at any time in a given environment is affected by their life cycle, by the presence of stressors that may force them outside of their normal reservoirs, and by the climate. The initiation of therapy can sometimes disrupt the life cycle of the infectious agent and may eradicate the infection. When a host and infectious agent come together at the right time and under the right conditions, disease transmission takes place.

Infectious agents may invade hosts through one of two basic mechanisms. The more common is direct transmission from person to person through a cough, sneeze, kiss, or sexual contact. The other mechanism, indirect transmission, can spread organisms in a number of ways. Infected persons often shed organisms into the environment. These organisms come to rest on doorknobs, handrails, computer keyboards, and so on. Other people who contact those surfaces are at risk for contracting the disease. Similarly, microorganisms may be transmitted via food products, water, or even through the soil.

Bloodborne diseases are transmitted by contact with the blood or body fluids of an infected person. They include AIDS, hepatitis B, hepatitis C, hepatitis D, and syphilis. The risk of transmission of bloodborne diseases increases if a patient has open wounds, active bleeding, or increased secretions. Assume that every patient has an infectious bloodborne disease and take precautions to avoid contact with blood and other body fluids.

Some infectious diseases may be transmitted through the air on droplets expelled during a productive cough or sneeze. They include tuberculosis, meningitis, mumps, measles, rubella, and chicken pox (varicella). Other, more common diseases such as the common cold, influenza, and respiratory syncytial virus (RSV) may also be transmitted by the **airborne** route.

Some infectious diseases are transmitted orally (primarily by eating) or by the **fecal-oral route,** in which enteric microorganisms (normally found in the GI system and the feces) are transmitted between potential hosts, as in shaking hands or other social customs, and then having the recipient somehow introduce the infectious agent into his mouth by scratching or eating with his hands. Fecal-oral diseases are prevalent in third world countries or in areas with unsanitary conditions. Hepatitis A, hepatitis E, and other viruses can be transmitted by this route. Foodborne illnesses include food poisoning, certain parasitic infections, and trichinosis.

The risk of infection is considered *theoretical* if transmission is acknowledged to be possible but has not actually been reported. It is considered *measurable* if factors in the infectious agent's transmission and their associated risks have been identified or deduced from reported data. Generally, the risk of disease transmission rises if a patient has open wounds, increased secretions, active coughing, or any ongoing invasive treatment where exposure to an infectious body fluid is likely (Table 11-1). In the prehospital setting, the unpredictable environment and behavior of patients increase the risk of exposure. For example, a patient with a

* **reservoir** any living creature or environment (water, soil, etc.) that can harbor an infectious agent.

* **bloodborne** transmitted by contact with blood or body fluids.

* **airborne** transmitted through the air by droplets or particles.

* **fecal-oral route** transmission of organisms picked up from the gastrointestinal tract (e.g., feces) into the mouth.

Generally, the risk of disease transmission rises if a patient has open wounds, increased secretions, active coughing, or any ongoing invasive treatment where exposure to an infectious body fluid is likely.

Table 11-1   MODES OF TRANSMISSION OF INFECTIOUS DISEASES

Disease	Blood Borne	Airborne	Sexual	Indirect	Opportunist	Oral-Fecal
Hepatitis A						✔
Hepatitis B	✔					
Hepatitis C						
HIV	✔		✔			
Influenza		✔	✔	✔		
Syphilis			✔			
Gonorrhea			✔			
Measles		✔				
Mumps		✔				
Strep throat		✔			✔	
Herpes virus	✔		✔	✔		
Food poisoning		✔		✔		✔
Lyme disease	✔					
Pneumonia		✔			✔	

closed head injury and multiple lacerations may be combative, thereby contaminating EMS personnel with blood or other body fluids. Broken windshield glass contaminated with blood may easily penetrate examination gloves and skin. Patients who are violent and aggressive may deliberately bite, scratch, or spit at rescuers. Many EMS patient care activities occur in a closed, poorly ventilated environment such as the back of an ambulance. Thus, you must have available, and routinely use, protective clothing and other barrier devices, as indicated.

Not all exposures to microorganisms from body fluids or infected patients will result in transmission of those agents. Nor are all infectious agents and diseases **communicable** (capable of being transmitted to another host). Communicability depends on several factors. Exposure to an infectious agent may just result in **contamination,** in which the agent exists only on the surface of the host without penetrating it. Penetration of the host implies that **infection** has occurred, but infection should never be equated with disease. Factors that affect the likelihood that an exposed individual will become infected and then actually develop disease include:

- *Correct mode of entry* Certain external barriers in hosts, particularly the skin, make it impossible for infectious agents to establish themselves. Mucous membranes, however, often present an effective point of entry.
- *Virulence* **Virulence** is an organism's strength or ability to infect or overcome the body's defenses. Some organisms, such as the hepatitis B virus (HBV), are very virulent and can remain infectious on a surface for weeks. Others, such as HIV and syphilis, die when exposed to air and light. Some bacteria (Clostridium) may remain dormant in the soil for months and be capable of causing disease if contracted. Infection generally occurs either when a highly virulent microorganism interacts with a normal, intact host or when a less virulent microorganism enters a host with impaired defenses (immunosuppression).

* **communicable** capable of being transmitted to another host.

* **contamination** presence of an agent only on the surface of the host without penetrating it.

* **infection** presence of an agent within the host, without necessarily causing disease.

Content Review

FACTORS AFFECTING DISEASE TRANSMISSION
- Mode of entry
- Virulence
- Number of organisms transmitted
- Host resistance

* **virulence** an organism's strength or ability to infect or overcome the body's defenses.

- *Number of Organisms Transmitted (Dose)* For most diseases, a minimum number of organisms must enter the host to cause infection. As a rule, the higher the number, the greater the likelihood of contracting the disease.
- *Host Resistance* **Resistance** is the host's the ability to fight off infection. Several factors affect the host's resistance. They include general health and fitness, genetic predisposition or resistance to infection, nutrition status, recent exposure to stressors, hygiene, and the presence of underlying disease processes. Persons with decreased immune function are at significantly increased risk for contracting infectious diseases. Cigarette smokers and those regularly exposed to secondhand cigarette smoke are also at increased risk.
- *Other Host Factors* The tendency of the host to travel or be in contact with other potential hosts, the age and socioeconomic status of the host, the characteristics of other hosts within the population of which the infected host is a member all effect the likelihood of contracting disease.

PHASES OF THE INFECTIOUS PROCESS

Disease progression varies greatly, depending on the infectious agent and the host. Conditions can manifest themselves in various ways. Once infected with an infectious agent, the host goes through a **latent period** when he cannot transmit the agent to someone else. Following the latent period is a **communicable period** when the host may exhibit signs of clinical disease and can transmit the infectious agent to another host.

The appearance of symptoms often lags after exposure to an infectious disease. The time between exposure and presentation, known as the **incubation period,** may range from a few days, as in the common cold, to months or years, as in HIV/AIDS or hepatitis. Thus, prehospital personnel must be notified if any patient for whom they provide care subsequently develops a life-threatening infectious disease.

Most viruses and bacteria have surface proteins, or **antigens,** that stimulate the body to produce **antibodies.** These antibodies react to or unite with the antigens. The antibodies' presence in the blood indicates exposure to the particular disease that they fight. Although testing for the presence of a specific disease antigen is difficult, laboratory tests can often spot antibodies that are specific for the disease or antigen. For example, they detect the human immunodeficiency virus (HIV) through the presence of antibodies specific to HIV. When a person develops antibodies after exposure to a disease, his previously negative test will be positive and **seroconversion** has occurred. The time between exposure to disease and seroconversion is referred to as the **window phase.** A person in the window phase may test negative even though he is infected. From the standpoint of the immune system response, the window phase is the period when antigen is present but antibody production has not reached detectable levels. The **disease period** is the duration from the onset of signs and symptoms of disease until the resolution of symptoms or death. Keep in mind that the resolution of symptoms does not necessarily imply that the infectious agent has been eradicated.

THE BODY'S DEFENSES AGAINST DISEASE

The body protects itself from disease in many ways. At the basic level, skin defends against invading infection and pathogens. Parts of the respiratory system assist by creating turbulent airflow and capturing foreign bodies with nasal hair.

* **resistance** a host's ability to fight off infection.

* **latent period** time when a host cannot transmit an infectious agent to someone else.

* **communicable period** time when a host can transmit an infectious agent to someone else.

* **incubation period** time between a host's exposure to infectious agent and the appearance of symptoms.

* **antigen** surface protein on most viruses and bacteria.

* **antibody** protein that attacks a disease antigen.

* **seroconversion** creation of antibodies after exposure to a disease.

* **window phase** time between exposure to a disease and seroconversion.

* **disease period** the duration from the onset of signs and symptoms of disease until the resolution of symptoms or death.

immune system the body's mechanism for defending against foreign invaders.

reticuloendothelial system (RES) the cells involved in the immune response.

antigen marker on the surface of a cell that identifies it as self or non-self.

leukocyte white blood cell.

neutrophil the most common phagocytic white blood cell.

macrophage after neutrophils, the most common phagocytic white blood cell.

phagocytosis process in which certain white blood cells ingest invaders.

cell-mediated immunity generalized, temporary defense against any invader.

humoral immunity specialized, permanent defense against a particular foreign antigen.

antibody a substance that is produced in response to and that destroys a particular antigen.

lymphocyte cell that attacks invader in immune response.

T lymphocytes cells that attack invaders in cell-mediated immune responses.

B lymphocytes cells that attack invaders in humoral immune responses.

immunoglobulin antibody.

Mucus can trap and kill foreign materials, transport them to the mouth and nose via the mucociliary escalator, and expel them as sputum. (Nicotine from cigarette smoke paralyzes the individual cilia of the escalator, making the expulsion of lower airway mucus, sometimes referred to as phlegm, difficult.) The urinary and gastrointestinal systems work cooperatively to eliminate pathogens via feces and urine. Three body systems that specifically protect against disease are the immune system, the complement system, and the lymphatic system.

THE IMMUNE SYSTEM

As you learned in Chapter 8 of Volume 1 and in Chapter 5 of this volume, the human body has a very sophisticated **immune system.** The various cells involved in the immune response are sometimes collectively referred to as the **reticuloendothelial system** (RES) because their locations are so widely scattered throughout the body. (*Reticulo* means "network"; *endothelial* refers to certain cells that line blood vessels, the heart, and various body cavities.)

The immune system fights disease by protecting the body from foreign invaders. To do this it must be able to differentiate "self" from "nonself." The immune system can recognize as foreign, or nonself, the **antigens** of most bacteria and viruses. Once the immune system identifies a material as nonself, it starts a series of actions intended to eliminate the foreign material. This series of mechanisms is initiated by the inflammatory response, which results from local tissue injury. Although this discussion focuses on infection, the initial injury may also be physical, chemical, or thermal.

The inflammatory response involves selected **leukocytes** (white blood cells), the functional units of blood in the immune response. The two types of white cells, **neutrophils** and **macrophages,** both attack the infectious agent by a combination of digestive enzymes and ingesting it in a process called **phagocytosis.** Neutrophils act first and are followed 12–24 hours later by the macrophages. Once phagocytosis occurs, the macrophages release chemicals called chemotactic factors, which trigger additional immune system responses.

Two types of immune system response are **cell-mediated immunity** and **humoral immunity.** Both are time-consuming processes that involve the actions of **lymphocytes,** which are another type of leukocyte. Cell-mediated immunity does not result in the formation of **antibodies** against the foreign antigens; humoral immunity does. The antibodies remain in the blood, ready to attack the same antigen upon any future reexposure.

Cell-mediated immunity generates various forms of **T lymphocytes** that react against specific antigens. Helper T-cells, suppressor T-cells, killer T-cells, and inflammatory T-cells work together against bacteria such as *M. tuberculosis,* the causative agent of tuberculosis, and viruses that have been taken up by host cells. This defense mechanism also responds to the presence of cancer cells and transplanted tissue. Humoral immunity, by contrast, results from the action of antibodies formed from mature **B lymphocytes** (plasma cells) in the lymph nodes and bone marrow. It aims primarily at toxins and pathogens not yet ingested by phagocytes. Humoral immunity is responsible for the immune system's properties of *memory* and *specificity.* These properties mean that a particular antigen is "remembered" when it enters the body again and, as a result, plasma cells produce antibodies that work specifically against that antigen. In this way, antibodies (also called **immunoglobulins**) protect against most infectious agents to which the body is repeatedly exposed.

Other classes of white blood cells, monocytes, eosinophils, basophils, and natural killer (NK) cells, also participate in the general immune system response. The five classes of human antibodies are:

- *IgG* The IgG antibody remembers an antigen and recognizes any repeated invasions. It is the principal immunoglobulin in human serum and is the major class of immunoglobulin in the immune response. It crosses the placental barrier from mother to fetus and is important in producing immunity prior to birth.
- *IgM* IgM is formed early in most immune responses.
- *IgA* The main immunoglobulin in exocrine secretions (milk, respiratory, saliva, and tears) is IgA.
- *IgD* Present on the surface of B lymphocytes, IgD acts as an antigen receptor.
- *IgE* IgE attaches to mast cells in the respiratory and intestinal tracts. It plays a major role in allergic reactions. Patients with allergies generally have increased levels of this immunoglobulin.

An unfortunate occasional aspect of humoral immunity is **autoimmunity,** the body's formation of antibodies against itself (autoantibodies). We do not completely understand autoimmunity, but it may be due in part to antigens that chemically "look like" the body's own tissues.

✱ **autoimmunity** the body's formation of antibodies against itself.

THE COMPLEMENT SYSTEM

Since cell-mediated and humoral immunity are time-consuming processes; the complement system provides an alternate pathway to react more quickly to foreign bodies. This system of at least 20 proteins works with antibody formation and the inflammatory reaction to combat infection. It responds by recognizing surface complex molecules (endotoxins) from gram-negative bacteria. Originally named because it "complemented" the action of antibodies so that foreign cell lysis could occur, complement is now known to start a cascade of biochemical events triggered by tissue injury. The number of reactions and products in this cascade increases almost exponentially. The net result is that complement is involved with the acute inflammatory response, helping phagocytosis, and the outright killing of certain bacteria such as *Neisseria* sp.

THE LYMPHATIC SYSTEM

The **lymphatic system** is a secondary circulatory system. It comprises the spleen, thymus, lymph nodes, and lymphatic ducts, a separate set of small, thin-walled vessels that collect overflow fluid from the tissue spaces and return it to the circulatory system. This fluid, known as **lymph,** has the same composition as normal interstitial fluid.

The lymphatic system is important in disease prevention. The lymph nodes filter the lymph before returning it to the circulatory system. They are lined with reticuloendothelial cells that attach to and destroy particulate matter, including microorganisms, through phagocytosis. The leftovers, usually amino acids and other cell fragments, return to the circulatory system to be used as building blocks in cellular metabolism.

✱ **lymphatic system** secondary circulatory system that collects overflow fluid from the tissue spaces and filters it before returning it to the circulatory system.

✱ **lymph** overflow circulatory fluid in spaces between tissues.

An essential organ in the lymphatic system is the spleen, a solid organ in the left upper abdominal quadrant. The spleen essentially functions as two separate organs. The white pulp of the spleen generates antibodies and produces B- and T-lymphocytes. The red pulp removes unwanted particulate matter such as old or damaged red blood cells and other blood elements. Blood loss from the spleen, which is very vulnerable to abdominal trauma, can be massive and rapidly fatal.

INDIVIDUAL HOST IMMUNITY

The interaction of cellular mediated immunity, humoral immunity, complement, the lymphatic system, the leukocytes, and all the cells of the RES result in *resistance*, the host's defense against present and future infection. An individual is said to have acquired **passive immunity** if he has received antibodies from the maternal circulation via the placenta (transplacental transmission) or from inoculation (injection). Passive immunity generally lasts from days to months. An individual who develops antibodies in response to inoculation by a killed or modified form of an infectious agent in an attenuated vaccine or its parts is said to have acquired **active immunity.** Active immunity is humoral immunity and generally lasts for years or the lifetime of the individual. After immunization or natural exposure to an antigen, an individual should *seroconvert* (show evidence of antibody response). The *assay,* or laboratory measure of the amount of antibodies against a particular antigen, is the *titer.* The measure of a particular vaccine's effectiveness is reported as the antibody titer. The titer most familiar to health care workers is the one reported after the Hepatitis B vaccination series.

The immune system's ability to develop antibodies is also used to classify microorganisms into serotypes. A serotype is determined by exposing a microorganism to known antibody solutions. When a reaction indicates the formation of an antigen-antibody complex, the antigens associated with that microorganism are then known, and the microorganism is thereafter designated as a certain serotype. The designation may be in letters, numbers, or alphanumerics and often depends on how the antigens are identified.

Immunizing against tetanus is common practice in emergency medicine. Tetanus is a rare, but frequently fatal, disease that results from a wound infected with the bacterium *Clostridium tetani.* This bacterium releases an exotoxin called tetanospasmin that causes the clinical signs and symptoms of the disease. Thus, the infection can be localized, but the patient will experience generalized symptoms because of the presence of the exotoxin in the circulation. Generalized tetanus causes pain and stiffness in the jaw muscles (hence the common name "lock jaw") and stiffness in the trunk muscles. This progresses to reflex convulsive spasms and tonic contractions of muscle groups. These are accompanied by autonomic nervous system dysfunction, laryngospasm, and other problems. As a rule, people in developed countries receive several doses of tetanus vaccine during their childhood. This is followed by periodic boosters every 5–10 years.

Occasionally, patients will present with a tetanus-prone wound who have never received any form of tetanus vaccination. This is a particular problem along the U.S.-Mexico border. In these cases, patients require passive antibodies until their immune system can begin to manufacture specific antibodies in response to the tetanus vaccine. Passive immunity is provided by injection of tetanus immune globulin (TIG) (Hypertet). This provides antibodies for immediate protection. Since the patient did not manufacture them, they are considered passive immunity. At the same time, the patient will receive a dose of tetanus toxoid. This will cause the patient's immune system to manufacture antibodies against tetanus, providing a form of active immunity. Since there is no specific treatment for tetanus, the best approach is to prevent it by aggressive immunization.

* **passive immunity** newborn's protection against disease that results from the mother's transferring some of her antibodies to the fetus.

* **active immunity** protection against disease developed after birth as a result of a direct exposure to the disease.

INFECTION CONTROL IN PREHOSPITAL CARE

To supplement the body's natural defenses against disease, EMS providers must protect themselves from infectious exposures (Figure 11-3). The four phases of infection control in prehospital care include preparation for response, response, patient contact, and recovery.

PREPARATION FOR RESPONSE

Infection control begins long before an emergency call. To ensure proper protection, the EMS agency should implement the following procedures:

- Establish and maintain written standard operating procedures (SOPs) for infection control, and monitor employee compliance.
- Prepare an infection control plan that includes a schedule of when and how to implement OSHA, NIOSH, and CDC pathogen standards and guidelines.
- Provide adequate original and ongoing infection control training to all personnel, including engineering and work practice controls.

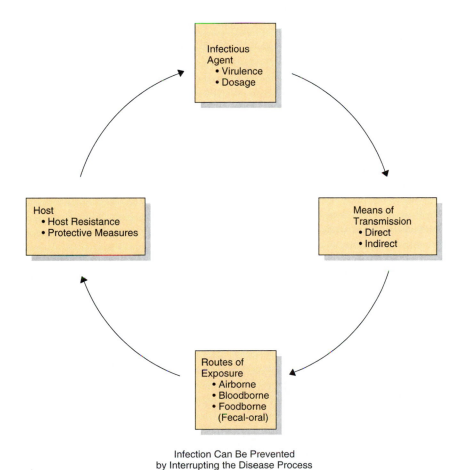

FIGURE 11-3 Interruption of infectious disease transmission is a role of prehospital personnel.

- Ensure that all employees are provided with personal protective equipment (PPE) and that it is fitted appropriately, checked regularly, maintained properly, and can be located easily.
- Ensure that all EMS personnel treat and bandage all personal wounds (e.g., open sores, cuts, or skin breaks) before any emergency response.
- Use disposable supplies and equipment whenever possible. The risk of transmitting disease is generally much lower than when reusing items, even though they have been cleaned or disinfected.
- Assure that all EMS personnel have access to the facilities and supplies needed to maintain a high level of personal hygiene.
- Do not allow EMS personnel to deliver patient care if they exhibit signs or symptoms of an infectious disease.
- Monitor all EMS personnel for compliance with vaccinations and appropriate diagnostic tests (e.g., **PPD**, antibody titers).
- Appoint a designated infectious disease control officer (IDCO) to serve as a contact person for personnel exposed to an infectious disease and monitor the infection control program.
- Identify specific job classifications and work processes in which the possibility of exposure exists.
- Provide haz-mat (hazardous materials) education for employees, including how to locate and interpret material safety data sheets (MSDS) regarding chemicals or chemical mixtures with information on the associated health hazards.

✱ PPD purified protein derivative, the substance used in a test for tuberculosis.

Do not assume that your EMS agency can protect you from exposure to all infectious agents. Your attitude toward protecting yourself against infectious agents is one measure of your professionalism.

RESPONSE

When responding to an EMS call, take the following infection control measures:

- Obtain as much information as possible from dispatch regarding the nature of the patient's illness or injury.
- Prepare for patient contact. Put on gloves and don eye and face protection before patient contact whenever practical.
- Prepare mentally for the call. Think *infection control!*

PATIENT CONTACT

Your contact with a patient, especially at an emergency scene, poses your highest risk for acquiring an infectious disease.

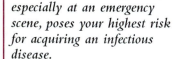

Your contact with a patient, especially at an emergency scene, poses your highest risk for acquiring an infectious disease. Have all personal protective equipment with you before leaving the emergency vehicle, and follow these guidelines:

- Isolate all body substances and avoid any contact with them.
- Wear appropriate personal protective equipment such as gowns, gloves, face shields, masks, protective eyewear, aprons, and similar items (Figure 11-4).

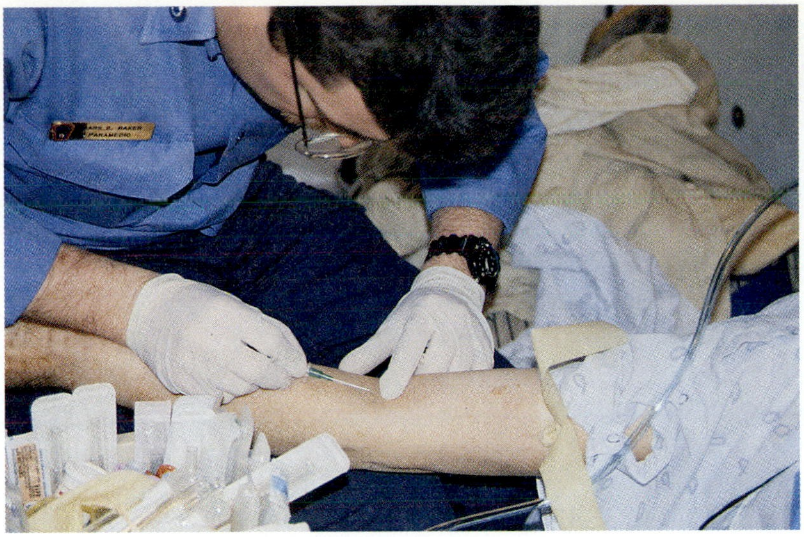

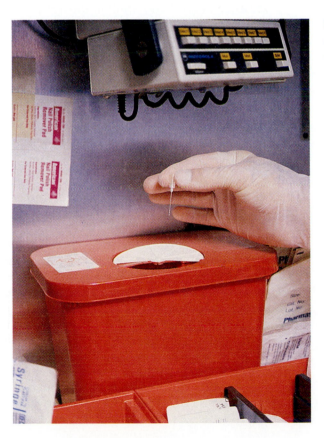

FIGURE 11-4 Always use the personal protection recommended for the degree of exposure anticipated.

- Allow only necessary personnel to make patient contact. Limit the risk to as few people as possible, thus minimizing exposure.
- Use airway adjuncts such as a pocket mask or bag-valve-mask unit to minimize exposure. Disposable items are preferable.
- Properly dispose of biohazardous waste.
- Use extreme caution with sharp instruments. Utilize retractable IV needles and needleless injection systems when possible. Never bend, recap, or remove contaminated needles. Dispose of all contaminated sharps in properly labeled puncture-resistant containers (Figure 11-5).

FIGURE 11-5 Dispose of needles and other sharp objects properly.

Task or Activity	Disposable Gloves	Gown	Mask	Protective Eyewear
Bleeding control with active bleeding	Yes	Yes	Yes	Yes
Bleeding control with minimal bleeding	Yes	No	No	No
Emergency childbirth	Yes	Yes	Yes	Yes
Blood drawing	Yes	No	No	No
IV insertion	Yes	No	No	No
Endotracheal intubation	Yes	No	Yes	Yes
EOA insertion	Yes	No	Yes	Yes
Oral/nasal suctioning; manually clearing airway	Yes	Yes	Yes	Yes
Handling/cleaning instruments with possible contamination	Yes	Yes	Yes	Yes
Measuring blood pressure	Yes	No	No	No
Giving an injection	Yes	No	No	No
Measuring temperature	Yes	No	No	No
Rescuing from a building fire	Yes	No	No	No
Cleaning back of ambulance after a medical call	Yes	No	No	No

- Never smoke, eat, or drink in the patient compartment of the ambulance. Each service should have strict guidelines regarding the presence of food and drink in the driver compartment during down times. Strictly adhere to OSHA guidelines.

- Do not apply cosmetics, lip balm, or handle contact lenses when a likelihood of exposure exists.

Table 11-2 details specific measures for protection against HIV (human immunodeficiency virus) and HBV (hepatitis B virus) infections.

RECOVERY

Infection control does not end when you deliver the patient to the emergency department.

Infection control does not end when you deliver the patient to the emergency department. Decontaminating the ambulance and equipment is essential. Take the following steps at the completion of each response:

- Wash hands immediately after patient contact (Figure 11-6). Ample data substantiate that *effective, vigorous* hand washing is superior to some disinfectants. On-scene, you can wipe your hands with a waterless hand-cleansing solution. However, this provides for only partial cleansing because it cannot grossly remove the particles to which microorganisms adhere. Only soap and water can do that. Upon returning to quarters, or at the earliest opportunity, thoroughly wash your hands with soap and warm water, paying attention to the webs between fingers. Overlooking this important habit may result in the inadvertent contamination of personal clothing or anything else that you contact. Such oversight can result in transmitting the disease to family and friends.

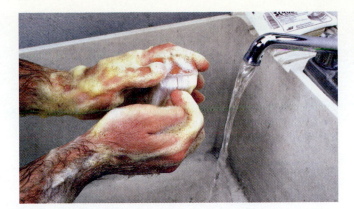

FIGURE 11-6   Hand washing is one of the most effective methods of preventing disease transmission.

- If you sustain a wound and are exposed to the body fluids of others, vigorously wash the wound with soap and warm water immediately, *before* contacting your employer or IDCO.
- Dispose of all biohazardous wastes in accordance with local laws and regulations.
- Place potentially infectious wastes in leak-proof biohazard bags. Bag any soiled linen and label for laundry personnel (Figure 11-7).
- Decontaminate all contaminated clothing and reusable equipment.
- Handle uniforms in accordance with the agency's standard procedures for personal protective equipment.

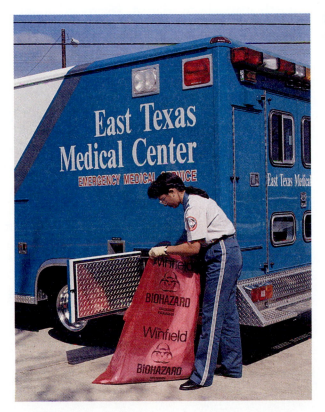

FIGURE 11-7   Bag all linen and label it infectious.

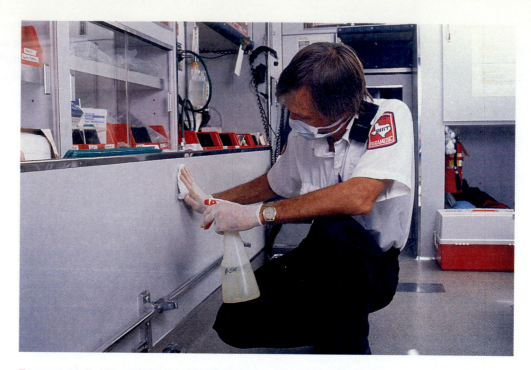

FIGURE 11-8   Complete routine cleaning and other housekeeping chores after each patient encounter.

Decontamination Methods and Procedures

✱ decontaminate to destroy or remove pathogens.

Content Review

DECONTAMINATION LEVELS
- Low-level disinfection
- Intermediate-level disinfection
- High-level disinfection
- Sterilization

✱ disinfect to destroy certain forms of microorganisms, but not all.

Decontaminate infected equipment according to local protocol and SOPs established by the EMS agency. Perform decontamination in a designated area that is properly marked and secured. The room should have a suitable ventilation system and adequate drainage. Be sure to wear gloves, gowns, boots, protective eyewear, and a face mask. To begin decontamination, remove surface dirt and debris with soap and water. Then disinfect and, if required, sterilize all items. The four levels of decontamination are low-level disinfection, intermediate-level disinfection, high-level disinfection, and sterilization.

Low-Level Disinfection Low-level **disinfection** destroys most bacteria and some viruses and fungi. It does not destroy *Mycobacterium tuberculosis* or bacterial spores. Use low-level disinfection for routine housekeeping and cleaning (Figure 11-8), as well as for removing visible body fluids. All EPA-registered disinfectants are suitable for low-level disinfection.

Intermediate-Level Disinfection Intermediate-level disinfection destroys *Mycobacterium tuberculosis* and most viruses and fungi. It does not, however, destroy bacterial spores. Use it for all equipment that has come into contact with intact skin such as stethoscopes, splints, and blood pressure cuffs. A 1:10 to 1:100 dilution of water and chlorine bleach is acceptable for intermediate-level disinfection. Hard-surface germicides and EPA-registered disinfectants/chemical germicides are also effective.

High-Level Disinfection High-level disinfection destroys all forms of microorganisms except certain bacterial spores. High-level disinfection is required for all reusable devices that have come into contact with mucous membranes, including laryngoscopes, Magill forceps, and airway adjuncts. For high-level disinfection, immerse objects in an EPA-approved chemical-sterilizing agent for

10 to 45 seconds (depending upon the manufacturer's instructions). Alternatively, immerse the device in hot water (176°–212°F) for 30 minutes.

Sterilization **Sterilization** destroys all microorganisms and is required for all contaminated invasive instruments. An autoclave that uses pressurized steam or ethylene-oxide gas effectively sterilizes equipment. These methods, however, are rarely available outside of a hospital setting. Alternatively, prolonged immersion (6–10 hours, depending on the manufacturer's instructions) in an EPA-approved chemical-sterilizing agent is usually adequate. Whenever possible, use disposable instruments for invasive procedures.

* **sterilize** to destroy all microorganisms.

INFECTIOUS DISEASE EXPOSURES

Infectious disease exposures occur during all hours of a work shift. Since you may not always be able to contact an agency administrator, you need a working knowledge of your agency's standard operating procedures, as well as of the laws and regulations applicable to exposures. The following recommendations will help to ensure that exposure management will protect you, other emergency responders and health care professionals, the agency, and the confidentiality of the patient's information.

Reporting an Infectious Disease Exposure Immediately report exposures of EMS personnel to the designated IDCO, according to local protocol. Report all exposures to blood, blood products, or any potentially infectious material, regardless of their perceived severity. This will permit immediate medical follow-up, including counseling for the EMS provider and identification of the infectious agent. It also enables the IDCO to evaluate the circumstances of the exposure and implement changes to prevent future exposures, if needed. Finally, it facilitates follow-up testing if the source individual consents.

Report all exposures to blood, blood products, or any potentially infectious material, regardless of their perceived severity.

The Ryan White Act The **Ryan White Act** is a federal law that outlines the rights and responsibilities of agencies and health care workers when an infectious disease exposure occurs. Under its provisions, the exposed employee has the right to ask the source patient's infection status, but neither the agency nor the employee can force the source individual to be tested. Employers must also tell their employees what to do if an exposure occurs.

* **Ryan White Act** federal law that outlines the rights and responsibilities of agencies and health care workers when an infectious disease exposure occurs.

Federal law further mandates that each agency designate an IDCO to whom exposures are reported. This officer coordinates implementation of the exposure control plan and follows local reporting requirements.

Postexposure Employers are required to provide a medical evaluation and treatment for any paramedic or other EMS provider exposed to an infectious disease. The nature of the exposure is assessed based on the route, dose, and nature of the infectious agent. As part of the medical evaluation, employees are entitled to receive counseling about alternatives for treatment, the risks of treatment, signs, symptoms, the possibility of developing disease, and preventing further spread of the potential infection. This includes the available medications, their potential side effects, and their contraindications. Treatment must be in line with current United States Public Health Service recommendations.

After a paramedic is exposed to an infectious disease, he has the option to submit a blood sample for baseline testing. If the employee does not consent to having his blood screened for specific diseases, the blood samples are normally maintained for 90 days in the event that he changes his mind.

The IDCO or other health care professional who specializes in occupational infectious diseases should counsel the exposed employee and obtain informed consent for post-exposure prophylaxis (PEP) based on CDC guidelines. All records related to employee counseling and PEP are forwarded to the IDCO. Vaccines may be made available to the employee if deemed appropriate by an occupational medicine physician.

Confidentiality The IDCO will maintain records of all exposures as required by law. All of these exposure records (like any medical records) are confidential. They must not be released to anyone without express written permission from the employee.

ASSESSMENT OF THE PATIENT WITH INFECTIOUS DISEASE

Approach every scene with a high index of suspicion that a patient may have an infectious disease.

When assessing a patient, always maintain a high index of suspicion that an infectious agent may be involved. Consider the dispatch information, evaluate the environment for its suitability for transmitting infectious agents, and maintain appropriate BSI. Gloves are the mandatory minimum level of personal protective equipment (PPE) required on every patient contact.

When approaching a patient with a possible infectious disease, look for general indicators of infection such as unusual skin signs, fever, weakness, profuse sweating, malaise, anorexia, and unexplained worsening of existing disease states. If an infection is localized, signs of inflammation may include redness, swelling, tenderness to palpation, capillary streaking, and warmth in the affected area. A rash or other diagnostic skin signs may make identifying an infectious disease much easier.

PAST MEDICAL HISTORY

The patient's past medical history (PMH) may provide valuable clues to his illness. Patients who have AIDS or are taking immunosuppressant medications such as steroids are particularly susceptible to infection. COPD patients, patients with autoimmune diseases, and transplant recipients frequently take steroids and immunosuppressants. Persons with diabetes and other endocrine disorders are also more likely to get infections due to additional stressors on their immune systems. Other conditions that increase the risk for developing infectious diseases include alcoholism, malnutrition, IV drug abuse, malignancy (cancer), and splenectomy (removal of the spleen), as well as artificial heart valves (aortic or mitral) or joints (hip or knee). Any significant increase in emotional stress may also increase a person's risk of significant illness, including infectious diseases.

A patient with a PMH of numerous untreated throat infections who suddenly develops a heart murmur, fever, and malaise may have rheumatic fever, a streptococcal infection that can affect the heart. Such patients are often found in medically underserved areas where access to primary care is difficult or nonexistent. Patients with cancer are at increased risk for acquiring numerous opportunistic infectious diseases. A recently transmitted sexual disease may precede systemic infection. Recent unfinished antibiotic treatment may lead to the proliferation of drug-resistant infectious agents, causing recurrent, persistent bacterial infections or development of other opportunistic infections.

In addition to determining past or current illnesses or diseases, thoroughly investigate the patient's chief complaint and any history of the present illness including:

- When did signs and symptoms begin?
- Is fever present? How has the temperature changed over time?
- Has the patient taken any aspirin, acetaminophen, or other medications?

- Does the patient have any neck pain or stiffness when his head is moved, especially during flexion?
- Has the patient had any difficulty swallowing?
- Has the patient had any previous symptoms or illnesses similar to this one?

THE PHYSICAL EXAMINATION

Physical examination of the patient whom you suspect of having an infectious disease follows the standard format for assessing a medical patient. Determine the patient's level of consciousness and vital signs early on. Increased temperature commonly indicates infection. Significant increases in pulse may occur due to the infection and as a result of elevated body temperature. As a consequence, metabolic needs will increase. The patient will require more oxygen and more nutrients to maintain normal physiologic function. This may be a serious problem for elderly, very young, or debilitated patients with concurrent illnesses that limit their cardiovascular and respiratory reserve.

Every EMS unit should have the capability of measuring and monitoring body temperature (e.g., a tympanic thermometer).

Hypotension in the patient with an infectious disease may result from dehydration, vasodilation, or both, as in septic shock. In rare cases, infections of the heart muscle (endocarditis) may result in decreased cardiac output (cardiogenic shock). In any case, assess the cause of hypotension and treat it promptly. If the lungs are clear, the judicious use of fluids may be beneficial; if fluid status is not a problem, vasopressors such as dopamine may be necessary.

Dehydration is a common consequence of infectious diseases. Increased body temperature is often accompanied by increased respiratory rate and concomitant fluid loss, of which the patient is often unaware (insensible fluid loss). Vomiting or diarrhea can quickly cause life-threatening dehydration, especially in pediatric patients who have large body surface areas relative to their volume. Electrolyte imbalances often occur with fluid loss. Advances in technology that may soon make the prehospital evaluation of electrolytes cost-effective may be indicated in the setting of significant dehydration. Clinically significant dehydration will usually cause tachycardia and hypotension, but you should be vigilant for more subtle signs that include thirst, poor skin turgor, and a shrunken and furrowed tongue. A history of decreased fluid intake, fever, vomiting, and/or diarrhea should trigger a thorough assessment of fluid status. While performing a physical exam similar to that for any patient with a medical emergency, assess the following:

- Skin for temperature, hydration, color, or rash
- Sclera for icterus
- Reaction to neck flexion (Is nuchal rigidity [neck stiffness] present?)
- Lymph nodes for swelling or tenderness (lymphadenopathy)
- Breath sounds (for adventitious sounds and evidence of consolidation)
- Hepatomegaly (enlargement of the liver)
- Purulent (pus-filled) lesions

SELECTED INFECTIOUS DISEASES

The following section profiles infectious diseases that either may be encountered in the prehospital setting or are commonly known by emergency health care practitioners. The first major category includes diseases of immediate concern to EMS. General profiles of other diseases follow. You should be familiar with the terminology of these profiles, realize which diseases you will more commonly encounter in patients, and know which BSI precautions to employ.

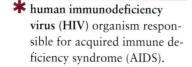

Content Review

DISEASES OF IMMEDIATE CONCERN TO EMS PROVIDERS

- HIV
- Hepatitis
- Tuberculosis
- Pneumonia
- Chickenpox
- Meningitis

DISEASES OF IMMEDIATE CONCERN TO EMS PROVIDERS

The diseases of immediate concern to EMS providers include HIV, hepatitis, tuberculosis, pneumonia, chickenpox, and bacterial meningitis. They are infectious diseases that have gained notoriety, pose a high risk for communicability and debilitating disease, or are relevant to direct patient care. While most attention focuses on reducing transmission from patient to health care worker, the profiles also consider reverse transmission, because responsible health care workers protect both themselves and their patients. The inclusion of chickenpox may surprise some EMS personnel, but the disease is highly communicable and poses a serious occupational risk for unvaccinated or previously unexposed health care workers.

Human Immunodeficiency Virus

* **human immunodeficiency virus (HIV)** organism responsible for acquired immune deficiency syndrome (AIDS).

The **human immunodeficiency virus (HIV)** is the most discussed and feared infectious agent of the modern era, especially of the last two decades. The clinical condition that it causes, acquired immune deficiency syndrome (AIDS), is not a disease *per se,* but a collection of signs and symptoms that share common anatomical, physiological, and biochemical derangements in the immune system. Like other viruses, HIV utilizes the host cell's reproductive apparatus to copy itself. HIV is a retrovirus, that is, it normally carries its genetic material in RNA (instead of DNA) and utilizes an enzyme called *reverse transcriptase* (hence the designation "*retro*virus") to use RNA to synthesize DNA. This is the reverse of the usual process of transcription of DNA into RNA. The action of reverse transcriptase enables genetic material from a retrovirus to become permanently incorporated into the DNA of an infected cell. Two types of HIV have been identified, HIV-1 and HIV-2. Most research targets the HIV-1 variant, which has proven much more pathogenic than HIV-2.

The emergence of HIV and AIDS, more than any other infectious process, has increased emergency and health care workers' awareness of the dangers of infectious disease. The worldwide research and educational activities resulting from concern about HIV and AIDS are effective models for teaching health care workers and lay persons about how other infectious diseases are transmitted and for providing personal and community action plans to prevent the spread of infectious agents. Although it is a worldwide epidemic, with an especially high mortality rate in sub-Saharan Africa, AIDS poses a significantly lower *occupational* risk to health care workers in developed countries than other infectious agents.

Pathogenesis In the past five years, we have learned about the dynamics of HIV infection and the development of AIDS. It was first assumed that the virus caused a cellular immune system response and then remained in a dormant phase. The humoral response was known to produce antibodies within one to three months after infection, with clinical disease developing in from one to ten years. For unexplained reasons, the virus would become active, and the worsening clinical signs were attributed to an increasing viral population. The extent of immune cell activity during the incubation phase, reported to be from months to ten years, was not immediately understood.

Research in the mid 1980s and early 1990s determined that HIV specifically targets T-lymphocytes with the CD4 marker, a surface molecule that attaches the virus to the cell, and a better understanding of the cellular immune response and CD4 markers emerged. A reasonably reliable correlation between disease progression and the decrease in CD4 T-lymphocyte count was developed. Physicians could predict the development of specific clinical events as the CD4 count decreased. For example, *Pneumocystis carinii* pneumonia (PCP), an opportunistic AIDS infection, frequently develops when CD4 counts drop to a certain level. The CD4 count thus became a guide to treatment. Its usefulness, however, was limited because it only reflected the immune system's destruction.

Recent advances in molecular biology and more reliable and cost-effective assays of proteins and other biochemical molecules have revealed a tremendous increase in virus production immediately after infection and have shown that the immune system increases its activity to counter it. Eventually the number of immune system cells (T-lymphocytes) offsets the viral load, reflected by the HIV RNA. This equilibrium, or "set point," may take years to establish. Even during the dynamic phase when the equilibrium has not yet been set, measurement of viral load is still the best available indicator of response to therapy and long-term clinical outcome.

Risk to the General Public HIV is transmitted through contact with blood, blood products, and body fluids. The virus has been noted in blood, semen, vaginal secretions, and breast milk. Although not yet reported, tears, amniotic fluid, urine, saliva, and bronchial secretions may theoretically transmit the disease.

The virus can enter the body through breaks in the skin, mucous membranes, the eyes, or by placental transmission. Reports of the transmission rate from mother to infant range from 13 to 30 percent. The virus is most commonly contracted through sexual contact or sharing contaminated needles. Before the initiation of stringent controls in screening donor blood and blood products, hemophiliacs and individuals needing frequent blood transfusions were at increased risk. Other groups initially identified at high risk included IV drug abusers and homosexual or bisexual males. The morbidity of heterosexual transmission of HIV has been steadily increasing, with vaginal and anal sex the primary concerns. The risk of oral sex has not been quantified but is believed to be low. Vector transmission by mosquitoes has been postulated but not yet reported. Coexisting sexually transmitted disease, especially with ulceration, appears to increase the risk of infection in sexual transmission. Ethnicity and gender are not established risk factors, and the period of maximum infectiousness cannot be effectively determined. No recovery from AIDS has ever been reported, although post-exposure prophylaxis has been demonstrated to decrease the severity of disease and delay mortality.

Risk to Health Care Workers Although contact with contaminated blood or body secretions potentially places health care workers at risk, infection from HIV-positive patients has been exceedingly rare, with an estimated probability of from 0.2 to 0.44 percent after exposure to virus-containing blood. Accidental needle-stick injuries are the most frequent source of infection in health care workers.

The risk for effective transmission of HIV to health care workers initially depends on whether the exposure to HIV was percutaneous, mucosal, or cutaneous (to intact skin). Within each of those categories, the risk depends on fluid type. Blood is the most dangerous, followed by fluids that may or may not contain blood: semen, vaginal secretions, and cerebrospinal, synovial, pleural, peritoneal, pericardial, and amniotic fluid. Urine and saliva, unlikely to contain blood, pose a very low risk. Source patients (those possibly infecting health care workers) who are HIV-positive or die within two months after the health care worker's exposure, are considered to increase the risk. The highest risk exposure involves a large volume of blood, high antibody titer against a retrovirus in the source patient, deep percutaneous injury, or actual intramuscular injection.

Clinical Presentation The Centers for Disease Control first established the case definition of what constituted AIDS in 1982. Since then, it has expanded the definition of the syndrome to include other diseases such as extrapulmonary and pulmonary tuberculosis, recurrent pneumonia, wasting syndrome, HIV dementia, and sensory neuropathy. The AIDS patient may first develop a mononucleosis-like syndrome with non-specific signs and symptoms such as fatigue, fever, sore throat, lymphadenopathy (lymph node disease), splenomegaly (enlarged spleen), rash, and diarrhea. Since not all of those signs are present, the situation may seem so trivial that the patient does not seek health care. Many patients develop purplish skin lesions known as Kaposi's sarcoma. Kaposi's sarcoma is a cancerous lesion that was quite rare until the HIV virus appeared. As the disease progresses, many patients develop life-threatening opportunistic infections such as *Pneumocystis carinii* pneumonia. Secondary infections caused by *Mycobacterium tuberculosis* may also be present (Figure 11-9). As AIDS progresses, it involves the central nervous system; dementia, psychosis, encephalopathy, and peripheral neurological disorders may develop.

Postexposure Prophylaxis There is no cure or vaccine for AIDS. After an exposure to a confirmed HIV-positive source patient, the health care worker should immediately seek evaluation and possible initiation of treatment by an occupational medicine or infectious disease physician. Current CDC recommendations establish two hours as the optimum time within which to start postexposure prophylaxis with triple therapy (two reverse transcriptase inhibitors [AZT and 3TC] and one protease inhibitor [IDV]) as the current standard for comparison. This is because early, aggressive treatment may decrease the viral load and alter the set point. Counseling by the ICDO or a trained occupational infectious disease specialist must supplement the postexposure evaluation as part of the agency's ex-

FIGURE 11-9 Clinical features of acquired immune deficiency syndrome (AIDS).

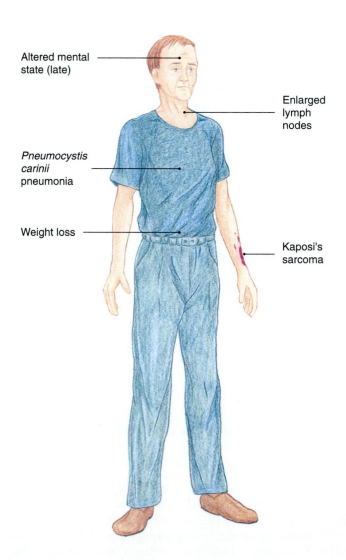

Altered mental state (late)

Enlarged lymph nodes

Pneumocystis carinii pneumonia

Weight loss

Kaposi's sarcoma

posure control plan. EMS personnel should not attempt to determine their own risk and need for postexposure prophylaxis. Health care workers have significantly underestimated their own risk and need for medical intervention regarding other infections, and the element of denial in HIV increases that tendency.

Summary of HIV HIV-positive patients generally do not present in life-threatening situations to EMS; however, they pose substantial psychosocial challenges. Despite changes in societal attitudes and increased tolerance of differences, HIV-positive individuals are often marginalized and shunned. Their subsequent feeling of social isolation is often worsened by depression. In spite of this, these patients are usually forthcoming about their infection status when dealing with health care workers. Although a paramedic generally has little to offer in terms of treatment, it is vitally important that care be compassionate, understanding, and nonjudgmental. Take appropriate precautions to prevent disease transmission, but if you truly understand the risk as it applies to you as a health care worker, it should be no barrier to your providing professional and emotionally supportive care, including a caring touch. In the EMS environment, physical isolation of the HIV-positive patient is unjustified.

Universal (Standard) Precautions The CDC, OSHA, and NIOSH recommend universal (standard) precautions for health care workers at increased risk for exposure to HIV and other bloodborne pathogens. Since reliably determining which patients have blood-borne infections is impossible, the following precautions are recommended for all patients.

- All health care workers should routinely use appropriate barrier precautions to prevent exposure of the skin and mucous membranes to any contact with blood, or other body fluids, from any patient. Wear disposable gloves whenever touching blood and body fluids, mucous membranes, or broken skin, handling items or surfaces soiled with blood or body fluids, and performing venipuncture or other vascular access procedures. Change and discard gloves after contact with each patient. To prevent exposure of the mucous membranes of the mouth, nose, and eyes, wear masks and protective eyewear or protective face shields during procedures likely to aerosolize blood or other body fluids. If a glove is torn or a needle-stick occurs, remove the glove and replace it as soon as possible. Discard the needle or instrument and obtain another. Wear gowns or aprons during any procedure likely to generate splashes of bloods or other body fluids.

- Wash your hands (including the webs between your fingers) and other skin surfaces thoroughly with soap and warm water after removal of gloves and especially after contamination with blood or other body fluids.

- Take precautions to prevent injuries caused by needles, scalpels, or other sharp instruments or devices whenever performing procedures, cleaning instruments, or disposing of instruments. To prevent needle-stick injuries, needles should not be recapped, purposely bent, broken by hand, removed from disposable syringes, or otherwise manipulated by hand. Position puncture-resistant containers as close as possible to work areas and place disposable syringes and needles, scalpel blades, and other sharp items in them for disposal.

- Although saliva has not been directly implicated in HIV transmission, use mouthpieces with one way valves or filters, bag-valve-mask devices, and other ventilation devices to avoid mouth-to-mouth contact. Place these resuscitation items where the need for resuscitation is predictable.

- Do not put gloved hands close to your mouth, and avoid wiping your face with your forearms or the backs of your gloved hands. Use clean towels to deal with perspiration.
- If you have exudative or weeping skin lesions, refrain from direct patient care and from handling patient care equipment until the condition resolves.
- Pregnant health care workers are not believed to be at greater risk of HIV infection than health care workers who are not pregnant. If a health care worker develops HIV infection during pregnancy, however, the infant is at risk for transplacental transmission. Therefore, pregnant health care workers should be especially familiar with, and strictly adhere to, precautions to minimize the risk of HIV transmission.
- Disinfection of diagnostic or therapeutic equipment and supplies is mandatory.

Hepatitis

✱ **hepatitis** inflammation of the liver characterized by diffuse or patchy tissue necrosis.

Hepatitis is an inflammation of the liver caused by viruses, bacteria, fungi, parasites, excessive alcohol consumption, or medications. Viruses are by far the most common cause of hepatitis. The clinical signs and symptoms of hepatitis secondary to viral infection are the same regardless of the type of virus. Initially they include headache, fever, weakness, joint pain, anorexia, nausea and vomiting, and in some cases, right upper quadrant abdominal pain. As disease progresses, the patient may become jaundiced, with fever often resolving at the onset of jaundice. This stage is sometimes marked by a darkened urine and the development of clay-colored stools. The various types of hepatitis are transmitted in specific ways. Hepatitis A, B, C, D, and E represent the greatest potential for communicable disease. Paramedics who practice universal precautions against blood-borne and fecal-oral transmission will drastically reduce their risk of contracting hepatitis through occupational exposure.

Hepatitis A Hepatitis A (infectious or viral hepatitis) is transmitted by the fecal-oral route. The causative agent, hepatitis A virus, is usually found in the stool of infected persons, who may not exercise suitable personal hygiene. After these individuals handle food or contact another individual even as casually as shaking hands, the virus can then be transmitted via contaminated hands, food, water, ice, and eating utensils. Furthermore, the virus can exist on unwashed hands for as long as four hours. Many hepatitis A infections are asymptomatic. They do not present with obvious signs like jaundice and are recognizable only by liver function studies. This is especially true of children, who represent most cases of infection and often transmit the virus to others by close social contact. Sexual contact can also spread the virus. Transmission by needle-stick injury is unlikely and has not been reported.

Diaper changing, especially in day care centers with an infected child, is known to increase risk. Travelers to areas with poor sanitary conditions are also at risk. Two inactivated hepatitis A vaccines (Havrix and Vaqta) provide effective active immunization. Health care workers serving on disaster medical teams to Africa, the Middle East, Central and South America, and Asia should be immunized. Immunization is not generally recommended for health care workers in the United States but may be advised in some areas where hepatitis A prevalence is unusually high. Passive preexposure immunization with immune globulin (gamma globulin) is therefore falling out of favor, but immunization may be used after exposure in selected incidents.

The hepatitis A virus's incubation period averages from three to five weeks, with the greatest probability of transmission in the latter half of that period. Afflicted individuals are most infectious during the first week of symptoms. The disease follows a mild course, is rarely serious, and lasts from two to six weeks.

Hepatitis B The hepatitis B (serum hepatitis) virus is transmitted through direct contact with contaminated body fluids (blood, semen, vaginal fluids, and saliva) and therefore represents a substantial risk to EMS providers. Hepatitis B is much more contagious than HIV. The potential for transmitting hepatitis B following exposure to infected blood ranges from 1.9 to 40.0 percent and by needle stick from 5.0 to 35.0 percent. The incidence of antibodies in hepatitis B in health care workers has been reported to be two to four times greater than in the community at large. Health care workers infected by hepatitis B can develop acute hepatitis, cirrhosis, and liver cancer. From 5.0 to 10.0 percent of infected health care workers may become asymptomatic chronic carriers and pose an infection risk to family and other intimate contacts. The effectiveness of the three series of immunizations has been reported to be close to 90.0 percent in adults and higher in children, but low rates of health care worker compliance with immunization are distressingly common. No clearly identifiable populations are at risk except for those individuals who are exposed to high-risk body fluids in the course of their employment.

In the general populace, sexual transmission of hepatitis B is common. Transmission has also been known to occur with transfusion, dialysis, needle and syringe sharing in IV drug use, tattooing, acupuncture, and communally used razors and toothbrushes. The virus is stable on surfaces with dried, visible blood for more than seven days. Infection of toddlers from household contacts with family member carriers has been reported. Transmission by insect vectors or the fecal-oral route has not been reported.

Serum markers that reflect amounts of antigen or antibody from surface or core molecules of the virus reliably reflect active infection, communicability, the window phase of infection, and peak virus replication levels. A detailed discussion of the clinical significance of these markers and how they guide therapy is beyond the scope of this text.

With as much as is known about hepatitis B's disease process and its consequences, combined with the fact that effective vaccines exist, the number of health care workers who have not been immunized or are unaware of their immune status is alarming. Two vaccines, Recombivax HB and Engerix B, both products of genetic recombinant technology, are available. They are reported to be as effective as the previously available Heptavax, derived from blood plasma, without the risk of HIV transmission or other viral infection. The immunization regimen is a series of three intramuscular injections. Following the initial dose, booster doses are administered at one and six months. After the immunization regimen, antibody assays are obtained to confirm active immunity.

All EMS workers should receive the hepatitis B vaccination series.

The target antibody titer is 10 milli-international units per ml (10 mIU/ml), with a recommendation to draw for antibody titer from 4 to 6 weeks after the series is completed. An additional booster may be necessary if the individual does not develop adequate antibody levels. The duration of protection is thought to be five years, perhaps longer. The vaccine is safe in pregnancy. Its side effects include local redness, occasional low grade fever, rash, nausea, joint pain, or mild fatigue.

Hepatitis B's incubation period lasts from eight to twenty-four weeks. Joint pain and rash are more common with hepatitis B infection than with other types of hepatitis, but 60 to 80 percent of hepatitis B infections are asymptomatic.

Hepatitis C The prevalence of hepatitis C (HCV) in the United States is believed to be 1.8 percent in the adult population and from 2.7 to 10.0 percent in health care workers. The virus is transmitted primarily by IV drug abuse and sexual contact. Sexual contact, however, does not appear to transmit hepatitis C as effectively as it does hepatitis B. After 1989, effective blood donor screening for hepatitis C practically eliminated the risk of transfusion-associated infection.

Fecal-oral transmission and household contact have not been reported as factors in transmission, and no specific groups have been identified to be at greater risk for hepatitis C infection.

Hepatitis C is a chronic condition in about 85 percent of infected people. Because of its chronic nature and its ability to cause active disease years later, it poses a great international public health problem. Antibodies can be produced against hepatitis C and provide the laboratory method for determining infection. However, the antibodies are not effective in eliminating the virus, and their presence does not indicate immunity. The ineffectiveness of antibodies is attributed to the virus's high mutation rate. Consequently, the cellular immune response, which results in the immune system's killing infected cells, is very aggressive and is believed, ironically, to cause most of the associated liver injury.

Hepatitis C infection, formerly called non-A, non-B hepatitis, often causes liver fibrosis, which progresses over decades to cirrhosis and is estimated to develop in about 20 percent of infected individuals. This progression is known to be accelerated in persons older than 50 at the time of initial infection, in those consuming more than 50 grams of alcohol per day, and in men. Cirrhosis has also been known to occur in those who have not consumed alcohol and can worsen to end-stage liver disease with jaundice, ascites, and esophageal varices.

No effective vaccination for hepatitis C exists. Treatment with alpha interferon has had limited success, with about 15–20 percent of patients responding positively, as defined by the liver enzymes' return to normal levels. Another drug, ribavirin (an antiviral), administered orally, is known to potentiate interferon's immune system effects, and researchers are now focusing their efforts on improving the results of combination therapy with ribavirin and alpha interferon.

Hepatitis D seems only to coexist with hepatitis B infection.

Hepatitis D The hepatitis D virus (HDV), formerly called delta hepatitis, depends on a surface antigen of the hepatitis B virus (HBV) to produce its structural protein shell. Thus, HDV infection seems to exist only with a coexisting HBV infection. Immunization against HBV therefore confers immunity to HDV. When a patient who has HBV infection with liver disease develops an overlying HDV infection, mortality rates are very high.

Parenteral HDV transmission occurs similarly to HBV in western Europe and North America. Fortunately, cases in health care workers are extremely rare. Frequent epidemics of nonparenteral transmission occur in central Africa, the Middle East, and the Mediterranean countries. HDV's incubation period has not been determined.

Hepatitis E Hepatitis E (HEV) is transmitted like hepatitis A virus (HAV), through the fecal-oral route, and seems to be associated with contaminated drinking water more commonly than HAV. It occurs primarily in young adults, with highest rates in pregnant women. First described in India, outbreaks have occurred in Russia, Nepal, Southeast Asia, the Middle East, Pakistan, and China. Only six cases were reported in the United States from 1989 to 1992, most likely because of more sanitary sources of drinking water.

Tuberculosis

* **tuberculosis (TB)** disease caused by a bacterium known as *Mycobacterium tuberculosis* that primarily affects the respiratory system.

Tuberculosis (TB) is the most common preventable adult infectious disease in the world. TB is caused by bacteria known collectively as the *Mycobacterium tuberculosis* complex, which includes *M. tuberculosis, M. bovis,* and *M. africanum.* Other bacteria in the *Mycobacterium* family can cause tuberculosis, particularly in immunocompromised patients. These other types of *Mycobacterium* are referred to as atypicals. It primarily affects the respiratory system, including a highly contagious form in the larynx. Untreated or undertreated, it may spread to other organ systems, causing extrapulmonary TB and other complications.

The disease appeared about 7,000 years ago and peaked in the eighteenth century. The number of new cases in the United States has increased steadily since 1985, in large part because of TB in AIDS patients and in recently arrived immigrants from countries where the disease is prevalent.

The development of multiple drug resistant tuberculosis (MDR-TB) has been known since the late 1940s. Drug resistance occurs when drug-resistant bacteria outgrow drug-susceptible bacteria. These bacteria acquire resistance either because of patient noncompliance with therapy or inadequate treatment regimens. Drug resistance occurs early in therapy, especially when only one drug is used. For this reason, most current CDC recommendations for the initiation of therapy in the United States involve several options for treatment, each calling for multiple medications, including isoniazid (INH), rifampin, pyrazinamide, ethambutol, and streptomycin, among others.

M. tuberculosis is most commonly transmitted through airborne respiratory droplets but may also be contracted by direct inoculation through mucous membranes and broken skin or by drinking contaminated milk. Animal reservoirs for the bacteria include cattle, swine, badgers, and primates. Coughing and other expiratory actions (sneezing, speaking, singing) create bacteria-containing droplets from 5 to 10 microns in size, which susceptible individuals inhale into the alveoli.

The risk of transmitting tuberculosis is not as high as measles. Although the average case infects only about a third of his close contacts, prolonged exposure to a person with active TB is always listed as a risk factor. Communicability varies from case to case. Although a single occupational exposure to a patient with active TB is highly unlikely to transmit the disease to a paramedic, universal precautions against TB should still be employed.

Skin Testing The commonly used purified protein derivative (PPD) skin test effectively identifies candidates for prophylactic drug therapy (to prevent active TB) in large groups of health care workers. It has limited value in guiding individual therapy in those with active TB because a positive PPD indicates previous infection but does not distinguish active from dormant disease. Another health care worker experienced in interpreting the results should read the skin test, rather than the worker tested, because health care workers are known to underinterpret positive results. In addition, the skin test must be interpreted on the basis of the disease's prevalence in the community. A negative test does not rule out active disease, particularly in immunosuppressed individuals or in those who were infected so recently that their immune systems have not yet had time to mount the cellular mediated response that causes a positive PPD.

Most EMS agencies require skin testing at least annually. This may be sufficient, but again, decisions about the frequency of testing should be based on the disease's prevalence in the community. For individuals who have not been previously skin tested or who have no documentation of a negative PPD in the last 12 months, two-step testing may be reasonable. In these individuals, an initial negative test may be due to weak reactivity to the PPD. A second skin test is administered from one to three weeks later. A positive reaction to the second test probably represents a boosted reaction, which means that the individual has been previously infected, and should be evaluated for possible prophylaxis. If the second test is negative, that individual is classified as uninfected. A positive reaction to any subsequent test would represent a new infection by *M. tuberculosis.*

Pathogenesis TB's incubation period is 4–12 weeks. In most people with subclinical infections, immediate disease (primary TB) does not develop because of a cell-mediated immune response. Development of disease normally occurs 6–12 months after infection. Susceptibility to primary infection is increased in persons who are malnourished and those persons whose immune systems are suppressed, such as the elderly, HIV patients, and people taking immunosuppressant drugs. Children less

TB is the most common preventable adult infectious disease in the world. Its incidence in the United States has been rising since 1985.

EMS workers should receive TB screening on an annual basis.

than three years old are at risk because of underdeveloped immune systems, with older children identified at lowest risk. As expected, the aged are at high risk, and the reactivation of latent infections in this age group implies that the immune system has difficulty dealing with the complex nature of the *M. tuberculosis* infection. Once the bacteria enter the lungs, alveolar macrophages attack them and attempt to "wall them off" (forming granulomas) in a localized immune response. For this reason most TB infections do not produce disease. Healed sites leave lesions of calcified areas known as Ghon foci. When Ghon foci combine with lymph nodes, they form a Ghon complex, which creates small, sharply defined shadows on a chest X-ray.

If the macrophages cannot destroy them, the bacteria lie dormant within the macrophages and are then distributed to other sites within the body. They remain dormant until some event, usually a depression of the immune system, triggers their reactivation into secondary TB. The sites of reactivation are greatest in areas of the lung with the highest oxygen tension, the apices or upper lobes. Reactivation in extrapulmonary sites such as lymph nodes, pleura, and pericardium are much more common in HIV-infected persons. In AIDS patients, the disease may spread to the thoracic and lumbar spine, destroying intervertebral disks and adjacent vertebral bodies. TB is also known to lead to subacute meningitis and granulomas in the brain.

Clinical Presentation The signs and symptoms of active TB can be very non-specific and can be manifestations of other clinical conditions. However, a typical list would include chills, fever, fatigue, productive or nonproductive chronic cough, and weight loss. Many patients report night sweats, leaving their bed linens drenched with perspiration. Hemoptysis (expectorating blood) is very suggestive of active TB. Reactivation of dormant TB manifests as signs and symptoms specific to the organ systems involved.

EMS Response Your acceptance of responsibility for protecting yourself from *M. tuberculosis* is the most important step in preventing disease transmission. A proactive, high-index-of-suspicion-driven response is essential. The factors that increase a paramedic's risk of transmission are close and sometimes prolonged contact with the patient. Care and transport are provided in a very small, often ineffectively ventilated, space, and the patient may affect various expiratory actions while in contact with EMS personnel. Placing a mask over the patient, when it does not create undue anxiety or dyspnea, effectively decreases the number of expectorated droplet nuclei. Also, nebulized medications may be administered more safely with a nebulization mask. Use appropriate respiratory precautions while performing CPR and intubation.

You should don a protective respirator upon contact with a patient you suspect may have TB. Your knowledge of the prevalence of TB and the most susceptible populations in your jurisdiction should reinforce your index of suspicion. The most current NIOSH/OSHA standards for protecting health care workers from TB call for N95 **respirators,** which are designed to prevent contaminated air from reaching the health care workers wearing them (Figure 11-10a). High efficiency particulate aspirator (HEPA) respirators (Figure 11-10b) are no longer required in TB, but EMS agencies may opt to continue their use. They are more expensive, bulky, and sometimes difficult to breathe through.

Masks, as opposed to respirators, work primarily as barriers against larger particles and are not certified to prevent contaminated air from reaching the paramedic. However, they effectively prevent the transmission of many airborne pathogens, especially when both provider and patient wear them. They also provide a more comfortable and cost-effective alternative to the routine use of respirators. The extensive terminology and guidelines relative to the design, construction, and classification of various respirators is beyond the scope of this text. EMS agencies and their ICDOs are responsible for educating their

* **respirator** an apparatus worn that cleanses or qualifies the air.

* **mask** a device for protecting the face.

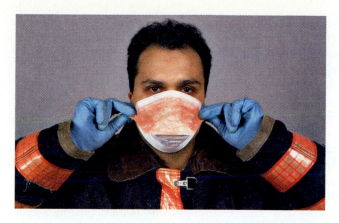

FIGURE 11-10A NIOSH/OSHA standards call for N95 **respirators** when caring for patients with tuberculosis.

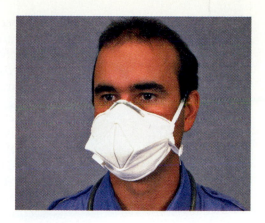

FIGURE 11-10B EMS agencies may opt to use high efficiency particulate aspirator (HEPA) respirators in TB.

personnel in the proper use and application of respirators and for ensuring proper fit and easy access. According to the NIOSH classification, N series respirators provide protection against non-oil-based aerosols, including the droplet nuclei from TB patients. These N type respirators must filter 95 percent of particles that are no larger than 0.3 microns in diameter, hence the designation N 95. This is a very safe standard since the diameter of TB aerosol droplets ranges from 5 to 10 microns. Health care workers' noncompliance causes most respirator failures.

Ventilation systems currently being marketed in selected ambulances claim to effectively recycle and filter enough air to ensure the expulsion of infected droplet nuclei. Such ventilation systems should include HEPA filtration in addition to recycling the patient compartment air volume according to OSHA standards. Do not open patient compartment windows to increase ventilation and dilute the concentration of droplet nuclei. The moving ambulance may create a Bernoulli effect that draws engine exhaust, including carbon monoxide, into the patient compartment.

Postexposure Identification and Management Early identification of exposure and drug prophylaxis, if deemed necessary, are the keys to effectively preventing active TB in health care workers. An occupational medicine physician should assess TB skin test results and determine the appropriateness of chest X-rays, sputum cultures, and a myriad of other diagnostic procedures to confirm infection or the presence of frank disease. The polymerase chain reaction (PCR) test, which eliminates the need to wait for cultures and provides a diagnosis in six hours, may soon become the gold standard for identifying the presence of *M. tuberculosis*.

Pneumonia

Patients with difficulty breathing often confront paramedics with the enigma of differentiating pneumonia from mild exacerbations of congestive heart failure and its more severe form, acute pulmonary edema. The mistaken assumption that a patient has CHF may lead to aggressive treatment that reduces the patient's respiratory drive, dries protective mucous secretions, and contributes to hypotension.

Pneumonia, an acute lung inflammation, is not a single disease but a family of diseases that result from respiratory infection by viruses, bacteria, or fungi. The infectious agent most often associated with pneumonia, and against which the

✻ **pneumonia** acute infection of the lung, including alveolar spaces and interstitial tissue.

pneumococcal vaccine is targeted, is *Streptococcus pneumoniae,* gram-positive spheres found in pairs or chains. Other microorganisms known to cause pneumonia are *Mycoplasma pneumoniae* (primary atypical pneumonia), *H. influenzae, Klebsiella pneumoniae, M. catarrhalis, Legionella, S. aureus* in nosocomial infections, and *P. carinii.* These agents are also known to cause meningitis, ear infections, and pharyngitis. In addition to droplet nuclei, the infectious agents are also spread by direct contact and through linens soiled with respiratory secretions.

Those at highest risk for pneumonia are the immunocompromised, patients with sickle cell disease, transplanted organs, cardiovascular disease, diabetes mellitus, kidney disease, multiple myeloma, lymphoma, Hodgkin's disease, those without functioning spleens, and the elderly, particularly those in common residential situations. Low-birth-weight neonates and malnourished infants are very susceptible. In otherwise healthy individuals, susceptibility is increased by a previous respiratory infection like influenza, exposure to inhaled toxins, chronic lung disease, and aspiration (post-alcohol ingestion, near drowning, ingested toxins, or gastric distention from BVM ventilation). When patients contract infectious agents of pneumonia outside of a hospital or other health care institution, they are referred to as cases of community-acquired pneumonia.

History and Assessment Always consider the possibility of community-acquired pneumonia. In geriatric communities where residents live in their own home but may share common social facilities, ask if neighbors recently have been diagnosed with pneumonia or other respiratory infections. Signs and symptoms in previously healthy individuals include an acute onset of chills, high-grade fever, dyspnea, pleuritic chest pain worsened by deep inspiration, and cough, which may be productive with phlegm of various colors. The absence of fever does not rule out pneumonia. Breath sounds may include adventitious lung sounds (crackles, wheezes) and signs of consolidation. When purulent fluids accumulate in many lobes of the lung because of inflammation, alveoli collapse and their acoustic properties change to those of solid tissue, hence the name *consolidation.* Consolidation causes the expiratory sounds in the peripheral lung fields to develop the same duration as inspiration and to be just as loud. Assessment with pulse oximetry may be useful. In geriatric patients, the only presenting sign may be an altered mental status; fever is often absent, and headache, aches and pain, nausea, diarrhea, and nonproductive cough, if present, do not allow you to rule out pneumonia. In children, fever, tachypnea, and retractions are ominous signs but are not specific to pneumonia; this triad of signs, however, reliably indicates respiratory distress secondary to an infectious process in pediatric patients.

Patient Management and PPE Management of the pneumonia patient aims at supporting adequate ventilation and oxygenation, with supplemental oxygen often providing relief. Always consider TB a possibility in any patient with pneumonia and place a mask either on yourself or on your patient.

Immunization and Postexposure Management An effective vaccination exists against most serotypes of *S. pneumoniae* known to cause disease. It is highly recommended for children two years old or younger, for adults over sixty-five years old, and for those without spleens. Routine vaccination of EMS workers is not necessary. In health care settings, health care workers who routinely treat elderly, immunocompromised, or other at-risk patients may be required to be immunized because they pose the risk of patient transmission. Because EMS workers are predominantly healthy, exposure to a single patient with pneumonia generally will not result in infection or disease. A number of antimicrobial agents are effective against the infectious agents known to cause pneumonia. However, multidrug resistant strains have been reported.

Chickenpox

Chickenpox is caused by the varicella zoster virus (VZV). The varicella zoster virus is in the herpesvirus family. Although chickenpox (**varicella**) in pediatrics is considered a self-limited disease that rarely causes severe complications, it is much more lethal in adults. It results in fewer than 100 deaths per year in the United States, but while adults represent only 2 percent of the morbidity, they account for 50 percent of the mortality. Thus, health care workers who have not been immunized against VZV or been exposed to it as children must increase their awareness of this infection and its consequences. It is estimated that 10 percent of adults have not contracted VZV during childhood. VZV is also the infectious agent of shingles (herpes zoster), a painful condition that causes skin lesions along the course of peripheral nerves and dermatome bands. Approximately 15 percent of patients with chickenpox will eventually develop shingles.

Clinical Presentation Chickenpox usually occurs in clusters during winter and spring and presents with respiratory symptoms, malaise, and low-grade fever, followed by a rash that starts on the face and trunk and progresses to the rest of the body, including mucous membranes. The rash may be the first sign of illness, and infected persons may have anywhere from a few to 500 lesions. It is more profuse on the trunk, with less distribution to the extremities and scalp. The fluid-filled vesicles that form the rash soon rupture, forming small ulcers that eventually scab over within one week, at which point the patient is no longer contagious. Transmission occurs through inhalation of airborne droplets and direct contact with weeping lesions and tainted linen. The incubation period is from ten to twenty-one days.

In adults, varicella's most common complication is a VZV pneumonia. A large percentage of adult deaths from VZV occur in immunocompromised patients. The most alarming aspect of adult epidemiology, however, is a significant death rate in previously healthy patients. Therefore, it is important for unexposed or unvaccinated paramedics to be immunized.

Assessing Immunity Most people develop immunity for life after recovery from childhood chickenpox infections. Thus, a history of chickenpox is considered adequate evidence of immunity. An available blood test can determine immunity in those who are unsure about their history or who have not had chickenpox.

Immunization A chickenpox vaccine, Varivax, has been licensed in the United States since 1995, and the Advisory Committee on Immunization Practices (ACIP) of CDC now recommends that all states require children entering day care facilities and elementary school to be vaccinated or have some other evidence of immunity. Such evidence would include a primary care provider's diagnosis of chickenpox, a reliable history of the disease, or blood test confirming immunity. Vaccination is also routinely recommended for all susceptible health care workers. ACIP has also strengthened its recommendations for all other susceptible persons 13 years old or younger to include any adolescents living in the same household with younger children.

The vaccine is administered as one subcutaneous dose in children under age 12 and as two doses in susceptible adolescents and adults. Among vaccinated people 13 years old or older, 78 percent developed protective antibodies, with 99 percent seroconverting after the second dose. Health care workers who receive the vaccination should have their antibody level checked six weeks after the second vaccination.

Patients with active TB, malignant conditions, or those being treated with immunosuppressants should not receive varicella vaccine. Its use in those taking steroids depends on a variety of factors beyond the scope of this discussion. Few

* **varicella** viral disease characterized by a rash of fluid-filled vesicles that rupture, forming small ulcers that eventually scab; commonly called *chickenpox*.

adverse effects have been reported through CDC's Vaccine Adverse Events Reporting System (VAERS). The most frequent was rash, with some cases of herpes zoster. No incidents of chickenpox have been reported. Although a few serious adverse effects were reported, no cause and effect relationship was clearly established with the vaccination. The vaccine manufacturer discourages taking aspirin within six weeks after receiving the vaccination.

EMS Response and Postexposure Observe universal precautions and place masks on patients. If a patient only has chickenpox, he should remain at home until the lesions are crusted and dry. If a susceptible paramedic is exposed to chickenpox, postexposure vaccination may be warranted. Recent data indicate that if used within three days, and possibly up to five days, Varivax may be effective in preventing chickenpox or lessening its severity. Varicella–zoster immune globulin (VZIG) is an alternative postexposure prophylaxis. Unlike Varivax, it provides passive immunity, and the most current recommendation for its use is in immunocompromised patients. The use of Acyclovir, which inhibits replication of the virus, within 24 hours of the onset of rash may decrease the disease's severity in adults and adolescents.

Meningitis

Meningitis is an inflammation of the meninges (the membranes protecting the brain and spinal cord) and cerebrospinal fluid, caused by bacterial and viral infections. Meningococcal meningitis (spinal meningitis), caused by *Neisseria meningitidis,* is the disease variant of greatest concern to EMS responders.

Other agents are, or have been, known to cause meningitis. *Streptococcus pneumoniae,* the primary infectious agent of concern in pneumonia, is the second most common cause of pneumonia in adults and the most common cause of otitis media in children. Vaccines have proven very effective, especially in children. *Haemophilus influenzae* type B, a gram-negative rod, was once the leading cause of meningitis in children aged six months to three years. However, with the implementation of effective childhood vaccination against *H. influenzae* since 1981, *N. meningitidis* has become the bacterium most commonly implicated in serious meningitis cases. Viruses and other microorganisms are known to cause meningitis, with similar disease profiles. Enteroviruses are implicated in 90 percent of patients with viral (aseptic) meningitis. In healthy individuals, viral meningitis is a self-limited disease that lasts about seven to ten days.

Transmission Factors *N. meningitidis* asymptomatically colonizes the upper respiratory tract of healthy individuals and is then transmitted by respiratory droplets. Up to 35 percent of the general population may be infected with the bacterium, which is prevented from gaining access to the CSF by the epithelial lining of the pharynx. Almost every human has probably been a carrier at some point in his life. Conversion from carrier to clinical disease is rare in developed countries and occurs in clusters in developing nations. The disease appears to peak in midwinter months with low temperature and humidity. This has been validated by observations of epidemic seasonal variations in the "meningitis belt" of sub-Saharan Africa. Epidemiologists have hypothesized that this pattern may represent a herd immunity, in which host resistance factors may be more a function of the population's general immunity than of the immunity of individuals within that population. One theory that could explain the phenomenon of herd immunity holds that another species within the genus *Neisseria* may be "mistaken" for *N. meningitidis* (a cross reaction), resulting in effective antibody production against the pathogen. Meningococcal meningitis occurs more commonly in some areas of the United States, and the world, for reasons not yet un-

EMS transport of a patient with chickenpox should be followed by extensive decontamination of the ambulance and any equipment used.

* meningitis inflammation of the meninges, usually caused by an infection.

derstood. Other factors that have been implicated in transmission of *N. meningitidis* include contacting oral secretions of the index case (kissing, sharing food or drink), crowding, close contact, smoking, and lower socioeconomic status. For the EMS responder, contact with secretions during mouth-to-mask ventilation, intubation, or suctioning would increase the probability of transmission.

Clinical Presentation The incubation period most commonly ranges from two to four days but may last as long as ten days. As with most bacterial infections, signs and symptoms develop rapidly within a few hours or one to two days of exposure and include fever, chills, headache, nuchal rigidity with flexion, arthralgia, lethargy, malaise, altered mental status, vomiting, and seizures. An upper respiratory or ear infection may precede the disease. A characteristic rash may appear and develop into hemorrhagic spots, or petechiae. Roughly 10 percent of patients may develop septic shock. Acute adrenal insufficiency, disseminated intravascular coagulation (DIC), and coma are other consequences. Death can ensue in six to eight hours.

Newborns and infants may seem slow or inactive, vomit, appear irritable, or feed poorly. Fever in newborns should be evaluated with a high index of suspicion for meningococcemia. Rarely, bulging of an open anterior fontanel is seen. In older children, assessment techniques that stretch the inflamed meninges and cause pain may reveal positive Brudzinski's and Kernig's signs. **Brudzinski's sign** is a physical exam finding suggestive of meningitis. Due to irritation of the meninges, flexion of the neck causes flexion of the hips and knees. To test for Brudzinski's sign, have the patient lie supine without a pillow. Flex the neck while observing the hips and knees. Flexion of the hips or knees when the neck is flexed is considered a positive Brudzinski's sign. **Kernig's sign** is likewise suggestive of meningitis. To elicit Kernig's sign, have the patient sit or lie and flex the hips. With the hips flexed, attempt to extend (straighten) the knee. Inability to fully extend the knee is due to meningeal irritation and is considered a positive Kernig's sign. Maternal antibodies protect newborns from meningitis and other infections until up to six months of age (slightly longer in breast fed children). Infants from six months to two years are especially susceptible to meningitis because they no longer have circulating maternal antibodies and their immune systems are immature and incompetent.

✳ Brudzinki's sign physical exam finding in which flexion of the neck causes flexion of the hips and knees.

✳ Kernig's sign inability to fully extend the knees with hips flexed.

Immunization *N. meningitidis* has several serotypes (A, B, C, X, Y, Z, 29-E, W-135), with B and C causing most disease outbreaks in the United States. The A serotype is the most common cause of epidemics in Africa and Asia. An effective vaccine has been developed against the A, C, Y, and W-135 serotypes. Attempts to develop one against the B serotype have so far resulted in weak immune responses. The meningococcal vaccine is not presently recommended for routine immunization of health care workers. Travelers to endemic areas and children younger than two years who are asplenic (without a spleen) or have a certain deficiency in their complement system are candidates for vaccination.

EMS Response and Postexposure Observing universal precautions and using masks on yourself and/or your patients with suspected meningococcal meningitis will adequately protect you against all the infectious agents of meningitis. Postexposure prophylaxis with rifampin, ciprofloxacin (Cipro), or ceftriaxone (Rocephin) is the primary means of preventing meningococcal disease. Prophylaxis should be started within 24 hours after exposure because the rate of effective transmission in close contacts (EMS responders) with the index-case patient has been estimated to be 500–800 times that of the general population. Initiation of chemoprophylaxis 14 days or more after the onset of illness in the index case is of limited or no value. All postexposure medications are easily complied with and have few side effects.

Content Review

OTHER JOB-RELATED AIRBORNE DISEASES

- Influenza and the common cold
- Measles
- Mumps
- Rubella
- Respiratory Syncytial Virus
- Pertussis

Effective, vigorous hand washing with soap and warm water after patient contact is the most important personal precaution against disease transmission.

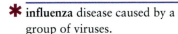 **influenza** disease caused by a group of viruses.

Other Job-Related Airborne Diseases

Influenza and colds, rubella, measles, mumps, and respiratory syncytial virus (RSV) are viral infections that may be contracted in the EMS environment. Pertussis, a highly contagious bacterial disease, also poses a risk. These diseases are transmitted by direct inhalation of infected droplets or through exposed mucosal surfaces. Handling contaminated surfaces or objects and subsequently introducing the virus by scratching, wiping, or other activities with unwashed hands (autoinoculation) is another route of transmission. Masks and ventilation are recommended for measles. Precautions against autoinoculation with RSV infections, influenza, and colds include masks, more practically placed on patients, and possibly gloves, gowns, and goggles. Avoid touching your face and areas of broken skin while in contact with the patient. Effective, vigorous hand washing with soap and warm water after patient contact is the most important personal precaution against disease transmission.

Influenza and the Common Cold Influenza is caused by viruses designated types A, B, and C. Within these types are various subtypes that mutate so often that they are identified on the basis of where they were isolated, the culture number, and year of isolation—for instance, A/Japan/305/57. Two glycoproteins, hemagglutinin and neuraminidase, on the outer membrane of an influenza virus determine its virulence. The letters H and N, which denote these two glycoproteins, are often seen in parentheses along with a number, as in A (H1N1). This method of classification helps epidemiologists to more specifically identify a flu virus, since it is based on the immune responses to hemagglutinin and neuraminidase.

Influenza is a leading cause of respiratory disease worldwide, and various strains cause epidemics, mainly during the winter months. It is easily transmittable in crowded spaces such as public transportation vehicles, and can be spread by direct contact. The virus can persist on environmental surfaces for hours, especially in low humidity and cold temperatures. Thus, it has a high potential for transmission by autoinoculation. It is much more serious than the common cold and has caused worldwide epidemics with high mortality rates. The last great epidemic was in 1918, and CDC and the World Health Organization (WHO) closely monitor worldwide disease outbreaks.

Influenza is characterized by the sudden onset of fever, chills, malaise, muscle aches, nasal discharge, and cough. The disease is more serious in the very young, the very old, and those with underlying disease. Its incubation period is from one to three days. Fever generally lasts three to five days. Signs include mild sore throat, nonproductive cough, and nasal discharge. The cough may be severe and of long duration. Secondary infections may occur as the virus damages respiratory epithelial cells, thereby decreasing resistance to other, primarily bacterial, disorders. Severe cases may result in pneumonia, hemorrhagic bronchitis, and death. The uncomplicated disease usually lasts two to seven days and full recovery is the norm.

Management is primarily supportive. Fever may increase body temperature to as high as 105°F. Begin cooling measures for patients with temperatures of 104°F or greater. Increased body temperature may lead to significant insensible fluid loss and dehydration. Determine hydration status early and begin fluid replacement if indicated.

Everyone is susceptible to influenza. Although infection confers resistance after recovery, the influenza viruses mutate so rapidly that protection is effective only against the particular strain or variant from which the person has just recovered. An immunization is available and is recommended for the elderly, those who live or work in correctional institutions, and military recruits. Patients should be immunized between early September and mid-November for maximum effectiveness. The CDC recommends vaccination for EMS personnel to reduce transmission of influenza to patients and to decrease worker absenteeism. EMS responders who are diabetics, especially those requiring frequent medical follow up, are strongly urged to be immunized. Three antiviral drugs, amantadine (Symmetrel), oseltamivir (Tambiflu), and rimantadine (Flumadine), are available for the prevention and treatment of influenza; however, they only work against the type A influenza virus. They are as effective as vaccines when used preventively, and they shorten the illness's duration when used as a treatment. A new agent, zanamavir (Relenza), which is effective against type B, was recently released. However, its use is limited because only 35 percent of influenza cases are type B and because it must be delivered by aerosol nebulizer.

The common cold, or viral rhinitis, is caused by the rhinoviruses, of which there are more than 100 serotypes. Its incidence in the United States rises in fall, winter, and spring, is highest in children younger than five years, and declines in older adults, displaced by more serious diseases. Transmission is by direct contact, airborne droplets, or more importantly, by hands and linen soiled with discharges from infected individuals. The incubation period ranges from 12 hours to 5 days and averages 48 hours. The disease's course is mild, often without fever and generally without muscle aching. Aside from severity, it is often difficult to differentiate from influenza. Mortality has not been reported, but a cold may lead to more serious complications such as otitis media and sinusitis.

Measles Measles (rubeola, hard measles), a systemic disease caused by the measles virus of the genus *Morbilli,* is highly communicable. It is most common in children but may affect older persons who have not had it. Immunity following disease is usually lifelong. Maternal antibodies protect neonates for about four to five months after birth.

> ✱ **measles** highly contagious, acute viral disease characterized by a reddish rash that appears on the fourth or fifth day of illness.

Measles is transmitted by inhalation of infective droplets and direct contact. The incubation period ranges from seven to fourteen days, averaging ten. The infected person presents prodromally like a severe cold, with fever, conjunctivitis, swelling of the eyelids, photophobia, malaise, cough, and nasopharyngeal congestion. The fever increases, rising to as high as 104°–106°F, when the rash reaches its maximum. A day or two before the rash develops, Koplik's spots (bluish-white specks with a red halo approximately 1 mm in diameter) appear on the oral mucosa. The red, bumpy (maculopapular) rash normally lasts about six days and spreads from head to feet by the third day. At that point, it appears to thicken on the head and shoulders and then disappear in the same direction as its progression.

Measles is so highly communicable that the slightest contact with an active case may infect a susceptible person. Infectivity is greatest before the prodrome and subsides about four days after the rash appears or as it fades. Everyone should be immunized. Immunization is 99 percent effective in children, for whom vaccination is mandatory since there is no specific treatment. Unimmunized or previously unexposed paramedics should mask their measles patients and be vigilant about handling linens and touching their face during and after the call. Postexposure hand washing is critical.

In otherwise healthy children or adults, uncomplicated measles has a low mortality rate. Potential complications include bacterial pneumonia, eye damage, and myocarditis. The most life-threatening sequela is encephalitis in children and adolescents that causes gradual decreases in mental capacity and muscle coordination.

Mumps The **mumps** virus, a member of the genus *Paramyxovirus,* is transmitted through respiratory droplets and direct contact with the saliva of infected patients. It is characterized by painful enlargement of the salivary glands. Most cases occur in the five- to fifteen-year age group. After a 12–25 day incubation period, mumps presents as a feverish cold that is soon followed by swelling and stiffening of the parotid salivary gland in front of the ear. The condition is often

> ✱ **mumps** acute viral disease characterized by painful enlargement of the salivary glands.

found bilaterally. The patient may also experience earache and difficulty chewing and swallowing. In most cases, the submaxillary and sublingual glands are very tender to palpation. Most cases resolve spontaneously within one week without intervention.

Mumps occurs in epidemics, with danger of transmission beginning one week before the infected person feels sick and lasting about two weeks. Lifelong immunity is generally conferred after infection, even in the absence of disease (subclinical infection).

Mumps is generally benign and self-limiting; however, complications may occur. In postpubescent patients, inflammation of the testicles (orchitis), breasts (mastitis), or ovaries (oophoritis) may occur, but is of short duration and of no serious consequence. Meningoencephalitis is fairly common but resolves without residual neurological sequelae.

A mumps live-virus vaccine is available and should be administered with measles and rubella vaccines to all children over one year old. Mumps is not easily transmitted, and with standard BSI precautions the risk of contracting the disease is minimal. For the benefit of their patients, EMS workers should not work without an established mumps/measles/rubella (MMR) immunity.

✱ rubella (German measles) systemic viral disease characterized by a fine pink rash that appears on the face, trunk, and extremities and fades quickly.

Rubella Rubella **(German measles)** is a systemic viral disease caused by the rubella virus, of the genus *Rubivirus,* transmitted by inhalation of infective droplets. Generally milder than measles, it is characterized by sore throat and low-grade fever, accompanied by a fine pink rash on the face, trunk, and extremities that lasts about 3 days. The incubation period is 12–19 days, with natural infection conferring lifelong immunity, as does immunization. Transfer of maternal antibodies does not confer lifelong immunity but does protect the neonate. There is no specific treatment for rubella. More serious complications that occur in measles do not occur in rubella, but young females sometimes develop a short course of arthritis.

Rubella is devastating to a developing fetus. Mothers infected during the first trimester are at risk for abnormal fetal development, with offspring often developing congenital rubella syndrome and shedding large quantities of virus in their secretions. An infant acquiring this infection *in utero* (in the uterus) is likely to be retarded and suffer eye inflammation, deafness, and congenital heart defects. All females, therefore, should be immunized against rubella before becoming pregnant.

Vaccines for measles, mumps, and rubella are commonly combined in an MMR vaccination, which can be given safely with the varicella vaccine. Immunization is 98–99 percent effective but is not recommended for pregnant women because of a theoretical possibility of birth defects. Health care workers have been identified as the source in numerous outbreaks. For this reason, and for their own protection, all EMS providers should be required to receive the MMR vaccination before they are allowed to work. Immunizations, along with placing a mask on the patient, are an effective method of preventing these diseases.

Paramedics should not be allowed to work until they have received the MMR vaccination.

✱ respiratory syncytial virus (RSV) common cause of pneumonia and bronchiolitis in children.

Respiratory Syncytial Virus Respiratory syncytial virus (RSV) is one of the most common causes of pneumonia and bronchiolitis in infants and young children. In this age group, RSV may be fatal. In older children and adults RSV is less common, and its symptoms are generally milder. RSV is often associated with outbreaks of lower respiratory infections from November to April. If a patient with pneumonia or bronchitis simultaneously contracts this virus, the disease becomes more severe. RSV commonly begins as an upper respiratory infection, and is often misdiagnosed as a simple cold. Children with RSV infection will initially develop a runny nose and nasal congestion. Later, this will spread to lower airway involvement evidenced by wheezing, tachypnea, and signs of respiratory distress. It is a common infection that can be diagnosed by a rapid assay using nasal washings. In winter months, wheezing in children under a year of age should be presumed to be due to RSV until proven otherwise. High-risk children (those with congenital heart conditions, prematurity, or cancers, for instance) can be treated with the antiviral agent ribavirin (Virazole). However, this treatment is quite expensive and poses a significant risk to unborn babies of pregnant health care workers. Postexposure prophylaxis with Respi-Gam (RSV immune globulin) is also an option.

Pertussis The word *pertussis* means "violent cough." **Pertussis** (whooping cough) is caused by the bacterium *Bordetella pertussis,* affecting the oropharynx in three clinical phases after an incubation period of from six to twenty days. The *catarrhal phase,* characterized by symptoms similar to those of the common cold, lasts from one to two weeks. The *paroxysmal phase,* during which the fever subsides, can last a month or longer. The patient develops a mild cough that quickly becomes severe and violent. Rapid consecutive coughs are followed by a deep, high-pitched inspiration. (This characteristic "whoop" often is not present in infants and adults.) The cough often produces large amounts of thick mucus, and vomiting may also occur. Sustained coughing may lead to increased intracranial pressure and intracerebral hemorrhage. Continually high intrapulmonary pressure and vigorous chest movement may cause pneumothorax. During the *convalescent phase* the frequency and severity of coughing attacks decrease, and the patient is not contagious.

The widespread vaccination of children in a combination diphtheria-pertussis-tetanus vaccine (DTP) caused a dramatic decrease in the incidence of pertussis until the early 1980s. Over the past 20 years, however, its incidence has steadily grown, with the greatest increase in persons aged 5 years or older. This has occurred in spite of unprecedented pertussis vaccination coverage. One factor in the increase may be a waning effectiveness of the vaccine among adolescents and adults vaccinated during childhood. Although disease is likely to confer immunity against pertussis, the duration of that immunity is unknown. Previously immunized and exposed adolescents and adults therefore may be at risk of infection. Thus, booster doses are recommended.

For patients with pertussis, EMS is most likely to be requested during the paroxysmal phase, when the primary treatment will be calming and oxygenating the patient. Anticipate the needs to intubate patients with respiratory failure and to perform chest decompression for those whose coughing paroxysms might have caused a pneumothorax. During the response, remember that pertussis is highly contagious. Fortunately, the communicable period is thought to be greatest before the paroxysmal phase. Transmission occurs via respiratory secretions or in an aerosolized form. Mask the patient and observe standard BSI precautions, including postexposure hand washing.

Everyone is susceptible to *B. pertussis* infection. Routine immunization of EMS workers against pertussis is not yet recommended. Evaluation of pertussis vaccination is ongoing, however, and considering the unknown duration of immunity with past immunization or exposure, adolescent and adult immunization may be recommended in the future. Erythromycin is known to decrease the period of communicability, but can reduce symptoms only if administered before the onset of violent coughing.

Viral Diseases Transmitted by Contact

Mononucleosis and herpex simplex type 1 infections pose little risk to EMS providers who observe BSI precautions and wash their hands after patient contact. Since these diseases cause relatively minor symptoms, patients may not even be aware of their infection status. The public is highly aware of these two diseases, however, so as health care providers, paramedics should be familiar with them.

Mononucleosis Mononucleosis is caused by the Epstein-Barr virus (EBV). It affects the oropharynx, tonsils, and the reticuloendothelial system (the phagocytes). A four- to six-week incubation period precedes the development of symptoms, which characteristically begin with fatigue. Fever, severe sore throat, oral discharges, and enlarged, tender lymph nodes generally follow several days to weeks later. Splenomegaly (enlargement of the spleen) is present in approximately one-half of patients. The disease is common; over 95 percent of the general population has antibodies to the virus. One half of all children will have contracted it before the age of five years. Infection by EBV generally confers immunity for life.

Mononucleosis is most commonly transmitted through oropharyngeal contact involving the exchange of saliva between an uninfected person and one who has the disease but who is asymptomatic. Kissing is implicated in adolescents and adults, and transmission from care givers to young children is common. Blood transfusions can be a mode of transmission, but with few cases of disease attributed to it. Active disease is most common in those between 15 and 25 years of age. The risk of contracting the disease without close facial contact is minimal. Symptoms generally dissipate within a few weeks, but full recuperation may take several months. There is no specific treatment for mononucleosis, and immunization is unavailable. Corticosteroids are occasionally administered to help minimize tonsillar swelling. Nonsteroidal antiinflammatory drugs (NSAIDs) may provide symptomatic relief.

Herpes Simplex Virus Type 1 There are two types of **herpes simplex virus,** herpes simplex virus type 1 (HSV-1) and herpes simplex virus type 2 (HSV-2). HSV-2 will be discussed in the section on sexually transmitted diseases. HSV-1 is transmitted in the saliva of carriers and commonly infects the oropharynx, face, lips, skin, fingers, and toes. Everyone is susceptible. Infections of health care workers' hands and fingers can result in herpetic whitlow, weeping inflammations at the distal fingers and toes. The incubation period following exposure ranges from two to twelve days. In the oral cavity, fluid-filled vesicles develop into cold sores or fever blisters that soon deteriorate into small ulcers. Fever, malaise, and dehydration may accompany these primary lesions. The lesions usually disappear in two to three weeks. They may recur spontaneously, especially following periods of stress or other illness. Recurrent HSV labialis (lip lesions) may cause problems for many years in some adults.

Although primarily recognized for causing skin and mucous membrane disorders, HSV-1 can cause meningoencephalitis in newborns and aseptic meningitis in adults. A high index of suspicion for HSV-1 in these situations may result in timely treatment with antiviral agents like acyclovir, which is somewhat effective against HSV-1.

Universal precautions, primarily gloves, are absolutely essential, especially if an intimate contact or family member of the EMS worker is afflicted. Breaks in the skin place everyone at greater risk, and may not be visible to the naked eye. Treatment with acylovir (Zovirax) provides relief when used topically or orally. Immunization is not available.

OTHER INFECTIOUS CONDITIONS OF THE RESPIRATORY SYSTEM

The majority of profiles in this section discuss pathological conditions of the airway caused by a variety of infectious agents. They are not diseases, per se. Volume 5, Chapter 2 on pediatrics discusses croup and epiglottitis in greater detail. Hantavirus is included here, although its sites of pathology extend beyond the airways.

Epiglottitis Epiglottitis is an inflammation of the epiglottis and may also involve the areas just above and below it. In children it is a true emergency, usually caused by *H. influenzae,* with an abrupt onset over several hours and without any immediate history of upper respiratory disease. Patients present with one or more of the "four Ds:" dysphonia, drooling, dysphagia, or distress. Epiglottitis can also occur in teenagers and adults. In the older age groups, stridor, sore throat, fever, and drooling usually develop over days, not hours. Due to natural immunity from initial infection, epiglottitis is not known to reoccur in any age group. Increased immunization against *H. influenzae* has reduced the incidence of epiglottitis caused by this bacterium. However, *S. pneumoniae* and *S. aureus* have been implicated as causative agents of epiglottitis.

Croup Croup (laryngotracheobronchitis) is a common cause of acute upper airway obstruction in children. A viral illness characterized by inspiratory and expiratory stridor and a seal-bark-like cough, it is most common in children under the age of three. Although generally not life threatening, croup may create panic in parents and children alike. Viruses implicated in croup include the parainfluenza viruses, rhinoviruses, and RSV. Croup is often preceded by an upper respiratory infection. The child commonly awakens during the night with acute respiratory distress, tachypnea, and retractions. Seasonal outbreaks of this disease are common. Total airway obstruction is rare.

* croup viral illness characterized by inspiratory and expiratory stridor and a seal-bark-like cough.

Pharyngitis Pharyngitis is a common infection of the pharynx and tonsils. It may be caused by a virus or bacteria and is characterized by a sudden onset of sore throat and fever. The tonsils and palate become red and swollen, and the cervical lymph nodes enlarge. Headache, neck pain, nausea, and vomiting may also be present. Most cases occur in late winter and early spring. Although this disease may occur in any age group, most cases are seen in five- to eleven-year-olds.

* pharyngitis infection of the pharynx and tonsils.

Group A streptococcus (strep throat) causes a particularly serious pharyngitis that, if left untreated, in certain cases, can progress to rheumatic fever. There are several sub-types of Group A streptococcus. One strain causes rheumatic fever. Another strain is responsible for scarlet fever (scarletina). Patients infected with this bacterium may present with a scarlet-colored rash. Because strep throat is very contagious, you should wear a mask when assessing and managing these patients. Although laboratory tests can easily determine which cases of pharyngitis are caused by strep, it is virtually impossible to tell clinically. Assume that all cases of pharyngitis are serious and contagious until proven otherwise. Antibiotics (penicillin, amoxicillin, erythromycin, azithromycin) effectively treat strep throat.

Sinusitis Sinusitis is an inflammation of the paranasal (ethmoid, frontal, maxillary, or sphenoid) sinuses. It occurs when mucus and pus cannot drain and become trapped in the sinus. Sinusitis is usually preceded by a viral upper respiratory infection or exposure to allergens, either of which may cause nasal congestion and blocked sinus passages. Postnasal drip may develop and nasal drainage may be blood-tinged and purulent. As fluids collect in the sinus, a sensation of pressure or fullness generally develops. If left untreated, the condition may become painful, and the infection can cause an abscess or spread into the cranium and attack the brain. Discomfort often worsens when the patient bends forward or when pressure is applied over the affected sinus. Sinusitis is occasionally a causative factor of meningitis. Management includes antibiotics, decongestants, and supportive care. Apply a heat pack directly over the affected sinus to help relieve pain and facilitate drainage.

* sinusitis inflammation of the paranasal sinuses.

Hantavirus Hantavirus is a family of viruses carried by rodents such as the deer mouse. Other known carriers are the rice and cotton rats in the southeastern United States and the white-footed mouse of the northeastern states. The common house mouse is not known to carry the virus. Most cases of hantavirus infection have occurred in the southwestern United States, particularly the Four Corners region. Transmission is primarily by inhalation of aerosols created by

* hantavirus family of viruses that are carried by the deer mouse and transmitted by ticks and other arthropods.

stirring up the dried urine, saliva, and fecal droppings of these rodents. Contamination of food and autoinoculation after handling objects tainted by rodent droppings may also cause transmission. Direct bites are possible routes, but are thought to be rare. Person-to-person transmission is not possible.

The virus causes hantavirus pulmonary syndrome (HPS), to which anyone is susceptible. The initial symptoms are fatigue, fever, and muscle aches, especially of large muscle groups. Headaches, nausea, vomiting, diarrhea, and abdominal pain are also common. Earache, sore throat, and rash are uncommon. Approximately four to ten days later, symptoms of pulmonary edema occur. Patients with fatal infections appear to have severe myocardial depression, which can progress to sinus bradycardia and subsequent electromechanical dissociation, ventricular tachycardia, or fibrillation. Hemodynamic compromise occurs a median of five days after symptoms' onset—usually dramatically within the first day of hospitalization. The only specific treatment is intensive supportive care, and no immunization is available.

EMS responders who find themselves in dusty, unoccupied buildings for extended times should wear face masks to prevent inhaling aerosolized rodent droppings.

GI SYSTEM INFECTIONS

Content Review

GI SYSTEM INFECTIONS
• Gastroenteritis
• Food Poisoning

You may on occasion respond to scenes with single or multiple cases of food-borne illness. Although you cannot determine the causative agent outside of the hospital, you must have a basic knowledge of the infectious process and guidelines for assessment, management, and safe handling of these patients. Many EMS personnel are being recruited and volunteering for domestic and international disaster medical teams. In these situations, when the sanitation infrastructure (water treatment and distribution, sewer, animal control, and so forth) are disrupted, GI system infections increase significantly.

Gastroenteritis

* gastroenteritis generalized disorder involving nausea, vomiting, gastrointestinal cramping or discomfort, and diarrhea.

Gastroenteritis is a gastrointestinal disorder manifested by nausea, vomiting, gastrointestinal cramping or discomfort, anorexia, and diarrhea. In more advanced cases, which are rare, it can cause lassitude and shock. It is a common disease that many of us in developed countries have experienced. The reference to "stomach flu" in these situations is incorrect, since an influenza of the GI system has not yet been identified. What this distressing and uncomfortable condition usually represents, at least in developed countries, is a viral gastroenteritis. The causative agents may be viruses (Norwalk virus, Rotavirus, and others), bacteria (*E. coli, K. pneumoniae, C. jejuni, E. aerogenes, V. cholerae, Shigella,* and *Salmonella*), and parasites (*G. lamblia, C. parvum, C. cayetensis*). Gastroenteritis is highly contagious via the fecal-oral route, including the ingestion of contaminated food and water. It is especially contagious during natural disasters in epidemic proportions. International travelers into endemic areas are very susceptible, while native populations are generally resistant.

In otherwise healthy persons, gastroenteritis is generally self-limiting and benign; however, in the very young, the very old, or those with preexisting disease, it can be serious and often fatal. Prolonged vomiting and/or diarrhea may result in dehydration and electrolyte disturbances. Patients generally experience painful and severe abdominal cramping, and some develop hypovolemic shock. Always consider dehydration in any patient who presents with signs of gastroenteritis. If a patient has vomited many times or is actively vomiting, has multiple medical problems, is debilitated, or at risk by virtue of age and general health, start an IV with isotonic saline. Pay careful attention to hydration status. If the patient is in shock, the management objectives are no different than for hemorrhagic shock. If the patient is not in shock, the judicious use of fluids is warranted. A good rule of thumb is to replace fluids at approximately the rate they are lost. The World Health Organization and other international disaster response agencies have found oral rehydration very effective in treating fluid loss, even with cholera. Do not feel compelled to pour in IV fluids. If prolonged vomiting or retching is present, administer an antiemetic such as droperidol (Inapsine), prochlorperazine (Compazine), or promethazine (Phenergan). Remember that vehicle movements often aggravate symptoms and increase the probability of vomiting.

With isolated cases of gastroenteritis, compliance with universal precautions and postexposure hand washing are critical to avoiding infection. In times of disaster, EMS responders must be more focused on environmental health and sanitation issues: preparing food, identifying clean sources of water, using mosquito netting while sleeping, and general sanitation. Eat hot foods only and drink hot beverages that have been brisk boiled. Be careful to avoid personal habits that facilitate fecal-oral transmission. Prevention is important because even though antimicrobials may be available to treat isolated cases, resources for treating gastroenteritis during disasters or in developing countries may be limited. In those situations, many people receive symptomatic treatment.

Food Poisoning

Food poisoning is a nonspecific term often applied to gastroenteritis. Food poisoning occurs suddenly and is caused by eating. Diarrhea, vomiting, and gastrointestinal discomfort characterize its more benign presentation. Most cases are caused by bacteria and their toxic products. In the majority of cases, only the GI system is affected, but other systems may be affected in some cases, as with botulism or *Escherichia coli* O157:H7, causing debilitating illness or death. *Clostridium botulinum* produces a very potent neurotoxin that causes flaccid paralysis by blocking the release of acetylcholine at motor end plates and preganglionic autonomic synapses.

E. coli O157:H7, transmitted by the ingestion of uncooked or undercooked ground beef, often causes severe bloody diarrhea and abdominal cramps; sometimes the infection causes nonbloody diarrhea or no symptoms. Drinking unpasteurized milk and swimming in or drinking sewage-contaminated water can also cause infection. Little or no fever is usually present, and the illness resolves in five to ten days. In some persons, particularly children under five years of age and the elderly, the infection can cause a complication called hemolytic uremic syndrome, in which the red blood cells are destroyed and the kidneys fail. About 2–7 percent of infections lead to this complication. In the United States, hemolytic uremic syndrome is the principal cause of acute kidney failure in children, and *E. coli* O157:H7 causes most cases of hemolytic uremic syndrome.

Other bacteria implicated in food poisoning include *Campylobacter, Salmonella, Shigella,* and *Vibrio cholerae.* Microorganisms may be transmitted in other meats that are insufficiently cooked. *Salmonella* is commonly transmitted through incompletely cooked poultry. It may also be spread through contaminated cookware and utensils used in preparation of poultry. Hepatitis A and Norwalk virus are known to have been ingested in undercooked seafood. Bacterial gastrointestinal infections tend to be much more severe than viral gastrointestinal infections. With bacterial infections, the patient will appear more toxic. There is often a history of bloody, foul-smelling diarrhea (especially with shigellosis). The presence of leukocytes in a fecal smear is suggestive of bacterial disease. Ultimately, stool cultures are required to confirm a bacterial cause of gastroenteritis.

Initiate standard advanced life support (ALS) protocols, including assessment of airway and ventilatory status, oxygenation, initiation of an IV, and cardiac

✳ **food poisoning** nonspecific term often applied to gastroenteritis that occurs suddenly and that is caused by the ingestion of food containing preformed toxins.

monitoring. Fluid resuscitation with isotonic crystalloids is often required. It is not uncommon for an adult with severe gastroenteritis to require 2–3 liters of fluid. In patients with significant vomiting or diarrhea, also consider antiemetics. Constant reassessment of ventilatory status is essential since the neurotoxin in *C. botulinum* ingestion may cause respiratory arrest. Observing universal precautions should protect against foodborne transmission of infectious agents. No immunization against these agents or their toxins exists.

Prevention efforts are the primary means of reducing foodborne illness. Advances in technology may provide better alternatives for food supply surveillance, an aspect of foodborne disease prevention that could be improved. Lawrence Berkeley National Laboratory has developed plastic strips that turn from blue to red in the presence of toxic strains of *E. coli*. This technology's basis could become a prototype for other simple reagent strips that can detect foodborne pathogens.

NERVOUS SYSTEM INFECTIONS

Encephalitis, rabies, tetanus, and Lyme disease all have significant effects on the nervous system. These infectious conditions or diseases do not necessarily pose occupational risks to EMS providers. They are well known to the general public, however, and are very much associated with recreational activities in which EMS responders participate.

Encephalitis

Encephalitis is an inflammation caused by infection of the brain and its structures, usually by viruses such as equine viruses, arboviruses, the rubella virus, or the mumps virus. These viral infections usually result in one of the following:

1. They cause no pathology until they are transported to cerebral neurons, which they invade, and then replicate (the rabies and arthropod-borne viruses, for instance).

2. They first injure nonnervous tissues and then, rarely, invade the cerebral neurons (for example, herpes simplex 1 and varicella-zoster virus).

Bacteria, fungi, or parasites may also cause encephalitis, but the viruses are the predominant infectious agents.

The clinical presentation of encephalitis is similar to that of meningitis since they often coexist. Signs and symptoms include decreased level of consciousness, fever, headache, drowsiness, coma, tremors, and a stiff neck and back. Seizures may occur in patients of any age but are most common in infants. Characteristic neurological signs include uncoordinated and involuntary movements, weakness of the arms, legs, or other portions of the body, or unusual sensitivity of the skin to various types of stimuli.

Treatment is difficult, even when the virus is known. Despite the severity of illness, many patients suffer no long-term neurological deficits; however, as many as 50 percent of children younger than one year may suffer irreversible brain damage after contracting eastern or western equine encephalitis, diseases of horses and mules transmitted to humans by mosquitoes.

Rabies

Rabies is transmitted by the rabies virus, a member of the Rhabdovirus family and *Lyssavirus* genus, which affects the nervous system. It exists in two epidemiological forms: *urban,* propagated chiefly through unimmunized domestic dogs and

Content Review

NERVOUS SYSTEM INFECTIONS

- Encephalitis
- Rabies
- Tetanus
- Lyme disease

✱ **encephalitis** acute infection of the brain, usually caused by a virus.

✱ **rabies** viral disorder that affects the nervous system.

cats, and *sylvatic,* propagated by skunks, foxes, raccoons, mongooses, coyotes, wolves, and bats. Humans are especially susceptible when bitten by infected animals. The virus is transmitted in the saliva of infected mammals by bites, an opening in the skin, or direct contact with a mucous membrane. It passes along motor and sensory fibers to the spinal ganglia corresponding to the site of invasion, and then to the brain, creating an *encephalomyelitis* that is almost always fatal. Although rare, transmission is also known to occur by inhalation of aerosolized virus, through nasal nerve fibers and mucosa, along the olfactory nerve, and then to the brain. Mammals are highly susceptible to infection. Transmission is known to be affected by the severity of the wound, abundance of the nerve supply close to the wound, the distance to the CNS, the amount and strain of virus, protective clothing, and other undetermined factors. The highly variable incubation period is usually from three to eight weeks but can be as short as nine days (rare) or as long as ten years. It is believed to be dependent on the bite site, with bites to the head and neck generally followed by shorter incubation periods.

Rabies is characterized by a non-specific *prodrome* (symptoms that precede the appearance of a disease) of malaise, headache, fever, chills, sore throat, myalgias, anorexia, nausea, vomiting, and diarrhea. The prodrome typically lasts from one to four days. The next phase, the *encephalitic phase,* begins with periods of excessive motor activity, excitation, and agitation. This is soon followed by confusion, hallucinations, combativeness, bizarre aberrations of thought, muscle twitches and tetany, and seizures. Soon, focal paralysis appears. When left untreated, it can cause death within two to six days. Attempts to drink water may produce laryngospasm, causing the characteristic profuse drooling commonly known as hydrophobia (fear of water).

Rabies in the United States has become more prevalent in the wild. From 1980 to 1999, 58 of the rabies cases diagnosed in the United States have been attributed to bat variants. It is not surprising then, that the CDC has identified wildlife as the most important potential source of infection for humans and domestic animals in this country. In Africa, Asia, and Latin America, dogs remain the major source. Human rabies is rare in the United States, but each year 16,000–39,000 people receive postexposure prophylaxis. This is not a matter of paranoia. The CDC estimates that up to one-third of persons who have contracted rabies cannot accurately relate a history of having been bitten by an animal. Thus, epidemiologists now believe that the inhalation route, once thought to be theoretical, may be more common than previously believed. Human-to-human transmission of rabies is not known to occur; however, paramedics should take BSI precautions to protect themselves from contact with infectious saliva. The use of masks in environments where a patient has been exposed may be prudent, judging from the recent epidemiological evidence in the United States with bats.

When caring for a bite patient, first inspect the site of the wound for bite pattern and the presence of saliva. Then rinse the wound with copious amounts of normal saline to remove saliva and blood. Do not bandage or dress the wound, but allow it to drain freely during transport. Irrigation en route from a 10- or 15-drop/ml IV administration set may be beneficial. If the patient refuses transport to the emergency department, you must inform him of the consequences of the bite and the importance of medical follow up. If time and circumstances permit, ensure that the suspect animal has been secured and contained for transport to the hospital or animal control shelter for subsequent postmortem examination of cerebral tissue.

If you are bitten or exposed to an animal you believe is rabid, take the following measures:

1. Vigorously wash the wound with soap and warm water.
2. Debride and irrigate the wound, and allow it to drain freely on the way to the emergency department.

3. Discuss postexposure prophylaxis with the physician. Consultation with public health officials may be necessary. Unless you have an actual bite from an animal whose behavior is consistent with rabies infection, exposure is a medical urgency, not emergency.

4. Consider the need for tetanus and other antibiotic therapy as the attending physician deems appropriate.

Several alternatives now exist for rabies immunization. Individuals who should be immunized include animal care workers and shelter personnel, those who work outdoors and have frequent contact with wild animals known to transmit rabies.

Tetanus

* **tetanus** acute bacterial infection of the central nervous system.

Tetanus is an acute bacterial infection of the central nervous system. It presents with musculoskeletal signs and symptoms caused by tetanospasmin, an exotoxin of the *Clostridium tetani* bacillus. *C. tetani* is present as extremely durable spores in the soil, street dust, and feces and is in the same genus as *C. perfringens,* the causative organism of gas gangrene. Since *Clostridium* species favor an anaerobic environment, the bacteria are particularly suited to colonizing dead or necrotic tissue. Infection has been contracted through wounds considered too minor to warrant medical attention and through burns. Although puncture wounds are classically associated with *C. tetani* infection, deep lacerations can also be suitable environments. Transmission can even occur by injection of contaminated drugs and surgical procedures, leading to the conclusion that *C. tetani* spores are found everywhere. The incubation period is variable (usually from three to twenty-one days, sometimes from one day to several months) and depends on the wound's severity and location. Generally, a shorter incubation period leads to a more severe illness. The mortality rate increases in direct proportion to age. The general population is susceptible, but incidence is highest in agricultural areas where unimmunized people are in frequent contact with animal feces. The disease is rare in the United States, with fewer than 100 cases reported each year.

Localized tetanus symptoms include rigidity of muscles in close proximity to the injury site. Subsequent generalized symptoms may include pain and stiffness in the jaw muscles and may progress to cause muscle spasm and rigidity of the entire body. Respiratory arrest may result. In children, abdominal rigidity may be the first sign. Rigidity occurs after the toxin is taken up at the myoneural junction and transported to the CNS. The toxin then acts upon inhibitory neurons, which normally suppress unnecessary efferent impulses and muscle movements. The reduction in inhibitory action results in the muscles' receiving more nervous impulses and tetany. Sometimes a sardonic grin, *risus sardonicus,* accompanies the lock jaw and conjures memories of the Cheshire Cat in *Alice in Wonderland.*

EMS responders will rarely encounter this disease, much less recognize its signs and symptoms until they are advanced to the point of tetany. A possible EMS scenario would be the transfer of a patient from a rural community hospital to an urban medical center for intensive care. Universal precautions should provide adequate protection. Masks probably are not necessary unless the infectious agent is unknown. Respiratory arrest is a possibility, so you should consider wearing masks while performing endotracheal intubation. If you incur a wound in the course of treating a patient, wash the wound thoroughly or, if warranted, have it inspected and debrided in the emergency department. Wounds that are cared for within six hours pose a lower risk for growth of anaerobic microorganisms. Consideration should be given to post exposure prophylaxis with tetanus immune globulin (TIG), diphtheria-tetanus toxoid (Td), or diphtheria-tetanus toxoid, pertussis (DTP).

Immunizations, which generally begin in childhood as DTP vaccinations, include boosters before entering elementary school and every ten years thereafter. A booster administered every ten years is believed to confer effective active immunity. Previous documented infection is not known to confer lifelong immunity.

Lyme Disease

Lyme disease is a recurrent inflammatory disorder accompanied by skin lesions, polyarthritis, and involvement of the heart and nervous system. Caused by the tickborne spirochete *Borrelia burgdorferi,* similar in shape to the causative organism of syphilis, it is the most commonly reported vector-borne disease in the United States. The tick that carries Lyme disease is very common in the Northeast, the Upper Midwest, and along the Pacific Coast. Deer and mice are both reservoirs of the tick, and the disease is common in people living and recreating near wooded areas with high deer populations. Most infections occur in spring and summer, when tick exposure is most likely. Everyone is susceptible, and natural infection does not appear to confer immunity. The incubation period ranges from three to thirty-two days.

Lyme disease progresses in three stages:

- *Early Localized Stage* A painless, flat, red lesion appears at the bite site. In some patients, a ring-like rash, *erythema migrans (EM),* develops and spreads outward. The outer border remains bright red, with the center becoming clear, blue, or even necrotic. The rash—often called a "bull's eye" rash—usually disappears in time, whether treated or not. At this stage, patients also may complain of headache, malaise, and muscle aches. Although uncommon, the patient's neck may be stiff.

- *Early Disseminated Stage* The spirochete spreads to the skin, nervous system, heart, and joints. More EM lesions develop. CNS sequelae include meningitis, seventh-cranial-nerve Bell's palsy, and peripheral neuropathy. Cardiac abnormalities include conduction defects and myopathy. Arthritis and myalgia are common months after infection. Approximately 8 percent of patients will have some cardiac involvement. The most common manifestations are varying degrees of atrioventricular block (first degree, Wenckebach, and complete heart block). Less commonly, myocarditis and left ventricular dysfunction are seen. Cardiac involvement typically lasts only a few weeks, but can recur.

- *Late Stage (persistent infection)* The late stage can occur months or years after the initial exposure. Although the incidence of cardiac problems is lower, it involves the same neurological complications as second stage, plus encephalopathy with cognitive deficits, depression, and sleep disorders. Monoarthritis of large joints and more than one joint concurrently (polyarthritis) is common.

Development of erythema migrans, the bull's eye rash, usually 3 to 30 days after tick exposure, is presumptive for the diagnosis.

The EMS response to Lyme disease will probably be to treat its clinical consequences, especially those of the disseminated and late stages. ALS treatment is directed toward those consequences, not the infection. Adhere to universal precautions. After responding to calls in heavily wooded areas infested by ticks, always check both your and the patient's clothing, shoes, socks, and body for ticks. Spray the ambulance compartment with an insecticide effective against arthropods. Available antibiotic therapies are effective for the stages of the disease progression.

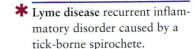

* **Lyme disease** recurrent inflammatory disorder caused by a tick-borne spirochete.

Content Review

STAGES OF LYME DISEASE
- Early localized
- Early disseminated
- Late

Content Review

SEXUALLY TRANSMITTED DISEASES

- Gonorrhea
- Syphilis
- Genital Warts
- Herpes simplex type 2
- Chlamydia
- Trichomoniasis
- Chancroid

✱ **sexually transmitted disease** (STD) illness most commonly transmitted through sexual contact.

✱ **gonorrhea** sexually transmitted disease caused by a gram-negative bacterium.

✱ **syphilis** blood-borne sexually transmitted disease caused by the spirochete *Treponema pallidum*.

Protection against Lyme disease (LYMErix) is now available as a series of three vaccinations, with the second dose given at one month and the third at twelve. It is recommended for persons aged 15–70 years whose activities result in frequent exposure to tick habitats, and for selected travelers to endemic areas where exposure to tick habitats is anticipated.

SEXUALLY TRANSMITTED DISEASES

Infectious diseases transmitted through sexual contact are known as **sexually transmitted diseases,** or **STDs.** They represent some of the most prevalent communicable diseases. A variety of bacterial (gonorrhea, syphilis, chancroid, chlamydia), viral (HIV, herpes), and parasitic (*Pediculosis, Trichomonas*) infections are spread by this route. Other illnesses that are generally not considered STDs, including hepatitis A, B, C, D, salmonella, and shigella, may also be transmitted through sexual contact. STDs affect the genital organs, often resulting in pathology to reproductive structures. Although EMS responders do not treat these diseases, other emergency health care personnel commonly know the information in the following profiles. Your knowledge of these diseases will put you on a "level playing field" with those other health care workers and bolster your credibility. When you treat or transport patients with STDs, observe universal precautions, avoid contact with lesions and exudates, and wash your hands vigorously after exposure.

Gonorrhea

Gonorrhea, caused by *Neisseria gonorrhoeae,* a gram-negative bacterium, is one of the most commonly diagnosed communicable diseases in the United States. Over one million cases are treated annually. Everyone is susceptible to infection, and although antibodies develop after exposure and confer immunity, they do so only for the specific serotype that caused the infection. Thus, persons contracting gonorrhea would not be immune to penicillinase-producing *N. gonorrhoeae* (PPNG), a strain of *N. gonorrhoeae* known by military personnel during the Vietnam War as black clap. Most commonly seen in males in their early twenties, gonorrhea is transmitted by direct contact with exudates of mucous membranes, primarily from direct sexual contact. In men, the disease presents as painful urination and a purulent urethral discharge. Untreated, it can lead to epididymitis, prostatitis, and urethral strictures. The majority of women contracting the disease have no pain and minimal discharge. In some cases, symptoms include urinary frequency, vaginal discharge, fever, and abdominal pain. Pelvic inflammatory disease (PID) often results after menstruation when bacteria spread from the cervix to the upper genital tract. Affected females are at increased risk for sterility, ectopic pregnancy, abscesses within reproductive structures, and peritonitis.

Gonorrhea may occasionally become systemic, causing sepsis or meningitis. Septic arthritis may result, presenting with fever, pain, swelling, and limited range of motion in one or two joints, sometimes leading to progressive deterioration. In the United States, single dosing is often effective in treating localized gonorrhea (genitourinary only). Treating systemic gonorrhea often involves additional chemotherapy. When gonorrhea infection coexists with chlamydial infections (as is estimated to occur in about 50 percent of gonorrhea patients), two-drug therapy is routinely advised. No immunization is available.

Syphilis

Syphilis is a disease caused by the spirochete *Treponema pallidum*. It is transmitted by direct contact with exudates from other syphilitic lesions of skin and mucous membranes, semen, blood, saliva, and vaginal discharges. It is therefore most commonly contracted through sexual intercourse but also may be transmitted by kissing or close contact with an open lesion. An estimated 30 percent of exposures result in infection. In congenital syphilis, infants contract the disease before birth from an infected mother. Everyone is susceptible to infection. Although the risk of transmission by blood transfusion or needle-stick injury is low, health care workers have been infected after physical examination involving manual contact with a lesion. A gradual immunity does develop after infection, but aggressive antimicrobial therapy may interfere with this natural antibody formation, especially during the primary and secondary stages.

Syphilis is characterized by lesions that may involve virtually any organ or tissue. It usually has cutaneous manifestations with frequent relapses, and it may remain latent for years. The incubation period is three weeks. Syphilis may occur in four stages, depending on how early and aggressively treatment is initiated:

Content Review

STAGES OF SYPHILIS
- Primary
- Secondary
- Latent
- Tertiary

- *Primary syphilis (first stage)* presents as a painless lesion, or chancre. In heterosexual men, the chancre is usually on the penis. In homosexual men, the chancre is often found on the anal canal, rectum, tongue, lips, or other point of entry. The chancre typically occurs three to six weeks after exposure. Nontender enlargement of regional lymph nodes may also occur.

- *Secondary syphilis (second stage),* or the bacteremic stage, begins five to six weeks after the chancre has healed. It is characterized by a maculopapular skin rash (small, red, flat lesions) on the palms and soles, condyloma latum (painless, wart-like lesions on warm, moist skin areas that are very infectious), and cutaneous infection in areas of hair growth causing loss of hair and/or eyebrows. These skin signs last for about six weeks. CNS disease (syphilitic meningitis) and arthritis may occur, as can infections of the eyes and kidneys.

- *Latent syphilis (third stage),* a period when symptoms improve or disappear completely, may last from months to many years. Twenty-five percent of cases may relapse with secondary stage symptoms; however, relapses usually do not occur after four years. Thirty-three percent of cases will progress to tertiary syphilis, and the rest will remain asymptomatic

- *Tertiary syphilis (fourth stage)* is the stage of syphilis that justifies its reputation as a "great imitator." Lesions with sharp borders, called gummas, may appear on skin and bones, causing a deep, gnawing pain. Cardiovascular syphilis may appear, usually ten years after the primary infection, resulting in aortic aneurysms that antibiotic therapy does not reverse. Neurosyphilis is diagnosed when there are neurological signs in seropositive patients. Meningitis may result, with possible spinal cord disease causing loss of reflexes, and reduced sensation of pain and temperature. The spirochetes can also invade the cerebral vessels, causing a stroke. A progressive dementia can also occur during this stage.

EMS responders may treat a variety of clinical complications of syphilis, often without being aware of infection as the primary etiology. ALS is directed toward treating the clinical presentation, which may include seizures, an acute onset of dementia, signs of a stroke, aortic aneurysm, or acute myocardial infarction. Avoid frequent contact with lesions on any part of the patient's body, and pay attention to handwashing technique after patient contact since *T. pallidum* is easily killed by heat, soap, and water.

For presumptive screening after exposure, rapid plasmin reagin (RPR) and venereal disease research labs (VDRL) tests are available. Because RPR or VDRL have fairly high rates of false-positive reactions, more specific tests should always follow. Treatment of primary syphilis is benzathine penicillin, with erythromycin and doxycycline (Vibramycin) as alternatives for patients allergic to penicillin. No immunization is available.

Genital Warts

Genital warts (condyloma acuminatum) are caused by the human papillomavirus (HPV), a DNA virus. To date, research has identified 70 HPV types, with most known to cause specific clinical manifestations. Some of the types known to cause genital warts are associated with cervical cancer. Genital warts are contagious and easily spread. In males, they generally appear as cauliflower-like, fleshy growths on the penis, anus, and mucosa of the anal canal. In females, they usually appear on the labial surfaces. Genital warts are sometimes difficult to distinguish from the condyloma latum seen in the secondary stage of syphilis. HPV has been implicated as a causative factor of cervical cancer in females.

Herpes Simplex Type 2

HSV-2 causes 70–90 percent of all genital herpes cases. Transmission is usually by sexual contact. Everyone is susceptible, but adolescents and young adults are most commonly afflicted. Neonates are often infected during passage down the birth canal. The prevalence of HSV-2 antibody, which does not confer immunity, is greater in lower socioeconomic groups and persons with multiple sex partners. The disease presents as vesicular lesions on the penis, anus, rectum, and mouth of the male depending on sexual activity. Females are sometimes asymptomatic, but can display lesions of the vagina, vulva, perineum, rectum, mouth, and cervix. Recurrent infections in females are often found on the vulva, buttocks, legs, and the perineum. Patients may present with fever and enlarged lymph nodes during the initial infection. Lesions may last up to several weeks before eventually crusting over and healing. The most serious consequence of HSV-2 infection is that painful lesions may recur periodically during the patient's lifetime, significantly diminishing quality of life. Recent evidence suggests that symptomatic treatment with the antiviral agent acyclovir orally, intravenously, or topically, may decrease the incidence of recurrences and lessen the severity of their symptoms. Other treatment alternatives include CO_2 laser removal, cryotherapy (freezing and removal) with liquid nitrogen, electrical cauterization, and interferon. Immunization is not currently available.

Chlamydia

* **chlamydia** group of intracellular parasites that cause sexually transmitted diseases.

Chlamydia is a genus of intracellular parasites most like gram-negative bacteria. Once thought to be viruses, the chlamydiae are now known to have an inner and outer membrane, to contain both DNA and RNA, and to be susceptible to numerous antibiotics. However, they lack peptidoglycan, a net of polysaccharides found in all true bacterial walls.

From the standpoint of STDs, *Chlamydia trachomatis* is the most clinically significant species, affecting the genital area, eyes, and respiratory system. Everyone is susceptible, and up to 25 percent of men may be carriers. *C. trachomatis* is responsible for roughly 50 percent of all cases of nongonococcal urethritis (NGU) in men, with dysuria and penile discharge common. It is transmitted by sexual activity and by hand-to-hand transfer of eye secretions, causing conjunctivitis. Internationally, this is the leading cause of preventable blindness. Because children are the major reservoir and the common use of infected linen can transmit chlamydia, child care center and school workers should exercise caution in handling blankets, sheets, and towels.

The symptoms are similar to gonorrhea's but less severe, often making the clinical differentiation difficult. In addition, the progression of disease in women is identical, with both causing a mucopurulent discharge that often accompanies cervicitis. Some women may have retrograde infections of the reproductive tract, causing pelvic inflammatory disease. Sterility may result. Newborns may be infected during passage through an infected birth canal, resulting in infant pneumonia or blindness.

No immunization is available, but *C. trachomatis* infection responds to a variety of antimicrobial agents such as tetracycline, doxycycline (Vibramycin), erythromycin (PCE), and orally administered azithromycin (Zithromax). Natural infection is not known to confer immunity.

Another species of Chlamydia, *C. pneumoniae*, has been found in atherosclerotic lesions of patients who have died of myocardial infarction. This has led to speculation about the relationship between *C. pneumoniae* infection and atherosclerosis as an inflammatory process.

Trichomoniasis

Trichomonas vaginalis, a protozoan parasite, is a common cause of vaginitis. In women, the symptoms of **trichomoniasis** include a greenish-yellow vaginal discharge, irritation of the perineum and thighs, and dysuria. This disease is frequently present with gonorrhea. Men are generally asymptomatic carriers of the disease. When present, symptoms include dysuria, urethral discharge, and discomfort in the perineum. The infection is currently treated with metronidazole (Flagyl).

* **trichomoniasis** sexually transmitted disease caused by the protozoan *Trichomonas vaginalis*.

Chancroid

Chancroid is a highly contagious ulcer caused by *Haemophilus ducreyi*, a gram-negative bacterium. It is more frequently diagnosed in men, particularly those who have sex with prostitutes. Uncircumcised men are at higher risk. It is spread by direct contact, mostly sexual, with open lesions and pus. Autoinoculation has occurred in infected persons. Its incubation period is typically 3–5 days but may be as long as 14 days.

* **chancroid** highly contagious sexually transmitted ulcer.

The disease begins with a painful, inflamed pustule or ulcer that may appear on the penis, anus, urethra, or vulva. It spreads easily to other sites such as breasts, fingers, and thighs. Lymph nodes may become swollen and tender, and fever may be present. Chancroid ulcer is linked with increased risk of HIV infection. Chancroid lesions in children beyond the neonatal period should alert EMS responders to the possibility of reportable child sexual abuse.

Health care workers have contracted the disease by contacting patients' ulcers. Immunization is not available, and infection does not appear to confer immunity. Several effective antimicrobials (for example, erythromycin) are available.

DISEASES OF THE SKIN

EMS responders' interactions with patients or the general public may expose them to contagious skin infections such as impetigo or the ectoparasites lice and scabies. Because the public frequently attempts to consult paramedics about general topics in personal and community health, your knowledge of ectoparasites may enable you to provide education and customer service. As always, use universal precautions and effective postexposure hand washing.

Content Review

DISEASES OF THE SKIN
- Impetigo
- Lice
- Scabies

Impetigo

impetigo infection of the skin caused by staphylococci or streptococci.

Impetigo is a very contagious infection of the skin caused by staphylococci or streptococci. The disease begins as a single vesicle that ruptures and forms a thick, honey-colored crust with a yellowish-red center. Lesions most commonly occur on the extremities and joints. Although few patients call an ambulance for this condition, it often appears on patients who seek EMS for other reasons. EMS responders who develop impetigo should not report for work until cleared by their physician. It is easily transmitted by direct skin-to-skin contact, so universal precautions should provide ample protection.

Lice

lice parasitic infestation of the skin of the scalp, trunk, or pubic area.

infestation presence of parasites that do not break the host's skin.

Lice (pediculosis) is a parasitic **infestation** of the skin of the scalp, trunk, or pubic area. Lice infest hosts rather than infect them because they do not break the skin. The three different varieties of infestations are *Pediculus humanus var. capitis* (head lice), *Pediculus humanus var. corporis* (body lice), and *Pthirus pubis* (pubic lice, or crabs). Historically, head lice have been involved in outbreaks of typhus, trench fever in World War I, and relapsing fever. Head and body lice appear similar, both being 3–4 mm long. Head lice are transmitted by sharing of combs or hats and are fairly common among young school-aged children regardless of socioeconomic status. Outbreaks in day care centers and schools are common. Head lice are easily diagnosed by the presence of small, white, oval-shaped eggs (nits) attached to the hair shafts. Nits can be seen with the naked eye but are more easily found with a magnifying glass. Lice themselves are rarely seen. They tend to leave febrile hosts, so high environmental temperatures and crowding favor transmission. Lice have a three-stage life cycle of eggs, nymphs, and adults. Eggs hatch in 7–10 days but cannot hatch below 72°F. The nymph stage lasts about 7–13 days, again depending on temperature, with a total egg to egg cycle of 3 weeks.

Anyone can be infested, and repeated infestations may cause an allergic response. Infestation often occurs on eyebrows and eyelashes, hair, mustaches, and beards. Symptoms are generally limited to severe itching. Body lice often infest clothing along seams close to skin surfaces and attach to the skin only to feed. They can be vectors of bacteria. Red macules, papules, and urticaria commonly appear on the shoulders, buttocks, and abdomen. Pubic lice infest through sexual contact by attaching to hair in the genital and anal regions but can also infest facial hair.

Any EMS responder exposed to a patient with lice may be treated with one of several nonprescription agents. Pyrethrin preparations such as RID are commonly used, but require two applications one week apart because they do not kill eggs. Permethrin agents such as Nix or Elimite theoretically require only a single application because they kill adults and eggs. Lindane 1% shampoo (Kwell) may be used, but it is available only by prescription and is more toxic than the other treatments. Eliminating the eggs by combing the hair is essential. Nits are more easily removed (nit picking) after soaking combs in a white vinegar solution or using a commercial preparation such as the Step 2 Nit Removal System. Separately bagging linen in an occupational setting is unnecessary. At home, however, isolating infested linen and clothing is advisable to avoid exposing uninfested laundry for extended periods. Lice are not known to jump great distances like fleas, so spraying the ambulance's interior close to the cot and the area by the patient's head with an insecticide, preferably one containing premethrin, should be sufficient after a call. Clean and wipe all sprayed areas to remove insecticide residues.

Scabies

Scabies is caused by infestation of a mite (*Sarcoptes scabiei*) that is barely visible without magnification. Exposure to the mite is through close personal contact, from hand holding to sexual relations. The mite can remain viable on clothing or in bedding for up to 48 hours.

Upon attaching to a new host, the female tunnels into the skin within 2.5 minutes and lays up to three eggs a day along the "burrow" in the epidermis. The larvae hatch shortly thereafter, leading to a full grown adult 10 to 20 days later. The adults remain near hair follicles and forage for nourishment with their jaws and the claws of their forelegs.

The primary symptom is intense itching (hence the name "seven-year itch"), usually at night. It generally occurs from two to six weeks after infestation. The irritation results from sensitization to the mite and its droppings. Inflammatory lesions appear as fine, wavy, dark lines, usually not more than one centimeter long. In males they most commonly occur on the webs of the fingers, wrists, elbows, armpits, belt line, thighs, and external genitalia. In females, they most often involve the areolae and nipples, abdomen, and lower portions of the buttocks. In infants, the head, neck, palms, and soles are frequently involved. Older children exhibit patterns similar to adults. Complications are generally due to infections of lesions that are broken by scratching.

Although everyone is susceptible to infection, immunocompromised patients sometimes develop Norwegian scabies, a more severe form of scabies. Persons with previous exposure appear to have fewer mites on subsequent exposures and develop symptoms much sooner (in from one to four days), suggesting an amnestic (remembered) immune system response. Outbreaks of scabies resistant to lindane (Kwell) have been reported in several nursing homes across the country.

Scabies remains communicable until all mites and eggs are destroyed. Because of the long incubation period, all household members and/or close contacts of infested EMS responders should be treated simultaneously. Although some experts recommend that clothing and uniforms worn within two days of treatment, along with towels and bed linen, should be washed in hot water or dry cleaned, this necessity is questionable for most infestations. It is essential, however, for articles contacting patients with Norwegian scabies. Bag and remove all linens from the ambulance immediately after you deliver the patient. To prevent spread of the mite, clean the stretcher and patient compartment as recommended for lice. Remove and decontaminate any clothing that may have contacted the patient.

The scabicides of choice are premethrin cream (Elimite) or lindane (Kwell), which is applied to the skin from the neck down, left on for 8 to 14 hours, and then washed off. This should be repeated within one week. If premethrin is ineffective, 10% crotamiton (Eurax) and ivermectin (Stromectol) are also available.

Nosocomial Infections

Hospitalized patients, especially those with compromised immune function, often acquire new infectious diseases. Especially virulent strains of microorganisms may cause these **nosocomial** (hospital acquired) diseases. Bacteria that resist antibiotics are of particular concern. Recently, vancomycin-resistant enterococcus (VRE) and methicillin-resistant *Staphylococcus aureus* (MRSA) have become especially alarming. Both of these organisms can cause severe host damage, and both are difficult to treat. They rapidly colonize patients in whom broad-spectrum antibiotics have eliminated normal flora. Hospitalized patients may also contract resistant strains of tuberculosis that spread easily from patient to patient if protective clothing and hand-washing precautions are not strictly observed.

* **scabies** skin disease caused by mite infestation and characterized by intense itching.

* **nosocomial** acquired while in the hospital.

PATIENT EDUCATION

In spite of increased emphasis in public education and extensive media attention in recent years, a lack of understanding of infectious diseases remains widespread among the public. The one exception may be HIV, due to its extensive and relatively objective media exposure. Media coverage of other infectious diseases such as hantavirus, Ebola, "flesh-eating bacteria," and others has been so sensational that it has accomplished little from an educational perspective and, in some cases, has spread misinformation and created undue fear.

As with more publicized topics in emergency medicine such as trauma and substance abuse, prevention is without question the most effective intervention in preventing transmission of infectious diseases. The key to effective prevention is education; however, because these diseases are less "glamorous" than other illnesses, attracting public attention is difficult, and influencing behavior poses a formidable challenge. Paramedics have an opportunity to assume a leadership role in this area. EMS personnel are often active in public and community education and are ideally positioned to influence the public's behavior. CPR and first aid classes offer a platform to also introduce and discuss issues related to disease transmission. Leading by example is extremely important. Paramedics, especially those working in rural and suburban areas, reflect the general community. They are in close contact with the people they serve, and are well respected in their communities. Taking an active part in public disease-prevention education will be among your most important roles as a paramedic.

Many of the diseases covered in this chapter are not emergencies and may not require emergency treatment. As out-of-hospital emergency medicine evolves from vocation to profession, however, it will require more education and greater knowledge in these areas. Infectious diseases' serious personal and public health implications require you to be knowledgeable in this area and take the lead in educating others.

PREVENTING DISEASE TRANSMISSION

Preventing or limiting exposure to infectious or communicable diseases cannot be overemphasized. While some infectious diseases are relatively minor with no long-term effects, others can be very serious and even life threatening. As a paramedic, you must be extremely vigilant during patient contact and take every step possible to ensure your health and safety. Personal accountability is important.

Do not go to work if you:

- Have diarrhea
- Have a draining wound or any type of wet lesions. Allow them to dry and crust over before returning to work.
- Are jaundiced
- Have mononucleosis
- Have been exposed to lice or scabies and have not yet been treated
- Have strep throat and have not been taking antibiotics for at least 24 hours
- Have a cold

Keep the following immunizations current: MMR, hepatitis A (if deemed appropriate in your jurisdiction), hepatitis B, DPT, polio, chickenpox, influenza (seasonal), and rabies (if appropriate).

Prevention is without question the best approach to infectious disease.

Infectious diseases have serious personal and public health implications; therefore, you must be knowledgeable in this area and take the lead in educating others.

As a paramedic, you must be extremely vigilant during your patient contact to take every step possible to ensure your health and safety.

Always approach the scene cautiously with a high index of suspicion. Upon arrival, control the scene to decrease the likelihood of body fluid exposure for everyone present. Observe BSI. Always wear gloves. If there is the remotest possibility of splashing or aerosolization of body fluids, wear protective eyewear or a mask with face shield. If large volumes of blood or other fluids may result from the response, don a gown. When contacting a patient who has or may have active TB, wear the appropriate N95 respirator.

Patients who have coughs, fever, headache, general weakness, recent weight loss, or nuchal rigidity or are taking certain medications may raise your awareness of the potential for contracting an infectious agent. With experience, you will develop your intuition and associate certain symptoms with infectious patients you have treated. Bolster your experience by increasing your knowledge, particularly your clinical acumen in recognizing the immunocompromised patient.

After a call, wash your hands first. Decontaminate and disinfect your equipment and the interior of the ambulance. Using commercially available disinfectants that certify bactericidal activity against *M. tuberculosis* should provide ample disinfection of those infectious agents that pose your greatest occupational risk. Remember that HIV is a fragile virus that any vigorous application of soap and water will kill. Utilize high-level disinfection on airway equipment. If the patient or the situation surrounding the response presents the possibility of lice, scabies, or ticks, spray the gurney and interior of the ambulance with the appropriate insecticide and wipe or mop up any residue. Ensure that linen will not be taken home. If practical, do not wear uniforms home. To discourage that practice, some EMS agencies consider uniforms as PPE. Report any infectious exposure to the IDCO, human resources director, or appropriate designated official.

The topics mandated by OSHA/NIOSH for compliance with published standards and guidelines (that is, bloodborne pathogens and TB) reflect the paramedic's minimum needed knowledge of infectious diseases. Proactive EMS agencies offer their personnel continuing education in infectious diseases that have high incidence or prevalence in the communities they serve. Continuing education sessions should include identification of causative agents, modes of transmission, epidemiological patterns within the community, signs and symptoms, methods to avoid infection, and special postexposure considerations, including postexposure prophylaxis, if appropriate.

To maintain a perspective on personal risk, always consider the interaction of three major factors: infectious agent, host, and environment. Are you aware of the infectious agent's virulence? Do you have some idea of the dose of the organism involved? For example, was a large volume of body fluid involved? How healthy are you? Do you have any chronic medical conditions or take any medications that would classify you as immunocompromised? What was the nature of the exposure? Is it significantly high? The probability of risk is sometimes just a measure of exposure. Not all infectious diseases are communicable. If they are communicable, they may not necessarily pose a high probability of developing disease. The risk and potential for HIV transmission to health care workers may be high, but the probability of transmission, which averages approximately 0.3 percent, is very low.

As you are promoted within your organization, your first additional responsibility may be as a preceptor for a new paramedic or student. You therefore assume responsibility for his well being. Are you familiar with your local protocols and procedures for reporting and recording an exposure? Can you adequately document the circumstances surrounding the exposure to facilitate review by the IDCO, physician, or agency administrator? If you cannot, what kind of a role model are you for that new employee or student?

Paramedics cannot allow their personal prejudices to interfere with providing optimum care for their patients. Patients should not be treated differently because they have an infectious disease that might reflect on their ethnicity, culture, sexual preference, or social status. You should not avoid certain procedures because you find a disease process or its consequences personally repulsive. It is sometimes helpful to think about doing things *for* patients, as opposed to doing things *to* them.

Paramedics work in a profession fraught with uncertainty. They make clinical decisions based upon limited data. They rarely deal with infectious disease emergencies but must constantly and consistently be vigilant to protect themselves, their patients, and other responders. The exposures are often unknown and involve intangible infectious agents. Thus, universal precautions, which are EMS practice standards, are predicated on the possibility that all body fluids, in any situation, are infectious. Adhering to those standards will markedly decrease your risk of occupational infection.

All body fluids are possibly infectious. Universal precautions should be followed at all times

SUMMARY

Over the past thirty years, medical science has made tremendous progress in diagnosing and treating infectious diseases. New vaccines and antibiotics are continually being developed. Advances in laboratory technology, notably the polymerase chain reaction (PCR), have made the presence and identification of microorganisms easier, quicker, and more accurate. Despite these tremendous advances, many infectious diseases cannot be effectively treated. Specific treatments for most viral diseases remain elusive, and each year countless people die from AIDS, hepatitis, pneumonia, sexually transmitted diseases, and other infectious diseases.

EMS can have a significant impact upon the incidence of infectious disease if providers remain knowledgeable, are leaders in public education, and are consistently alert in protecting themselves and their patients. The title of the International Association of Fire Fighters (IAFF) hepatitis B curriculum, *The Silent War,* provides a metaphor for the dilemma of infectious diseases in EMS: EMS personnel deal with few infectious disease emergencies; however, when we do respond to such emergencies, we often are unaware of the disease's presence until after the call. Standard (universal) precautions, often written for clinical and research facilities with more predictable hazards and risks, are increased to body substance isolation (BSI) for emergency health care providers because of the uncertainties of our profession. Constant vigilance and personal accountability are the keys to reducing those risks.

YOU MAKE THE CALL

Early on a wintry December morning, you and your partner, Dennis Murphy, respond to a call for a 27-year-old male patient complaining of shortness of breath and weakness. Upon your arrival at the scene, you discover a frail, emaciated male lying in bed. A registered nurse is caring for him. The RN tells you that the young man has AIDS and has been ill for several weeks, worsening over the past three hours. He is reluctant to accept transportation to the hospital but feels he has no choice.

Wearing latex gloves, you and your partner approach the victim. He immediately says, "What's the deal with the gloves? You can't catch it that way! Nobody wants to even touch me anymore!" Surprised, you explain that the need for the gloves exists with every patient and that it is for his protection as well as yours.

An initial assessment reveals that the patient has a patent airway, labored respirations of 22, and a heart rate of 100/regular. You place the patient on high-flow oxygen via a nonrebreather mask. Pulse oximetry reading prior to oxygen is 87%. Temperature is 101°F. The patient has a peripheral in-dwelling catheter that was placed by his physician. As you consult with the RN, you determine that you will have to ask medical direction for approval to access the peripheral catheter and provide the patient with hydrating fluids. As soon as you have contacted medical direction, you plan to transport the patient to the nearest emergency facility.

1. What essential BSI precautions should you take?
2. What are your primary concerns for this patient?
3. How would your care or BSI precautions differ for patients without AIDS?

See Suggested Responses at the back of this book.

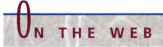

FURTHER READING

Benenson, Abram S., ed. *Control of Communicable Diseases Manual.* 16th ed. Washington, D.C.: American Public Health Association, 1995.

Brillman, Judith C. and Ronald W. Quenzer. *Infectious Disease in Emergency Medicine.* 2nd ed. Philadelphia: Lippincott, Williams, and Wilkins, 1998.

Brooks, Geo. F., Janet S. Butel, and Stephen A. Morse. *Jawetz, Melnick, and Adelberg's Medical Microbiology.* 21st ed. Stanford, Conn.: Appleton and Lange, 1998.

Ewald, Paul W. *Evolution of Infectious Disease.* New York: Oxford University Press, 1994.

Gates, Robert H. *Infectious Disease Secrets.* Philadelphia, Pa.: Hanley and Belfus, 1998.

Gorbach, Sherwood, John Bartlett, and Neil Blacklow. *Infectious Diseases.* 2nd ed. Philadelphia: Saunders, 1998.

Isada, Carlos M., et. al. *Infectious Diseases Handbook.* 3rd ed. Hudson, Oh.: Lexi-Comp Inc., 1999.

Isselbacher, Kurt J., et al. *Harrison's Principles of Internal Medicine.* 14th ed. New York: McGraw-Hill, 1998.

Manian, Farrin A. *Mosby's Curbside Clinician: Infectious Diseases.* St. Louis: Mosby, 1998.

ON THE WEB

Visit Brady's Paramedic Website at www.bradybooks.com/paramedic.

CHAPTER 12

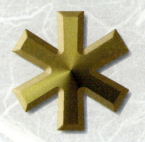

Psychiatric and Behavioral Disorders

Objectives

After reading this chapter, you should be able to:

1. Define behavior and distinguish among normal behavior, abnormal behavior, and the behavioral emergency. (pp. 608–609)
2. Discuss the prevalence of behavioral and psychiatric disorders. (p. 609)
3. Discuss the pathophysiology of behavioral and psychiatric disorders. (pp. 609–610)
4. Discuss the factors that may alter the behavioral or emotional status of an ill or injured individual. (pp. 609–610)
5. Describe the medical legal considerations for management of emotionally disturbed patients. (pp. 627–628)

6. Describe the overt behaviors associated with behavioral and psychiatric disorders. (pp. 614–625)
7. Define the following terms:
   - Affect (p. 611)
   - Anger (p. 617)
   - Anxiety (pp. 616–617)
   - Confusion (p. 611)
   - Depression (pp. 618–619)
   - Fear (p. 611)
   - Mental status (p. 611)
   - Open-ended question (p. 612)
   - Posture (p. 611)
8. Describe verbal techniques useful in managing the emotionally disturbed patient. (pp. 611–613)

Continued

Objectives Continued

9. List the appropriate measures to ensure the safety of the paramedic, the patient, and others. (pp. 610–612, 627–631)
10. Describe the circumstances when relatives, bystanders, and others should be removed from the scene. (p. 611)
11. Describe techniques to systematically gather information from the disturbed patient. (pp. 611–613, 627)
12. Identify techniques for physical assessment in a patient with behavioral problems. (pp. 611–613, 627–631)
13. List situations in which you are expected to transport a patient forcibly and against his will. (pp. 627–631)
14. Describe restraint methods necessary in managing the emotionally disturbed patient. (pp. 628–631)
15. List the risk factors and behaviors that indicate a patient is at risk for suicide. (p. 624)
16. Use the assessment and patient history to differentiate between the various behavioral and psychiatric disorders. (pp. 610–625)
17. Given several preprogrammed behavioral emergency patients, provide the appropriate scene size-up, initial assessment, focused assessment, and detailed assessment, then provide the appropriate care and patient transport. (pp. 608–631)

CASE STUDY

On a hot August night, paramedic ambulance crew Kelly Underwood and Charles Bear have been dispatched to a possible psychiatric emergency at a local supermarket. They carefully approach the scene and observe a man standing in front of the store with his back to them. The manager approaches the ambulance and tells Kelly and Charles that the man came to the store and announced that the produce was poisonous. The manager also warns them that the man's behavior is somewhat bizarre. The man turns and begins shouting loudly, "Don't come in here! They're selling poison. They're trying to kill us all!" Charles radios for police assistance. He and Kelly remain in the ambulance and observe the patient until police arrive.

When the police arrive, Kelly quickly briefs them on the situation and the patient's status. The officers recognize the man as a psychiatric patient with whom they have recently had contact at a local motel. The man begins yelling and says he is working for the government. He yells at the top of his voice, "We'll close this place down!" The police ask Kelly and Charles to prepare the stretcher and restraints as a precaution. As the police approach the man, he calls them "poisoners." His agitation continues to escalate despite the efforts of the crew and officers to calm him. It becomes obvious that restraint is

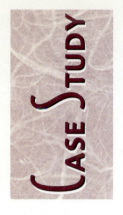

needed. The officers make the initial approach and control the patient's arms. Kelly is able to safely control the man's legs while Charles moves the stretcher into place. After moving the patient to the stretcher, they restrain his arms and legs using wide roller bandages. Kelly performs an assessment to rule out medical or traumatic causes of the patient's altered mental status. He monitors the man carefully en route to the emergency department. From there the patient is eventually transferred to the psychiatric center.

INTRODUCTION

Many of the topics you have studied up to this point have had objective diagnostic criteria. For example, you know that a tachycardia is a heart rate of over 100 beats per minute, and a bradycardia is a rate of under 60. Behavioral and psychiatric emergencies, however, are not so clear-cut. Nonetheless, they include patient presentations that require a complete patient history, physical exam, and a skilled approach to the situation.

Another significant difference between behavioral and psychiatric conditions and other types of medical emergencies is that most of your assessment and care will depend on your people skills. You can evaluate a bradycardia with a cardiac monitor and treat it with atropine or a pacing unit. You provide psychological care for the cardiac patient to reduce anxiety and offer emotional support. You evaluate the psychiatric patient, on the other hand, by observing his behavior, by gathering information from his family and bystanders, and by interviewing him. Your care, which includes support, calming reassurance, and occasionally restraint, requires interpersonal skills more than diagnostic equipment.

BEHAVIORAL EMERGENCIES

✱ **behavior** a person's observable conduct and activity.

✱ **behavioral emergency** situation in which a patient's behavior becomes so unusual that it alarms the patient or another person and requires intervention.

Behavior is a person's observable conduct and activity. A **behavioral emergency** is a situation in which a patient's behavior becomes so unusual, bizarre, threatening, or dangerous that it alarms the patient or another person such as a family member or bystander and requires the intervention of emergency service and/or mental health personnel.

Notice that the definition of behavioral emergency does not use the word *abnormal*. Saying that a behavioral emergency involves "abnormal behavior" would be easy, but the differentiation between normal and abnormal is largely subjective. What is normal varies based on culture, ethnic group, socioeconomic class, and personal interpretation and opinion. What one person considers normal, another might consider highly abnormal. Generally, however, normal behavior can be defined as behavior that is readily acceptable in a society.

Objective factors that may indicate a behavioral or psychological condition include actions or situations that

- Interfere with core life functions (eating, sleeping, ability to maintain housing, interpersonal or sexual relations)

- Pose a threat to the life or well-being of the patient or others
- Significantly deviate from society's expectations or norms

We will discuss specific diseases and conditions later in the chapter.

PATHOPHYSIOLOGY OF PSYCHIATRIC DISORDERS

Experts estimate that up to 20 percent of the population has some type of mental health problem and that as many as one person in seven will actually require treatment for an emotional disturbance. These problems may be severely disabling and require inpatient care, or the patient may quietly tolerate them with no outward symptoms. That all people with psychiatric conditions exhibit bizarre or unusual behavior is a misconception. The small percentage of patients with psychiatric disorders who publicly exhibit bizarre behavior tends to create this misconception among lay people. In reality, most patients who suffer from disorders such as anxiety, depression, eating disorders, or mild personality disorders function normally on a daily basis, going unnoticed in society. Nonetheless, behavioral and psychiatric disorders incapacitate more people than all other health problems combined. Most patients with mental illness are cared for in outpatient settings such as public mental health centers. Only those with severe psychiatric illnesses remain institutionalized. Because of this, EMS providers are increasingly being called to care for patients with behavioral complaints. A common reason for EMS intervention in psychiatric illness is patients' failure to take their psychiatric medications. When mental health patients such as schizophrenics begin to deteriorate and develop bizarre behavior, more often than not they have not been adhering to their psychiatric medication regimen.

Another common misconception is that all mental patients are unstable and dangerous and that their conditions are incurable. This is simply not true. Research in psychiatry, like other areas in medicine, has made great strides in determining causes and treatments for many psychiatric conditions. Suffering from a mental disorder is not reason for embarrassment or shame, although society often stigmatizes these patients unfairly. The general causes of behavioral emergencies are biological (or organic), psychosocial, and sociocultural. Each of these three possible causes should guide your questioning during the patient interview. Keep in mind, however, that a patient's condition may result from more than one pathological process.

BIOLOGICAL

For many years, medical practitioners have used the terms *biological* and *organic* interchangeably when discussing certain types of psychiatric disorders whose causes are physical rather than purely psychological. They result from disease processes such as infections and tumors or from structural changes in the brain such as those brought on by the abuse of alcohol or drugs (including over-the-counter and prescription medications). It could be argued, however, that even purely psychological conditions originate in the brain and for that very reason are organic. Indeed, many psychiatric conditions do originate from alterations in brain chemistry.

Behavioral emergencies frequently involve biological conditions. Never assume a patient with an altered mental status or unusual behavior is suffering

Most patients who suffer from disorders such as anxiety, depression, eating disorders, or mild personality disorders function normally on a daily basis, going unnoticed in society.

Content Review

GENERAL CAUSES OF BEHAVIORAL EMERGENCIES
Biological (organic)
Psychosocial (personal)
Social (situational)

* **biological/organic** related to disease processes or structural changes.

Never assume a patient with an altered mental status or unusual behavioral is suffering from a purely psychological condition or disease until you have completely ruled out medical conditions and substance abuse.

from a purely psychological condition or disease until you have completely ruled out medical conditions and substance abuse.

PSYCHOSOCIAL

* **psychosocial** related to a patient's personality style, dynamics of unresolved conflict, or crisis management methods.

Psychosocial (personal) conditions are related to a patient's personality style, dynamics of unresolved conflict, or crisis management methods. These disorders are not attributable to substance abuse or medical conditions.

Environment plays a large part in psychosocial development. Traumatic childhood incidents may affect a person throughout life. Parents or other persons in positions of authority can have a tremendous impact on a child's development. Dysfunctional families, abusive parents, alcohol or drug abuse by parents, or neglect can cause behavioral problems from childhood through adulthood. Such conditions, in addition to—or in combination with genetic predisposition and brain chemistry—form the basis for psychosocial conditions.

SOCIOCULTURAL

* **sociocultural** related to the patient's actions and interactions within society.

Sociocultural (situational) causes of behavioral disorders are related to the patient's actions and interactions within society and to factors such as socioeconomic status, social habits, social skills, and values. These problems are usually attributable to events that change the patient's social space (relationships, support systems), social isolation, or otherwise have an impact on socialization.

Some events in the lives of children and adults that may cause a profound psychological change are rape, assault, witnessing the victimization of another, death of a loved one, and acts of violence such as war or riots. Events that occur over time may also have an impact on the individual. These include the loss of a job, economic problems such as poverty, and ongoing prejudice or discrimination. Sometimes simply doing anything outside the norms of society can lead to stress and psychological changes.

ASSESSMENT OF BEHAVIORAL EMERGENCY PATIENTS

The assessment and care of behavioral emergency patients is similar to that for other medical conditions. The order of assessment (scene size-up, initial assessment, focused history and physical examination) remains unchanged. Potential medical conditions that mimic behavioral emergencies require you to perform a thorough medical assessment.

Among the differences between your assessment and care of a patient with a medical condition and one with a behavioral emergency is that, as already noted, you actually begin your care at the same time you begin your assessment by developing a rapport with the patient. Interpersonal skills are important for all patients, but perhaps never more than for one who is experiencing a behavioral emergency. Additionally, the focused history and physical exam for a behavioral emergency includes a mental status examination.

SCENE SIZE-UP

As with any call, determining scene safety is of the utmost importance. Approach the scene carefully. If a patient is experiencing a behavioral emergency that is significant enough to warrant EMS, it is most likely significant enough to have law enforcement authorities respond. Most patients experiencing behavioral emer-

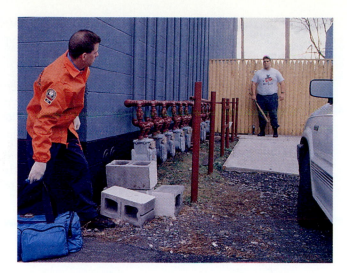

FIGURE 12-1 Approach every patient cautiously. If you determine a potential for violence, request police assistance.

gencies or crises will not attack you; however, those who are behaving unusually, experiencing hallucinations or delusions, or are under the effect of a substance may become violent. Approach every patient cautiously to protect yourself and your crew from injury (Figure 12-1).

The scene size-up also includes making observations that relate to patient care. Look for evidence of substance use or abuse, for therapeutic medications that may indicate an underlying medical condition (or abuse of that medication), and for signs of violence or destruction of property. Examine the general environmental condition and, when possible, observe the patient from a distance to note any visible behavior patterns or violent behavior.

Approach every patient cautiously to protect yourself and your crew from injury.

INITIAL ASSESSMENT

Because many behavioral emergencies are caused by or concurrent with medical conditions, you should be acutely suspicious of life-threatening emergencies. As with any other injury or condition, assess the ABCs and intervene when necessary. Continue to observe the patient for any clues to his underlying condition. Be cautious of any overt behavior such as **posture** or hand gestures. Note any emotional response such as rage, **fear,** anxiety, **confusion,** or anger. Early in the evaluation try to determine the patient's **mental status,** the state of his cerebral functioning. Continue assessing mental status throughout the patient encounter by evaluating his awareness, orientation, cognitive abilities, and **affect** (visible indicators of mood).

Control the scene as soon as possible. Remove anyone who agitates the patient or adds confusion to the scene. Generally, a limited number of people around the patient is best. At times, performing an effective assessment and care may necessitate totally clearing a room or moving the patient to a quiet area. Finally, observe the patient's affect in greater detail. To avoid being grabbed or struck by the patient, stay alert for signs of aggression.

✱ **posture** position, attitude, or bearing of the body.

✱ **fear** feeling of alarm and discontentment in the expectation of danger.

✱ **confusion** state of being unclear or unable to make a decision easily.

✱ **mental status** the state of the patient's cerebral functioning.

✱ **affect** visible indicators of mood.

FOCUSED HISTORY AND PHYSICAL EXAMINATION

Your examination of a patient experiencing a behavioral emergency is largely conversational. This makes your interpersonal technique very important. Just as starting an IV with poor technique most likely will not establish a patent IV line, interviewing with poor interpersonal skills most likely will not obtain significant

Stay alert for signs of aggression.

information. Remove the patient from the crisis area and limit interruptions. Focus your questioning and assessment on the immediate problem and follow these guidelines:

- *Listen.* Ask open-ended questions (those that require more than a yes or no response). These will encourage your patient to respond in detail and share important information. Listen to the answer. Pay attention. No one likes being ignored. When you need information from a patient, listen.

- *Spend time.* Rushing the patient's answers, cutting him off, or appearing hurried will cause him to "shut down" and stop answering questions.

- *Be assured.* Communicate self-confidence, honesty, and professionalism.

- *Do not threaten.* Avoid rapid or sudden movements or questions that the patient might interpret as threats. Approach him slowly and confidently.

- *Do not fear silence.* Silence can be appropriate. Encourage the patient to tell his or her story, but do not be forceful or antagonizing.

- *Place yourself at the patient's level.* Standing over the patient may be intimidating. Unless you are intentionally attempting to gain a position of authority, crouch, kneel, or sit near the patient. Do not position yourself where you cannot respond appropriately to danger or attack.

- *Keep a safe and proper distance.* The surest way to make a behavioral emergency patient violent is to invade his "personal space" (Figure 12-2). This is an area within an approximately three-foot radius around every person; encroaching upon it causes anxiety. If appropriate, however, you may touch the patient's shoulder or use another consoling touch when he allows.

- *Appear comfortable.* Do not appear uncomfortable—even if you are. Talking to patients about suicide, self-mutilation, or other psychological conditions is difficult. If the patient sees that you are uncomfortable, however, he is unlikely to open up to you. Would you expect a patient to tell you his reasons for attempting suicide when you appear uncomfortable even saying the word? To help, use terms the patient has used. If he says he wanted to "end it all," begin with that. Caregivers

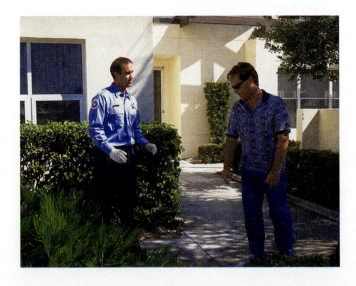

FIGURE 12-2 Avoid invading the patient's personal space, the area within about three feet of the patient.

sometimes hesitate to use the word *suicide* because it might give the patient ideas of suicide. If you are there to care for a suicidal or potentially suicidal patient, however, he has already had those thoughts.

- *Avoid appearing judgmental.* Patients who are experiencing behavioral emergencies may feel strong emotions toward their caregivers. The patient should believe that you are interested in his condition and welfare. Be supportive and empathetic, and avoid judgments, pity, anger, or any other emotions that may damage your relationship with the patient.

- *Never lie to the patient.* Honesty is the best policy. Do not reinforce false beliefs or hallucinations or mislead the patient in any way.

MENTAL STATUS EXAMINATION

As part of the focused history and physical examination for behavioral emergencies, do not overlook any physical or medical complaint. In addition to the medical evaluation, which is covered in depth throughout this and the other volumes of this program, your examination of the patient with psychiatric or behavioral disorders should include a psychological evaluation, also known as a **mental status examination** (MSE). The components of the MSE include:

✱ mental status examination (MSE), a structured exam designed to quickly evaluate a patient's level of mental functioning.

- *General Appearance.* The patient's appearance can provide important information when looking at his "big picture." Observe hygiene, clothing, and overall appearance.

- *Behavioral Observations.* Observe verbal or nonverbal behavior, strange or threatening appearance, or facial expressions. Note tone of voice, rate, volume, and quality.

- *Orientation.* Does the patient know who he is and who others are? Is he oriented to current events? Can he concentrate on simple questions and answer them?

- *Memory.* Is the patient's memory intact for recent and long-term events?

- *Sensorium.* Is the patient focused? Paying attention? What is his level of awareness?

- *Perceptual Processes.* Are the patient's thought patterns ordered? Does he appear to have any hallucinations, delusions, or phobias?

- *Mood and Affect.* Observe for indicators of the patient's mood. Is it appropriate? What is his prevailing emotion? Depression, elation, anxiety, or agitation? Other?

- *Intelligence.* Evaluate the patient's speech. What is his level of vocabulary? His ability to formulate an idea?

- *Thought Processes.* What is the patient's apparent form of thought? Are his thoughts logical and coherent?

- *Insight.* Does the patient have insight into his own problem? Does he recognize that a problem exists? Does he deny or blame others for his problem?

- *Judgment.* Does the patient base his life decisions on sound, reasonable judgments? Does he approach problems thoughtfully, carefully, and rationally?

- *Psychomotor.* Does the patient exhibit an unusual posture or is he making unusual movements? Patients with hallucinations may react to them. For example, a patient who believes he is covered with insects may be picking at his skin to remove the "bugs."

PSYCHIATRIC MEDICATIONS

Many patients who suffer from psychiatric or behavioral disorders are under the care of a mental health professional and may be taking prescription medications. During the interview and history-taking process, determine whether the patient is taking medications and, if so, what type. The patient's use of such medications can provide clues to his underlying condition. Additionally, if a patient is not taking a medication as directed, his condition may deteriorate. Some schizophrenic patients may receive periodic injections of extremely long-acting antipsychotics (for example, haloperidol deconoate) because of poor compliance. They will often carry an identification card or may report that they "go to the clinic every three weeks for a shot." Types of psychiatric medications are discussed in the pharmacology chapter, Volume 1, Chapter 9.

SPECIFIC PSYCHIATRIC DISORDERS

Almost all psychiatric disorders have two diagnostic elements: symptoms of the disease or disorder and indications that the disease or disorder has impaired major life functions resulting in loss of relationships, a job, or housing or in another significant social problem. To define specific conditions, mental health professionals use the *Diagnostic and Statistical Manual of Mental Disorders,* Fourth Edition (DSM-IV). Published by the American Psychiatric Association (APA), the DSM-IV details diagnostic criteria for all currently defined psychiatric disorders, which are grouped according to the patient's signs and symptoms. The recognized types of behavioral and psychiatric disorders include:

- Cognitive disorders
- Schizophrenia
- Anxiety disorders
- Mood disorders
- Substance-related disorders
- Somatoform disorders
- Factitious disorders
- Dissociative disorders
- Eating disorders
- Personality disorders
- Impulse control disorders

The following summaries of these illnesses' major criteria do not imply that you should diagnose behavioral disorders. Even for skilled psychologists and psychiatrists, diagnosis is complicated by the considerable overlap in symptoms from one disease to another. A patient may actually fit into several categories. You should use the information here only as a guide to better understanding the science of psychiatry and the criteria applied to patients with behavioral emergencies. Knowledge of these terms and conditions will also allow you to communicate better with psychiatric care providers.

COGNITIVE DISORDERS

Psychiatric disorders with organic causes such as brain injury or disease are known as cognitive disorders. This family of disorders includes conditions caused by metabolic disease, infections, neoplasm, endocrine disease, degenerative neurological disease, and cardiovascular disease. They might also be caused by physical or chemical injuries due to trauma, drug abuse, or reactions to prescribed drugs. The specific brain pathology will differ based on the type of disease. Two types of cognitive disorders are delirium and dementia.

Delirium Delirium is characterized by a relatively rapid onset of widespread disorganized thought. These patients suffer from inattention, memory impairment, disorientation, and a general clouding of consciousness. In some cases, individuals may experience vivid visual hallucinations. Delirium is characterized by a fairly acute onset (hours or days) and may be reversible. Delirium may be due to a medical condition, substance intoxication, substance withdrawal, or multiple etiologies. Confusion is a hallmark of delirium.

Dementia Dementia may be due to several medical problems. Included among the more common causes of dementia are Alzheimer's disease (both early and late onset), vascular problems, AIDS, head trauma, Parkinson's disease, substance abuse, and other chronic problems. Regardless of its cause, dementia involves memory impairment, cognitive disturbance, and pervasive impairment of abstract thinking and judgment. Unlike delirium, dementia usually develops over months and, in many cases, is irreversible.

Dementia involves cognitive deficits manifested by both memory impairment (diminished ability to learn new information or to recall previously learned information) and one or more of the following cognitive disturbances:

* *Aphasia.* Impaired ability to communicate.
* *Apraxia.* Impaired ability to carry out motor activities despite intact sensory function.
* *Agnosia.* Failure to recognize objects or stimuli despite intact sensory function.
* *Disturbance in executive functioning.* Impaired ability to plan, organize, or sequence.

These conditions must significantly impair social or occupational functioning and represent a significant decline from a previous level of functioning. Your approach to patients with either of these conditions should be supportive. Assess and manage any medical complaints or conditions and transport to an appropriate medical facility.

SCHIZOPHRENIA

Schizophrenia is a common mental health problem, affecting an estimated one percent of the United States population. Its hallmark is a significant change in behavior and a loss of contact with reality. Signs and symptoms often include hallucinations, delusions, and depression. The schizophrenic patient may live in his "own world" and be preoccupied with inner fantasies. Although several biological and psychosocial theories attempt to explain the condition and its manifestations, its definitive cause is unknown.

The symptoms of schizophrenia include:

* *Delusions.* Fixed, false beliefs that are not widely held within the context of the individual's cultural or religious group.
* *Hallucinations.* Sensory perceptions with no basis in reality. These are often auditory ("hearing voices").
* *Disorganized speech.* Frequent derailment or incoherence.
* *Grossly disorganized* or *catatonic behavior.*
* *Negative symptoms* (**flat affect**).

* **delirium** condition characterized by relatively rapid onset of widespread disorganized thought.

* **dementia** condition involving gradual development of memory impairment and cognitive disturbance.

* **schizophrenia** common disorder involving significant change in behavior often including hallucinations, delusions, and depression.

* **delusions** fixed, false beliefs not widely held within the individual's cultural or religious group.

* **hallucinations** sensory perceptions with no basis in reality.

* **catatonia** condition characterized by immobility and stupor, often a sign of schizophrenia.

* **flat affect** appearance of being disinterested, often lacking facial expression.

A diagnosis of schizophrenia requires that two or more symptoms must each be present for a significant portion of each month over the course of six months. The symptoms must cause a social or occupational dysfunction (decline in social relations or work from the predisease state). Most schizophrenics are diagnosed in early adulthood.

The DSM-IV defines several major types of schizophrenia:

Content Review

MAJOR TYPES
OF SCHIZOPHRENIA
Paranoid
Disorganized
Catatonic
Undifferentiated

- *Paranoid.* The patient is preoccupied with a feeling of persecution and may suffer delusions or auditory hallucinations.
- *Disorganized.* The patient often displays disorganized behavior, dress, or speech.
- *Catatonic.* The patient exhibits catatonic rigidity, immobility, stupor, or peculiar voluntary movements. Catatonic schizophrenia is exceedingly rare.
- *Undifferentiated.* The patient does not readily fit into one of the categories above.

Your approach to the schizophrenic patient should be supportive and nonjudgmental. Do not reinforce the patient's hallucinations, but understand that he considers them real. Speak openly and honestly with him. Be encouraging yet realistic. Remain alert for aggressive behavior, and restrain the patient if he becomes violent or presents a danger to you, to himself, or to others.

ANXIETY AND RELATED DISORDERS

* **anxiety disorder** condition characterized by dominating apprehension and fear.

* **anxiety** state of uneasiness, discomfort, apprehension, and restlessness.

* **panic attack** extreme period of anxiety resulting in great emotional distress.

The group of illnesses known as **anxiety disorders** is characterized by dominating apprehension and fear. These disorders affect approximately two to four percent of the population. Broadly defined, **anxiety** is a state of uneasiness, discomfort, apprehension, and restlessness. More specifically, anxiety disorders fall into three categories: panic disorder, phobia, and posttraumatic stress syndrome.

Panic Attack The DSM-IV does not list **panic attacks** in themselves as a disease. Characterized by recurrent, extreme periods of anxiety resulting in great emotional distress, they are symptoms of disease and are included among the criteria for other disorders (panic disorder, agoraphobia). Panic attacks differ from generalized feelings of anxiety in their acute nature. They are usually unprovoked, peaking within 10 minutes of their onset and dissipating in less than one hour.

The presentation of panic and anxiety may resemble a cardiac or respiratory condition. This presents a dilemma for EMS personnel. Ruling out those conditions is difficult in the prehospital setting; psychiatrists usually diagnose anxiety or panic disorders by excluding known medical conditions. Keys to identifying panic or anxiety in the field are the patient's having a history of the condition and being outside the expected age range for certain cardiac or respiratory illnesses. This, of course, is not to say that young people cannot have myocardial infarction. Many symptoms of panic resemble those of hyperventilation, and some do appear to be correlated, such as the paresthesia from panic being due largely to hyperventilation.

The diagnostic criteria for a panic attack require a discrete period of intense fear or discomfort, during which four or more of the following symptoms develop abruptly and reach a peak within ten minutes:

Content Review

ANXIETY RELATED
DISORDERS
Panic attack
Phobia
Posttraumatic stress
  syndrome

- Palpitations, pounding heart, or accelerated heart rate
- Sweating
- Trembling or shaking

- Sensations of shortness of breath or smothering
- Feeling of choking
- Chest pain or discomfort
- Nausea or abdominal distress
- Feeling dizzy, unsteady, lightheaded, or faint
- Derealization (feelings of unreality) or depersonalization (being detached from oneself)
- Fear of losing control or going crazy
- Fear of dying
- Paresthesia (numbness or tingling sensations)
- Chills or hot flashes

Management for anxiety disorders is generally simple and supportive. Show empathy. Assess any medical complaints and manage them appropriately. If the patient experiences hyperventilation, calm and reassure him in order to decrease his respiratory rate to normal. Patients with severe or incapacitating symptoms may benefit from the administration of a sedative. Benzodiazepines, such as diazepam (Valium) and lorazepam (Ativan) can be administered in the prehospital setting. In addition, antihistamines, such as hydroxyzine (Vistaril) and diphenhydramine (Benadryl), have sedative effects and are useful in treating patients with significant anxiety. Consult medical direction in accordance with local protocol and transport to an appropriate medical facility.

Phobias Everyone has some source of fear or anxiety that they consciously avoid. When this fear becomes excessive and interferes with functioning, it is a **phobia**. A phobia, generally considered an intense, irrational fear, may be due to animals, the sight of blood (or injection or injury), situational factors (elevators, enclosed spaces), or environmental conditions (heights or water). Exposure to the situation or item will induce anxiety or a panic attack. Some patients experience extreme phobias that prevent or limit their normal daily activities. For example, a patient suffering from agoraphobia (fear of crowds) may confine himself to his home and avoid ever venturing outdoors. In most patients, however, the phobia is less severe; the patient realizes that his fear is unreasonable, and the anxiety dissipates.

> *** phobia** excessive fear that interferes with functioning.

Management for a patient with a phobia is supportive. Understand that the patient's fear is very real. Do not force him to do anything that he opposes. Manage any underlying problems and transport for evaluation.

Posttraumatic Stress Syndrome EMS providers often are particularly interested in **posttraumatic stress syndrome** because their responsibilities may make them susceptible to it. Originally recognized on the battlefields of war, posttraumatic stress syndrome is a reaction to an extreme, usually life-threatening, stressor such as a natural disaster, victimization (rape, for instance), or other emotionally taxing situation. It is characterized by a desire to avoid similar situations, recurrent intrusive thoughts, depression, sleep disturbances, nightmares, and persistent symptoms of increased arousal. The patient may feel guilty for having survived the incident, and substance abuse may frequently complicate his condition.

> *** posttraumatic stress syndrome** reaction to an extreme stressor.

Treat any posttraumatic stress syndrome patient with respect, empathy, and support, and transport him to an appropriate facility for evaluation.

Mood Disorders

The DSM-IV defines mood as "a pervasive and sustained emotion that colors a person's perception of the world." Common examples of mood alterations include depression, elation, **anger,** and anxiety. The main **mood disorders** are depression and bipolar disorder.

> *** anger** hostility or rage to compensate for an underlying feeling of anxiety.

> *** mood disorder** pervasive and sustained emotion that colors a person's perception of the world.

Depression Depression is characterized by a profound sadness or feeling of melancholy. It is common in everyday life and is to be expected following the break-up of a relationship or the loss of a loved one. Most of us have experienced some sort of depression, at least in its mildest form. It is one of the most prevalent psychiatric conditions, affecting from 10 to 15 percent of the population. When depression becomes prolonged or severe, however, it is diagnosed as a *major depressive episode.*

The symptoms of major depressive disorder include:

- Depressed mood most of the day, nearly every day, as indicated by subjective report or observation by others.
- Markedly diminished interest in pleasure in all, or almost all, activities most of the day nearly every day.
- Significant weight loss (without dieting) or weight gain. A five-percent change in body weight is considered significant.
- Insomnia or hypersomnia nearly every day.
- Psychomotor agitation or retardation every day (observable by others, not just the subjective feeling of the patient).
- Feelings of worthlessness or excessive inappropriate guilt (may be delusional) nearly every day.
- Diminished ability to think or concentrate, or indecisiveness nearly every day.
- Recurrent thoughts of death (not just fear of dying), recurrent suicidal ideation without a specific plan, or a suicide attempt or a specific plan for committing suicide. (Depression greatly increases the risk of suicide.)

The diagnostic criteria for major depressive disorder require that five or more of the symptoms have been present during the same two-week period and represent a change from previous functioning; at least one of the symptoms must be either a depressed mood or loss of interest in pleasure. The condition must cause clinically significant distress or impairment in social, occupational, or other important functions. Further, it must not meet the criteria for a mixed episode (mixtures of mania and depression); it must not be due to the direct physiological effects of a substance such as drug abuse or a medication, or to a general medical condition such as hypothyroidism; finally, it must not be better accounted for by **bereavement.** The acronym *In SAD CAGES* provides a screening mnemonic for major depression.

- *In*terest
- *S*leep
- *A*ppetite
- *D*epressed mood
- *C*oncentration
- *A*ctivity
- *G*uilt
- *E*nergy
- *S*uicide

Depression may occur as an isolated condition, but it is often accompanied by other disorders such as substance abuse, anxiety disorders, and schizophrenia. Depression can also affect a patient without meeting all of the identified clinical criteria. It can affect different people in different ways and is often atypical. Bereavement is one of the situations in which depression is expected. If the depression lasts longer than two months or is accompanied by suicidal ideation or marked functional impairment, it could be classified as a major depressive episode. Depression is more prevalent in females and is spread evenly throughout the life span.

Bipolar Disorder Bipolar disorder is characterized by one or more **manic** episodes (periods of elation), with or without subsequent or alternating periods of depression. In the past, the term *manic-depressive* was used to describe this condition. Bipolar disorder is not particularly common, affecting approximately less than one percent of the population.

Manic-depressive episodes are not the "Jeckyl and Hyde" transformations that television and the movies often portray. However, they often begin suddenly and escalate rapidly over a few days. In contrast to major depressive disorders, bipolar disorders usually develop in adolescence or early adulthood and occur as often in males as in females. Some patients with major depressive episodes will eventually develop a bipolar disorder and experience manic episodes. Commonly patients have several depressive episodes before having a manic episode.

The diagnostic criteria for a manic episode require a distinct period of abnormally and persistently elevated, expansive, or irritable mood lasting for at least one week (or for any duration when hospitalization is necessary). Three or more (four or more if the mood is only irritable) of the following symptoms must have been present to a certain degree and must have persisted during that time:

- Inflated self-esteem or grandiosity
- Decreased need for sleep
- More talkative than usual or pressure to keep talking
- Flight of ideas or subjective experience that thoughts are racing
- Distractibility
- Increase in goal directed activity (socially, at work or school, or sexually) or psychomotor agitation
- Excessive involvement in pleasurable activities that have a high potential for painful consequences (buying sprees, sexual indiscretions, foolish business investments)
- Delusional thoughts (grandiose ideas or unrealistic plans)

The symptoms must not meet the criteria for a mixed episode. The mood disturbance must be severe enough to markedly impair occupational or social functioning, to require hospitalizing the patient to prevent harm to himself or others, or present with psychotic features. As with depression, the symptoms must not be due to the direct physiological effects of a substance or a general medical condition. Patients with bipolar illness are often prescribed lithium (Lithobid, Eskalith) for treatment.

Management of these patients includes maintaining a calm, protective environment. Avoid confronting the manic patient. Never leave a depressed or suicidal patient alone. Assess and manage any other coexisting medical problems, and transport to an appropriate medical facility. Bipolar patients in an extreme manic phase may be overtly psychotic. In these cases, medication with an antipsychotic medication such as haloperidol may be indicated. Always contact medical directionl for treatment options.

✳ **bipolar disorder** condition characterized by one or more manic episodes, with or without periods of depression.

✳ **manic** characterized by excessive excitement or activity (mania).

Many patients with bipolar disorder are treated with lithium. Lithium has a very narrow therapeutic index, making lithium toxicity a significant complicating factor.

SUBSTANCE RELATED DISORDERS

Substance abuse is a common disorder. Any patient exhibiting symptoms of a psychiatric or behavioral disorder should be screened for substance use and/or abuse. Substance abuse patients may present as being depressed, psychotic, or delirious, and their signs and symptoms may mimic those of many behavioral disorders. The DSM-IV lists substance abuse as a psychiatric disorder; you should consider it a serious condition. Any mood-altering chemical has the potential for abuse. Alcohol is a common part of our culture, but can be abused. The user of a substance may be intoxicated from the effects of the chemical or may be ill from addiction or withdrawal of the chemical. Intoxication, in and of itself, may cause behavioral problems.

Repetitive use of a mood-altering chemical may lead to dependence or addiction. Dependence on a substance is characterized by repeated use of the substance. Dependence may be either psychological, physical, or both. Psychological dependence is a compelling desire to use the substance, inability to reduce or stop use, and repeated efforts to quit. Physical dependence is characterized by the need for increased amounts of the chemical to obtain the desired effect. Also, the presence of withdrawal symptoms when the substance is reduced or stopped is characteristic of physical dependence. All drugs have the potential to cause psychological dependence; many have the potential to cause physical dependence as well.

SOMATOFORM DISORDERS

* **somatoform disorder** condition characterized by physical symptoms that have no apparent physiological cause and are attributable to psychological factors.

Somatoform disorders are characterized by physical symptoms that have no apparent physiological cause. They are believed to be attributable to psychological factors. People who suffer from somatoform disorders believe their symptoms are serious and real. The major types of somatoform disorder are:

- *Somatization disorder.* The patient is preoccupied with physical symptoms.
- *Conversion disorder.* The patient sustains a loss of function, usually involving the nervous system (for instance, blindness or paralysis), unexplained by any medical illness.
- *Hypochondriasis.* Exaggerated interpretation of physical symptoms as a serious illness.
- *Body dysmorphic disorder.* A person believes he or she has a defect in physical appearance.
- *Pain disorder.* The patient suffers from pain, usually severe, that is unexplained by a physical ailment.

Somatoform disorders are often difficult to identify and diagnose. They can mimic and be confused with various bona fide physical conditions. Never attribute physical symptoms to a behavioral disorder until medical conditions have been ruled out.

FACTITIOUS DISORDERS

* **factitious disorder** condition in which the patient feigns illness in order to assume the sick role.

Factitious disorders are sometimes confused with somatoform disorders. They are characterized by the following three criteria:

- An intentional production of physical or psychological signs or symptoms.

- Motivation for the behavior is to assume the "sick role."
- External incentives for the behavior (e.g., economic gain, avoiding work, avoiding police) are absent.

While patients suffering from factitious disorders essentially feign their illnesses, that does not preclude the possibility of true physical or psychological symptoms. The disorder is apparently more common in males than in females. In severe cases, patients will go to great length to obtain medical or psychological treatment. Patients with factitious disorders often will voluntarily produce symptoms and will present with a very plausible history. They often have an extensive knowledge of medical terminology and can be very demanding and disruptive. In severe cases (Munchausen syndrome), patients will undergo multiple surgical operations and other painful procedures.

DISSOCIATIVE DISORDERS

Like somatoform disorders, **dissociative disorders** are attempts to avoid stressful situations while still gratifying needs. In a manner, they permit the person to deny personal responsibility for unacceptable behavior. The individual avoids stress by *dissociating* from his core personality. These behavior patterns can be complex but are quite rare. The disorders include:

Psychogenic Amnesia While amnesia is a partial or total *inability* to recall or identify past events, **psychogenic amnesia** is a *failure* to recall. The "forgotten" material is present but "hidden" beneath the level of consciousness.

Fugue State An amnesic individual may withdraw even further by retreating in what is known as a **fugue state.** A patient in a fugue state actually flees as a defense mechanism and may travel hundreds of miles from home.

Multiple Personality Disorder In **multiple personality disorder** the patient reacts to an identifiable stress by manifesting two or more complete systems of personality. While such disorders have received a great deal of attention in television, film, and novels, they are actually quite rare.

Depersonalization Depersonalization is a relatively more frequent dissociative disorder that occurs predominantly in young adults. Patients experience a loss of the sense of one's self. Such individuals suddenly feel "different"—that they are someone else or that their body has taken on a different form. The disorder is often precipitated by acute stress.

EATING DISORDERS

The two classifications of eating disorders are anorexia nervosa and bulimia nervosa. Both generally occur between adolescence and the age of 25. The condition afflicts women more than men at a rate of 20:1.

Anorexia Nervosa Anorexia is the loss of appetite. **Anorexia nervosa** is a disorder marked by excessive fasting. Individuals with this disorder have an intense fear of obesity and often complain of being fat even though their body weight is low. They suffer from weight loss (25 percent of body weight or more), refusal to maintain body weight, and often a cessation of menstruation from severe malnutrition.

Bulimia Nervosa Recurrent episodes of seemingly uncontrollable binge eating with compensatory self-induced vomiting or diarrhea, excessive exercise, or dieting and with a full awareness of the behavior's abnormality characterize **bulimia nervosa.** Individuals often display personality traits of perfectionism, low self-esteem, and social withdrawal.

* **dissociative disorder** condition in which the individual avoids stress by separating from his core personality.

Content Review

DISSOCIATIVE DISORDERS
Psychogenic amnesia
Fugue state
Multiple personality disorder
Depersonalization

* **psychogenic amnesia** failure to recall, as opposed to inability to recall.

* **fugue state** condition in which an amnesiac patient physically flees.

* **multiple personality disorder** manifestation of two or more complete systems of personality.

* **depersonalization** feeling detached from oneself.

Content Review

EATING DISORDERS
Anorexia nervosa
Bulimia nervosa

* **anorexia nervosa** psychological disorder characterized by voluntary refusal to eat.

* **bulimia nervosa** recurrent episodes of binge eating.

The weight loss and body changes experienced by anorexic and bulimic patients can lead to serious physical problems. Starvation and attempts to purge can have drastic consequences such as anemia, dehydration, vitamin deficiencies, hypoglycemia, and cardiovascular problems. In addition to psychological support, prehospital care is likely to include treatment for dehydration and physical problems. Both disorders have a high potential morbidity and mortality.

PERSONALITY DISORDERS

* **personality disorder** condition that results in persistently maladaptive behavior.

Most adults' personalities are attuned to social demands. Some individuals, however, often seem ill-equipped to function adequately in society. These people might be suffering from a **personality disorder.** Stemming largely from immature and distorted personality development, these personality, or character, disorders result in persistently maladaptive ways of perceiving, thinking, and relating to the world.

The broad category of personality disorder includes problems that vary greatly in form and severity. Although others might describe them as "eccentric" or "troublesome," some patients with personality disorders function adequately. In extreme cases, patients act out against or attempt to manipulate society.

Personality Disorder Clusters

The DSM-IV groups similar personality disorders into three broad types, Cluster A, Cluster B, and Cluster C.

Cluster A These individuals often act odd or eccentric. Their unusual behavior can take drastically different forms. This cluster includes the following:

- *Paranoid personality disorder.* Pattern of distrust and suspiciousness.
- *Schizoid personality disorder.* Pattern of detachment from social relationships.
- *Schizotypal personality disorder.* Pattern of acute discomfort in close relationships, cognitive distortions, and eccentric behavior.

Cluster B Individuals often appear dramatic, emotional, or fearful. This cluster includes the following:

- *Antisocial personality disorder.* Pattern of disregard for the rights of others.
- *Borderline personality disorder.* Pattern of instability in interpersonal relationships, self-image, and impulsivity.
- *Histrionic personality disorder.* Pattern of excessive emotions and attention seeking.
- *Narcissistic personality disorder.* Pattern of grandiosity, need for admiration, and lack of empathy.

Cluster C Individuals often appear anxious or fearful. This cluster includes the following:

- *Avoidant personality disorder.* Pattern of social inhibition, feelings of inadequacy, and hypersensitivity to criticism.
- *Dependent personality disorder.* Pattern of submissive and clinging behavior related to an excessive need to be cared for.
- *Obsessive-compulsive disorder.* Pattern of preoccupation with orderliness, perfectionism, and control.

Content Review

PERSONALITY DISORDER CLUSTERS

- Cluster A personality disorders
  —Paranoid
  —Schizoid
  —Schizotypal
- Cluster B personality disorders
  —Antisocial
  —Borderline
  —Histrionic
  —Narcissistic
- Cluster C personality disorders
  —Avoidant
  —Dependent
  —Obsessive-compulsive

Diagnosing a personality disorder requires evaluating the individual's long-term functioning and behavior. In many cases, the individual suffers from multiple disorders. A complete interview, history, and assessment will assist you in determining your approach. Your prehospital care will vary based on the patient's chief complaint and overall presentation.

IMPULSE CONTROL DISORDERS

Related to the personality disorders are the **impulse control disorders.** Recurrent impulses and the patient's failure to control them characterize these disorders. Examples of impulse control disorders include:

* *Kleptomania.* A recurrent failure to resist impulses to steal objects not for immediate use or for their monetary value
* *Pyromania.* A recurrent failure to resist impulses to set fires
* *Pathological gambling.* A chronic and progressive preoccupation with gambling and the urge to gamble
* *Trichotillomania.* A recurrent impulse to pull out one's own hair
* *Intermittent explosive disorder.* Recurrent and paroxysmal episodes of significant loss of control of aggressive responses

Disorders of impulse control may be harmful to the patient and others. Prior to committing the act the patient will have an increasing sense of tension. After the act, he will either have pleasure gratification or release.

* **impulse control disorder** condition characterized by the patient's failure to control recurrent impulses.

SUICIDE

Suicide, simply stated, is when a person intentionally takes his or her own life. Suicide is alarmingly common. It is the ninth leading cause of death overall, and it is the third leading cause in the 15–24-year age group. Suicide rates have risen dramatically in the younger age groups and have also increased significantly in the elderly population. Women attempt suicide more than men, but men—especially those over 55 years of age—are more likely to succeed. Statistically, suicide successes and methods vary widely by race, sex, and culture. The most common methods of suicide (1992) are:

1. Bullet wound (60 percent)
2. Poisoning (18 percent)
3. Strangulation (15 percent)
4. Cutting (1 percent)
5. Other, or unspecified (6 percent)

Assessing Potentially Suicidal Patients

In cases of attempted suicide, many focus on whether the patient really wanted to kill himself. Indeed this question will be at the heart of the patient's future psychiatric care, and information from the paramedic will be crucial to making that determination. But never lose sight of patient care while probing the psychological nature of attempted suicide.

Perform an appropriate focused history and physical exam concurrently with providing sound psychological care. Mental health professionals are rarely on the scene. It is up to you to document observations at the scene, especially any detailed suicide plans, any suicide notes, and any statements of the patient and bystanders. This information may not be available after the event when the patient receives psychiatric screening at the hospital. Such care and observations at the

Document observations at the scene of an attempted suicide, especially any detailed suicide plans, suicide notes, and statements by the patient and bystanders.

scene, combined with detailed documentation, are critical to the patient's long-term psychological care.

Risk Factors for Suicide

The risk factors for suicide are numerous. When assessing a patient who has indicated suicidal intentions, screen for any of these risk factors:

- Previous attempts (Eighty percent of persons who successfully commit suicide have made a previous attempt.)
- Depression (Suicide is 500 times more common among patients who are severely depressed than those who are not.)
- Age (Incidence is high between the ages of 15 and 24 years and over the age of 40.)
- Alcohol or drug abuse
- Divorced or widowed (The rate is five times higher than among other groups.)
- Giving away personal belongings, especially cherished possessions
- Living alone or in increased isolation
- The presence of **psychosis** with depression (for example, suicidal or destructive thoughts or hallucinations about killing or death)
- Homosexuality (especially homosexuals who are depressed, aging, alcoholic, or HIV-infected)
- Major separation trauma (mate, loved one, job, money)
- Major physical stresses (surgery, childbirth, sleep deprivation)
- Loss of independence (disabling illness)
- Lack of goals and plans for the future
- Suicide of same-sexed parent
- Expression of a plan for committing suicide
- Possession of the mechanism for suicide (gun, pills, rope)

psychosis extreme response to stress characterized by impaired ability to deal with reality.

Patients who have attempted suicide must be evaluated in a hospital or psychiatric facility. Many people assume that "they were just looking for attention." Applied to the wrong patient, that conjecture may contribute to his death.

AGE-RELATED CONDITIONS

Some behavioral disorders are particularly common among patients at the ends of the age spectrum—the young and the elderly. Your awareness of age-related conditions will help you to assess and interact with these patients.

Crisis in the Geriatric Patient

Common physical problems among the elderly include dementia, chronic illness, and diminished eyesight and hearing. The elderly also experience depression that is often mistaken for dementia. When confronted with an elderly person in a crisis, take the following steps:

- Assess the patient's ability to communicate.
- Provide continual reassurance.
- Compensate for the patient's loss of sight and hearing with reassuring physical contact.

- Treat the patient with respect. Call the patient by name and title, such as "Mrs. Jones." Avoid such terms as "dear," "honey," and "babe."
- Avoid administering medication.
- Describe what you are going to do before you do it.
- Take your time. Do not convey the impression that you are in a hurry.
- Allow family members and friends to remain with the patient if possible.

Crisis in the Pediatric Patient

Behavioral emergencies are not limited to adults. Children also have behavioral crises. While the child's developmental stage will affect his or her behavior, these general guidelines will assist you when confronting an emotionally distraught or disruptive child.

- Avoid separating a young child from his parent.
- Attempt to prevent the child from seeing things that will increase his distress.
- Make all explanations brief and simple, and repeat them often.
- Be calm and speak slowly.
- Identify yourself by giving both your name and your function.
- Be truthful with the child. Telling the truth will develop trust.
- Encourage the child to help with his care.
- Reassure the child by carrying out all interventions gently.
- Do not discourage the child from crying or showing emotion.
- If you must be separated from the child, introduce the person who will assume responsibility for his care.
- Allow the child to keep a favorite blanket or toy.
- Do not leave the child alone, even for a short period.

Always be mindful of every young or elderly patient's uniqueness. Treat him equally and fairly, as you would any other patient.

MANAGEMENT OF BEHAVIORAL EMERGENCIES

Patients who are experiencing behavioral emergencies require both medical and psychological care. In general, take the following measures when you treat a patient who is experiencing a behavioral emergency:

1. Assure scene safety and BSI precautions.
2. Provide a supportive and calm environment.
3. Treat any existing medical conditions.
4. Do not allow the suicidal patient to be alone.
5. Do not confront or argue with the patient.
6. Provide realistic reassurance.
7. Respond to the patient in a direct, simple manner.
8. Transport to an appropriate receiving facility.

Remember to treat the whole patient. Never overlook any serious, or potentially serious, medical complaints while focusing on the psychiatric assessment.

MEDICAL

Patients who are experiencing apparent behavioral emergencies often have concurrent medical conditions—some of which may be responsible for the behavioral problem. Current literature indicates that medical conditions and/or substance abuse cause a much higher proportion of behavioral emergencies than previously believed. Medical care may include treatment for overdose, lacerations, toxic inhalation, hypoxia, or metabolic conditions. Many patients with chronic psychiatric conditions take medications for their illnesses; when abused, those medications have extremely toxic side effects. (See the pharmacology chapter, Volume 1, Chapter 9.) Additionally these patients often live in conditions ranging from substandard housing to the street. This existence may predispose them to other medical problems such as exposure, infections, and untreated illnesses.

PSYCHOLOGICAL

Patients who present with an apparent behavioral emergency also require psychological care. The time you spend developing a rapport with the patient—before, during, and after assessment—is actually a part of the care you provide. In effect, when you begin an assessment you are also beginning your care, and you will continue to perform psychological assessment and care concurrently with medical assessment and care. Be calm and reassuring while you interview your patient.

Since much of your care will be aimed at the psychological problem, you should steer your conversation and actions in that direction. Visualize your patients on a continuum ranging from agitated and out-of-control to introverted and depressed (Figure 12-3). As a paramedic, you will need to defuse the agitated pa-

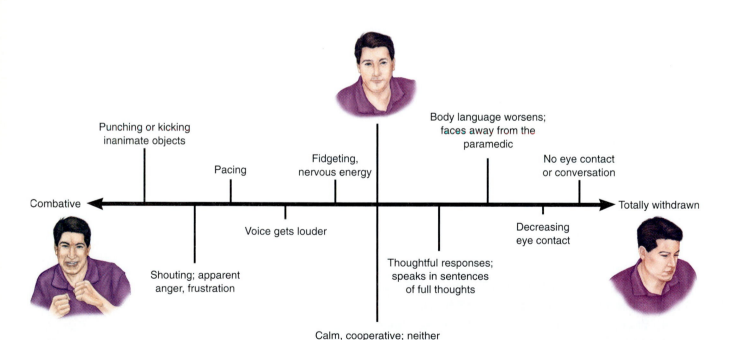

FIGURE 12-3 Continuum of patient responses during behavioral emergency. Whether dealing with an agitated or withdrawn patient, you will use your interpersonal skills to bring him to the calm, cooperative state in the middle of the continuum.

tient and attempt to communicate with the withdrawn patient. These situations especially will require the interviewing skills you learned earlier in this chapter.

As you approach the patient, introduce yourself and state that you want to help, since this might not be intuitively clear to a person with distorted perceptions. As you begin to converse, note how the patient reacts to you. Generally, if he responds appropriately to your actions, you should continue what you are doing. If the patient becomes more agitated or further withdrawn, rethink. Perhaps you are getting too close, talking too fast, or addressing difficult topics too early. Be sure your exit path is not blocked.

Your approach to these patients requires excellent people skills—especially listening and observing. If you do not use these skills, or if you rush or seem disinterested, your care will likely fail. Therapeutic communication, as this interaction has been called, is an art. "Talking down" the behavioral emergency patient requires effort and skill. Some patients, however, will not react favorably even to the best people skills. Extremely withdrawn patients or those with severe psychotic symptoms may never fully respond during the time you spend with them out of the hospital. These patients still deserve quality care and compassion, even when they are uncommunicative or restrained.

Talking down the behavioral emergency patient is an art that requires effort and skill.

Just as we must observe the patient, the patient observes us. Patients may actually be able to "read" us as accurately (or more accurately) than we read them. Perform your assessment and care confidently and competently. If patients sense uneasiness or indecision, they are more likely to act out. Never play along with a patient's hallucinations or delusions. It may seem to be the easiest route, but ultimately it may be harmful. Often the patient will recognize that you are patronizing him. Or the patient may talk of hallucinations or appear delusional, but not fully believe what he says. If you play along, you will lose credibility.

VIOLENT PATIENTS AND RESTRAINT

Who should be responsible for restraining a patient at an emergency scene is sometimes controversial. Many argue that physical restraint is clearly a police responsibility and EMS should not be involved. Others point out the gray areas, such as when the police are 30 minutes away, when only one officer is available, or when a patient is in imminent danger and paramedics must choose to act. One thing is certain: you should know how to control violent situations and restrain patients safely and effectively. Your agency's policies, your safety, and your patient's safety and needs will dictate how you handle individual emergencies. No EMS personnel should ever perform an unsafe act.

No EMS personnel should ever perform an unsafe act.

Most patients will respond to your care and therefore consent to treatment. Still, you will have patients whom the best interpersonal techniques cannot calm or reassure. If a patient must be legally transported against his will or if he becomes violent en route, restraint may be necessary.

The laws of consent state that no competent person may be transported against his will. A person who is in imminent danger of harming himself or others is not considered competent to refuse transport. Most states have laws that allow persons fitting this criterion to be transported against their will to a hospital or approved psychiatric facility. Who has the authority to determine this varies from state to state. In some areas it is the police, in others a physician.

Patients who are suicidal or homicidal clearly meet this criterion. No one will dispute that the patient with a knife to his wrist or the patient standing on a high ledge about to jump are both potential dangers to themselves. The many others who are on the border require careful evaluation. The patient who stripped off all his clothes in sub-zero weather or the patient who is not oriented enough to stay on the sidewalk and wanders into traffic may also meet the criterion.

Paramedics must be intimately familiar with local laws and protocols that apply to patient restraint.

Follow medical direction or local protocol when determining who can order a patient transported against his will. Protocols or agency rules may also state whether you should be involved in restraining violent patients. Finally, scene size-up may uncover dangers that you will decide to leave for the police to defuse before providing care. In general, be guided by what is best for the patient.

METHODS OF RESTRAINT

The main objective in restraint is to restrict the patient's movement in order to stop dangerous behaviors and prevent him from harming himself.

The main objective in restraint is to restrict the patient's movement in order to stop dangerous behaviors and prevent him from harming himself. Consider the following general guidelines during restraint:

- Use the minimum force needed to restrain the patient. When verbal techniques will work, physical restraint may not be necessary.
- Use appropriate devices to perform restraint. Metal handcuffs may cause injury; approved leather restraints and wide roller bandages are generally considered safer.
- Restraint is not punitive. Patients who are agitated frequently insult you, your partner, even your mother. This is not personal. The patient would make the same comments to anyone else in your position. Remain calm.
- Patients who have been restrained require careful monitoring. Assessment and care are not over when the patient is restrained; they are just beginning.

There are many techniques and devices for restraining the violent patient. Before restraining a person, consider the normal range of motion for the major joints. The arms cannot flail backwards, the legs cannot kick backwards, and the spinal column cannot double over backwards. Also consider the power of each major muscle group. For example, the flexor muscles of the arm are much stronger than the extensor muscles. Whenever possible, position the patient to limit his or her strength and range of motion.

Become familiar with your EMS system's restraint devices. Commercial leather restraints, jacket restraints, and soft restraints are optimal, but you can also improvise restraints from common materials:

- Small towels, cravats, or triangular bandages can be wrapped around a wrist or ankle and secured to the cot with strong tape.
- Webbed straps, ordinarily used with spine boards, can be used as restraints.
- Roll bandage (Kling) can be used to restrict movement of the patient's extremities and thus restrain him.

When you must restrain a patient, do not attempt to hold him for a long period. This sets up a confrontation and aggravates the situation. It also limits care, because you will be too busy holding the patient to treat him. Continuous restraint also requires more than one paramedic or assistant per patient. Following this sequence of actions will help you to restrain an unarmed patient:

1. Make certain you have adequate assistance; this will reduce the likelihood of injury both to you and to the patient. Prepare your stretcher and restraint equipment in advance. Keep restraints out of the patient's view until you need them.

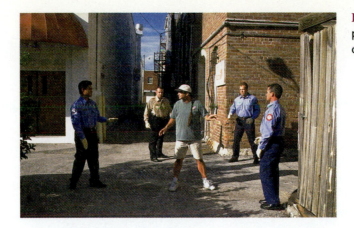

FIGURE 12-4A Encircle the patient and give him one last opportunity to cooperate.

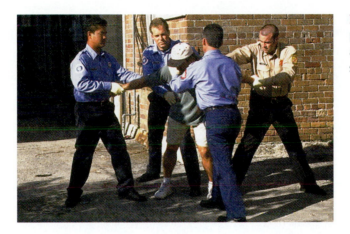

FIGURE 12-4B Assign one person to each limb and approach the patient at the same time.

2. Offer the patient one final opportunity to cooperate (Figure 12-4A).

3. If the patient does not respond to this request, at least two persons, preferably three or four, should move swiftly towards him. He cannot simultaneously focus on multiple paramedics (Figure 12-4B). When four rescuers are present, one person can control each extremity. This prevents the patient from striking and kicking. Keep away from the patient's mouth to avoid being bitten. Your swiftness will minimize the accuracy of a patient's kick or blow. Attempting to restrain a patient with too many rescuers can be confusing and inefficient. Someone should continue talking with the patient throughout the restraining process.

4. When the patient's extremities are physically restrained, move him to a prone or laterally recumbent position on the stretcher, where he can be secured. This prevents him from using his strong abdominal and leg muscles to break free from restraint. If your agency uses the Reeves stretcher to secure patients, be sure that the circumferential wrapping does not restrict the patient's respiratory efforts.

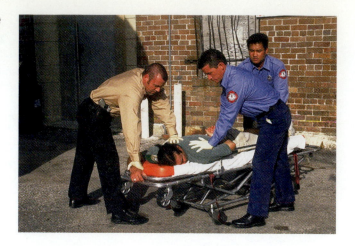

FIGURE 12-4C After you have subdued the patient, position him prone or on his side.

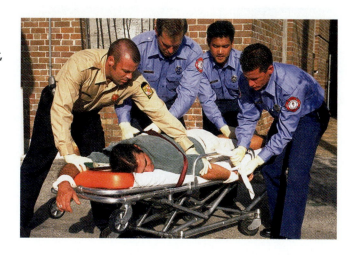

FIGURE 12-4D To prevent the patient's large muscle groups from working together, restrain one arm at his side and the other above his head.

5. Generally once a patient is restrained, keeping him restrained is best. The thought of regaining control of a patient in a moving ambulance by yourself is not pleasant. If the patient calms down, you may try to reduce the discomforts caused by the restraints, but you must keep adequate restraints in place.

6. Monitor the patient carefully during transport.

POSITIONING AND RESTRAINING PATIENTS FOR TRANSPORT

Once the patient is subdued, position him prone or on his side (Figure 12-4C). This dramatically reduces resistance and allows continued airway assessment and maintenance. Adjust the cot to its lowest position to improve stability, avoid lifting, and shorten the distance to the ground in case the patient falls. Do not allow the patient's large muscle groups to work together. For example, restrain one arm at the patient's side and the other above his head (Figure 12-4D). Place a

Patients who are physically restrained must receive frequent and close monitoring. Ideally this should include continuous ECG monitoring and pulse oximetry. Vital signs should be taken at least every 15 minutes, or every 5 minutes if the patient's condition is critical.

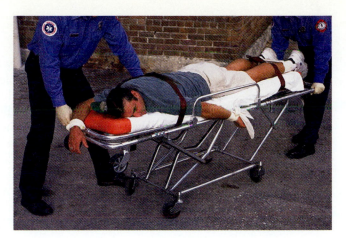

FIGURE 12–4E Continually monitor the restrained patient's airway, breathing, and circulation.

webbed strap across the patient's lumbar region, but do not cinch it too tightly. After applying restraints to the ankles and securing the cot, tie the ankle restraints to one another. Do not remove the restraints until enough personnel are present to control the patient. Always check the distal pulses after placing restraints.

Restraint is not without risk either to the paramedic or to the patient. Improper restraint threatens injury to everyone involved. Occasionally a restrained patient dies. The term for this phenomenon is **positional asphyxia**. The most common scenario in these cases involves a patient who has struggled violently, either during the restraint process or during a foot pursuit or struggle with police. The patient is eventually captured, restrained, and placed in a hog-tie or hobble restraint. He struggles for a time, then becomes quiet. While police and EMS crews think he is calming down, he is actually in cardiac arrest. Resuscitation attempts are usually unsuccessful. Some experts believe the restraint itself causes the patient's death. Others believe the combination of restraint, exertion, hyperthermia, and drug or alcohol abuse causes it. To prevent these deaths (and the liability they will bring), never use hog-tie or hobble restraints. Monitor all restrained patients carefully (Figure 12-4E), as noted earlier. Be alert for mental status changes from agitated to calm or sleepy—they may mean hypoxia. Monitor respiratory rate and depth frequently.

✱ **positional asphyxia** death from positioning that prevents sufficient intake of oxygen.

Never use hog-tie or hobble restraints.

CHEMICAL RESTRAINT

Some EMS systems allow the use of antipsychotic medications for controlling acutely psychotic and combative patients. This is especially important for long transports or for aeromedical operations. The most commonly used antipsychotics include haloperidol (Haldol), chlorpromazine (Thorazine) and others. These medications can be very effective in sedating patients who are agitated or hostile. Remember that medications in this class may cause an extrapyramidal system (EPS) reaction. Be prepared for EPS reactions and, if indicated, administer diphenhydramine (Benadryl) or a similar agent. Always consult and follow local protocol regarding use of antipsychotic agents or chemical restraint.

SUMMARY

Calls involving psychiatric and behavioral emergencies will challenge your skills as a paramedic. Differentiating physiological and psychological conditions will try your diagnostic skills, and developing the interview abilities that form the basis of psychiatric assessment and care will test your people skills. Ultimately, you will be called upon to help patients in a time of great need—the time of crisis. Once you determine that the patient is experiencing a purely behavioral emergency your compassion and communication skills rather than medications and procedures will benefit him most.

Situations involving crisis can drain your emotions. Observing a suicide or attempted suicide or struggling with or restraining a patient can take its toll. Take care of yourself before, during, and after these calls.

YOU MAKE THE CALL

You are called for a behavioral emergency in an office building parking lot on a cold February day. You arrive to find the police watching over a man in a car. They tell you he is a psychiatric patient who has crashed his car into several others in the parking lot. The crashes were low speed and you do not suspect spinal injuries. Your initial assessment is unremarkable. The patient responds verbally but is not alert. He is talking about "the coming of the Lord." He is nonviolent and does not resist your assessment. He has no obvious injuries. Religious literature and several Bibles are scattered about the car. You note the patient is wearing only a shirt in below-zero temperatures and is sweating profusely.

1. What do you suspect this patient's problem is? What are the possibilities?
2. Is the sweating significant? The religious literature? The car crashes?
3. Should this patient be treated as a psychiatric emergency?

See Suggested Responses at the back of this book.

FURTHER READING

American Psychiatric Association. *Diagnostic and Statistical Manual of Mental Disorders.* 4th ed. (DSM-IV). Washington, D.C.: American Psychiatric Press, 1995.

Dernocoeur, K.B. *Streetsense: Communication, Safety, and Control.* 3rd ed. Redmond, WA: Laing Research Services, 1996.

Frances, Allen, Michael B. First, and Harold Allen Pincus. *DSM-IV Guidebook.* Washington, D.C.: American Psychiatric Press, 1995.

Kachur, S. Patrick, et al. *Suicide in the United States, 1980–1992.* Violence Surveillance Summary Series, No. 1. Atlanta: Centers for Disease Control and Prevention, National Center for Injury Prevention and Control, 1995.

Marcus, Eric. *Why Suicide?* San Francisco: Harper Collins, 1996.

Soreff, Stephen M. and Robert T. Cadigan. *EMS Street Strategies: Effective Patient Interaction.* Philadelphia: F.A. Davis, 1992.

Spitzer, Robert L., et al. *DSM-IV Casebook.* Washington, D.C.: American Psychiatric Press, 1995.

ON THE WEB

Visit Brady's Paramedic Website at www.bradybooks.com/paramedic.

CHAPTER 13

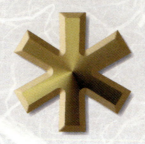

Gynecology

Objectives

After reading this chapter, you should be able to:

1. Review the anatomic structures and physiology of the female reproductive system. (pp. 637–641)
2. Identify the normal events of the menstrual cycle. (pp. 641–643)
3. Describe how to assess a patient with a gynecological complaint. (pp. 643–646)
4. Explain how to recognize a gynecological emergency. (pp. 643–646)
5. Describe the general care for any patient experiencing a gynecological emergency. (pp. 646–647, 649)
6. Describe the pathophysiology, assessment, and management of the following gynecological emergencies.
   a. Pelvic inflammatory disease (pp. 647–648)
   b. Ruptured ovarian cyst (p. 648)
   c. Cystitis (p. 648)
   d. Mittelschmertz (p. 648)
   e. Endometritis (p. 648)
   f. Endometriosis (pp. 648–649)
   g. Ectopic pregnancy (p. 649)
   h. Vaginal hemorrhage (p. 649)
7. Describe the assessment, care and emotional support of the sexual assault patient. (pp. 650–652)
8. Given several preprogrammed gynecological patients, provide the appropriate assessment, management, and transportation. (pp. 650–652)

CASE STUDY

It is near dusk on a warm summer evening when you and your partner, Sam Rusk, are dispatched from quarters to a nearby community park for an "assault." Within four minutes, you are pulling up to the park access gate near the security office, where you are met by a police officer and the park security supervisor. The police officer tells you that your 28-year-old female patient was found wandering in the park by a security officer just as the park was closing. He tells you that the Crime Scene Unit is en route. The supervisor reports that the officer who found her is sitting with her in the office.

You enter the security office as Sam gets the stretcher and jump kit from the back of the medic unit. The patient is seated on a cot facing away from the door. The security officer is sitting on a chair next to the cot, talking quietly to her. The patient has a white cotton blanket, provided by the officer, wrapped tightly over her shoulders and around her body. You observe that her hair is tangled and matted with leaves and small twigs sticking from it. As you approach her, you identify yourself, and introduce Sam, as paramedics who are there to help her. She turns her tear-stained, battered face toward you and nods, saying "I know" so quietly that you can barely hear her. The park officer stands and tells you that your patient's name is Stephanie. He then excuses himself, telling her that she's in good hands and that he'll be right outside.

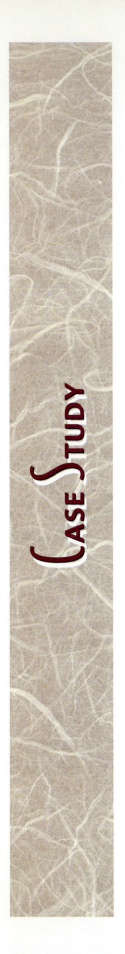

You pull up the chair that had been used by the officer and position it in front of Stephanie to complete your initial assessment. Although your priority is the assessment of her ABCs, you cannot ignore her obvious injuries. She has dried blood on her nose and mouth and her left eye is bruised and nearly swollen shut. You tell her that you need to perform some simple procedures to make sure that she's okay and ask her permission to do so. Again she nods, her eyes never leaving your face. In a soft hoarse voice, she says quietly, "He raped me, even though I begged him not to."

Stephanie's airway is open and her breathing is regular in rate and depth. You ask her if you can check her pulse, and she unwraps the blanket just enough to let her right forearm extend toward you. You find that her pulse is strong but rapid and her skin is cool and dry. You notice an abrasion around her wrist that makes you wonder if she had been tied down. You also observe that she has several broken nails on the trembling hand she extends toward you. Again with her permission you gently unwrap the blanket to reveal a torn, dirty T-shirt which is splattered with blood. She is wearing nothing else. Her inner thighs are covered with dried blood, as well as dirt and leaves. You limit your rapid trauma assessment to merely a search for life-threatening injuries, since Stephanie will undergo a thorough exam by the Sexual Assault Nurse Examiner (SANE). Stephanie's blood pressure is 108/70. Her pulse is strong and regular at 110 beats per minute. Her breathing is quiet and non-labored at a rate of 24 breaths per minute with a pulse oximeter reading of 99 percent on room air.

Explaining all the while exactly what you're going to do and asking her permission to do so, you and Sam help her stand and then pivot her onto the stretcher, leaving her wrapped in the blanket in which you found her. You move her to the medic unit. As you get her settled, and before beginning the short drive to the hospital, Sam contacts medical direction and requests that the SANE meet you at the hospital.

En route you complete Stephanie's SAMPLE history. She denies allergies and reports that the only medication she takes is a multivitamin tablet daily. Stephanie denies any significant past medical history. She ate a chef's salad for lunch about mid-afternoon. Stephanie says that she was grabbed from behind while she was jogging and that she was dragged off the path and into the woods. You reassure her that she is safe now and no one will hurt her. Within minutes you arrive at the hospital.

Emma Cannise, RN, the SANE coordinator, meets you at the emergency entrance to the hospital. You introduce Stephanie to Emma, who then accompanies you to the evaluation unit located behind the main emergency department. You give her a brief report, and she signs off on your patient care report.

Returning to quarters, you and Sam discuss how ironic it was that this month's continuing medical education (CME) program was a presentation by Emma Cannise on caring for victims of sexual assault.

INTRODUCTION

The term **gynecology** is derived from Greek, *gynaik,* meaning "woman." Gynecology is the branch of medicine that deals with the health maintenance and the diseases of women and primarily of their reproductive organs. **Obstetrics** is the branch of medicine that deals with the care of women throughout pregnancy. Most of the gynecological emergency patients that you will encounter will be experiencing either abdominal pain or vaginal bleeding. This chapter focuses on the assessment and care of non-pregnant patients with problems of the reproductive system. The assessment and care of the obstetrical patient is the subject of the next chapter.

* **gynecology** the branch of medicine that deals with the health maintenance and the diseases of women, primarily of the reproductive organs.

* **obstetrics** the branch of medicine that deals with the care of women throughout pregnancy.

ANATOMY AND PHYSIOLOGY

It is essential that you have a thorough understanding of the anatomy and physiology of the female reproductive system. This knowledge will allow you to better understand, recognize, and treat gynecological emergencies when they arise.

FEMALE REPRODUCTIVE ORGANS

The most important female reproductive organs are internal and are located within the pelvic cavity. These include the ovaries, fallopian tubes, uterus, and vagina, which are essential to reproduction. The external genitalia have accessory functions, in that they protect body openings and play an important role in sexual functioning.

External Genitalia

The female external genitalia are known collectively as the *vulva,* or *pudendum* (Figure 13–1).

Perineum The *perineum* is a roughly diamond-shaped, skin-covered muscular tissue that separates the vagina and the anus. These tissues form a sling-like structure supporting the internal pelvic organs and are able to stretch during childbirth. This area is sometimes torn as a result of sexual assault or during childbirth. An *episiotomy,* or incision of the perineum, may be done to facilitate delivery of the baby and to prevent spontaneous tearing, which may cause significant injury to the perineum and adjacent structures. Sometimes the term *perineum* is used to include the entire vulvar area.

Mons Pubis The *mons pubis* is a fatty layer of tissue over the *pubic symphysis,* the junction of pubic bones. During puberty, the hormone *estrogen* causes fat to be deposited under the skin, giving it a mound-like shape. This serves as a cushion that protects the pubic symphysis during intercourse. Also during puberty, the mons becomes covered with pubic hair and its sebaceous and sweat glands become more active.

Labia The *labia* are the structures that protect the vagina and the urethra. There are two distinct sets of labia. The *labia majora* are located laterally, while the *labia minora* are more medial. Both sets of labia are subject to injury during trauma to the vulvar area, such as occurs with sexual assault.

The *labia majora* are two folds of fatty tissue that arise from the mons pubis and extend to the perineum, forming a cleft. During puberty, pubic hair grows on the lateral surface, and sebaceous glands on the hairless medial

FIGURE 13-1   The vulva.

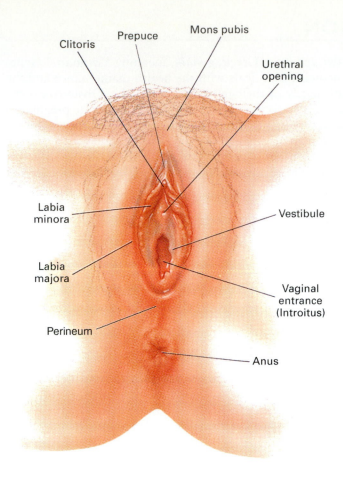

Clitoris   Prepuce   Mons pubis

Urethral opening

Labia minora

Vestibule

Labia majora

Vaginal entrance (Introitus)

Perineum

Anus

surface begin to secrete lubricants. The labia majora serve to protect the inner structures of the vulva. The *labia minora*, lying medially within the labia majora, are two smaller, thinner folds of highly vascular tissue, well supplied with nerves and sebaceous glands, which secrete lubricating fluid. During sexual arousal the labia minora become engorged with blood.

The area protected by the labia minora is called the *vestibule*. The vestibule contains the urethral opening and the external opening of the vagina called the vaginal orifice, or *introitus*. The secretions of two pairs of glands (Skene and Bartholin) lubricate these structures during sexual stimulation. Located within the vestibule is the *hymen*. It is a thin fold of mucous membrane that forms the external border of the vagina, partly closing it.

Clitoris   The *clitoris* is highly innervated and richly vascular erectile tissue that lies anterior to the labia minora. This cylindrical structure is a major site of sexual stimulation and orgasm in women. The *prepuce* is a fold of the labia minora that covers the clitoris.

Urethra   Although not truly a part of the female reproductive system the *urethra,* which drains the urinary bladder, is superior and anterior to the vagina. In the human female, the urethra is only 2 to 3 centimeters in length, which enables bacteria to travel more easily to the bladder than in the male. For this reason, the female is more susceptible to bladder infections than the male. As a rule, bladder infections occur more often in females once they become sexually active. In fact, after periods of prolonged sexual activity, it is not uncommon

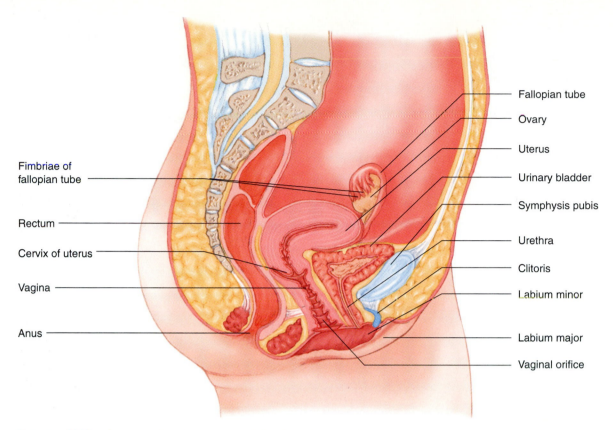

Fimbriae of fallopian tube

Rectum

Cervix of uterus

Vagina

Anus

Fallopian tube

Ovary

Uterus

Urinary bladder

Symphysis pubis

Urethra

Clitoris

Labium minor

Labium major

Vaginal orifice

FIGURE 13-2   Cross-sectional anatomy of the female reproductive system.

for women to develop a bladder infection. Sometimes this is referred to as "honeymoon cystitis."

Internal Genitalia

The internal female reproductive organs are the vagina, the uterus, the fallopian tubes, and the ovaries (Figures 13–2 and 13–3).

Vagina The *vagina* is an elastic canal made up primarily of smooth muscle, 9 to 10 centimeters in length, that connects the external genitalia to the uterus. It lies between the urethra/bladder and the anus/rectum. Lined with mucous membrane, the vagina extends up and back from the vaginal orifice to the lower end of the uterus (cervix). The vaginal walls are crisscrossed with ridges that allow it to stretch during childbirth, allowing passage of the fetus. The vagina's primary blood supply is the vaginal artery. The pudendal nerve innervates the lower third of the vagina and the external genitalia. The vagina has three functions:

- It is the female organ of copulation and receives the penis during sexual intercourse.
- Often called the birth canal, it forms the final passageway for the infant during childbirth.
- It provides an outlet for menstrual blood and tissue to leave the body.

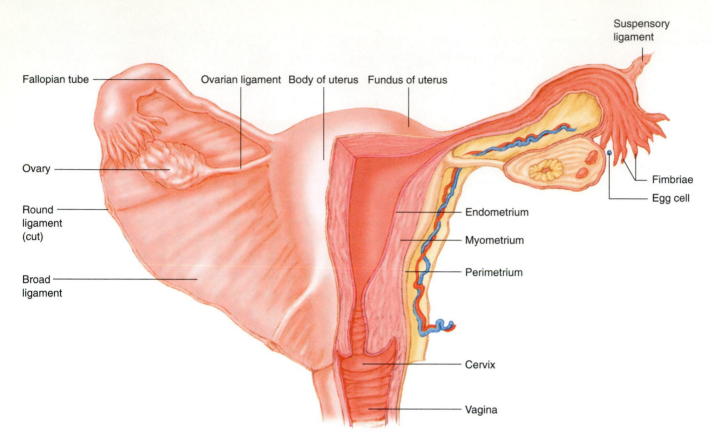

FIGURE 13-3 The uterus, fallopian tubes, and ovaries.

Labels in figure:
Fallopian tube
Ovarian ligament   Body of uterus   Fundus of uterus
Suspensory ligament
Ovary
Fimbriae
Egg cell
Round ligament (cut)
Endometrium
Myometrium
Perimetrium
Broad ligament
Cervix
Vagina

Uterus The *uterus* is a hollow, thick-walled, muscular, inverted-pear-shaped organ that connects with the vagina. It lies in the center of the pelvis and is flexed forward between the bladder and rectum above the vagina. Approximately 7.5 centimeters (three inches) long and 5 centimeters (two inches) wide, the uterus is held loosely in position by ligaments, peritoneal folds, and the pressure of adjacent abdominal structures. The primary function of the uterus is to provide a site for fetal development. During pregnancy, the uterus stretches to a size capable of containing the fetus, placenta, and the associated membranes and amniotic fluid. At term, the gravid uterus measures approximately 40 centimeters (16 inches) in length. The uterus has an extensive blood supply, primarily from the uterine arteries which are branches of the internal iliac artery. The autonomic nervous system innervates the uterus. In a non-pregnant state, the uterine cavity is flat and triangular.

The uterus has two major parts: the *body* (or corpus) and the *cervix,* or neck. The upper two-thirds of the uterus forms the body and is comprised of smooth muscle layers. The lower third is the cervix.

The rounded uppermost portion of the body of the uterus is the *fundus,* which lies above the point where the fallopian tubes attach. Measurement of fundal height (distance from the symphysis pubis to the fundus) may be used to estimate gestational age during pregnancy. The fundal height measured in centimeters is generally comparable to the weeks of gestation. For instance, if the fundal height is 30 centimeters, the gestational age is about 30 weeks. This method of assessing uterine size is most accurate from 22 to 34 weeks.

The body of the uterus has three layers of tissue that make up the uterine wall. The innermost layer or lining is called the **endometrium.** Each month, stimulated by estrogen and progesterone, the endometrium builds up in preparation for the implantation of a fertilized ovum. If fertilization does not occur, the lining degenerates and sloughs off. This sloughing of the uterine lining is referred to as the *menses,* or menstrual period.

The thick middle layer of the uterine wall, called the **myometrium** is made up of three distinct layers of smooth muscle fibers. In the outer layer, primarily over the fundus, the fibers run longitudinally, which allows expulsion of the fetus following cervical dilation. The middle (and thicker) layer is made up of figure-eight patterns of interlaced muscle fibers which surround large blood vessels. The contraction of these fibers helps control post-delivery bleeding. The myometrial fibers also contract during menstruation to maximize the sloughing of the endometrium. It has been suggested that menstrual cramps are due to fatigue of the myometrial fibers. The innermost layer of the myometrium is comprised of circular smooth muscle fibers that form sphincters at the point of fallopian tube attachment and at the internal opening of the cervix.

The outermost layer of the uterine wall is a serous membrane called the **perimetrium** that partially covers the corpus of the uterus. The perimetrium, which is a layer of the visceral peritoneum that lines the abdominal cavity and abdominal organs, does not extend to the cervix. The most significant aspect of this partial coverage is that it allows surgical access to the uterus without the risk of infection that is associated with peritoneal incisions.

The cervix, or neck of the uterus, extends from the narrowest portion of the uterus to connect with the vagina. That distance forms the cervical canal and is only approximately 2.5 centimeters (1 inch) in length. Elasticity characterizes the cervix. During labor, it dilates to a diameter of approximately 10 centimeters to allow delivery of the fetus.

Fallopian Tubes The two *fallopian tubes,* also called uterine tubes, are thin flexible tubes that extend laterally from the uterus and curve up and over each ovary on either side. Each tube is approximately 10 centimeters (4 inches) in length and about 1 centimeter in diameter (about the size of a pencil lead), except at its ovarian end which is trumpet-shaped. Each fallopian tube has two openings, a fimbriated (fringed) end that opens into the abdominal cavity in the area adjacent to the ovaries and a minute opening into the uterus. The function of the tubes is to conduct the egg from the space around the ovaries into the uterine cavity via peristalsis (wavelike muscular contractions). Fertilization usually occurs in the distal third of the fallopian tube.

Ovaries The *ovaries* are the primary female gonads, or sex glands. Almond-shaped, the ovaries are situated laterally on either side of the uterus in the upper portion of the pelvic cavity. They have two functions One function is the secretion of the hormones estrogen and progesterone in response to stimulation from follicle stimulating hormone (FSH) and luteinizing hormone (LH) secreted from the anterior pituitary gland. The second function of the ovaries is the development and release of eggs (ova) for reproduction.

THE MENSTRUAL CYCLE

The female undergoes a monthly hormonal cycle, generally every 28 days, that prepares the uterus to receive a fertilized egg. The onset of the menstrual cycle, that is, the onset of ovulation at puberty, establishes female sexual maturity. This onset, known as **menarche,** usually begins between the ages of 10 and 14. At first, the periods are irregular. Later they become more regular and predictable. The

✱ **endometrium** the inner layer of the uterine wall where the fertilized egg implants.

✱ **myometrium** the thick middle layer of the uterine wall made up of smooth muscle fibers.

✱ **perimetrium** the serosal peritoneal membrane which forms the outermost layer of the uterine wall.

✱ **menarche** the onset of menses, usually occurring between ages 10 and 14.

length of the menstrual cycle may vary from 21 to 32 days. A "normal" menstrual cycle is what is normal for the woman in question. Because of this, it is important to inquire as to the normal length of the patient's menstrual cycle. Regardless of the length of the menstrual cycle, the period of time from ovulation to menstruation is always 14 days. Any variance in cycle length occurs during the pre-ovulatory phase.

From puberty to menopause, the female sex hormones (estrogen and progesterone) control the ovarian-menstrual cycle, pregnancy, and lactation. These hormones are not produced at a constant rate, but rather their production surges and diminishes in a cyclical fashion. The secretion of estrogen and progesterone by the ovaries is controlled by the secretion of FSH and LH.

THE PROLIFERATIVE PHASE

The first two weeks of the menstrual cycle, known as the proliferative phase, are dominated by estrogen, which causes the uterine lining (endometrium) to thicken and become engorged with blood. In response to a surge of LH at approximately day 14, **ovulation** (release of an egg) takes place.

At birth, each female's ovary contains some 200,000 ova within immature ovarian follicles known as graafian follicles. This is the female's lifetime supply of ova, which are gradually "used up" through ovulation during her lifetime.

In response to FSH and increased estrogen levels, once during every menstrual cycle, a follicle reaches maturation and ruptures, discharging its egg through the ovary's outer covering into the abdominal cavity. The ruptured follicle, under the influence of LH, develops the corpus luteum, a small yellowish body of cells, which produces progesterone during the second half of the menstrual cycle. If the egg is not fertilized, the corpus luteum will atrophy about 3 days prior to the onset of the menstrual phase. If the egg is fertilized, the corpus luteum will produce progesterone until the placenta takes over that function.

The cilia (fine, hairlike structures) on the fimbriated ends of the fallopian tubes draw the egg into the tube and sweep it toward the uterus. If the woman has had sexual intercourse within approximately 24 hours of ovulation, fertilization may take place. If the egg is fertilized, it normally implants in the thickened lining of the uterus, where the fetus subsequently develops. If it is not fertilized, it passes into the uterine cavity and is expelled.

THE SECRETORY PHASE

The stage of the menstrual cycle immediately surrounding ovulation is referred to as the secretory phase. If the egg is not fertilized, the woman's estrogen level drops sharply while the progesterone level dominates. Uterine vascularity increases during this phase in anticipation of implantation of a fertilized egg.

THE ISCHEMIC PHASE

If fertilization doesn't occur, estrogen and progesterone levels fall. Vascular changes cause the endometrium to become pale and small blood vessels to rupture.

THE MENSTRUAL PHASE

During the menstrual phase, the ischemic endometrium is shed, along with a discharge of blood, mucus, and cellular debris. This is known as **menstruation**. A "normal" menstrual cycle depends upon the regular pattern in the individual woman. The first day of the menstrual cycle is the day on which bleeding begins

✱ ovulation the release of an egg from the ovary.

✱ menstruation sloughing of the uterine lining (endometrium) if a fertilized egg is not implanted. It is controlled by the cyclical release of hormones. Menstruation is also called a *period*.

and the menstrual flow usually lasts from 3 to 5 days, although this varies from woman to woman. An average blood loss of about 50 ml is common. The absence of a menstrual period in any woman in the childbearing years (generally ages 12 to 55) who is sexually active and whose periods are usually regular should raise the suspicion of pregnancy.

Some women regularly experience marked physical signs and symptoms immediately prior to the onset of their menstrual period. These are collectively known as **premenstrual syndrome (PMS)**. Although you may hear crude jokes made about PMS, there is no denying the reality of the physical changes that accompany the changing hormonal levels. It is not uncommon for women to report breast tenderness or engorgement, transient weight gain or bloating as a result of fluid retention, excessive fatigue, and/or cravings for specific foods. Women who are prone to migraine headaches may see them increase during the premenstrual period. Other women may have only minimal physical symptoms, but are more affected by emotional responses such as irritability, anxiety, or depression. The severity of PMS varies with each individual and may require treatment focused on relief of symptoms.

Menopause, the cessation of menses, marks the cessation of ovarian function and the cessation of estrogen secretion. Menstrual periods generally continue to occur until a woman is 45 to 55, at which time they begin to decline in frequency and length until they ultimately stop. The end of reproductive life is also known as the "climacteric," which is derived from Greek meaning "critical time of life." Occasionally, physicians use the term *surgical menopause,* which means that a woman's periods have stopped because of surgical removal of her uterus, ovaries, or both. The decrease in estrogen levels causes many women to experience hot flashes, night sweats, and mood swings during menopause. It is not uncommon for hormone replacement therapy (oral estrogen, or estrogen and progesterone) to be prescribed to help relieve these complaints and to provide other health benefits associated with continuing adequate levels of these hormones.

* **premenstrual syndrome (PMS)** a variety of signs and symptoms, such as weight gain, irritability, or specific food cravings associated with the changing hormonal levels that precede menstruation.

* **menopause** the cessation of menses and ovarian function due to decreased secretion of estrogen.

ASSESSMENT OF THE GYNECOLOGICAL PATIENT

Beyond labor and delivery, the most common emergency complaints of women in the childbearing years are abdominal pain and vaginal bleeding. Abdominal pain in women in the childbearing years is often due to problems of the reproductive organs. Complete the initial assessment in the usual manner. Then proceed with the focused history and physical exam. In addition to the usual history and physical assessment activities, you will need to ask specific questions pertinent to reproductive function and dysfunction. However, don't allow yourself to get distracted from getting complete past medical histories including chronic medical problems, medications, and allergies.

You may feel uncomfortable asking a patient about her reproductive history, but remember that you are a health care professional who is trying to obtain pertinent information in order to provide the best possible care for your patient. If you conduct yourself in this manner, it should not be uncomfortable for you or your patient. Assess your patient's emotional state. If she is reluctant to discuss her complaint in detail, respect her wishes and transport her to the emergency department where a more thorough assessment can be done.

Content Review

MOST COMMON EMERGENCY GYNECOLOGICAL COMPLAINTS
Abdominal pain
Vaginal bleeding

HISTORY

Once you have completed your initial assessment, use the SAMPLE approach for obtaining additional information about the history of the present illness.

dysmenorrhea painful menstruation.

dyspareunia painful sexual intercourse.

If the chief complaint is pain, then use the mnemonic OPQRST to gather more information. Is the patient's pain abdominal or in the pelvic region? Is it localized in a specific quadrant of the pelvis? Is she having her menstrual period? If so, how does the pain she is having now compare with how she usually feels? Some women have severe discomfort during their menstrual periods. This is called **dysmenorrhea**. Others may experience **dyspareunia**, painful sexual intercourse. Does walking or defecation aggravate her pain? What, if anything, alleviates her pain? Does positioning herself on her back or side with her knees bent relieve her discomfort?

You need to determine if there are any associated signs or symptoms that will be helpful in determining what is wrong with your patient. For instance, does your patient report a fever or chills? Is she reporting signs of gastrointestinal problems, such as nausea, vomiting, diarrhea, or constipation? Or perhaps she's complaining of urinary problems, such as frequency, painful urination, or "colicky" urinary cramping. Does she report a vaginal discharge or bleeding? If so, you should obtain information about the color, amount, frequency, or odors associated with either vaginal bleeding or discharge. If she reports vaginal bleeding, how does the amount compare with the volume of her usual menstrual period? Does she report dizziness with changes in position (orthostatic hypotension), syncope, or diaphoresis?

You will need to obtain specific information about her obstetric history. Has she ever been pregnant? *Gravida (G)* is the term used to describe the number of times a woman has been pregnant, including this one if she is pregnant. How many of those pregnancies ended in the delivery of a viable infant? *Para or parity (P)* refers to the number of deliveries. *Abortion* (Ab) refers to any pregnancy that ends before 20 weeks of gestation, regardless of cause. You may see this information recorded in "shorthand," for example, $G_3 P_2 Ab_1$, or gravida 3, para 2, ab 1. This means that she has been pregnant 3 times and had 2 prior deliveries and 1 pregnancy that ended before 20 weeks gestation. These terms refer to the number of pregnancies and deliveries, not the number of infants delivered, so even twins or triplets counts only as one pregnancy and one delivery.

You will also need to obtain a gynecological history. Question the patient about previous ectopic pregnancies, infections, cesarean sections, pelvic surgeries such as tubal ligation, abortions (either elective or therapeutic), and dilation and curettage (D&C) procedures. Also ask the patient about any prior history of trauma to the reproductive tract. It is often helpful to find out whether the patient, if sexually active, has had pain or bleeding during or after sexual intercourse.

In the female patient of childbearing age, always document the LMP.

It is important to document the date of the patient's last menstrual period, commonly abbreviated LMP (or LNMP for "last normal menstrual period"). Ask whether the period was of a normal length and whether the flow was heavier or lighter than usual. An easy way for women to estimate menstrual flow is by the number of pads or tampons used. She can easily compare this number to her routine usage. It is also important to inquire how regular the patient's periods tend to be. Ask her what form of birth control, if any, she uses. Also, find out if she uses it regularly. Direct questions such as "Could you be pregnant?" are generally unlikely to get an accurate response. Indirect questioning is often more helpful in determining the likelihood of pregnancy, such as "When did your last menstrual period start?" If you suspect pregnancy, inquire about other signs, including a late or missed period, breast tenderness, bloating, urinary frequency, or nausea and vomiting. Until proven otherwise, you should assume that any missed or late period is due to pregnancy even though your patient may deny it.

Any patient of reproductive age who still has her uterus should be considered to be pregnant until proven otherwise.

Contraception, or the prevention of pregnancy, takes many forms with variable degrees of effectiveness. You should have some familiarity with the various forms, their method of action, and their reliability (Table 13–1). Remember that

| Table 13-1 | CONTRACEPTIVES |

Type of Contraceptive	Method of Action	Effectiveness
Rhythm Method	Abstinence during fertile phase—follows 6 to 8 months of monitoring the menstrual cycle to determine fertile phase	Effective if abstinent during fertile phase; however, this is difficult to judge with precision
Coitus interruptus (withdrawal)	Penis withdrawn prior to ejaculation	Oldest and least reliable form of contraception
Condom	Barrier prevents transport of sperm	Reliable if used consistently and properly; additional benefit is that latex condoms prevent disease transmission.
Diaphragm	Barrier covers cervix to prevent entry of sperm	Reliable if proper fit and used consistently.
Spermicide	Destroys sperm or neutralizes vaginal secretions to immobilize sperm	Limited effectiveness, but increases when used with a barrier device
Intrauterine device (IUD)	Unclear; either prevents implantation of fertilized egg or affects sperm motility through cervix	Highly effective
Oral contraceptives (birth control pill)	Combination of estrogen and progesterone inhibits release of egg	Highly effective
Norplant	Progestin-containing capsules cause changes in cervical mucus to inhibit sperm penetration	Highly effective and continuous (up to six years) but requires surgical implantation
Depo-Provera	Suppresses ovulation	Highly effective and continuous (3 months)
Tubal ligation	Prevents egg from being fertilized by blocking tube	Highly effective but requires surgery

many contraceptives are medications, so don't forget to ask about their use. With the exception of oral contraceptives ("the pill") and intrauterine devices (IUDs), side effects caused by contraceptives are relatively rare. Oral contraceptives have been associated with hypertension, rare incidents of stroke and heart attack, and possibly pulmonary embolism. IUDs can cause perforation of the uterus, uterine infection, or irregular uterine bleeding. This is especially true for IUDs that have remained in place longer than the time recommended by the manufacturer, which rarely exceeds 2 years.

PHYSICAL EXAM

Physical examination of the gynecological patient is limited in the field. More than at any other time, the patient's comfort level should guide your actions. Respect your patient's modesty and maintain her privacy. This may mean that you need to exclude parents from the room when assessing adolescent patients or that you need to exclude spouses of married patients. Recognizing that most people are not comfortable discussing matters related to sexuality or reproductive organs, take your cues from the patient. Maintain a professional demeanor. Explain all procedures thoroughly so that your patient can understand them prior to initiating any care. Some women may feel more comfortable if they can be cared for by a female paramedic.

As always, the level of consciousness is the best indicator of your patient's status. Assess your patient's general appearance, paying particular attention to the color of her skin and mucous membranes. Cyanosis and pallor may indicate shock or a gas-exchange problem, while a flushed appearance is more indicative of fever.

Remember that vital signs are useful clues to the nature of your patient's problem. Pain and fever tend to cause an increase in pulse and respiratory rates along with a slight increase in blood pressure. Significant bleeding will cause increased pulse and respiratory rates as well as narrowing pulse pressures (the difference between systolic and diastolic pressures). Perform a tilt test to assess for orthostatic changes in her vital signs (a decrease in blood pressure and an increase in pulse rate when the patient rises from a supine or seated position), which again points to significant blood loss.

Do not perform an internal vaginal exam in the field.

Assess your patient for evidence of vaginal bleeding or discharge. If possible estimate blood loss. The use of more than two sanitary pads per hour is considered significant bleeding. If serious bleeding is reported or evident, it may be necessary to inspect the patient's perineum. Document the color and character of the discharge, as well as the amount, and the presence or absence of clots. *Do not perform an internal vaginal exam in the field.*

Pay particular attention to the abdominal examination. Auscultate the abdomen and note whether bowel sounds are absent or hyperactive. Gently palpate the abdomen. Document and report any masses, distention, guarding, localized tenderness, or rebound tenderness. In thin patients, a palpable mass in the lower abdomen may be an intrauterine pregnancy. At three months, the uterus is barely palpable above the symphysis pubis. At four months, the uterus is palpable midway between the umbilicus and the symphysis pubis. At five months (approximately 20 weeks), the uterus is palpable at the level of the umbilicus.

MANAGEMENT OF GYNECOLOGICAL EMERGENCIES

General management of gynecological emergencies is focused on supportive care.

In general, the management of the patient experiencing a gynecological emergency is focused on supportive care. Rely on your initial assessment to guide your decision-making about the need for oxygen therapy or intravenous access. If your patient's status warrants it, administer oxygen or assist ventilation as necessary. As a rule, intravenous access and fluid replacement is usually not indicated. However, if your patient has excessive bleeding or demonstrates signs of shock, then establish at least one large bore IV and administer normal saline at a rate indicated by the patient's presentation. You may also want to initiate cardiac monitoring if your patient is unstable.

Do not pack dressings in the vagina.

Continue to monitor and evaluate serious bleeding. *Do not pack dressings in the vagina.* Discourage the use of tampons to absorb blood flow. If your patient is bleeding heavily, count and document the number of sanitary pads used. If your patient demonstrates signs of impending shock, you may elect to place her in the Trendelenburg position (head lower than feet). The use of a pneumatic anti-shock garment in this situation should be governed by your local protocol. If shock is not a consideration, then position your patient for comfort in the left lateral recumbent position or supine with her knees bent, as this decreases tension on the peritoneum. Analgesics (pain-control medications) are not usually given in the field for gynecological complaints because these drugs tend to mask signs and symptoms of a deteriorating condition and make assessment and diagnosis difficult.

Since it is not appropriate to perform an internal vaginal exam in the field, most patients with gynecological complaints will be transported to be evaluated by a physician. Some problems may require surgical intervention, so you should consider emergency transport to the appropriate facility based on your local protocols.

Psychological support is particularly important when caring for patients with gynecological complaints. Keep calm. Maintain your patient's modesty and privacy. Remember that this is likely to be a very stressful situation for your patient, and she will appreciate your gentle, considerate care.

SPECIFIC GYNECOLOGICAL EMERGENCIES

Gynecological emergencies can be generally divided into two categories—medical and traumatic.

MEDICAL GYNECOLOGICAL EMERGENCIES

Gynecological emergencies of a medical nature are often hard to diagnose in the field. The most common symptoms of a medical gynecological emergency are abdominal pain and/or vaginal bleeding.

Gynecological Abdominal Pain

Pelvic Inflammatory Disease Probably the most common cause of non-traumatic abdominal pain is **pelvic inflammatory disease (PID)**. Pelvic inflammatory disease (PID) is an infection of the female reproductive tract that can be caused by a bacterium, virus, or fungus. The organs most commonly involved are the uterus, fallopian tubes, and ovaries. Occasionally the adjoining structures, such as the peritoneum and intestines, also become involved. PID is the most common cause of abdominal pain in women in the childbearing years, occurring in one percent of that population. The highest rate of infection occurs in sexually active women ages 15 to 24. The most common causes of PID are gonorrhea *(Neisseria gonorrhoeae)* or chlamydia *(Chlamydia trachomatis),* although rarely streptococcus or staphylococcus bacteria may cause it. Commonly, gonorrhea or chlamydia progresses undetected in a female until frank PID develops.

> * **pelvic inflammatory disease (PID)** an acute infection of the reproductive organs that can be caused by a bacteria, virus, or fungus.

Predisposing factors include multiple sexual partners, prior history of PID, recent gynecological procedure, or an IUD. Post-infection damage to the fallopian tubes is a common cause for infertility. PID may be either acute or chronic. If it is allowed to progress untreated, sepsis may develop. Additionally, PID may cause adhesions, in which the pelvic organs "stick together." Adhesions are a common cause of chronic pelvic pain and increase the frequency of infertility and ectopic pregnancies.

> *PID is a major risk factor for pelvic adhesions.*
>
>

While it is possible for a patient with pelvic inflammatory disease to be asymptomatic, most patients with PID complain of abdominal pain. It is often diffuse and located in the lower abdomen. It may be moderate to severe, which occasionally makes it difficult to distinguish it from appendicitis. Pain may intensify either before or after the menstrual period. It may also worsen during sexual intercourse, as movement of the cervix tends to cause increased discomfort. Patients with PID tend to walk with a shuffling gait, since walking often intensifies their pain. In severe cases, fever, chills, nausea, vomiting, or even sepsis may accompany PID. Occasionally, patients have a foul-smelling vaginal discharge, often yellow in color, as well as irregular menses. It is common also to have mid-cycle bleeding.

Generally, on physical examination, the patient with PID appears acutely ill or toxic. The blood pressure is normal, although the pulse rate may be slightly increased. Fever may or may not be present. Palpation of the lower abdomen generally elicits moderate to severe pain. Occasionally, in severe cases, the abdomen will be tense with obvious rebound tenderness. Such cases may be impossible to distinguish from appendicitis in the prehospital setting.

The primary treatment for PID is antibiotics, often administered intravenously over an extended period. Once the causative organism is determined, the sexual partner may also require treatment. In the field, the primary goal is to make the patient as comfortable as possible. Place the patient on the ambulance stretcher in the position in which she is most comfortable. She may wish to draw her knees up toward her chest, as this decreases tension on the peritoneum. *Do not perform a vaginal examination.* If your patient has signs of sepsis, administer oxygen and establish intravenous access.

Ruptured Ovarian Cyst *Cysts* are fluid-filled pockets. When they develop in the ovary, they can rupture and be a source of abdominal pain. When an egg is released from the ovary, a cyst, known as a corpus luteum cyst, is often left in its place. Occasionally, cysts develop independent of ovulation. When the cysts rupture, a small amount of blood is spilled into the abdomen. Because blood irritates the peritoneum, it can cause abdominal pain and rebound tenderness. Ovarian cysts may be found during a routine pelvic examination. However, in the field setting, your patient is likely to complain of moderate to severe unilateral abdominal pain, which may radiate to her back. She may also report a history of dyspareunia, irregular bleeding, or a delayed menstrual period. It is not uncommon for patients to rupture ovarian cysts during intercourse or physical activity. This often results in immediate, severe abdominal pain causing the patient to immediately stop intercourse or other physical activity. Ruptured ovarian cysts may be associated with vaginal bleeding.

✱ **cystitis** infection of the urinary bladder.

Cystitis Urinary bladder infection, or **cystitis,** is a common cause of abdominal pain. Bacteria usually enter the urinary tract via the urethra, ascending into the bladder and ureters. The bladder lies anterior to the reproductive organs and, when inflamed, causes pain, generally immediately above the symphysis pubis. If untreated, the infection can progress to the kidneys. In addition to abdominal pain, your patient may report urinary frequency, pain or burning with urination (**dysuria**), and a low-grade fever. Occasionally the urine may be blood-tinged.

✱ **dysuria** painful urination often associated with cystitis.

Mittelschmerz Occasionally, ovulation is accompanied by mid-cycle abdominal pain known as **mittelschmerz.** It is thought that the pain is related to peritoneal irritation due to follicle rupture or bleeding at the time of ovulation. The unilateral lower quadrant pain is usually self-limited and may be accompanied by mid-cycle spotting. While some women may report a low-grade fever, it should be noted that body temperature normally increases at the time of ovulation and remains elevated until the day prior to the onset of the menstrual period. Treatment is symptomatic.

✱ **mittelschmerz** abdominal pain associated with ovulation.

✱ **endometritis** infection of the endometrium.

Endometritis An infection of the uterine lining called **endometritis** is an occasional complication of **miscarriage,** childbirth, or gynecological procedures such as dilatation and curettage (D & C). Commonly reported signs and symptoms include mild to severe lower abdominal pain, a bloody, foul-smelling discharge, and fever (101° to 104° F). The onset of symptoms is usually 48 to 72 hours after the gynecological procedure or miscarriage. These infections often mimic the presentation of PID and can be quite serious if not quickly treated with the appropriate antibiotics. Complications of endometritis may include sterility, sepsis, or even death.

✱ **miscarriage** commonly used term to describe a pregnancy which ends before 20 weeks gestation; may also be called spontaneous abortion.

✱ **endometriosis** condition in which endometrial tissue grows outside of the uterus.

Endometriosis Endometriosis is a condition in which endometrial tissue is found outside of the uterus. Most commonly it is found in the abdomen and pelvis, although it has been found virtually everywhere in the body, including the central nervous system and lungs. Regardless of its site, the tissue responds to the hormonal changes associated with the menstrual cycle and thus bleeds in a cyclic manner. This bleeding causes inflammation, scarring of adjacent tissues, and the subsequent development of adhesions, particularly in the pelvic cavity.

Endometriosis is usually seen in women between the ages of 30 to 40 and is rarely seen in postmenopausal women. The exact cause is unknown. The most common symptom is dull, cramping pelvic pain that is usually related to menstruation. Dyspareunia and abnormal uterine bleeding is also commonly reported. Painful bowel movements have also been reported when the endometrial tissue has invaded the gastrointestinal tract. It is not uncommon for endometriosis to be diagnosed when the patient is being evaluated for infertility. Definitive treatment may include medical management with hormones, analgesics, and anti-inflammatory drugs, and/or surgery to remove the excessive endometrial tissue or adhesions from other organs.

Ectopic Pregnancy An **ectopic pregnancy** is the implantation of a fetus outside of the uterus. The most common site is within the fallopian tubes. This is a surgical emergency, because the tube can rupture, triggering a massive hemorrhage. Patients with ectopic pregnancy often have severe unilateral abdominal pain which may radiate to the shoulder on the affected side, a late or missed menstrual period, and, occasionally, vaginal bleeding. Additional discussion of ectopic pregnancy is presented in the next chapter.

Management of Gynecological Abdominal Pain

Any woman with significant abdominal pain should be treated and transported to the hospital for evaluation. Administer oxygen and establish intravenous access if indicated. Refer to the earlier section on management of gynecological emergencies for additional information.

Non-traumatic Vaginal Bleeding

Non-traumatic vaginal bleeding is rarely seen in the field unless it is severe. Refer to the earlier section in this chapter on completing a patient history. You should not presume that vaginal bleeding is due to normal menstruation. Occasionally a woman will experience **menorrhagia,** or excessive menstrual flow, but rarely is it the cause for a 911 call. Hemorrhage, regardless of cause, is always potentially life threatening, so be alert for signs of impending shock.

The most common cause of non-traumatic vaginal bleeding is a spontaneous abortion (miscarriage). If it has been more than 60 days since your patient's LMP, you should assume that this is the cause. Vaginal bleeding due to miscarriage is often associated with cramping abdominal pain and the passage of clots and tissue. The loss of a pregnancy, even at a very early phase, is a significant emotional event for your patient, so your kind and considerate care is important. Spontaneous abortion and other causes of bleeding in the obstetric patient will be discussed further in the next chapter. Other potential causes of vaginal bleeding include cancerous lesions, PID, or the onset of labor.

Management of Non-traumatic Vaginal Bleeding

Your field management of patients suffering non-traumatic vaginal bleeding will depend on the severity of the situation and your assessment of the patient's status. Absorb the blood flow. *Do not pack the vagina.* If your patient is passing clots or tissue, save these for evaluation by a physician. Transport your patient in a position of comfort. The initiation of oxygen therapy and intravenous access should be guided by the patient's condition.

* **ectopic pregnancy** the implantation of a developing fetus outside of the uterus, often in a fallopian tubes.

Ectopic pregnancy is a life-threatening condition.

Content Review

TREATMENT FOR ABDOMINAL PAIN

Make the patient comfortable.
Transport.

* **menorrhagia** excessive menstrual flow.

The most common cause of nontraumatic vaginal bleeding is spontaneous abortion (miscarriage).

Content Review

TREATMENT FOR VAGINAL BLEEDING

Absorb blood flow, but do not pack the vagina.
Transport.
Initiate oxygen therapy and IV access based on the patient's condition.

TRAUMATIC GYNECOLOGICAL EMERGENCIES

Most cases of vaginal bleeding result from obstetrical problems or are related to the menstrual period. However, trauma to the vagina and perineum can also cause bleeding and abdominal pain.

Causes of Gynecological Trauma

The incidence of genital trauma is increasing, with vaginal injury occurring far more commonly than male genital injury. Gynecological trauma may occur at any age. Blunt trauma occurs more frequently than penetrating trauma. Straddle injury (such as may occur with riding a bicycle) is the most common form of blunt trauma. Vaginal injuries are most often lacerations due to sexual assault. Other causes of gynecological trauma include blunt force to the lower abdomen due to assault or seat-belt injuries, direct blows to the perineal area, foreign bodies inserted into the vagina, self-attempts at abortion, and lacerations following childbirth.

Management of Gynecological Trauma

Injuries to the external genitalia should be managed by direct pressure over the laceration or a chemical cold pack applied to a hematoma. In most cases of vaginal bleeding, the source is not readily apparent. If bleeding is severe or your patient demonstrates signs of shock, establish IV access to maintain intravascular volume and monitor vital signs closely. Blunt force may cause organ rupture leading to the development of peritonitis or sepsis. *Never* pack the vagina with any material or dressing, regardless of the severity of the bleeding. Expedite transport to the emergency department since surgical intervention is often required.

Sexual Assault

Sexual assault continues to represent the most rapidly growing violent crime in America. Over 700,000 women are sexually assaulted annually. Unfortunately, it is estimated that more than 60 percent of all sexual assaults are never reported to authorities. Male victims represent 5 percent of reported sexual assaults. Sexual abuse of children is reported even less frequently. It is estimated that the incidence of sexual abuse in children ranges from 50,000 to350,000/year. There is no "typical victim" of sexual assault. Nobody, from small children to aged adults, is immune.

Most victims of sexual assault know their assailants. Friends, acquaintances, intimates, and family members commit the vast majority (80 percent) of sexual assaults against women. Acquaintance rape is particularly common among adolescent victims. Sexual assault is a crime of violence, not passion, that is motivated by aggression and a need to control, humiliate, or inflict pain. There are very few predictors of who is capable of committing sexual assault, as age, economic status, and ethnic origins vary widely. Common behavioral characteristics found among rapists include poor impulse control, the need to achieve sexual satisfaction within the context of violence, and immaturity.

The definition of sexual assault varies from state to state. The common element of any definition is sexual contact without consent. Generally, rape is defined as penetration of the vagina or rectum of an unwilling female or the rectum in an unwilling male. In most states, penetration must occur for an act to be classified as rape. Sexual assault also includes oral-genital sex. Regardless of the legal definition, sexual assault is a crime of violence with serious physical and psychological implications.

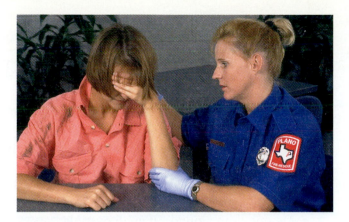

FIGURE 13–4 If possible, have a female EMT or paramedic accompany the sexual assault victim to the hospital.

Assessment The victim of sexual assault is a unique patient with unique needs. Your patient needs emergency medical treatment and psychological support. Your patient also needs to have legal evidence gathered. *Your* objectivity is essential, as your attitude may affect long-term psychological recovery. As a rule, victims of sexual abuse *should not* be questioned about the incident in the field. Don't ask questions about specific details of the assault. It is not important, from the standpoint of prehospital care, to determine whether penetration took place. Do not inquire about the patient's sexual practices. Confine your questions to the physical injuries the patient received. Even well-intentioned questions may lead to guilt feelings in the patient. Don't ask questions, such as why did you go with him or get in his car.

The psychological response of sexual assault victims is widely variable. The victim of sexual assault may be withdrawn or hysterical. Some use denial, anger, or fear as defense mechanisms. Approach the patient calmly and professionally. Allay the patient's fear and anxiety. Respond to the patient's feelings but be aware of your own. If the patient is incompletely dressed, a cover should be offered. Respect the patient's modesty. Explain all procedures and obtain the patient's permission before beginning them. Avoid touching the patient other than to take vital signs or examine other physical injuries. *Do not* examine the genitalia unless there is life-threatening hemorrhage.

Management In most situations, psychological and emotional support is the most important help you can offer. Maintain a nonjudgmental attitude and assure the patient of confidentiality. If the patient is female, allow her to be cared for by a female EMT or paramedic (if available). If the patient desires, have a female accompany her to the hospital (Figure 13–4). Provide a safe environment, such as the back of a well-lit ambulance. Respond to the patient's feelings and respect the patient's wishes. Unless your patient is unconscious, do not touch the patient unless given permission. Even when your patient appears to have an altered level of consciousness, explain what's going to be done before initiating any treatment.

Preservation of physical evidence is important. When the patient arrives at the hospital, a physician or sexual assault nurse examiner will complete a sexual assault examination to gather physical evidence. To protect this evidence, it is important that you adhere to the following guidelines:

- Consider the patient a crime scene and protect that scene.
- Handle clothing as little as possible, if at all.
- If you must remove clothing, bag separately each item that must be bagged.
- Do not cut through any tears or holes in the clothing.

Do not ask about specific details of a sexual assault.

Do not examine the external genitalia of a sexual assault victim unless there is a life-threatening hemorrhage.

Psychological and emotional support are the most important elements of care for the sexual assault victim.

- Place bloody articles in brown paper bags.
- Do not examine the perineal area.
- If the assault took place within the hour or the patient is bleeding, put an absorbent underpad (e.g., Chux) under the patient's hips to collect that evidence.
- If you cover the patient with a sheet or blanket, turn that over to the hospital as evidence.
- Do not allow patients to change their clothes, bathe, or douche (if female) before the medical examination.
- Do not allow patients to comb their hair, brush their teeth, or clean their fingernails.
- Do not clean wounds, if at all possible.
- If you must initiate care on scene, avoid disruption of the crime scene.

Documentation When completing your patient care report, keep the following documentation guidelines in mind:

- State patient remarks accurately.
- Objectively state your observations of the patient's physical condition, environment, or torn clothing.
- Document any evidence (e.g., clothing, sheets) turned over to the hospital staff and the name of the individual to whom you gave it.
- Do NOT include your opinions as to whether rape occurred.

SUMMARY

Most gynecological emergency patients have either abdominal pain or vaginal bleeding. The patient with abdominal pain should be made comfortable and transported to the emergency department. The management of vaginal bleeding depends on the severity. Minor bleeding should be simply monitored. Severe bleeding should be treated with IV fluids, if indicated.

In the case of sexual assault, you should first determine if any life-threatening physical injuries exist. Second, respect the patient's wishes and offer emotional support. Third, in treating victims of sexual assault, make every effort to preserve physical evidence. As with any type of emergency care, the primary concern is the patient.

YOU MAKE THE CALL

Late one evening in early winter, you are dispatched to a dormitory at the local university for a female with abdominal pain. When you arrive, the resident assistant escorts you to the room of your 17-year-old patient. There, the resident assistant introduces you to your patient and tells her that she'll wait in the other room. Your patient is a slightly built young female who appears to be acutely ill. She is lying on her left side with her knees drawn up to her chest, crying quietly. Her skin is slightly flushed and diaphoretic. The tearful patient complains of excruciating lower abdominal pain that has increased in intensity over the past several hours. She says that she has not eaten today because she was too nauseated, but she denies vomiting or diarrhea.

The patient's blood pressure is 82/64. Her pulse is 116 and thready. Respirations are 24 per minute with a pulse oximetry reading of 95 percent. Her temperature is 104°F. Lung sounds are clear and equal bilaterally. The abdominal exam reveals diffuse tenderness over both lower quadrants. She denies any past medical problems and says that she takes no medications, including birth control pills. She denies any allergies. Her LMP was seven weeks ago, but reports that earlier this evening she noticed a foul-smelling, bloody discharge. After questioning, she admits that she found out she was pregnant a week ago, but when she told her boyfriend, he told her to "get rid of it." She reports that three days ago she had an abortion at a local clinic. Her obstetric history is gravida 1, para 0, ab 1.

1. What is your first priority?
2. What else should you do?
3. What do you suspect is the likely cause of her signs and symptoms?
4. Since your patient is a minor, do you have any legal requirements to notify her parents or obtain their consent before treating her?

See Suggested Responses at the back of this book.

FURTHER READING

Card, Dolores E. "What Every EMT Needs to Know About Rape." *Emergency Medical Services* 23 (4) (April 1994), 46–49, 85.

Greenspan, Francis S. and Gordon J. Strewler. *Basic & Clinical Endocrinology.* 5th ed. Stamford, CT: Appleton & Lange, 1997.

Ladewig, Patricia Wieland, Marcia L. London and Sally B. Olds. *Maternal-Newborn Maternal Care.* 4th ed. Menlo Park, CA: Addison Wesley Longman, Inc., 1998.

McCance, Kathryn L. and Sue E. Huether. *Pathophysiology: The Biologic Basis for Disease in Adults and Children.* 3rd ed. St. Louis, MO: C.V. Mosby Company, 1998.

National Crime Center and Crime Victims Research and Treatment Center. *Rape in America: A Report to the Nation.* Arlington, VA, 1992:1–16.

Neff, Janet A. and Pamela Stinson Kidd. *Trauma Nursing: The Art and Science.* St. Louis, MO: Mosby-Year Book, 1993.

Stewart, Charles E. "Sexually Related Trauma: Female Injuries." *Emergency Medical Services* 24 (4) (April 1995), 48–53.

Thibodeau, Gary A. and Kevin T. Patton. *Anatomy & Physiology.* 4th ed. St. Louis, MO: Mosby-Year Book, 1999.

Tortora, Gerard J. and Sandra Reynolds Grabowski. *Principles of Anatomy and Physiology.* 9th ed. New York, NY: John Wiley and Sons, 1999.

ON THE WEB

Visit Brady's Paramedic Website at www.bradybooks.com/paramedic.

CHAPTER 14

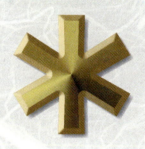

Obstetrics

Objectives

After reading this chapter, you should be able to:

1. Describe the anatomic structures and physiology of the reproductive system during pregnancy. (pp. 656–661)
2. Identify the normal events of pregnancy. (pp. 661–664)
3. Describe how to assess an obstetrical patient. (pp. 664–667)
4. Identify the stages of labor and the paramedic's role in each stage. (pp. 680–683)
5. Differentiate between normal and abnormal delivery. (pp. 689–694)
6. Identify and describe complications associated with pregnancy and delivery. (pp. 668–679, 687–696)
7. Identify predelivery emergencies. (pp. 668–679)
8. State indications of an imminent delivery. (pp. 681–682)
9. Identify the contents of an obstetrical kit and explain the use of each item. (pp. 683–686)
10. Differentiate the management of a patient with predelivery emergencies from a normal delivery. (pp. 667–679)

Continued

Objectives Continued

11. State the steps in the predelivery preparation of the mother. (p. 683)
12. Establish the relationship between body substance isolation and childbirth. (p. 683)
13. State the steps to assist in the delivery of a newborn. (pp. 683–686)
14. Describe how to care for the newborn. (pp. 686–689)
15. Describe how and when to cut the umbilical cord. (pp. 683, 686)
16. Discuss the steps in the delivery of the placenta. (p. 686)
17. Describe the management of the mother post-delivery. (pp. 686, 694–696)
18. Summarize neonatal resuscitation procedures. (pp. 688–689)
19. Describe the procedures for handling abnormal deliveries, complications of pregnancy, and maternal complications of labor. (pp. 668–679, 681–683, 689–696)
20. Describe special considerations when meconium is present in amniotic fluid or during delivery. (p. 694)
21. Describe special considerations of a premature baby. (pp. 678–679)
22. Given several simulated delivery situations, provide the appropriate assessment, management, and transport for the mother and child. (pp. 656–696)

CASE STUDY

The crew members of Fire Station 32 are relaxing in the television room when, suddenly, they hear an automobile screech to a halt at the station door. The captain rushes to the door and finds an old station wagon parked out front with a man standing beside it yelling, "Help! My wife needs help!"

The whole crew spills out the door. In the back seat of the station wagon, they see a pregnant female. She keeps saying, "The baby is coming, the baby is coming!" The ambulance normally based at Station 32 has gone out for gas. The captain notifies fire dispatch, which orders the ambulance to return. Meanwhile, the paramedics assigned to the engine learn that the patient is 29 years old and that this is her sixth pregnancy. She exclaims that she feels as if she has to move her bowels.

Now the patient begins to scream. "I've got to push, I've got to push," she yells. The paramedics don gloves and goggles and the senior paramedic checks for crowning. He easily spots the top of the baby's head during a contraction. One member of the crew retrieves an OB kit and an oxygen bottle from the medic box on the fire engine. Shortly thereafter, the patient gives birth to a baby girl in the back of the station wagon.

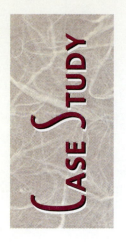

CASE **S**TUDY

At the time of delivery, the ambulance crew arrives. They assist the engine crew in cutting the cord, then dry and wrap the baby in a warming blanket. APGAR scores are 8 at 1 minute and 9 at 5 minutes. The mother receives fundal massage, oxygen, and an IV of normal saline solution. The paramedics then transport both mother and daughter to the hospital without incident. The father follows in the station wagon.

The next morning, as the Station 32 crew members are walking to their cars, they see a stork artfully painted on the window of the car belonging to the paramedic who delivered the baby.

INTRODUCTION

Pregnancy and childbirth are normal, natural events, usually requiring only basic assistance and care. However, it is important to be able to recognize and care for complications that occasionally occur.

Pregnancy, childbirth, and the potential complications of each are the focus of this chapter. Pregnancy is a normal, natural process of life that results from ovulation and fertilization. Complications of pregnancy are uncommon, but when they do occur, you must be prepared to recognize them quickly and manage them appropriately. Complications such as hypertension or eclampsia may result from the pregnancy itself. In addition, complications such as diabetes or cardiac diseases may result from the body's responses to the pregnancy. In some cases complications are a consequence of trauma.

Childbirth occurs daily, usually requiring only the most basic assistance, although childbirth complications do occasionally occur. These include preterm labor, multiple births, abnormal presentations, bleeding, or distressed neonates, to name but a few.

This chapter will prepare you to assess and care for the female patient throughout her pregnancy and delivery of her child.

THE PRENATAL PERIOD

The *prenatal period* (literally "prebirth period") is the time from conception until delivery of the fetus. During this period, fetal development takes place. In addition, significant physiological changes occur in the mother. Health care visits during pregnancy are referred to as "prenatal visits" or "prenatal care."

ANATOMY AND PHYSIOLOGY OF THE OBSTETRIC PATIENT

As you learned in the previous chapter, the first two weeks of the menstrual cycle are dominated by the hormone estrogen, which causes the endometrium (the inner lining of the uterus) to thicken and become engorged with blood. In response to a surge of luteinizing hormone (LH) and follicle stimulating hormone (FSH), **ovulation,** or release of an egg (ovum) from the ovary, takes place. The egg travels down the fallopian tube to the uterus. If the egg has been fertilized, it becomes implanted in the uterus and pregnancy begins. If the egg has not been fertilized, menstruation (discharge of blood, mucus, and cellular debris from the endometrium) takes place 14 days after ovulation. (The time from ovulation to menstruation is always exactly 14 days. However, the time from menstruation to

* **ovulation** the release of an egg from the ovary.

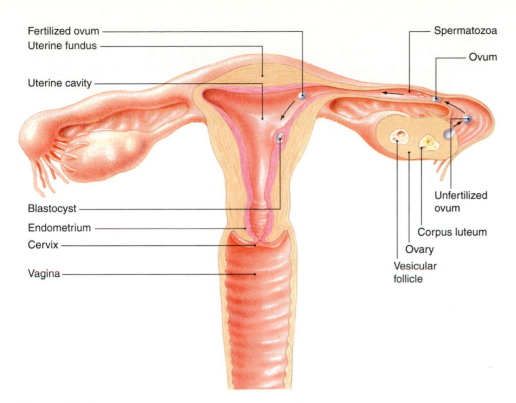

FIGURE 14-1   Fertilization and implantation of the ovum.

Labels (clockwise from top left):
Fertilized ovum
Uterine fundus
Uterine cavity
Spermatozoa
Ovum
Unfertilized ovum
Corpus luteum
Ovary
Vesicular follicle
Vagina
Cervix
Endometrium
Blastocyst

the next ovulation may vary by several days from the average of 14 days, which is why it can be difficult for couples to find the optimum time of the month to conceive, or to avoid conceiving, a baby.)

If the woman has had intercourse within 24 to 48 hours before ovulation, fertilization may occur. The male's seminal fluid carrying numerous spermatozoa, or male sex cells, enters the vagina and uterus and travels toward the fallopian tubes. Fertilization, which usually takes place in the distal third of the fallopian tube, occurs when a male spermatozoon fuses with the female ovum (Figure 14-1). After fertilization, the ovum begins cellular division immediately, which continues as it moves through the fallopian tube to the uterus. The ovum then becomes a *blastocyst* (a hollow ball of cells). The blastocyst normally implants in the thickened uterine lining, which has been prepared for implantation by the hormone progesterone, where the fetus and placenta subsequently develop.

Approximately three weeks after fertilization, the placenta develops on the uterine wall at the site where the blastocyst attached (Figure 14-2). The **placenta,** known as the "organ of pregnancy," is a temporary, blood-rich structure that serves as the lifeline for the developing fetus. It transfers heat while exchanging oxygen and carbon dioxide, delivering nutrients such as glucose, potassium, sodium, and chloride, and carrying away wastes such as urea, uric acid, and creatinine. The placenta also serves as an endocrine gland throughout pregnancy, secreting hormones necessary for fetal survival as well as the estrogen and progesterone required to maintain the pregnancy. Additionally, the placenta serves as a protective barrier against harmful substances. (However, some drugs such as narcotics, steroids, and some antibiotics, are able to cross the placental membrane from the mother to the fetus.) When expelled from the uterus following birth of the child, the placenta and accompanying membranes are called the **afterbirth.**

✳ **placenta** the organ that serves as a lifeline for the developing fetus. The placenta is attached to the wall of the uterus and the umbilical cord.

✳ **afterbirth** the placenta and accompanying membranes that are expelled from the uterus after the birth of a child.

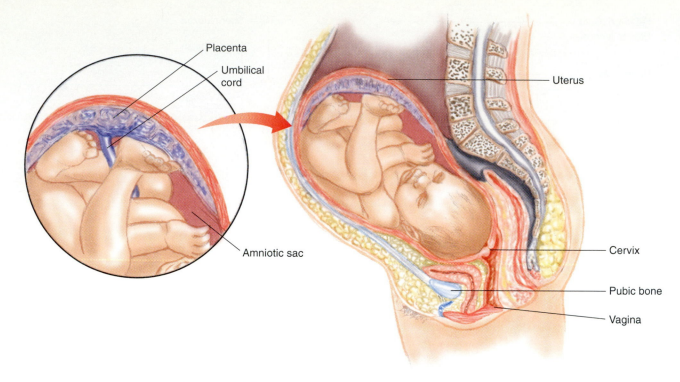

FIGURE 14-2 Anatomy of the placenta.

The placenta is connected to the fetus by the **umbilical cord,** a flexible, rope-like structure approximately two feet in length and three-quarters of an inch in diameter. Normally, the umbilical cord contains two arteries and one vein. The umbilical vein transports oxygenated blood to the fetus, while the umbilical arteries return relatively deoxygenated blood to the placenta.

The fetus develops within the **amniotic sac,** sometimes called the "bag of waters" (BOW). This thin-walled membranous covering holds the **amniotic fluid** that surrounds and protects the fetus during intrauterine development. The amniotic fluid increases in volume throughout the course of the pregnancy. After the 20th week of gestation, the volume varies from 500 to 1000 cc. The presence of amniotic fluid allows for fetal movement within the uterus and serves to cushion and protect the fetus from trauma. The volume changes constantly as amniotic fluid moves back and forth across the placental membrane. During the latter part of the pregnancy, the fetus contributes to the volume by secretions from the lungs and urination. Although it may rupture earlier, the amniotic sac usually breaks during labor, and the amniotic fluid or "water" flows out of the vagina. This is called *rupture of the membranes (ROM).* It is what has happened when the pregnant woman says, "My water has broken."

Physiologic Changes of Pregnancy

The physiologic changes associated with pregnancy are due to an altered hormonal state, the mechanical effects of the enlarging uterus and its significant vascularity, and the increasing metabolic demands on the maternal system. It is important for you to understand the physiologic changes associated with pregnancy so that you can better assess your pregnant patients.

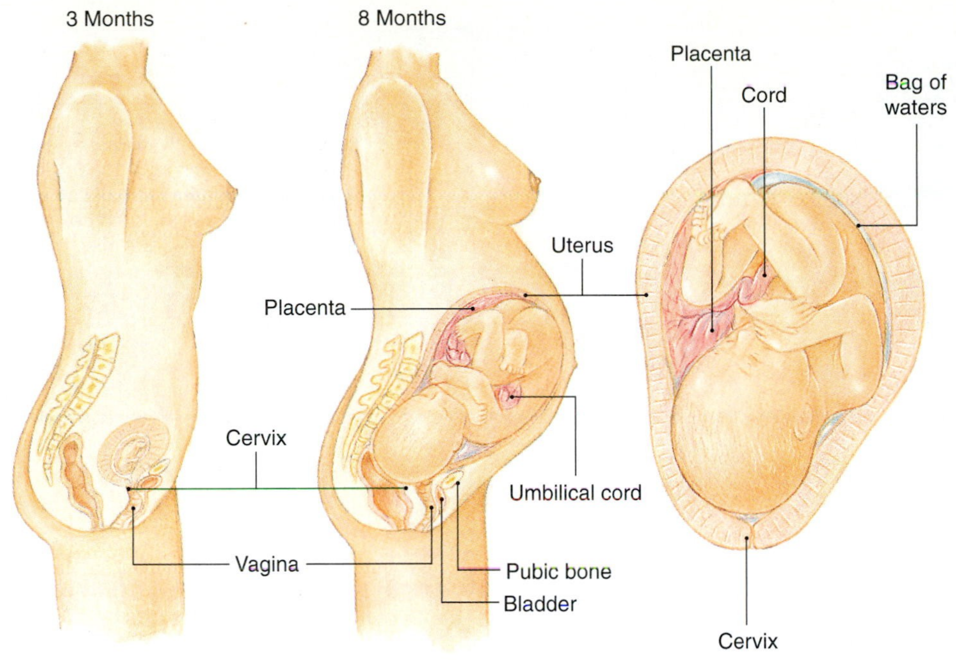

FIGURE 14-3 Uterine changes associated with pregnancy.

Labels on figure: 3 Months, 8 Months, Placenta, Cord, Bag of waters, Uterus, Placenta, Cervix, Umbilical cord, Vagina, Pubic bone, Bladder, Cervix

Reproductive System It is understandable that the most significant pregnancy-related changes occur in the uterus. In its non-pregnant state, the uterus is a small pear-shaped organ weighing about 60 g (2 ounces) with a capacity of approximately 10 cc. By the end of pregnancy, its weight has increased to 1000 g (slightly more than 2 pounds) while its capacity is now approximately 5,000 ml (Figure 14-3). Another notable change is that during pregnancy the vascular system of the uterus contains about one-sixth (16 percent) of the mother's total blood volume.

Other changes occurring in the reproductive system include the formation of a mucous plug in the cervix that protects the developing fetus and helps to prevent infection. This plug will be expelled when cervical dilatation begins prior to delivery. Estrogen causes the vaginal mucosa to thicken, vaginal secretions to increase, and the connective tissue to loosen to allow for delivery. The breasts enlarge and become more nodular as the mammary glands increase in number and size in preparation for lactation.

Respiratory System During pregnancy, maternal oxygen demands increase. To meet this need, progesterone causes a decrease in airway resistance. This results in a 20 percent increase in oxygen consumption and a 40 percent increase in tidal volume. There is only a slight increase in respiratory rate. The diaphragm is pushed up by the enlarging uterus, resulting in flaring of the rib margins to maintain intrathoracic volume.

Cardiovascular System Various changes take place in the cardiovascular system during pregnancy (Figure 14-4). Cardiac output increases throughout pregnancy, peaking at 6–7 liters/minute by the time the fetus is fully developed. The maternal blood volume increases by 45 percent and, although both red blood cells and plasma increase, there is slightly more plasma, resulting in a relative anemia. To combat this anemia, pregnant women receive supplemental iron to increase the oxygen-carrying capacity of their red blood cells. Due to the increase in blood volume, the pregnant female may suffer an acute blood loss of

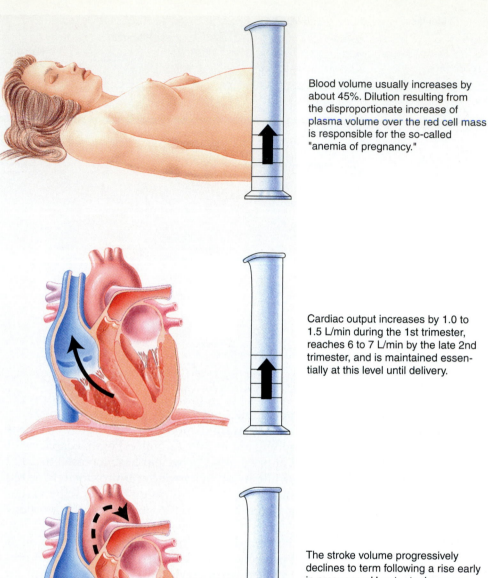

Blood volume usually increases by about 45%. Dilution resulting from the disproportionate increase of plasma volume over the red cell mass is responsible for the so-called "anemia of pregnancy."

Cardiac output increases by 1.0 to 1.5 L/min during the 1st trimester, reaches 6 to 7 L/min by the late 2nd trimester, and is maintained essentially at this level until delivery.

The stroke volume progressively declines to term following a rise early in pregnancy. Heart rate, however, increases by an average of 10 to 15 beats/min.

FIGURE 14-4   The hemodynamic changes of pregnancy.

30–35 percent without a significant change in vital signs. The maternal heart rate increases by 10–15 beats/minute. Blood pressure decreases slightly during the first two trimesters of pregnancy and then rises to near non-pregnant levels during the third trimester.

Supine hypotensive syndrome occurs when the gravid uterus compresses the inferior vena cava when the mother lies in a supine position, causing decreased venous return to the right atrium, which lowers blood pressure. Current research suggests that the abdominal aorta may also be compressed. The enlarging uterus also may press on the pelvic and femoral vessels, causing impaired venous return from the legs and venous stasis. This may lead to the development of varicose veins, dependent edema, and postural hypotension. Some patients are predisposed to this problem because of an overall decrease in circulating blood volume or because of anemia. Assessment and management of supine hypotensive syndrome will be discussed later in this chapter.

Gastrointestinal System Nausea and vomiting are common in the first trimester as a result of hormone levels and changed carbohydrate needs. Peristalsis is slowed, so delayed gastric emptying is likely and bloating or constipation is common. As the uterus enlarges, abdominal organs are compressed, and the resulting compartmentalization of abdominal organs makes assessment difficult.

Urinary System Renal blood flow increases during pregnancy. The glomerular filtration rate increases by nearly 50 percent in the second trimester and remains elevated throughout the remainder of the pregnancy. As a result, the renal tubular absorption also increases. Occasionally glucosuria (large amounts of sugar in the urine) may result from the kidney's inability to reabsorb all of the glucose being filtered. Glucosuria may be normal or may indicate the development of gestational diabetes. The urinary bladder gets displaced anteriorly and superiorly increasing the potential for rupture. Urinary frequency is common, particularly in the first and third trimesters, due to uterine compression of the bladder.

Musculoskeletal System Loosened pelvic joints caused by hormonal influences account for the waddling gait that is often associated with pregnancy. As the uterus enlarges and the mother's center of gravity changes, postural changes take place to compensate for anterior growth, causing low back pain.

FETAL DEVELOPMENT

Fetal development begins immediately after fertilization and is quite complex. The time at which fertilization occurs is called *conception*. Since conception occurs approximately 14 days after the first day of the last menstrual period, it is possible to calculate, with fair accuracy, the approximate date the baby should be born. This estimate is usually made during the mother's first prenatal visit. The normal duration of pregnancy is 40 weeks from the first day of the mother's last menstrual period. This is equal to 280 days, which is 10 lunar months or, roughly, 9 calendar months. This estimated birth date is commonly called the *due date*. Medically, it is known as the **estimated date of confinement (EDC)**. Generally, pregnancy is divided into *trimesters*. Each trimester is approximately 13 weeks, or 3 calendar months, long.

During the course of pregnancy, several different terms are used to describe the stages of development. The *pre-embryonic stage* covers the first 14 days following conception. The *embryonic stage* begins at day 15 and ends at approximately 8 weeks. The period from 8 weeks until delivery is known as the *fetal stage*. As a paramedic you should be familiar with some of the significant developmental milestones that occur during these three periods (Table 14-1).

During normal fetal development, the sex of the infant can usually be determined by 16 weeks gestation. By the 20th week, *fetal heart tones (FHTs)* can be detected by stethoscope. The mother also has generally felt fetal movement. By 24 weeks, the baby may be able to survive if born prematurely. Fetuses born after 28 weeks have an excellent chance of survival. By the 38th week the baby is considered *term,* or fully developed.

✱ **estimated date of confinement (EDC)** the approximate day the infant will be born. This date is usually set at 40 weeks after the date of the mother's last menstrual period (LMP).

Table 14-1	SIGNIFICANT FETAL DEVELOPMENTAL MILESTONES
Pre-embryonic Stage	
2 weeks	Rapid cellular multiplication and differentiation
Embryonic Stage	
4 weeks	Fetal heart begins to beat
8 weeks	All body systems and external structures are formed
	Size: approximately 3 centimeters (1.2 inches)
Fetal Stage	
8–12 weeks	Fetal heart tones audible with Doppler
	Kidneys begin to produce urine
	Size: 8 centimeters (3.2 inches), weight about 1.6 ounces
	Fetus most vulnerable to toxins
16 weeks	Sex can be determined visually
	Swallowing amniotic fluid and producing meconium
	Looks like a baby, although thin
20 weeks	Fetal heart tones audible with stethoscope
	Mother able to feel fetal movement
	Baby develops schedule of sucking, kicking, and sleeping
	Hair, eyebrows, and eyelashes present
	Size: 19 centimeters (8 inches), weight approximately 16 ounces
24 weeks	Increased activity
	Begins respiratory movement
	Size: 28 centimeters (11.2 inches), weight 1 pound 10 ounces.
28 weeks	Surfactant necessary for lung function is formed
	Eyes begin to open and close
	Weighs 2 to 3 pounds
32 weeks	Bones are fully developed but soft and flexible
	Subcutaneous fat being deposited
	Fingernails and toenails present
38–40 weeks	Considered to be full-term
	Baby fills uterine cavity
	Baby receives maternal antibodies

Most of the fetus's organ systems develop during the first trimester. Therefore, this is when the fetus is most vulnerable to the development of birth defects.

FETAL CIRCULATION

The fetus receives its oxygen and nutrients from its mother through the placenta. Thus, while in the uterus, the fetus does not need to use its respiratory system or its gastrointestinal tract. Because of this, the fetal circulation shunts blood around the lungs and gastrointestinal tract.

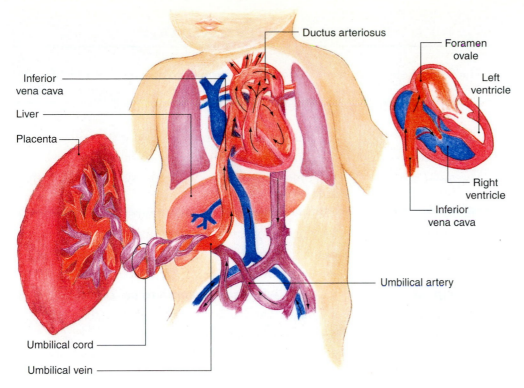

Inferior
vena cava

Liver

Placenta

Umbilical cord

Umbilical vein

Ductus arteriosus

Foramen
ovale

Left
ventricle

Right
ventricle

Inferior
vena cava

Umbilical artery

FIGURE 14-5   The maternal-fetal circulation.

The infant receives its blood from the placenta by means of the umbilical vein (Figure 14-5). The umbilical vein connects directly to the inferior vena cava by a specialized structure called the *ductus venosus*. Blood then travels through the inferior vena cava to the heart. The blood enters the right atrium and passes through the tricuspid valve into the right ventricle. It then exits the right ventricle, through the pulmonic valve, into the pulmonary artery. The fetus's heart has a hole between the right and left atria, termed the *foramen ovale*, which allows mixing of the oxygenated blood in the right atrium with that leaving the left ventricle bound for the aorta.

At this time, the blood is still oxygenated. Once in the pulmonary artery, the blood enters the *ductus arteriosus*, which connects the pulmonary artery with the aorta. The ductus arteriosus causes blood to bypass the uninflated lungs. Once in the aorta, blood flow is basically the same as in extrauterine life. Deoxygenated blood containing waste products exits the fetus, after passage through the liver, via the umbilical arteries.

The fetal circulation changes immediately at birth. As soon as the baby takes its first breath, the lungs inflate, greatly decreasing pulmonary vascular resistance to blood flow. Also, the ductus arteriosus closes, diverting blood to the lungs. In addition, the ductus venosus closes, stopping blood flow from the placenta. The foramen ovale also closes as a result of pressure changes in the heart, which stops blood flow from the right to left atrium.

OBSTETRIC TERMINOLOGY

The field of obstetrics has its own unique terminology. You should be familiar with this terminology, since patient documentation and communications with other health care workers and physicians often require it.

antepartum	the time interval prior to delivery of the fetus
postpartum	the time interval after delivery of the fetus
prenatal	the time interval prior to birth, synonymous with antepartum
natal	relating to birth or the date of birth
*gravidity**	the number of times a woman has been pregnant
*parity**	number of pregnancies carried to full term
primigravida	a woman who is pregnant for the first time
primipara	a woman who has given birth to her first child
multigravida	a woman who has been pregnant more than once
nulligravida	a woman who has not been pregnant
multipara	a woman who has delivered more than one baby
nullipara	a woman who has yet to deliver her first child
grand multiparity	a woman who has delivered at least seven babies
gestation	period of time for intrauterine fetal development

*The gravidity and parity of a woman is expressed in the following "shorthand": G4P2. "G" refers to the gravidity, and "P" refers to the parity. The woman in this example would have had 4 pregnancies and 2 births.

GENERAL ASSESSMENT OF THE OBSTETRIC PATIENT

INITIAL ASSESSMENT

The initial approach to the obstetrical patient should be the same as for the non-obstetrical patient, with special attention paid to the developing fetus. Complete initial assessment quickly. Next, obtain essential obstetric information.

HISTORY

The SAMPLE history will allow you to gain specific information about the mother's situation as well as her pertinent medical history.

General Information

Obtain information about the pregnancy Ask about gravidity, parity, length of gestation, and EDC. Ask about past gynecological or obstetrical complications and prenatal care. Determine current medications and any drug allergies.

You will want to obtain information about the pregnancy, such as the mother's gravidity and parity, the length of gestation, and the estimated date of confinement (EDC), if known. In addition, you should determine whether the patient has had any cesarean sections or any gynecological or obstetrical complications in the past. It is also important to ascertain whether the patient has had any prenatal care. Determine what type of health care professional (physician or nurse midwife) is providing her care and when she was last evaluated. Ask the patient whether a sonogram examination was done. A sonogram reveals the age of the fetus, the presence of more than one fetus, abnormal presentations, and certain birth defects. A general overview of the patient's current state of health is important. Pay particular attention to current medications and drug and/or medication allergies.

Pre-existing or Aggravated Medical Conditions

Pregnancy aggravates many pre-existing medical conditions and may trigger new ones.

Diabetes Previously diagnosed diabetes can become unstable during pregnancy due to altered insulin requirements. Diabetics are at increased risk of developing preeclampsia and hypertension (discussed later in this chapter). Pregnancy may also accelerate the progression of vascular disease complications of diabetes. It is not uncommon for pregnant diabetics to have problems with fluctuating blood sugar levels, causing hypoglycemic or hyperglycemic episodes. Also, many patients develop diabetes during pregnancy *(gestational diabetes)*. Pregnant diabetics cannot be managed with oral hypoglycemic agents because these drugs tend to cross the placenta and affect the fetus. Therefore, all pregnant diabetics are placed on insulin, if their blood sugar levels cannot be controlled by diet alone. It has been shown that maintaining careful control of the mother's blood sugar between 70 and 120 mg/dl reduces risks to mother and fetus.

Diabetes also affects the infant. Infants of diabetic mothers, especially those with poorly controlled blood sugar levels, tend to be large. This complicates delivery. Such infants also may have trouble maintaining body temperature after birth and may be subject to hypoglycemia. Babies born to diabetic mothers are also at increased risk of congenital anomalies (birth defects).

Heart Disease During pregnancy, cardiac output increases up to 30 percent. Patients who have serious pre-existing heart disease may develop congestive heart failure in pregnancy. When confronted by a pregnant patient in obvious or suspected heart failure, inquire about pre-existing heart disease or murmurs. It is important to be aware, however, that most patients develop a quiet systolic flow murmur during pregnancy. This is caused by increased cardiac output and is rarely a source of concern.

Hypertension Hypertension is also aggravated by pregnancy. Generally, blood pressure is lower in pregnancy than in the non-pregnant state. However, women who were borderline hypertensive before becoming pregnant may become dangerously hypertensive when pregnant. Also, many common blood pressure medications cannot be used during pregnancy. In addition, preeclampsia (discussed later in this chapter) may contribute to maternal hypertension. Persistent hypertension may adversely affect the placenta, thus compromising the fetus as well as placing the mother at increased risk for stroke, seizure, or renal failure.

Seizure Disorders Most women with a history of seizure disorders controlled by medication have uneventful pregnancies and deliver healthy babies. However, women who have poorly controlled seizure disorders are likely to have increased seizure activity during pregnancy. Medications to control seizures are commonly administered throughout the pregnancy.

Pregnancy can aggravate pre-existing medical conditions such as diabetes, heart disease, hypertension, seizure disorders, and neuromuscular disorders, and may trigger new ones. (However, a remission of neurological disorder symptoms during pregnancy is not unusual.)

Neuromuscular Disorders Disabilities associated with neuromuscular disorders, such as multiple sclerosis, may be aggravated by pregnancy. However, it is more common that pregnant women enjoy remission of symptoms during pregnancy and a slight increase in relapse rate during the postpartum period. The strength of uterine contractions is not diminished in these patients. Also, their subjective sensation of pain is often less than seen in other patients.

Pain

When the patient complains of pain, determine onset, character, and especially the regularity of occurrence.

If the patient is in pain, try to determine when the pain started and whether its onset was sudden or slow. Also, attempt to define the character of the pain—its duration, location, and radiation, if any. It is especially important to determine whether the pain is occurring on a regular basis.

Vaginal Bleeding

If there is vaginal bleeding, determine events prior to its start. Assess the amount by the number of sanitary pads used and save any clots or passed tissue.

The presence of vaginal bleeding or spotting is a major concern in an obstetrical patient. Ask about events immediately prior to the start of bleeding. You also need to gain information about the color, amount, and duration. To assess the amount of bleeding, count the number of sanitary pads used. If your patient is passing clots or tissue, save this material for evaluation. In addition, question the patient about the presence of other vaginal discharges, as well as the color, amount, and duration.

Active Labor

For a patient in labor, determine if she feels the need to push or move her bowels or if her membranes have ruptured (her "water broke")—all signs of possible imminent delivery.

When confronted with a patient in active labor, assess whether the mother feels the need to push or has the urge to move her bowels. Determine whether the patient thinks her membranes have ruptured. Patients often sense this as a dribbling of water or, in some cases, a true gush of water.

PHYSICAL EXAMINATION

Always protect the patient's modesty.

Physical examination of the obstetric patient is essentially the same as for any emergency patient. However, you should be particularly careful to protect the patient's modesty as well as to maintain her dignity and privacy.

When examining a pregnant patient, first estimate the date of the pregnancy by measuring the *fundal height*. The fundal height is the distance from the symphysis pubis to the top of the uterine fundus. Each centimeter of fundal height roughly corresponds to a week of gestation. For example, a woman with a fundal height of 24 centimeters has a gestational age of approximately 24 weeks. If the fundus is just palpable above the symphysis pubis, the pregnancy is about 12–16 weeks gestation. When the uterine fundus reaches the umbilicus, the pregnancy is about 20 weeks. As pregnancy reaches term, the fundus is palpable near the xiphoid process. If fetal movement is felt when the abdomen is palpated, the pregnancy is at least 20 weeks. Fetal heart tones can be heard by stethoscope at approximately 18–20 weeks. The normal fetal heart rate ranges from 140–160 beats per minute.

Generally, vital signs in the pregnant patient should be taken with the patient lying on her left side. As noted earlier, as pregnancy progresses, the uterus increases in size. Ultimately, when the patient is supine, the weight of the uterus compresses the inferior vena cava, severely compromising venous blood return from the lower extremities. Turning the patient to her left side alleviates this problem. Occasionally, it may be helpful to perform orthostatic vital signs. First, obtain the blood pressure and pulse rate after the patient has rested for five minutes in the left lateral recumbent position. Then repeat the vital signs with the patient sitting up or standing. A drop in the blood pressure level of 15 mmHg or more, or an increase in the pulse rate of 20 beats per minute or more, is considered significant and should be reported and documented. When performing this maneuver, it is always important to be alert for syncope. This procedure should *not* be performed if the patient is in obvious shock.

You may need to examine the genitals to evaluate any vaginal discharge, the progression of labor, or the presence of a *prolapsed cord,* an umbilical cord that comes out of the uterus ahead of the fetus. This can be accomplished simply by looking at the perineum. If, during the physical examination, the patient reports that she feels the need to push, or if she feels as though she must move her bowels, examine her for crowning. **Crowning** is the bulging of the fetal head past the opening of the vagina during a contraction. Crowning is an indication of impending delivery. Examine for crowning only during a contraction. *Do not perform an internal vaginal examination in the field.*

* **crowning** the bulging of the fetal head past the opening of the vagina during a contraction. Crowning is an indication of impending delivery.

Do not perform an internal vaginal examination in the field.

GENERAL MANAGEMENT OF THE OBSTETRIC PATIENT

The first consideration for managing emergencies in obstetric patients is to remember that you are in fact caring for two patients, the mother and the fetus. Fetal well-being is dependent on maternal well-being. Also keep in mind that your calm, professional demeanor and caring attitude will go a long way in reducing the emotional stress during any obstetric emergency. Remember to protect your patient's privacy and maintain her modesty.

The physiologic priorities for obstetric emergencies are identical to those for any other emergency situation. Focus your efforts on maintaining the airway, breathing, and circulation. Administer high-flow, high-concentration oxygen as needed based on the patient's condition. Initiate intravenous access by using a large bore catheter in a large vein and consider fluid resuscitation based on your local protocols. If your patient is bleeding or showing signs of shock, establish two IV lines. Cardiac monitoring is also appropriate. Place your patient in a position of comfort, but remember that left lateral recumbent is preferred after the 24th week.

If pain is the primary complaint, administer analgesics such as morphine. However, analgesics should be used with caution since they can alter your ability to assess a deteriorating condition as well as other changes in patient status and may negatively affect the fetus. Nitrous oxide is the preferred analgesic in pregnancy, but narcotics are acceptable.

When transport is indicated, transport immediately to a hospital that is capable of managing emergency obstetric and neonatal care. Report the situation to the receiving hospital prior to your arrival, as emergency department personnel may want to summon obstetrics department staff to assist with patient care.

Always remember that you are caring for two patients, the mother and the fetus.

Focus on airway, breathing, and circulation. Monitor for shock. As needed, administer oxygen, initiate IV access, consider fluid resuscitation, and monitor the heart. Place the patient in a position of comfort. The left lateral recumbent position is preferred after the 24th week.

COMPLICATIONS OF PREGNANCY

Pregnancy is a normal process. However, women who are pregnant are not immune from injury or other health problems. There may also be complications associated with the pregnancy itself.

TRAUMA

Paramedics frequently receive calls to help a pregnant woman who has been in a motor vehicle accident or who has sustained a fall. In pregnancy, syncope occurs frequently. The syncope of pregnancy often results from compression of the inferior vena cava, as described earlier, or from normal changes in the cardiovascular system associated with pregnancy. Also, the weight of the gravid uterus alters the patient's balance, making her more susceptible to falls.

Pregnant victims of major trauma are more susceptible to life-threatening injury than are non-pregnant victims because of the increased vascularity of the gravid uterus. Trauma is the most frequent, non-obstetric cause of death in pregnant women. Some form of trauma, usually a motor vehicle crash or a fall but sometimes physical abuse, occurs in 6–7 percent of all pregnancies. Since the primary cause for fetal mortality is maternal mortality, the pregnant trauma patient presents a unique challenge. The later in the pregnancy, the larger the uterus and the greater the likelihood of injury. All patients at 20 weeks (or more) gestation with a history of direct or indirect injury should be transported for evaluation by a physician.

Paramedics should *anticipate* the development of shock based on the mechanism of injury rather than waiting for overt signs and symptoms. Due to the cardiovascular changes of pregnancy, overt signs of shock are late and inconsistent. Trauma significant enough to cause maternal shock is associated with a 70–80 percent fetal mortality. In the face of acute blood loss, significant vasoconstriction will occur in response to catecholamine release, resulting in maintenance of a normotensive state for the mother. However, this causes significant uterine hypoperfusion (20–30 percent decrease in cardiac output) and fetal bradycardia.

Generally, the amniotic fluid cushions the fetus from blunt trauma fairly well. However, in direct abdominal trauma, the pregnant patient may suffer premature separation of the placenta from the uterine wall, premature labor, abortion, uterine rupture, and possibly fetal death. The presence of vaginal bleeding or a tender abdomen in a pregnant patient should increase your suspicion of serious injury. Fetal death may result from death of the mother, separation of the placenta from the uterine wall, maternal shock, uterine rupture, or fetal head injury. Any pregnant patient who has suffered trauma should be immediately transported to the emergency department and evaluated by a physician. Trauma management essentials include the following:

- Apply a C-collar to provide cervical stabilization and immobilize on a long backboard.
- Administer high-flow, high-concentration oxygen.
- Initiate two large bore IVs for crystalloid administration per protocol.

Transport all trauma patients at 20 weeks or more gestation. Anticipate the development of shock.

- Transport tilted to the left to minimize supine hypotension.
- Reassess frequently.
- Monitor the fetus.

MEDICAL CONDITIONS

The pregnant patient is subject to all of the medical problems that occur in the non-pregnant state. Abdominal pain is a common complaint. It is often caused by the stretching of the ligaments that support the uterus. However, appendicitis and cholecystitis can also occur. Pregnant women are at increased risk of developing gallstones as a result of hormonal influences that delay emptying of the gall bladder. In pregnancy, the abdominal organs are displaced because of the increased mass of the gravid uterus in the abdomen, which makes assessment more difficult. The pregnant patient with appendicitis may complain of right upper quadrant pain or even back pain. The symptoms of acute cholecystitis may also differ from those in non-pregnant patients. Any pregnant patient with abdominal pain should be evaluated by a physician.

Any pregnant patient with abdominal pain should be evaluated by a physician.

BLEEDING IN PREGNANCY

Vaginal bleeding may occur at any time during pregnancy. Bleeding is usually due to abortion, ectopic pregnancy, placenta previa, or abruptio placentae. Generally, the exact etiology of vaginal bleeding during pregnancy cannot be determined in the field. Refer to the earlier discussion in this chapter and your own local protocols for management of obstetric emergencies. Vaginal bleeding is associated with potential fetal loss. Keep in mind that this is a very emotionally stressful situation for your patient, so a professional, caring demeanor is imperative.

Content Review

CAUSES OF BLEEDING DURING PREGNANCY

Abortion
Ectopic pregnancy
Placenta previa
Abruptio placentae

Abortion

Abortion, the expulsion of the fetus prior to 20 weeks gestation, is the most common cause of bleeding in the first and second trimesters of pregnancy. The terms "abortion" and "miscarriage" can be used interchangeably. Generally, the lay public think of abortion as termination of pregnancy at maternal request and of miscarriage as an accident of nature. Medically, the term abortion applies to both kinds of fetal loss. Spontaneous abortion, the naturally occurring termination of pregnancy that is often called miscarriage, is most commonly seen between the 12th and 14th weeks of gestation. It is estimated that 10 to 20 percent of all pregnancies end in spontaneous abortion. If the pregnancy has not yet been confirmed, the mother often assumes she is merely having a period with unusually heavy flow.

About half of all abortions are due to fetal chromosomal anomalies. Other causes include maternal reproductive system abnormalities, maternal use of drugs, placental defects, or maternal infections. Although many people believe that trauma and psychological stress can cause abortion, research does not support that belief.

* **abortion** termination of pregnancy before the 20th week of gestation. The term "abortion" refers to both miscarriage and induced abortion. Commonly, "abortion" is used for elective termination of pregnancy and "miscarriage" for the loss of a fetus by natural means. A miscarriage is sometimes called a "spontaneous abortion."

CLASSIFICATIONS OF ABORTION

Since you will be interacting with other health care professionals, you should be familiar with the variety of terms used to describe the classifications of abortion.

complete abortion	an abortion in which all of the uterine contents including the fetus and placenta have been expelled.
incomeplete abortion	an abortion in which some, but not all, fetal tissue has been passed. Incomplete abortions are associated with a high incidence of infection.
threatened abortion	a potential abortion characterized by unexplained vaginal bleeding during the first half of pregnancy in which the cervix is slightly open and the fetus remains in the uterus and is still alive. In some cases of threatened abortion, the fetus still can be saved.
inevitable abortion	a potential abortion, characterized by vaginal bleeding accompanied by severe abdominal cramping and cervical dilatation, in which the fetus has not yet passed from the uterus, but the fetus cannot be saved.
spontaneous abortion	naturally occurring expulsion of the fetus prior to viability, generally as a result of chromosomal abnormalities. Most spontaneous abortions occur before the twelfth week of pregnancy. Many occur within two weeks after conception and are mistaken for menstrual periods. Commonly called a *miscarriage*.
elective abortion	an abortion in which the termination of pregnancy is desired and requested by the mother. Elective abortions during the first and second trimesters of pregnancy have been legal in the United States since 1973. Most elective abortions are performed during the first trimester. Some clinics perform second-trimester abortions. Second-trimester abortions have a higher complication rate than first-trimester abortions. Third-trimester elective abortions are generally illegal in this country.
criminal abortion	intentional termination of a pregnancy under any condition not allowed by law. It is usually the attempt to destroy a fetus by a person who is not licensed or permitted to do so. Criminal abortions often are attempted by amateurs and they are rarely performed in aseptic surroundings.
therapeutic abortion	termination of a pregnancy deemed necessary by a physician, usually to protect maternal health and well-being.
missed abortion	an abortion in which fetal death occurs but the fetus is not expelled. This poses a potential threat to the life of the mother if the fetus is retained beyond six weeks.
habitual abortion	spontaneous abortions that occur in three or more consecutive pregnancies.

Assessment The patient experiencing an abortion is likely to report cramping abdominal pain and a backache. She is also likely to report vaginal bleeding, which is often accompanied by the passage of clots and tissue. If the abortion was not recent, then frank signs and symptoms of infection may be present. In addition to your routine emergency assessments, assess for orthostatic vital sign changes and ascertain the amount of vaginal bleeding.

Management Place the patient who is experiencing an abortion in a position of comfort. Treat for shock with oxygen therapy and IV access for fluid resuscitation. As mentioned earlier, any tissue or large clots should be retained and given to emergency department personnel. If the abortion occurs during the late first trimester or later, a fetus may be passed. Often, the placenta does not detach, and the fetus is suspended by the umbilical cord. In such a case, place the umbilical clamps from the OB kit on the cord and cut it. Carefully wrap the fetus in linen or other suitable material and transport it to the hospital with the mother.

An abortion is generally a very sad occurrence. Provide emotional support to the parents. This can be a devastating psychological experience for the mother, so avoid saying trite but inaccurate phrases meant to provide comfort. Inappropriate remarks include "You can always get pregnant again" or "This is nature's way of dealing with a defective fetus." Parents who wish to view the fetus should be allowed to do so. Occasionally, Roman Catholic parents may request baptism of the fetus. You can perform this by making the sign of a cross and stating, "I baptize you in the name of the father, the son, and the holy spirit. Amen."

Signs and symptoms of an abortion include cramping abdominal pain, backache, and vaginal bleeding, often accompanied by passage of clots and tissue.

Treat the patient suffering an abortion as you would any patient at risk for hypovolemic shock. Provide emotional support to the parents.

Ectopic Pregnancy

As you learned earlier, the fertilized egg normally is implanted in the endometrial lining of the uterine wall. The term *ectopic pregnancy* refers to the abnormal implantation of the fertilized egg outside of the uterus. Approximately 95 percent are implanted in the fallopian tube. Occasionally (< one percent), the egg is implanted in the abdominal cavity. Current research indicates that the incidence of ectopic pregnancy is one for every 44 live births. Improved diagnostic technology is credited with an increased incidence, as most are detected between the 2nd and 12th week. Ectopic pregnancy accounts for approximately 10 percent of maternal mortality.

Predisposing factors in the development of ectopic pregnancy include scarring of the fallopian tubes due to pelvic inflammatory disease (PID), a previous ectopic pregnancy, or previous pelvic or tubal surgery, such as a tubal ligation. Other factors include endometriosis or use of an intrauterine device (IUD) for birth control.

Assessment Ectopic pregnancy most often presents as abdominal pain, which starts out as diffuse tenderness and then localizes as a sharp pain in the lower abdominal quadrant on the affected side. This pain is due to rupture of the fallopian tube when the fetus outgrows the available space. The woman often reports that she missed a period or that her LMP occurred 4 to 6 weeks ago, but with decreased menstrual flow that was brownish in color and of shorter duration than usual. As the intra-abdominal bleeding continues, the abdomen becomes rigid and the pain intensifies and is often referred to the shoulder on the affected side. The pain is often accompanied by syncope, vaginal bleeding, and shock.

Assume that any female of childbearing age with lower abdominal pain is experiencing an ectopic pregnancy.

Assume that any female of childbearing age with lower abdominal pain is experiencing an ectopic pregnancy.

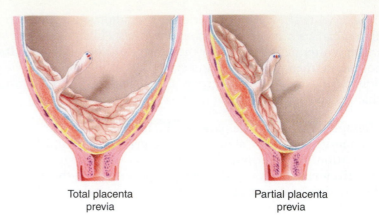

Total placenta
previa

Partial placenta
previa

FIGURE 14-6   Placenta previa (abnormal implantation).

Ectopic pregnancy is life-threatening. Transport the patient immediately.

Management   Ectopic pregnancy poses a significant life threat to the mother. Transport this patient immediately, since surgery is often required to resolve the situation. Interim care measures should include oxygen therapy and IV access for fluid resuscitation. Trendelenburg position or the use of a pneumatic anti-shock garment may be indicated by your local protocols.

Placenta Previa

Placenta previa occurs as a result of abnormal implantation of the placenta on the lower half of the uterine wall, resulting in partial or complete coverage of the cervical opening (Figure 14–6). Vaginal bleeding, which may initially be intermittent, occurs after the 7th month of the pregnancy as the lower uterus begins to contract and dilate in preparation for the onset of labor. This process pulls the placenta away from the uterine wall, causing bright red vaginal bleeding. Placenta previa occurs in about one of every 250 live births. It is classified as complete, partial, or marginal, depending on whether the placenta covers all or part of the cervical opening or is merely in close proximity to the opening.

Third-trimester bleeding should be attributed to either placenta previa or abruptio placentae until proven otherwise. Placenta previa usually presents with painless bleeding. Abruptio placentae usually presents with sharp pain, with or without bleeding.

Although the exact cause of placenta previa is unknown, certain predisposing factors are commonly seen. These factors include a previous history of placenta previa, multiparity, or increased maternal age. Other factors include the presence of uterine scars from cesarean sections, a large placenta, or defective development of blood vessels in the uterine wall.

Assessment   The patient with placenta previa is usually a multigravida in her third trimester of pregnancy. She may have a history of prior placenta previa or of bleeding early in the current pregnancy. She may report a recent episode of sexual intercourse or vaginal examination just before vaginal bleeding began, or she may not bleed until the onset of labor. The onset of painless bright red vaginal bleeding, which may occur as spotting or recurrent hemorrhage, is the hallmark of placenta previa. In fact, any painless bleeding in pregnancy is considered placenta previa until proven otherwise. The bleeding may or may not be associated with uterine contractions. The uterus is usually soft, and the fetus may be in an unusual presentation. *Vaginal examination should never be attempted, as an examining finger can puncture the placenta, causing fatal hemorrhage.*

Never attempt vaginal examination since an examining finger can puncture the placenta and cause fatal hemorrhage.

The presence of placenta previa may already have been diagnosed with an ultrasound during prenatal care, in which case the mother is anticipating the onset of symptoms. The prognosis for the fetus is dependent on the extent of the previa. Obviously, in profuse hemorrhage the fetus is at risk of severe hypoxia

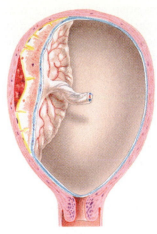
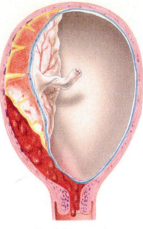
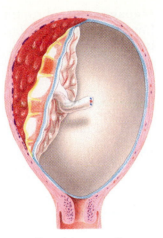

Partial separation
(concealed hemorrhage)

Partial separation
(apparent hemorrhage)

Complete separation
(concealed hemorrhage)

FIGURE 14-7   Abruptio placentae (premature separation).

and the viability of the placenta is compromised. You should perform your assessment and physical exam as discussed earlier in this chapter.

Management   If the placenta previa was previously diagnosed, your patient may already have been managed by placing her on bed rest. Because of the potential for profuse hemorrhage, you should treat for shock. Administer oxygen and initiate intravenous access. Additionally, continue to monitor the maternal vital signs and FHTs. Since the definitive treatment is delivery of the fetus by cesarean section, it is imperative to transport the patient to a hospital with obstetric surgical capability.

Abruptio Placentae

Abruptio placentae, or the premature separation (abruption) of a normally implanted placenta from the uterine wall, poses a potential life threat for both mother and fetus (Figure 14-7). The incidence of abruptio placentae is one in 120 live births. It is associated with 20 to 30 percent fetal mortality, which rises to 100 percent in cases where the majority of the placenta has separated. Maternal mortality is relatively uncommon, although it rises markedly if shock is inadequately treated. Abruptio placentae is classified as marginal (or partial), central (severe), or complete, as explained below.

Although the cause of abruptio placentae is unknown, predisposing factors include multiparity, maternal hypertension, trauma, cocaine use, increasing maternal age, and history of abruption in previous pregnancy.

Assessment   The presenting signs and symptoms of abruptio placentae vary depending on the extent and character of the abruption. Partial abruptions can be marginal or central. Marginal abruptio is characterized by vaginal bleeding but no increase in pain. In central abruptio, the placenta separates centrally and the bleeding is trapped between the placenta and the uterine wall, or "concealed," so there is no vaginal bleeding. However, there is a sudden sharp, tearing pain and development of a stiff, boardlike abdomen. In complete abruptio placentae there is massive vaginal bleeding and profound maternal hypotension. If the patient is in labor at the time of the abruptio, separation of the placenta from the uterine wall will progress rapidly, with fetal distress versus fetal demise dependent on percentage of separation.

Because of the potential for profuse hemorrhage, always treat the patient with suspected placenta previa for shock. Transport immediately since definitive treatment is delivery by cesarean section.

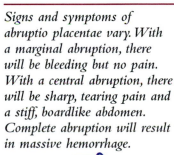

Signs and symptoms of abruptio placentae vary. With a marginal abruption, there will be bleeding but no pain. With a central abruption, there will be sharp, tearing pain and a stiff, boardlike abdomen. Complete abruption will result in massive hemorrhage.

Abruptio placentae is a life-threatening emergency. Treat for shock, including fluid resuscitation, and transport immediately in the left lateral recumbent position.

Management Abruptio placentae is a life-threatening obstetrical emergency. Immediate intervention to maintain maternal oxygenation and perfusion is imperative. Immediately place two large bore intravenous lines and begin fluid resuscitation. Position your patient in the left lateral recumbent position. Transport immediately to a hospital with available surgical obstetric and high-risk neonatal care.

MEDICAL COMPLICATIONS OF PREGNANCY

As discussed earlier, pregnancy can exacerbate pre-existing medical conditions such as diabetes, heart disease, hypertension, and seizure or neuromuscular disorder.

Hypertensive Disorders

The American College of Obstetricians and Gynecologists has identified four classifications of *hypertensive disorders of pregnancy* (formerly called "toxemia of pregnancy"). They include the following:

- *Preeclampsia and eclampsia*

  Pregnancy-induced hypertension (PIH), which includes preeclampsia and eclampsia, occurs in approximately 5 percent of all pregnancies. Preeclampsia is the most common hypertensive disorder seen in pregnancy. There is a higher incidence among primigravidas, particularly if they are teenagers or over the age of 35. Others at increased risk are diabetics, women with a history of preeclampsia, and those who are carrying multiple fetuses.

  Preeclampsia is a progressive disorder that is usually categorized as mild or severe. Seizures (or coma) develop in its most severe form, known as eclampsia. Preeclampsia is defined as an increase in systolic blood pressure by 30 mmHg and/or a diastolic increase of 15 mmHg over baseline on at least two occasions at least six hours apart. Remember that maternal blood pressure normally drops during pregnancy, so a woman may be hypertensive at 120/80 if her baseline in early pregnancy was 90/66. If there is no baseline blood pressure available then a reading ≥ 140/90 is considered to be hypertensive.

  Preeclampsia is most commonly seen in the last ten weeks of gestation, during labor, or in the first 48 hours postpartum. The exact cause of preeclampsia is unknown. It is thought to be caused by abnormal vasospasm, which results in increased maternal blood pressure and other associated symptoms. Additionally, the vasospasm causes decreased placental perfusion, contributing to fetal growth retardation and chronic fetal hypoxia.

  Mild preeclampsia is characterized by hypertension, edema, and protein in the urine. Severe preeclampsia progresses rapidly with maternal blood pressures reaching 160/110 or higher, while the edema becomes generalized and the amount of protein in the urine increases significantly. Other commonly seen signs and symptoms in the severe state include headache, visual disturbances, hyperactive reflexes, and the development of pulmonary edema, along with a dramatic decrease in urine output.

  Patients who are preeclamptic have intravascular volume depletion, since a great deal of their body fluid is in the third space. Those who develop severe preeclampsia and eclampsia are at increased risk for cerebral hemorrhage, pulmonary embolism, abruptio placentae, disseminated intravascular coagulopathy (DIC), and the development of renal failure.

Content Review

MEDICAL COMPLICATIONS OF PREGNANCY

Hypertensive disorders
Supine hypotensive syndrome
Gestational diabetes

Eclampsia, the most serious manifestation of pregnancy-induced hypertension, is characterized by grand mal (major motor) seizure activity. Eclampsia is often preceded by visual disturbances, such as flashing lights or spots before the eyes. Also, the development of epigastric pain or pain in the right upper abdominal quadrant often indicates impending seizure. Eclampsia can often be distinguished from epilepsy by the history and physical appearance of the patient. Patients who become eclamptic are usually grossly edematous and have markedly elevated blood pressure, while epileptics usually have a prior history of seizures and are usually taking anticonvulsant medications. If eclampsia develops, death of the mother and fetus frequently results. The risk of fetal mortality increases by 10 percent with each maternal seizure.

- *Chronic hypertension*

  Hypertension is considered chronic when the blood pressure is ≥ 140/90 before pregnancy or prior to the 20th week of gestation, or if it persists for more than 42 days postpartum. As a general rule, if the diastolic pressure exceeds 80 mmHg during the second trimester, chronic hypertension is likely. The cause of chronic hypertension is unknown. The goal of management is to prevent the development of preeclampsia.

- *Chronic hypertension superimposed with preeclampsia*

  It is not uncommon for the chronic hypertensive who develops preeclampsia to progress rapidly to eclampsia even prior to the 30th week of gestation. The same diagnostic criteria for preeclampsia are used (systolic blood pressure increases > 30 mmHg over baseline, edema, and protein in the urine).

- *Transient hypertension*

  Transient hypertension is defined as a temporary rise in blood pressure which occurs during labor or early in postpartum and which normalizes within ten days.

Assessment Obtaining an accurate history is extremely important whenever you suspect one of the hypertensive disorders of pregnancy. Question the patient about excessive weight gain, headaches, visual problems, epigastric or right upper quadrant abdominal pain, apprehension, or seizures. On physical exam, patients with PIH or preeclampsia are usually markedly edematous. They are often pale and apprehensive. The reflexes are hyperactive. The blood pressure, which is usually elevated, should be taken after the patient has rested for 5 minutes in the left lateral recumbent position.

Management Definitive treatment of the hypertensive disorders of pregnancy is delivery of the fetus. However, in the field, use the following management tactics to prevent dangerously high blood pressures or seizure activity.

- *Hypertension*

  Closely monitor the patient who is pregnant and has elevated blood pressure without edema or other signs of preeclampsia. Record the fetal heart tones and the mother's blood pressure level.

- *Preeclampsia*

  The patient who is hypertensive and shows other signs and symptoms of preeclampsia, such as edema, headaches, and visual disturbances, should be treated quickly. Keep the patient calm and dim the lights. Place the patient in the left lateral recumbent position and quickly carry out the initial assessment. Begin an IV of normal saline.

With suspected hypertensive disorder, it is critical to obtain an accurate history, including information about weight gain, headaches, visual problems, epigastric or right upper quadrant abdominal pain, apprehension, or seizures.

Preeclampsia and eclampsia are life-threatening. Keep the patient calm. Dim the lights. Place patient in left lateral recumbent position and transport quickly without lights or sirens. Administer magnesium sulfate to control seizures if they occur. Medical direction may request administration of antihypertensive or sedative drugs.

Transport the patient rapidly, without lights or sirens. If the blood pressure is dangerously high (diastolic > 110), medical direction may request the administration of hydralazine (Apresoline) or similar anti-hypertensives that are safe for use in pregnancy. If the transport time is long, the administration of magnesium sulfate may also be ordered.

- *Eclampsia*

    If the patient has already suffered a seizure or a seizure appears to be imminent, then, in addition to the above measures, administer oxygen and manage the airway appropriately. Administer a bolus dose of magnesium sulfate (2 to 5 g diluted in 50 to 100 mL slow IV push) to control the seizures. If you are unable to control the seizures with magnesium sulfate, you may consider diazepam (Valium) or other sedative. It is important to keep calcium gluconate available for use as an antidote to magnesium sulfate. Also monitor your patient closely for signs (vaginal bleeding or abdominal rigidity) of abruptio placentae or developing pulmonary edema. Transport immediately to a hospital with surgical obstetric and neonatal care availability.

Supine-Hypotensive Syndrome

Supine-hypotensive syndrome usually occurs in the third trimester of pregnancy. Also known as vena caval syndrome, supine hypotensive syndrome occurs when the gravid uterus compresses the inferior vena cava when the mother lies in a supine position (Figure 14-8).

Assessment Supine-hypotensive syndrome usually occurs in a patient late in her pregnancy who has been supine for a period of time. The patient may complain of dizziness, which results from the decrease in venous return to the right atrium and

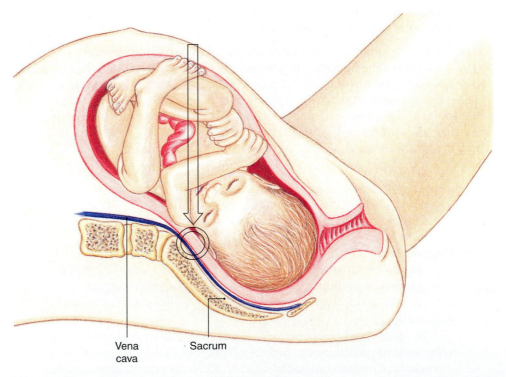

Vena cava   Sacrum

FIGURE 14-8 The supine-hypotensive syndrome results from compression of the inferior vena cava by the gravid uterus.

consequent lowering of the patient's blood pressure. Question the patient about prior episodes of a similar nature and about any recent hemorrhage or fluid loss. Direct the physical examination at determining whether the patient is volume depleted.

Management If there are no indications of volume depletion, such as decreased skin turgor or thirst, place the patient in the left lateral recumbent position or elevate her right hip. Monitor the fetal heart tones and maternal vital signs frequently. If there is clinical evidence of volume depletion, administer oxygen and start an IV of normal saline. Check for orthostatic changes (a decrease in blood pressure and increase in heart rate when rising from the supine position) and place electrodes for cardiac monitoring. Transport the patient promptly in the left lateral recumbent position

Treat supine hypotensive syndrome by placing the patient in the left lateral recumbent position or elevating her right hip. Monitor fetal heart tones and maternal vital signs. If volume depletion is evident, initiate an IV of normal saline.

Gestational Diabetes

Diabetes mellitus occurs in approximately 4 percent of all pregnancies. Hormonal influences cause an increase in insulin production as well as an increased tissue response to insulin during the first 20 weeks of gestation. However, during the last 20 weeks placental hormones cause an increased resistance to insulin and a decreased glucose tolerance. This causes catabolism (the "breaking down" phase of metabolism) between meals and during the night. At these times, ketones may be present in the urine because fats are metabolized more rapidly. Further, maternal glucose stores are used up, as they are the sole source of glucose to meet the energy needs of the growing fetus. This is known as the *diabetogenic* (diabetes-causing) *effect of pregnancy*. Gestational diabetes usually subsides after pregnancy.

Routine prenatal care includes screening to detect diabetes throughout the pregnancy. Women who are considered to be at high risk for developing gestational diabetes are given a glucose tolerance test at their first prenatal visit. High risk is associated with maternal age (over 35), obesity, hypertension, family history of diabetes, and history of prior stillbirth.

Management of gestational diabetes requires good prenatal care. The mother will be instructed on diabetic management and the importance of balancing diet and exercise as well as how to monitor her glucose levels and administer insulin. Fetal development will be monitored on an ongoing basis throughout the pregnancy.

Assessment When you encounter a pregnant patient with an altered mental status, consider hypoglycemia as a likely cause. Remember that the clinical signs and symptoms of hypoglycemia are many and varied. An abnormal mental status is the most important. Physical signs may include diaphoresis and tachycardia. If the blood sugar falls to a critically low level, she may sustain a hypoglycemic seizure or become comatose, which poses a potential life threat to the mother and fetus. Obtaining an accurate history of associated signs and symptoms, such as nausea, vomiting, abdominal pain, increased urination, or a recent infection, will allow you to ascertain whether diabetic ketoacidosis might be the cause of your patient's altered mental status. Determine the blood glucose level in addition to obtaining baseline vital signs and FHTs.

Consider hypoglycemia when encountering a pregnant patient with altered mental status.

Management If the blood glucose level is noted to be less that 60 mg/dl, draw a red-top tube of blood and start an IV of normal saline. Next, administer 50–100 ml (25–50 g) of 50 percent dextrose intravenously. If the patient is conscious and able to swallow, complete glucose administration with orange juice, sugared soft drinks, or commercially available glucose pastes.

If the blood glucose level is in excess of 200 mg/dl, draw a red-top tube (or the tube specified by local protocols) of blood and then establish IV access to administer one to two liters of 0.9 percent sodium chloride per protocol. If transport time is lengthy, medical direction may request intravenous or subcutaneous administration of regular insulin.

If blood glucose is below 60 mg/dl, draw a red-top tube of blood, start an IV of normal saline, and administer 25 grams of 50 percent dextrose. If blood glucose is above 200 mg/dl, draw a red-top tube of blood and administer 1 to 2 liters of normal saline by IV per protocol.

BRAXTON-HICKS CONTRACTIONS

It is occasionally difficult to determine the onset of labor. As early as the 13th week of gestation, the uterus contracts intermittently, thus conditioning itself for the birth process. It is also believed that these contractions enhance placental circulation. These painless, irregular contractions are known as Braxton-Hicks contractions. As the EDC approaches, these contractions become more frequent. Ultimately, the contractions become stronger and more regular, signaling the onset of labor. Labor consists of uterine contractions that cause the dilation and **effacement** (thinning and shortening) of the cervix. The contractions of labor are firm, fairly regular, and quite painful. Prior to the onset of labor Braxton-Hicks contractions, occasionally called *false labor,* increase in intensity and frequency but do not cause cervical changes.

It is virtually impossible to distinguish false labor from true labor in the field. Distinguishing the two requires repeated vaginal examinations, over time, to determine whether the cervix is effacing and dilating. *Remember: Internal vaginal exams should not be performed in the field.* Therefore, all patients with uterine contractions should be transported to the hospital for additional evaluation.

Braxton-Hicks contractions do not require treatment by the paramedic aside from reassurance of the patient and, if necessary, transport for evaluation by a physician.

PRETERM LABOR

As you have already learned, normal gestation is 40 weeks and, in terms of fetal development, the fetus is not considered to be full term until the 38th week. True labor that begins before the 38th week of gestation is called *preterm labor* and frequently requires medical intervention. A variety of maternal, fetal, or placental factors may cause this potentially life-threatening situation for the mother and fetus.

- Maternal Factors
  - Cardiovascular disease
  - Renal disease
  - Pregnancy-induced hypertension (PIH)
  - Diabetes
  - Abdominal surgery during gestation
  - Uterine and cervical abnormalities
  - Maternal infection
  - Trauma, particularly blows to the abdomen
  - Contributory factors: history of preterm birth, smoking, and cocaine abuse
- Placental Factors
  - Placenta previa
  - Abruptio placentae
- Fetal Factors
  - Multiple gestation
  - Excessive amniotic fluid
  - Fetal infection

In many cases, physicians attempt to stop preterm labor to give the fetus additional time to develop in the uterus. Prematurity is the primary neonatal health problem in the nation and occurs in 7 to 10 percent of all live births. All of the preterm infant's organ systems are immature to some degree, but lung development is of greatest concern. Although technological advances in the care of

* **effacement** the thinning and shortening of the cervix during labor.

preterm infants have improved the prognosis dramatically, the consequences of a preterm birth can last a lifetime.

Assessment When confronted by a patient with uterine contractions, first determine the approximate gestational age of the fetus. If it is less than 38 weeks, then suspect preterm labor. If gestational age is greater than 38 weeks, treat the patient as a term patient, as described later in this chapter.

After determining gestational age, obtain a brief obstetrical history. Then question the mother about the urge to push or the need to move her bowels or urinate. Also ask if her membranes have ruptured. Any sensation of fluid leakage or "gushing" from the vagina should be interpreted as ruptured membranes until proven otherwise. Next, palpate the contractions by placing your hand on the patient's abdomen. Note the intensity and length of the contractions, as well as the interval between contractions.

Commonly reported signs and symptoms of preterm labor include contractions that occur every 10 minutes or less, low abdominal cramping that is similar to menstrual cramps, or a sensation of pelvic pressure. Other complaints such as low backache, changes in vaginal discharge, and abdominal cramping with or without diarrhea may also be reported. Rupture of the membranes is confirmatory for preterm labor.

Management Preterm labor, especially if quite early in the pregnancy, should be stopped if possible. The process of stopping labor, or **tocolysis**, is frequently practiced in obstetrics. However, it is infrequently done in the field.

There are three general approaches to tocolysis. The first is to sedate the patient, often with narcotics or barbiturates, thus allowing her to rest. Often, after a period of rest, the contractions stop on their own. The second approach is to administer a fluid bolus intravenously. The administration of approximately 1 liter of fluid intravenously increases the intravascular fluid volume, thus inhibiting ADH secretion from the posterior pituitary. Since oxytocin and ADH are secreted from the same area of the pituitary gland, the inhibition of ADH secretion also inhibits oxytocin release, often causing cessation of uterine contractions. Ultimately, if the above methods fail, a beta agonist, such as terbutaline or ritodrine, or magnesium sulfate may be administered to stop labor by inhibiting uterine smooth muscle contraction. Current research in tocolysis includes the administration of calcium channel blockers, such as nifedipine, and prostaglandin inhibitors, such as indomethacin. You may also find that a patient with preterm labor has been given corticosteroids to accelerate fetal lung maturity.

As a rule, tocolysis in the field is limited to sedation and hydration, especially if transport time is long. Paramedics may, however, transport a patient from one medical facility to another with beta agonist administration underway. You should therefore be familiar with its use. Commonly associated side effects include being jittery, tachycardia usually described by the patient as palpitations, and occasionally abdominal pain. You will, of course, want to transport your patient to the nearest facility that has neonatal intensive care capabilities. Careful and frequent monitoring of maternal vital signs and FHTs is imperative during tocolysis.

The patient with suspected preterm labor should be transported immediately.

* **tocolysis** the process of stopping labor.

THE PUERPERIUM

The **puerperium** is the time period surrounding birth of the fetus. Childbirth generally occurs in a hospital or similar facility with appropriate equipment. Occasionally, prehospital personnel may be called upon to attend a delivery in the field. Therefore, you should be familiar with the birth process and some of the complications that may be associated with it.

* **puerperium** the time period surrounding the birth of the fetus.

LABOR

Childbirth, or the delivery of the fetus, is the culmination of pregnancy. The process by which delivery occurs is called **labor,** the physiologic and mechanical process in which the baby, placenta, and amniotic sac are expelled through the birth canal. The duration of labor is widely variable.

Prior to the onset of true labor, the head of the fetus descends into the bony pelvis area. The frequency and intensity of the Braxton-Hicks contractions increase in preparation for true labor. Increased vaginal secretions and softening of the cervix occur. Bloody show, pink-tinged secretions, is generally considered a sign of imminent labor as the mucous plug is expelled from the cervix. Labor then usually begins within 24 to 48 hours. Many people also consider the rupture of the membranes as a sign of impending labor. If labor does not begin spontaneously within 12 to 24 hours after rupture, labor will likely require induction because of the risk of infection.

Pressure exerted by the fetus on the cervix causes changes that lead to the subsequent expulsion of the fetus. Muscular uterine contractions increase in frequency, strength, and duration. You can assess the frequency and duration of contractions by placing one hand on the fundus of the uterus. Time contractions from the beginning of one contraction until the beginning of the next. It is important to note whether the uterus relaxes completely between contractions. It is also desirable to monitor fetal heart tones during and between contractions. Occasional fetal bradycardia occurs during contractions, but the heart rate should increase to a normal rate (120-160) after the contraction ends. Failure of the heart rate to return to normal between contractions is a sign of fetal distress.

Labor is generally divided into three stages (Figure 14-9):

- **Stage One (Dilatation Stage)**
  The first stage of labor begins with the onset of true labor contractions and ends with the complete dilatation and effacement of the cervix. Early in pregnancy the cervix is quite thick and long, but after complete *effacement* it is short and paper-thin. Effacement usually begins several days before active labor ensues. *Dilatation* is the progressive stretching of the cervical opening. The cervix dilates from its closed position to 10 centimeters, which is considered complete dilation. This stage lasts approximately 8 to 10 hours for the woman in her first labor, the nullipara, and about 5 to 7 hours in the woman who has given birth previously, the multipara. Early in this stage the contractions are usually mild, lasting for 15 to 20 seconds with a frequency of 10 to 20 minutes. As labor progresses, the contractions increase in intensity and occur approximately every 2 to 3 minutes with duration of 60 seconds.

- **Stage Two (Expulsion Stage)**
  The second stage of labor begins with the complete dilatation of the cervix and ends with the delivery of the fetus. In the nullipara, this stage lasts 50 to 60 minutes, while it takes about half that amount of time for the multipara. The contractions are very strong, occurring every 2 minutes and lasting for 60 to 75 seconds. Often, the patient feels pain in her lower back as the fetus descends into the pelvis. The urge to push or "bear down" usually begins in the second stage. The membranes usually rupture at this time, if they have not ruptured previously. Crowning during contractions is evident as the delivery of the fetus nears. Crowning occurs when the head (or other presenting part of the fetus) is visible at the vaginal opening during a contraction and is the definitive sign that birth is imminent. The

Content Review

STAGES OF LABOR
Stage one: dilatation
Stage two: expulsion
Stage three: placental

First stage: beginning of contractions to full cervical dilation

Second stage: baby enters birth canal and is born

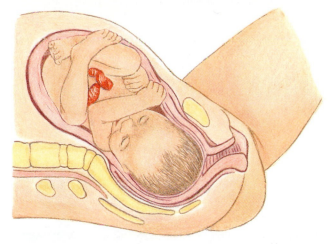
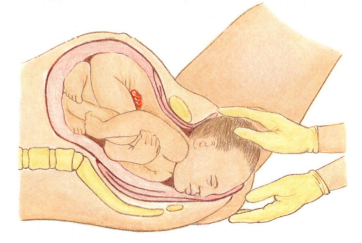

Third stage: delivery of the placenta

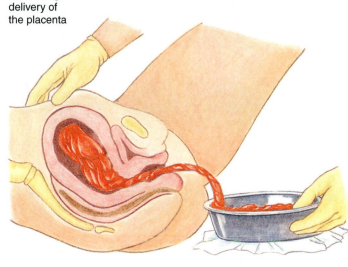

FIGURE 14-9   Stages of labor.

most common presentation is for the infant to be delivered headfirst, face down (vertex position).

- *Stage Three (Placental Stage)*

   The third and final stage of labor begins immediately after the birth of the infant and ends with the delivery of the placenta. The placenta generally delivers within 5 to 20 minutes. There is no need to delay transport to wait for its delivery. Classic signs of placental separation include a gush of blood from the vagina; a change in size, shape or consistency of the uterus; lengthening of the umbilical cord protruding from the vagina; and the mother's report that she has the urge to push.

MANAGEMENT OF A PATIENT IN LABOR

Probably one of the most important decisions you must make with a patient in labor is whether to attempt to deliver the infant at the scene or to transport the patient to the hospital (Figure 14-10). It is generally preferable to transport the mother unless delivery is imminent. There are several factors to take into consideration when making this decision. They include the patient's number of previous

Transport the patient in labor unless delivery is imminent. Maternal urge to push or the presence of crowning indicates imminent delivery. Delivery at the scene or in the ambulance will be necessary.

The Puerperium   **681**

FIGURE 14-10 The decision
to deliver at the scene or to
attempt transport is often a
difficult one.

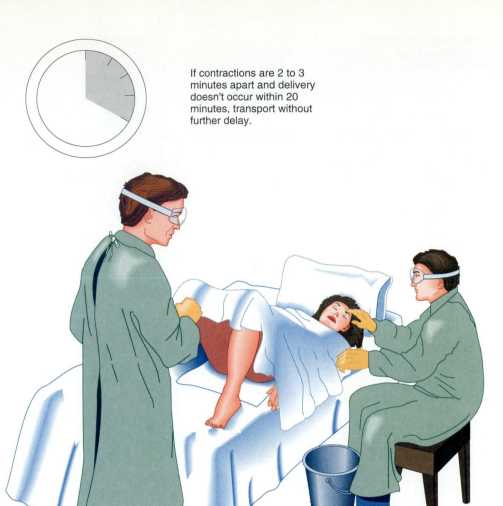

If contractions are 2 to 3
minutes apart and delivery
doesn't occur within 20
minutes, transport without
further delay.

pregnancies, the length of labor during the previous pregnancies, the frequency of contractions, the maternal urge to push, and the presence of crowning. Some women have rapid labors and may be completely dilated in a short period of time. Also, as mentioned above, multiparas generally have shorter labors than nulliparas. The maternal urge to push or the presence of crowning indicates that delivery is imminent. In such cases, the infant should be delivered at the scene or in the ambulance.

Traditionally, a woman who had previously delivered by a cesarean section was advised to deliver all subsequent infants by cesarean sections. However, current thinking encourages women to attempt vaginal birth after cesarean (VBAC). If your patient has had prenatal care during this pregnancy she has probably already discussed this with her health care provider. The only absolute contraindication for VBAC is a classic vertical uterine incision. However, most cesarean sections done today are done using a low transverse uterine incision. (Note that a horizontal skin incision does not assure that the uterine incision is horizontal.) A labor patient who is opting for VBAC requires no more special care than any other labor patient does.

However, certain factors should prompt immediate transport, despite the threat of delivery. These include prolonged rupture of membranes (> 24 hours), since prolonged time between rupture and delivery often leads to fetal infection; abnormal presentation, such as breech or transverse; prolapsed cord; or fetal distress, as evidenced by fetal bradycardia or meconium staining (the presence of meconium, the first fetal stools, in the amniotic fluid). The presence of multiple fetuses may also contribute to your decision to transport. You will read more about these conditions later in this chapter.

FIELD DELIVERY

If delivery is imminent, you can assist the mother to deliver the baby in the field (Procedure 14-1 and Figures 14-11 through 14-19). Equipment and facilities must be quickly prepared. Set up a delivery area. This should be out of public view, such as in a bedroom or the back of the ambulance. Administer oxygen to the mother via nasal cannula or nonrebreather mask. If time permits, establish intravenous access and administer normal saline at a keep-open rate. Place the patient on her back with knees and hips flexed and buttocks slightly elevated. It should be noted that this position is easier on you than the mother. She may prefer to squat or lie in a semi-Fowler's position with her knees and hips flexed. Either of these positions enables gravity to facilitate the delivery. If time permits, drape the mother with toweling from the OB kit. Place one towel under the buttocks, another below the vaginal opening, and another across the lower abdomen.

Until delivery, the fetal heart rate should be monitored frequently. A drop in the fetal heart rate to less than 90 beats per minute indicates fetal distress and should prompt immediate transport with the mother in the left lateral recumbent position. Coach the mother to breathe deeply between contractions and to push with contractions. If the baby does not deliver after 20 minutes of contractions every 2–3 minutes, *transport immediately*.

Prepare the OB equipment and don sterile gloves, gown, and goggles. If time permits, wash your hands and forearms prior to gloving. As the head crowns, control it with gentle pressure. Providing support to the head and perineum decreases the likelihood of vaginal and perineal tearing and decreases the potential for rapid expulsion of the baby's skull through the birth canal which may cause intracranial injury. Support the head as it emerges from the vagina and begins to turn. If it is still enclosed in the amniotic sac, tear the sac open to permit escape of the amniotic fluid and enable the baby to breathe.

Gently slide your finger along the head and neck to ensure that the umbilical cord is not wrapped around the baby's neck. If it is, try to gently slip it over the shoulder and head. If this cannot be done and it is so wrapped tightly as to inhibit labor, carefully place two umbilical cord clamps approximately 2 inches apart and cut the cord between the clamps. As soon as the infant's head is clear of the vagina, instruct the mother to stop pushing. While supporting the head, suction the baby's mouth, then nose, using a bulb syringe. If meconium-stained fluid is noted, suction the mouth, nares, and pharynx with mechanical suction to prevent aspiration. Then tell the mother to resume pushing, while you support the infant's head as it rotates.

Gently guide the baby's head downward to allow delivery of the upper shoulder. Do not pull! Gently guide the baby's body upward to allow delivery of the lower shoulder. Once the head and shoulders have been delivered, the rest of the body will follow rapidly. Be prepared to support the infant's body as it emerges. Remember to keep the baby at the level of the vagina to prevent over- or undertransfusion of blood from the cord. Never "milk" the cord. Clamp and cut the

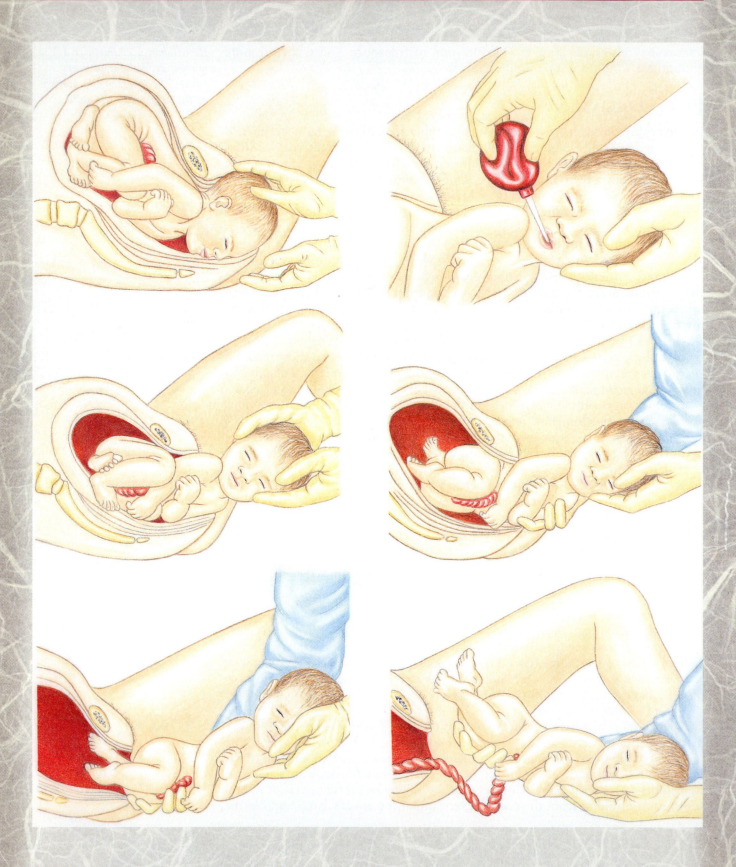

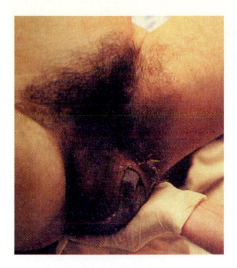

FIGURE 14-11 Crowning.

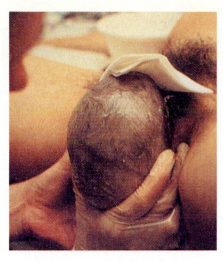

FIGURE 14-12 Delivery of the head.

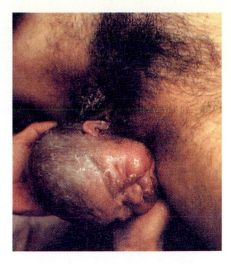

FIGURE 14-13 External rotation of the head.

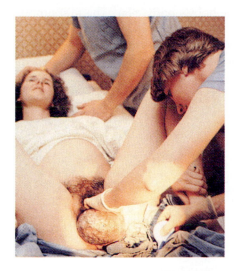

FIGURE 14-14 As soon as possible, suction the mouth, then the nose.

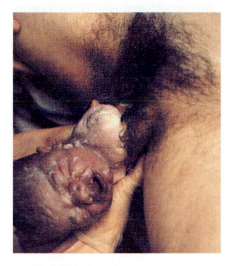

FIGURE 14-15 Delivery of the anterior shoulder.

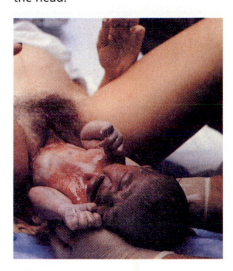

FIGURE 14-16 Complete delivery of the infant.

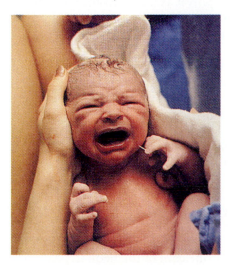

FIGURE 14-17 Dry the infant.

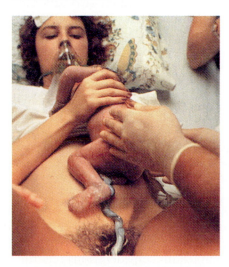

FIGURE 14-18 Place the infant on the mother's stomach.

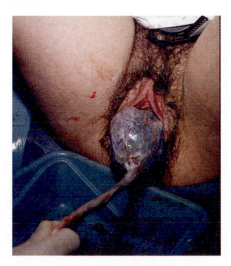

FIGURE 14-19 Deliver the placenta and save for transport with the mother and infant.

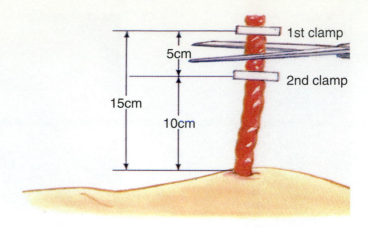

FIGURE 14-20   Clamp and cut the cord.

cord as follows (Figure 14-20). Supporting the baby's body, place the first umbilical clamp approximately 10 centimeters from the baby. Place the second clamp approximately 5 centimeters above the first. Then carefully cut the umbilical cord between the clamps. Wipe the baby's face clean of blood and mucus and repeat suctioning of the mouth and nose until the airway is clear. Dry the infant thoroughly and then cover with warm, dry blankets or towels, and position on his side. Record the time of birth.

Usual maternal blood loss with delivery is 1 pint (about 500 cc). Following delivery, if the uterus is contracting normally, the fundus should be at the level of the umbilicus and have the size and consistency of a grapefruit. After birth, the mother's vagina should continue to ooze blood. Do not pull on the umbilical cord. Eventually, the cord will appear to lengthen, which indicates separation of the placenta. The placenta should be delivered and transported with the mother to the hospital. If it does deliver, place it in a plastic biohazard bag and bring it to the hospital for evaluation. Retained placenta may cause maternal hemorrhage or become a source of infection. However, there is no need to delay transport for delivery of the placenta. At this time, massage the uterine fundus by placing one hand immediately above the symphysis pubis and the other on the uterine fundus. Cup the uterus between the two hands and support it as it is massaged. Continue massage until the uterus assumes a woody hardness. Avoid overmassage. Putting the baby to the mother's breast also stimulates uterine contractions, which will further decrease bleeding.

Following delivery, inspect the mother's perineum for tears. If any tears are present, apply direct pressure. Continuously monitor vital signs. Note the presence of continued hemorrhage and report it to medical direction. In some systems, paramedics may administer oxytocin (Pitocin) to facilitate uterine contraction in the control of postpartum hemorrhage. Oxytocin should only be administered *after* delivery of the placenta has been confirmed. Following stabilization, transport the mother and infant to the hospital.

NEONATAL CARE

* **neonate** newborn infant

Care of the **neonate** will be discussed in detail in Volume 5, Chapter 1. Initial care of the neonate has been described in the preceding section. Several additional important considerations regarding routine care of the neonate, APGAR scoring, and neonatal resuscitation are briefly discussed in the following sections.

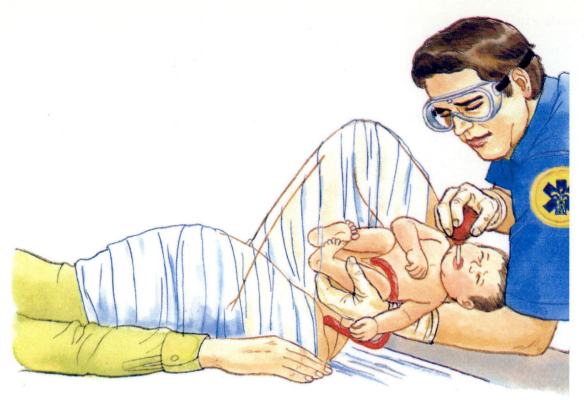

FIGURE 14-21   Re-suction the airway as needed.

Routine Care of the Neonate

Newborns are slippery and will require both hands to support the head and torso. Position yourself so that you can work close to the surface where you have placed the infant.

Maintain warmth! Cold infants rapidly become distressed infants. Quickly dry the infant with towels, discarding each as it becomes wet. Then cover the infant with a dry receiving blanket or use a commercial warming blanket made of a material such as Thinsulate™.

Repeat suctioning of the mouth and nose as needed until the infant's airway is clear (Figure 14-21). Generally, suctioning and drying the baby will stimulate respirations, crying, and activity. This should cause the infant to "pink up." (Do not be alarmed if the extremities remain dusky. This is known as *acrocyanosis* and is very common in the first hours of life.) If this is not effective, you may try flicking your finger against the soles of the feet or rubbing gently in a circular motion in the middle of the back (Figure 14-22).

Assess the neonate as soon as possible after birth. The normal neonatal respiratory rate should average 30–60 breaths per minute while the heart rate should be between 100–180 beats per minute. If resuscitation is not indicated, assign APGAR scores. Do not however, delay resuscitative efforts and transport in order to complete APGAR scoring.

APGAR Scoring

Named for Dr. Virginia Apgar, who developed the assessment tool, the APGAR scoring system is a means of evaluating the status of a newborn's vital functions at 1 minute and 5 minutes after delivery. There are five parameters and each is given

Support the infant's head and torso, using both hands. Maintain warmth, repeat suctioning of the mouth and nose as needed, and assess using APGAR scoring.

FIGURE 14-22 Stimulate the infant as required.

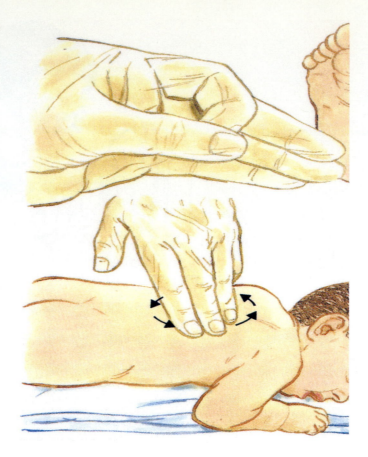

a score from a low value of 0 to a normal value of 2. APGAR is an acronym for the names of the five parameters, which are *a*ppearance (skin color), *p*ulse rate, *g*rimace (irritability), *a*ctivity (muscle tone), and *r*espiratory effort (Table 14-2).

The majority of infants are healthy and active and have total scores between 7–10, requiring only routine care. Infants scoring between 4–6 are moderately depressed and require oxygen and stimulation to breathe. Infants scoring 0–3 are severely depressed and require immediate ventilatory and circulatory assistance. By repeating the score at 1 and 5 minutes, it is possible to determine whether intervention has caused a change in infant status.

Neonatal Resuscitation

It is estimated that approximately 6 percent of all neonates born in a hospital require resuscitation. It is likely that this percentage is higher for out-of-hospital deliveries, although the exact numbers are not available. Factors that contribute to the need for resuscitation include prematurity, pregnancy and delivery complications, maternal health problems, or inadequate prenatal care.

If tactile stimulation does not increase the neonate's respiratory rate, immediately assist ventilations using a pediatric bag-valve-mask device attached to high-flow oxygen. Reassess after 15 to 30 seconds. If the respiratory rate is now within normal limits, assess the heart rate. If not, continue ventilations.

Assess the heart rate using a stethoscope to auscultate the apical pulse, by feeling the pulse at the base of the umbilical cord, or by palpating the brachial or femoral artery. The heart rate should normally be between 100 and 180 beats per minute with a range of 140 to 160 beats per minute being optimal. If

If the infant's respirations are below 30 per minute and tactile stimulation does not increase the rate to a normal range, immediately assist ventilations using a pediatric bag-valve-mask with high-flow oxygen. If the heart rate is below 80 and does not respond to ventilations, initiate chest compressions. Transport to a facility with neonatal intensive care capabilities.

Table 14-2	THE APGAR SCORE			
Element	0	1	2	Score
Appearance (skin color)	Body and extremities blue, pale	Body pink, extremities blue	Completely pink	
Pulse rate	Absent	Below 100/min	100/min or above	
Grimace (Irritability)	No response	Grimace	Cough, sneeze, cry	
Activity (Muscle tone)	Limp	Some flexion of extremities	Active motion	
Respiratory effort	Absent	Slow and irregular	Strong cry	
			TOTAL SCORE =	

the pulse is 100 or greater with spontaneous respirations, continue your assessment. If the rate is less than 100, continue positive pressure ventilations. Initiate chest compressions if the heart rate is less than 80 beats per minute and is not responding to ventilations. Continue to reassess respiratory status and heart rate frequently.

Make every effort to expedite transport to a facility capable of providing neonatal intensive care while you continue resuscitative efforts. If you have a long transport time, it may be necessary to initiate vascular access in order to administer medications or fluid resuscitation. The most logical (and easiest) access is the umbilical vein. If this is not feasible, consider peripheral veins or an intraosseous access. While many medications (epinephrine, atropine, lidocaine, and naloxone) can be administered via the endotracheal route, this route is not suitable for fluid resuscitation. During transport, continue to maintain warmth while supporting ventilations, oxygenation, and circulation. Refer to Volume 5, Chapter 1 for more information regarding neonatal resuscitation.

ABNORMAL DELIVERY SITUATIONS

Breech Presentation

Most infants present head first and face down, which is called the vertex position. Breech presentation is the term used to describe the situation in which either the buttocks or both feet present first. This occurs in approximately 4 percent of all live births. In such presentations, there is an increased risk for delivery trauma to the mother, as well as an increased potential for cord prolapse, cord compression, or anoxic insult for the infant. Although the cause is unknown, breech presentations are most commonly associated with preterm birth, placenta previa, multiple gestation, and uterine and fetal anomalies.

Management Because cesarean section is often required, delivery of the breech presentation is best accomplished at the hospital. However, if field delivery is unavoidable, the following maneuvers are recommended. First, position the mother with her buttocks at the edge of a firm bed. Ask her to hold her legs in a flexed

Content Review

ABNORMAL DELIVERIES
Breech presentation
Prolapsed cord
Limb presentation
Occiput posterior

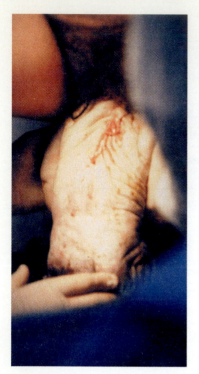

FIGURE 14-23 Breech delivery.

> *If the infant starts to breathe with its face pressed against the vaginal wall, form a "V" with the index and middle fingers on either side of the infant's nose and push the vaginal wall away from the infant's face. If necessary, continue during transport.*

position. She will often require assistance in doing this. As the infant delivers, do not pull on the infant's legs. Simply support them. Allow the entire body to be delivered with contractions while you merely continue to support the infant's body (Figure 14-23).

As the head passes the pubis, apply gentle upward traction until the mouth appears over the perineum. If the head does not deliver, and the baby begins to breathe spontaneously with its face pressed against the vaginal wall, place a gloved hand in the vagina with the palm toward the infant's face. Form a "V" with the index and middle fingers on either side of the infant's nose, and push the vaginal wall away from the infant's face to allow unrestricted respiration (Figure 14-24). If necessary, continue during transport.

Alternatively, you may find that the shoulders, not the head, are the most difficult part to deliver. In that case, allow the body to deliver to the level of the umbilicus. Support the infant's body in your palm while gently extracting approximately 4 to 6 inches of umbilical cord. Be very careful that you do not compress the cord during this extraction. Gently rotate the infant's body so that the shoulders are now in an anterior-posterior position. Apply gentle traction to the body until the axilla become visible. Guide the infant's body upward to deliver the posterior shoulder. Then, guide the neonate downward to facilitate delivery of the anterior shoulder. Now gently ease the head through the birth canal. Continue your care of the mother and infant as you would with a normal delivery.

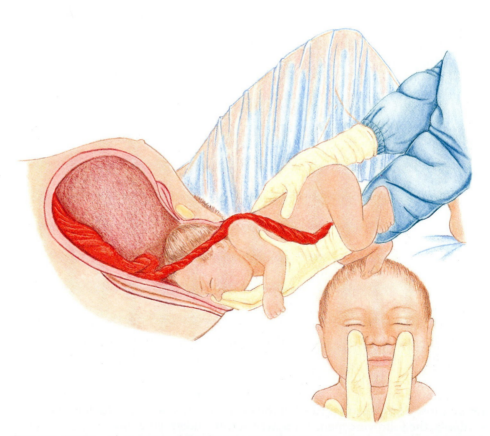

FIGURE 14-24 Placement of the fingers to maintain the airway in a breech birth.

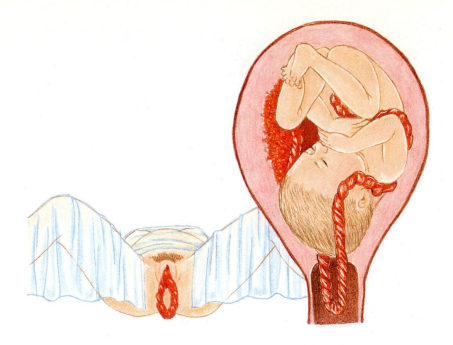

- Elevate hips, administer oxygen and keep warm
- Keep baby's head away from cord
- Do not attempt to push cord back
- Wrap cord in sterile moist towel
- Transport mother to hospital, continuing pressure on baby's head

FIGURE 14-25   Prolapsed cord.

Prolapsed Cord

A *prolapsed cord* occurs when the umbilical cord precedes the fetal presenting part. This causes the cord to be compressed between the fetus and the bony pelvis, shutting off fetal circulation (Figure 14-25). This occurs once in every 250 deliveries. Predisposing factors include prematurity, multiple births, and premature rupture of the membranes before the head is fully engaged. It is a serious emergency, and fetal death will occur quickly without prompt intervention.

Management If the umbilical cord is seen in the vagina, insert two fingers of a gloved hand to raise the presenting part of the fetus off the cord. At the same time, gently check the cord for pulsations, but take great care to insure that you do not compress the cord. Place the mother in a Trendelenburg or knee-chest

If the umbilical cord is seen in the vagina, insert two gloved fingers to raise the fetus off the cord. Place the mother in Trendelenburg or knee-chest position, administer oxygen, and transport immediately. Do not attempt delivery.

FIGURE 14-26 Patient positioning for prolapsed cord.

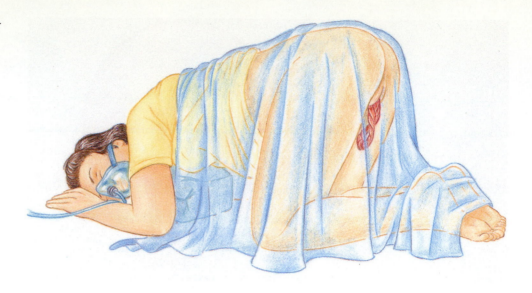

position (Figure 14-26). Administer high-flow oxygen to the mother and transport her immediately, with the fingers continuing to hold the presenting part off the umbilical cord. If assistance is available, apply a dressing moistened with sterile saline to the exposed cord. *Do not attempt delivery! Do not pull on the cord! Do not attempt to push the cord back into the vagina!*

Limb Presentation

Sometimes, if the baby is in a transverse lie across the uterus, an arm or leg is the presenting part protruding from the vagina. This is seen in less than one percent of births and is more commonly associated with preterm birth and multiple gestation.

Management When examination of the perineum reveals a single arm or leg protruding from the birth canal, a cesarean section is necessary. Under no circumstance should you attempt a field delivery. Do not touch the extremity, as to do so may stimulate the infant to gasp, risking inhalation and aspiration of amniotic fluid. *Do not pull on the extremity or attempt to push it back into vagina!*

Assist the mother into a knee-chest position as is also done when there is a prolapsed cord and administer oxygen via nonrebreather mask. Provide reassurance to the mother. Transport immediately (still in knee-chest position) for emergency cesarean section.

With limb presentation, place the mother in knee-chest position, administer oxygen, and transport immediately. Do not attempt delivery.

Other Abnormal Presentations

Other abnormal presentations can complicate delivery. One of the most common is the *occiput posterior position.* Normally, as the infant descends into the pelvis, its face is turned posteriorly. This is important, as extension of the head assists delivery. However, if the infant descends facing forward, or occiput posterior, its passage through the pelvis is delayed. This presentation occurs most frequently in primigravidas. In multigravidas it usually resolves spontaneously.

The presenting part may also be the face or brow, rather than the crown of the head. Occasionally, during these presentations, the face or brow can be seen high in the pelvis during a contraction. Usually, vaginal delivery is impossible in these cases.

As described earlier for a limb presentation, the fetus can lie transversely in the uterus. In such a case, the fetus cannot enter the pelvis for delivery. If the membranes rupture, the umbilical cord can prolapse, or an arm or leg can enter the vagina. Vaginal delivery is impossible.

Management Early recognition of an abnormal presentation is important. If one is suspected, the mother should be reassured, placed on oxygen, and transported immediately, since forceps or cesarean delivery is often required.

OTHER DELIVERY COMPLICATIONS

Although most deliveries proceed without incident, complications can arise. Therefore, you should be prepared to deal with them.

Multiple Births

Multiple births are fairly rare, with twins occurring approximately once in every 90 deliveries, about 40 percent of those being preterm. Usually, the mother knows or at least suspects the presence of more than one fetus. Multiple births should also be suspected if the mother's abdomen remains large after delivery of one baby and labor continues.

Management Manage this situation with the normal delivery guidelines, recognizing that you will need additional personnel and equipment to manage a multiple birth. In twin births, labor often begins earlier than expected, and the infants are generally smaller than babies born singly. Usually, one twin presents vertex and the other breech. There may be one shared placenta or two placentas. After delivery of the first baby, clamp and cut the cord. Then deliver the second baby. Because prematurity is common in multiple births, low birth weight is common and prevention of hypothermia is even more crucial.

Cephalopelvic Disproportion

Cephalopelvic disproportion occurs when the infant's head is too big to pass through the maternal pelvis easily. This may be caused by an oversized fetus. Large fetuses are associated with diabetes, multiparity, or post-maturity. Fetal abnormalities such as hydrocephalus, conjoined twins, or fetal tumors may make vaginal delivery impossible. Women of short stature or women with contracted pelvises are at increased risk for this problem. If cephalopelvic disproportion is not recognized and managed appropriately, fetal demise or uterine rupture may occur.

Cephalopelvic disproportion tends to develop most frequently in the primigravida. There may be strong contractions for an extended period of time. On physical examination, the fetus may feel large. Also, labor generally does not progress. The fetus may be in distress, as evidenced by fetal bradycardia or meconium staining.

Management The usual management of cephalopelvic disproportion is cesarean section. Administer oxygen to the mother and establish intravenous access. Transport should be immediate and rapid.

Precipitous Delivery

A *precipitous delivery* is a delivery that occurs after less than 3 hours of labor. This type of delivery occurs most frequently in the grand multipara and is associated with a higher-than-normal incidence of fetal trauma, tearing of the umbilical cord, or maternal lacerations.

Management The best way to handle precipitous delivery is to be prepared. Do not turn your attention from the mother. Be ready for a rapid delivery, and

Whenever an abnormal presentation or position of the fetus makes normal delivery impossible, reassure the mother, administer oxygen, and transport immediately. Do not attempt field delivery in these circumstances.

Content Review

OTHER DELIVERY COMPLICATIONS
Multiple births
Cephalopelvic disproportion
Precipitous delivery
Shoulder dystocia
Meconium staining

attempt to control the infant's head. Once delivered, the baby may have some difficulty with temperature regulation and must be kept warm.

Shoulder Dystocia

A *shoulder dystocia* occurs when the infant's shoulders are larger than its head. This occurs most frequently with diabetic and obese mothers and in post-term pregnancies. In shoulder dystocia, labor progresses normally and the head is delivered routinely. However, immediately after the head is delivered, it retracts back into the perineum because the shoulders are trapped between the symphysis pubis and the sacrum ("turtle sign").

Management If a shoulder dystocia occurs, *do not pull on the infant's head*. Administer oxygen to the mother and have her drop her buttocks off the end of the bed. Then flex her thighs upward to facilitate delivery and apply firm pressure with an open hand immediately above the symphysis pubis. If delivery does not occur, transport the patient immediately.

Meconium Staining

Meconium staining occurs when the fetus passes feces into the amniotic fluid. Between 10 and 30 percent of all deliveries have meconium-stained fluid. It is always indicative of a fetal hypoxic incident. Hypoxia causes an increase in fetal peristalsis along with relaxation of the anal sphincter, causing meconium to pass into the amniotic fluid. In addition to the stress that caused the incident, there is a risk of aspiration of the meconium-stained fluid.

Meconium staining is often associated with prolonged labor but may be seen in term, post-term, and low birth weight infants. The incident may occur a few days prior to delivery or during labor. Some meconium staining is virtually always associated with breech deliveries. This is due to vagal stimulation, which occurs as a result of the pressure of the contracting uterus on the fetus's head.

Evidence of meconium staining is readily observable. Normally the amniotic fluid is clear or possibly light straw-colored. When meconium is present, the color varies from a light yellowish-green to light green or worst case, dark green, which is sometimes described as "pea soup." As a rule, the thicker and darker the color, the higher the risk of fetal morbidity.

If meconium is thick, visualize the infant's glottis and suction the hypopharynx and trachea using an endotracheal tube until all meconium has been cleared from the airway.

Management As noted earlier, once the head of the newborn is out of the birth canal you should suction the mouth and nose on the perineum. If the meconium is thin and light colored no further treatment is required, and you should continue with the delivery and routine care. However, if the meconium is thick, visualize the glottis and suction the hypopharynx and trachea using an endotracheal tube until you have cleared all of the meconium from the newborn's airway. Failure to do so will cause the meconium to be pushed farther into the airway and down into the lungs during the delivery process.

MATERNAL COMPLICATIONS OF LABOR AND DELIVERY

Several maternal problems can arise during and after delivery. These include postpartum hemorrhage, uterine rupture, uterine inversion, and pulmonary embolism.

Postpartum Hemorrhage

Postpartum hemorrhage is the loss of more than 500 cc of blood immediately following delivery. It occurs in approximately 5 percent of deliveries. The most common

Content Review

MATERNAL COMPLICATIONS
Postpartum hemorrhage
Uterine rupture
Uterine inversion
Pulmonary embolism

cause of postpartum hemorrhage is *uterine atony*, or lack of uterine muscle tone. This tends to occur most frequently in the multigravida and is most common following multiple births or births of large infants. Uterine atony also occurs after precipitous deliveries and prolonged labors. In addition to uterine atony, postpartum hemorrhage can be caused by placenta previa, abruptio placentae, retained placental parts, clotting disorders in the mother, or vaginal and cervical tears. Occasionally, the uterus fails to return to its normal size during the postpartum period, and postpartum hemorrhage occurs long after the birth, potentially as much as two weeks postpartum.

Assessment of the patient with postpartum hemorrhage should focus on the history and the predisposing factors described above. You must rely heavily on the clinical appearance of the patient and her vital signs. Often, the uterus will feel boggy and soft on physical examination. Vaginal bleeding is usually obvious as a steady, free flow of blood. Counting the number of sanitary pads used is a good way to monitor the bleeding. When postpartum bleeding takes place in the hospital setting the pads are often weighed, since 500 cc of blood weighs approximately one pound. You should also examine the perineum for evidence of traumatic injury, which may be the source of the bleeding.

Management When confronted by a patient with postpartum hemorrhage, complete the initial assessment immediately. Administer oxygen and begin fundal massage. Establish at least one, preferably two, large-bore IVs of normal saline. If shock is evident, apply anti-shock trousers according to your local protocols. Never attempt to force delivery of the placenta or pack the vagina with dressings. In severe cases, medical direction may request the administration of oxytocin (Pitocin). The usual dose is 10 to 20 USP units (20 mg) oxytocin in one liter of normal saline to run at 125 cc/hr titrated to response. If IV access cannot be obtained, an alternative therapy is to administer 10 USP units intramuscularly.

When there is a loss of more than 500 cc of blood immediately following delivery, administer oxygen and begin fundal massage. Establish two large-bore IVs of normal saline. Treat for shock as necessary. Follow local protocols regarding application of anti-shock trousers.

Uterine Rupture

Uterine rupture is the actual tearing, or rupture, of the uterus. It usually occurs with the onset of labor. However, it can also occur before labor as a result of blunt abdominal trauma. During labor, it often results from prolonged uterine contractions or a surgically scarred uterus, such as occurs from previous cesarean sections, especially in those with the classic vertical incision. It can also occur following a prolonged or obstructed labor, as in the case of cephalopelvic disproportion or in conjunction with abnormal presentations. Although it is a rare occurrence, it carries with it an extremely high maternal and fetal mortality rate.

The patient with uterine rupture will complain of excruciating abdominal pain and will often be in shock. Uterine rupture is virtually always associated with the cessation of labor contractions. If the rupture is complete, the pain usually subsides. On physical examination, there is often profound shock without evidence of external hemorrhage, although it is sometimes associated with vaginal bleeding. Fetal heart tones are absent. The abdomen is often tender and rigid and may exhibit rebound tenderness. It is often possible to palpate the uterus as a separate hard mass found next to the fetus.

Management Management is the same as for any patient in shock. Administer oxygen at high concentration. Next, establish two large-bore IVs with normal saline and begin fluid resuscitation. Monitor vital signs and fetal heart tones continuously. Transport the patient rapidly. If the fetus is still viable, the definitive treatment is cesarean section with subsequent repair or removal of the uterus.

Uterine Inversion

Uterine inversion is a rare emergency occurring only once in every 2,500 live births. It occurs when the uterus turns inside out after delivery and extends through the cervix. When uterine inversion occurs, the supporting ligaments and blood vessels supplying blood to the uterus are torn, usually causing profound shock. The average blood loss associated with uterine inversion ranges from 800 to 1,800 cc. Uterine inversion usually results from pulling on the umbilical cord while awaiting delivery of the placenta or from attempts to express the placenta when the uterus is relaxed.

In the rare occurrence of uterine inversion, begin fluid resuscitation, then make one attempt to replace the uterus. If this fails, cover the uterus with towels moistened with saline and transport immediately.

Management If uterine inversion occurs, you must act quickly. First, place the patient in a supine position and begin oxygen administration. *Do not* attempt to detach the placenta or pull on the cord. Initiate two large bore IVs of normal saline and begin fluid resuscitation. Make one attempt to replace the uterus, using the following technique. With the palm of the hand, push the fundus of the inverted uterus toward the vagina. If this single attempt is unsuccessful, cover the uterus with towels moistened with saline and transport the patient immediately.

Pulmonary Embolism

Pulmonary embolism is the presence of a blood clot in the pulmonary vascular system (see Chapter 1). It can occur after pregnancy, usually as a result of venous thromboembolism. It is one of the most common causes of maternal death and appears to occur more frequently following cesarean section than vaginal delivery. Pulmonary embolism may occur at any time during pregnancy. There is usually a sudden onset of severe dyspnea accompanied by sharp chest pain. Some patients also report a sense of impending doom. On physical examination, the patient may show tachycardia, tachypnea, jugular vein distention, and, in severe cases, hypotension.

Pulmonary embolism usually presents with sudden severe dyspnea and sharp chest pain. Administer high-flow oxygen and support ventilations as needed. Establish an IV of normal saline. Transport immediately, monitoring the heart, vital signs, and oxygen saturation.

Management Management of pulmonary embolism consists of administration of high-flow oxygen and ventilatory support as needed. Also establish an IV of normal saline at a keep-open rate. Initiate cardiac monitoring and carefully monitor the patient's vital signs and oxygen saturation while transporting her immediately.

SUMMARY

Childbirth is a normal process and obstetrical emergencies are fairly uncommon. However, all pregnant patients are at risk for developing complications, and it is impossible to predict which ones will actually occur. It is therefore important to recognize these complications and act accordingly. Keep in mind that you are caring for two patients, and as long as you remember the priorities of patient care, the situation should go smoothly. Relax and enjoy the opportunity to help bring a new life into the world.

YOU MAKE THE CALL

It is 9 A.M. and you and your partner are participating in an in-station drill when you are dispatched for a "possible stroke." You soon arrive at a garden apartment where you are met by a very anxious man. He reports that he just arrived home from working the night shift and found his pregnant wife semi-conscious on the living room floor. He says that he talked to her about an hour ago and she was "fine."

Your assessment reveals a 25-year-old pregnant female who responds to verbal stimuli with incoherent muttering. Her airway is patent and her respirations are non-labored at a rate of 20 per minute. Lung sounds are clear bilaterally. Her pulse is strong and regular at 96 per minute. Her flushed skin is warm to the touch. She is diaphoretic. You observe that her ankles are markedly edematous. Her blood pressure is 158/100. There are no obvious signs of traumatic injury.

Your partner starts her on high-flow oxygen with a nonrebreather mask and initiates an IV of normal saline at a keep-open rate. He also checks her blood glucose level and finds that it is >120 mg/dl. You obtain her obstetric history, learning that she is a G1P0 who is at 32 weeks gestation. She has had good prenatal care and is scheduled for an appointment at 4 o'clock this afternoon. Her husband tells you that she has been taking prenatal vitamins with iron throughout her pregnancy. He denies any other medical problems other than the fact that her doctor has been "watching" her blood pressure for the past couple of months. He denies any alcohol or recreational drug use by his wife.

1. What is your first priority?
2. What do you suspect is the likely cause of the patient's signs and symptoms?
3. Your patient's husband is very concerned about the well-being of his wife and baby. What should you tell him?
4. How should this patient be transported to the hospital?

See Suggested Responses at the back of this book.

FURTHER READING

Cunningham, F., et. al. *Williams Obstetrics*, 20th ed. New York: McGraw-Hill, 1996.

Davis, Robert B. and Donna Vinal. "When Things Go Wrong at Home: Obstetrical Emergencies Outside the Hospital." *JEMS* 20(5): 30–38.

Flatum-Riemers, Jan. "OB Emergencies." *Emergency Medical Services* 23(4): 51–57.

Greenspan, Francis S. and Gordon J. Strewler. *Basic and Clinical Endocrinology.* 5th Ed. Stamford, Conn.: Appleton and Lange, 1997.

Kupas, Douglas E., Scott C. Harter, and Arno Vosk. "Out-of-Hospital Perimortem Cesarean Section." *Prehospital Emergency Care* 2(3), 206–208.

Ladewig, Patricia Wieland, Marcia L. London, and Sally B. Olds. *Essentials of Newborn Nursing.* 4th ed. Menlo Park, Calif.: Addison Wesley Longman, 1998.

Mattera, Connie J. "Emergency Childbirth: Part 1." *JEMS* 23(6), 74–85.

_____. "Emergency Childbirth: Part 2." *JEMS* 23(77), 60–74.

McCance, Kathryn L. and Sue E. Huether. *Pathophysiology: The Biologic Basis for Disease in Adults and Children.* 3rd ed. St. Louis: Mosby, 1998.

Neff, Janet A. and Pamela Stinson Kidd. *Trauma Nursing: The Art and Science.* St. Louis: Mosby-Year Book, 1992.

Shah, Kayur H., Richard K. Simons, Troy Holbrook, Dale Fortlage, Robert J. Winchell, and David B. Hoyt. "Trauma in Pregnancy: Maternal and Fetal Outcomes." *The Journal of Trauma* 45(1), 83–86.

Thibodeau, Gary A. and Kevin T. Patton. *Anatomy and Physiology.* 4th ed. St. Louis: Mosby-Year Book, 1999.

Tortora, Gerard J. et. al. *Principles of Anatomy and Physiology.* 9th ed. John Wiley & Sons, 1999.

Vilke, Gary M., Glenn Mahoney, and Theodore C. Chan. "Postpartum Coronary Artery Dissection." *Annals of Emergency Medicine* 32(2), 260–262.

ON THE WEB

Visit Brady's Paramedic Website at www.bradybooks.com/paramedic.

Suggested Responses to "You Make the Call"

The following are suggested responses to the "You Make the Call" scenarios presented in each chapter of Paramedic Care, Volume 3, Medical Emergencies. *Each represents an acceptable response to the scenario but should not be interpreted as the only correct response.*

Chapter 1—Pulmonology

1. What pathophysiologic abnormality of the respiratory system do you suspect?

The patient is suffering from a disorder of ventilation as the result of COPD. The destruction of the elastic properties of the lungs traps air and makes exhalation more difficult, requiring more energy. In addition, both COPD and lung cancer involve a disorder of lung perfusion, although through different mechanisms. This prevents oxygen from entering the pulmonary capillaries.

2. How would you initially manage this patient?

The patient's airway should be assessed for patency and high-flow supplemental oxygen should be administered by nonrebreather mask. The patient should be closely observed for signs of carbon dioxide retention (lethargy, confusion, hypoventilation) as patients with COPD depend on low levels of oxygen to stimulate breathing (hypoxic drive). Supplemental oxygen should *not* be withheld. The patient should be closely monitored for respiratory depression.

3. Why is the finding of cough and fever significant in this patient?

Upper respiratory tract infection and pneumonia are common in patients with underlying lung disorders because their normal defenses, including mucus production and cilia action, are limited. These conditions also worsen underlying diseases such as COPD and pneumonia.

Chapter 2—Cardiology

1. What is your assessment of the patient's condition?

This patient appears acutely ill. There are significant compensatory mechanisms at work to maintain end-organ perfusion as evidenced by the rapid heart rate and peripheral vasoconstriction. The clinical picture is most consistent with a dissecting abdominal aortic aneurysm. Most of these begin below the level of the renal arteries and can be quite large. The mortality rate is very high, even with prompt care and emergent surgery.

2. What prehospital care should be provided?

This gentleman will benefit most from emergency transport with care provided en route. He should be immediately moved to the ambulance. As soon as possible, high-flow oxygen therapy should be initiated with a nonrebreather mask. En route, 1–2 large bore IV lines should be started and isotonic crystalloids infused to help support the blood pressure. The PASG can have a role in these cases. You should always follow local medical direction guidelines.

3. What is the pathological cause and what are the risk factors associated with the problem?

The pathological cause is a small tear in the inner layer of the aorta (*tunica intima*) that allows a false passage to develop within the layers of the aorta. The initial tear is usually due to *cystic medial necrosis*. This is a complication of hypertension. In addition to hypertension, other risk factors include age, male gender, diabetes, and family history. Surgery to correct an abdominal aneurysm is fairly routine if detected before dissection and rupture occur.

Chapter 3—Neurology

1. Based on the clinical symptoms present, what might be wrong with this patient?

Based on the presence of the signs and symptoms (elevated blood pressure, headache, and slurred speech) stroke (brain attack) or TIA should be suspected.

2. What would account for the quickly dissipating symptoms?

The speed of recovery and resolution of symptoms would narrow the diagnosis further to TIA.

3. What is the priority in managing this patient's care?

Protecting the patient's airway and providing oxygen are the priorities.

4. What are the appropriate steps in caring for this patient?

Assure scene safety; BSI precautions. Establish and maintain airway. Provide positive pressure ventilations at 20/min if breathing is inadequate or absent; provide oxygen by nonrebreather at 15 lpm if breathing is adequate. Take a patient history. Position patient supine or semi-upright if congestive heart failure is present or in left lateral recumbent position if mental status is altered or airway compromised. Determine blood glucose level. Start an IV of normal saline or lactated Ringer's at a keep-open rate. (If patient is hypoglycemic, medical direction may order 50% dextrose by IV push.) Monitor cardiac rhythm. Protect paralyzed extremities. Reassure the patient. Rapidly transport, without excessive movement or noise, to appropriate facility.

Chapter 4—Endocrinology

1. What is your first priority?

As always, maintenance of the patient's airway has the highest priority, and you should address that first. Position your patient to maximize her respiratory effort and then initiate oxygen therapy with a nonrebreather mask at 100 percent concentration.

2. What additional intervention is needed?

Your assessment reveals that she is dehydrated and hypoglycemic. You should establish intravenous access and begin fluid resuscitation per protocol. At the time that you start your IV, obtain a blood sample in a red top tube (or as designated by your local protocol), and administer 50 ml (25 grams) of 50 percent dextrose. Obtain a 12-lead ECG and continue cardiac monitoring.

3. What do you suspect is the likely cause of her signs and symptoms?

The sudden cessation of her glucocorticoid (prednisone) therapy has triggered Addisonian crisis (acute adrenal insufficiency).

4. Should you transport this patient to the hospital or could her husband take her in their private vehicle?

This is a life-threatening emergency and she should be transported immediately to the hospital for definitive care. Under no circumstances should she be allowed to go by car because she is already hypotensive with orthostatic changes. The presence of peaked T waves on her ECG indicates that she is hyperkalemic and is at great risk of potentially serious cardiac dysrhythmias.

Chapter 5—Allergies and Anaphylaxis

1. What is the most likely explanation of the patient's emergency?

Despite the fact that the catfish is poisonous, it appears most likely that the patient is suffering a severe allergic reaction to the toxin or to another substance transmitted during the puncture. Hardhead catfish toxins generally cause localized burning and pain. They rarely cause systemic symptoms except in cases where patients are hypersensitive to the toxin.

2. How would you treat this patient?

The approach to this patient would be similar to any patient with an allergic or anaphylactic reaction. First, the patient should receive supplemental oxygen via a nonrebreather mask. IV access should be obtained. If the patient has normal vital signs and adequate perfusion, consider treating with 0.3–0.5 mg of epinephrine 1:1,000 subcutaneously. If the patient exhibits signs of cardiovascular collapse characterized by hypotension and inadequate tissue perfusion, consider the intravenous administration of 0.3–0.5 mg of epinephrine 1:10,000. Either regimen should be followed by 25–50 mg of diphenhydramine (Benadryl) intravenously. Consideration should also be given to intravenous corticosteroids. As the patient has pain and inflammation from the catfish toxin, apply heat to the puncture area. Heat helps to deactivate the toxin and provides localized pain relief. If the patient's pain is severe, and he has normal vital signs, consider administering an analgesic agent for pain control.

3. Should the local marine institute be advised of a potentially toxic strain of hardhead catfish?

Not immediately. This is most likely an allergic reaction to a standard catfish. Most likely, the patient has been exposed to the catfish toxin at some time in the past. Thus, he was sensitized to the antigen and, following another exposure, developed an allergic reaction to the toxin. The fish in question was probably no more toxic than similar fish in the area.

Chapter 6—Gastroenterology

1. What are your first steps in caring for this patient?

The first priority would be to carefully lower the patient to the floor to prevent any injury from a fall. Quickly assess the ABCs and initiate high flow oxygen or positive pressure ventilation if needed.

2. What are some of the possible causes for the patient's condition?

The possible causes of this patient's illness include shock of indeterminate cause, hemorrhagic shock from GI bleed, syncope from severe pain (such as a kidney stone), and simple syncope.

3. What information would you attempt to ascertain from the patient's wife?

Information that could be ascertained includes a SAMPLE and OPQRST history.

4. What physical clues might you identify in this situation?

Physical information that might be present includes vomitus in the toilet, blood in the toilet from a lower GI bleed, melena, medication bottles, or similar signs.

Chapter 7—Urology and Nephrology

1. What is your first management priority?

Your first priority is stabilizing airway, breathing, and circulation. The patient shows evidence of severe dehydration (hypovolemia) with cardiac stress (tachycardia) and possible early hypovolemic shock. Mentation appears to be acutely impaired.

2. *What risk factors, if any, might the patient have for a renal complication to his condition? Which renal complication, if any?*

He is elderly, may have underlying hypertension (diuretic), is at risk for shock, and may already have compromised cardiac function (possible arrhythmia). In light of possible oliguria or even anuria by history, his profile puts him at risk for acute renal failure (prerenal failure).

3. *Should you agree to the neighbor's driving the patient to the hospital after he finishes dressing? If not, why?*

No. He should be treated for hypovolemic shock (with cardiac function monitored by ECG). He should be transported gently but expediently to the nearest appropriate facility. Because of the possibility of ARF, all of his medicines should be gathered and brought along to see if the antibiotic or any other drug might be nephrotoxic.

Chapter 8—Toxicology

1. *What class of toxin are you dealing with?*

With the history you have obtained, the patient appears to have been exposed to a pesticide. These chemicals are typically organophosphates, which can be extremely toxic in large amounts. They can cause pathology by inhalation or absorption through the skin and eyes. Although rare, occasionally ingestions do occur but primarily by curious children playing in the garage who don't recognize the potential danger.

2. *What toxidrome will you expect to find when you make a further assessment of the patient?*

Organophosphates are associated with the acetylcholinesterase inhibition toxidrome. The signs and symptoms can be subdivided into autonomic nervous system (ANS) and central nervous system (CNS) effects. ANS effects include sweating, small pupils, profuse production of saliva and tears, wheezing, cramps, vomiting, diarrhea, urinary incontinence, bradycardia, hypotension, muscle fasciculations, weakness, paralysis, and respiratory failure. CNS effects vary but usually involve anxiety, ataxia, seizures, and suppression of reflexes, respiration, and circulation.

3. *What are your priorities in managing this situation?*

Obviously rapid intervention is needed in this potentially lethal situation. However, do not forget the importance of rescuer safety. The "spill" in the garage, where there is usually insufficient ventilation, has been enough to incapacitate one person (the patient) already. Proceed with caution. Use the proper equipment to prevent inhalation and skin contact with the organophosphates. With safety in mind, remove the patient from the garage to minimize further intake of poison. If there is contamination of the patient's clothes, remove them and wipe the patient down with soap and water to remove any chemical left on the skin. Proceed with your usual initial assessment and management. With excess secretions caused by organophosphates, this patient will have airway difficulty. Suction along with high-flow oxygen and bag-valve-mask assisstance will be needed. Bronchospasm may be present and may need treatment. Proceed to intubation if airway control is not adequate with simpler methods. Establish an IV line with normal saline as soon as possible and give fluids generously. The patient will usually be in early dehydration because of the profuse sweating, salivation, lacrimation, and urinary output. Contact Poison Control and assign a high priority for transporting this patient.

4. Beyond standard supportive measures, what other intervention will help treat this patient?

Organophosphate poisoning is one of the toxidromes for which an antidote is available. Atropine is effective in countering some of the toxic effects, but be aware that the quantity of atropine needed is usually well beyond the usual use of atropine. Give atropine 2 mg IV push every 5–15 minutes until you note improvement in the bradycardia, excessive moisture production, and so on. Patients with severe poisonings can deplete a hospital's supply of atropine, requiring hundreds of milligrams of atropine. Pralidoxime will counter the nicotinic effects, but this will usually be given in the hospital rather than in the prehospital setting.

Chapter 9—Hematology

1. What hemostatic responses will seek to control this blood loss?

Vascular spasm, platelet aggregation, and blood coagulation.

2. Why are the heart rate and respiratory rate elevated?

Loss of red blood cells leads to a degree of hypoxia. The body will attempt to compensate by increasing pulse and respirations to quickly deliver what oxygen can be carried by the red blood cells.

3. What will the body do about replacing red blood cells?

The hypoxia triggered by the red blood cell loss will stimulate the kidneys to release erythropoietin. This will stimulate the red bone marrow to release red blood cells into circulation.

4. What body mechanisms will fight off an infection?

A variety of white blood cells will attempt to prevent an infection. The neutrophils will travel to the infection site and engulf any foreign matter. Monocytes will mature into macrophages and dispose of the dead or dying neutrophils. Lymphocytes will begin a two-pronged attack with T cells releasing chemical messengers to "turn on" the immune system and B cells producing antibodies that surround and inactivate a foreign protein.

Chapter 10—Environmental Emergencies

1. What illness are you dealing with?

This condition is known as High Altitude Pulmonary Edema (HAPE), the most lethal of the high altitude illnesses. The exact mechanism that produces this condition is not clear. In general, high altitude causes increases in pulmonary pressure as blood is shunted to the central circulation to maximize oxygen to the essential core structures (heart and brain). This pulmonary hypertension, along with individual susceptibility, causes fluid to leak out into the lung tissue, greatly compromising respiratory function.

2. What predisposing factors lead to this illness?

Children are more susceptible than adults to HAPE. Men are more susceptible than women. Other risk factors include cold weather, use of sleeping medicine, too much salt intake, strenuous activity, and rapid ascent to high elevations without a period of acclimatization.

3. What is the definitive treatment for this condition?

HAPE is easily and rapidly reversible so early recognition of the problem is critical. Immediate descent to lower altitude is the treatment of choice. The patient should be transported so that he is not required to make any undue exertion during descent. In our case study, evacuation to sea level would be ideal since "Biff" is experiencing severe symptoms including neurological impairment.

4. If definitive treatment is not possible, what other measures can be used?

In certain cases descent or evacuation is not possible. There may be a snowstorm or other factors making it dangerous. In these situations several possibilities exist. Supplemental oxygen can reverse HAPE over 36 to 72 hours. If there is sufficient oxygen supply and the patient is stable this may be enough. At least, oxygen can be used as a temporizing measure. In addition, the patient with HAPE can be placed in a portable hyperbaric bag. These bags inflate to a pressure of 2 psi, simulating a descent of several thousand feet. A valve system keeps oxygen and carbon dioxide proportions correct. Finally, some medications may be helpful. Morphine, furosemide (a diuretic), and nifedipine (antihypertensive) have all been used successfully in the past.

Chapter 11—Infectious Disease

1. What essential BSI precautions should you take?

Gloves are required on every patient contact. Explain, as the paramedics in the scenario did, that gloves are required to protect the patient as well as the EMS providers. This is the standard regardless of the presence of a disease. If any possibility exists of the spread of respiratory droplets, another BSI precaution with this patient is a HEPA mask. Tuberculosis and other respiratory diseases may accompany AIDS patients. In addition, if splashing or splattering of blood is possible, wear a face mask with a shield and a gown.

2. What are your primary concerns for this patient?

AIDS patients are susceptible to many diseases and conditions. Your priority (once you have taken the proper BSI precautions) is to manage the patient's airway, breathing, and circulation. Assure an open airway, provide supplemental oxygen, and then consider fluids to manage the presence of hypovolemia.

3. How would your care or BSI precautions differ for patients without AIDS?

Your care should be similar regardless of the presence of disease. Obviously, knowing a patient has a particular disease should prompt you to be exceptionally attentive to appropriate BSI precautions; however, you should never believe that a patient is disease-free simply because he or she says so. Assume that every patient's body fluids are contagious, and treat them with the utmost caution.

Chapter 12—Psychiatric and Behavioral Disorders

1. What do you suspect this patient's problem is? What are the possibilities?

In the broad scheme, the paramedic must explore three major categories to determine the patient's problem: psychiatric condition, medical condition, or traumatic condition caused by the accident. Any of those conditions, either alone or in combination, could explain the current behavior. The possibilities include psychiatric emergency; medical conditions such as hypoglycemia or hypoxia; and traumatic conditions such as head injury. Consider the patient to have an altered mental status until you can rule out any medical and traumatic conditions that might cause it.

2. Is the sweating significant? The religious literature? The car crashes?

Every item seen and heard at a scene is a piece of the puzzle. The religious literature is notable but not conclusive. Is this a psychiatric patient with religious delusions or a religious person with hypoglycemia? Sweating, especially in frigid temperatures, is more notable. In fact, this sign caused the paramedics to look further.

3. Should this patient be treated as a psychiatric emergency?

  This patient was a diabetic. It was later determined (after 2 amps of 50% dextrose and orange juice) that the patient had not calibrated his home glucometer that morning. It gave a reading to "700," causing him to take extra insulin. He got about 30 minutes from his house when he began feeling faint and pulled off the highway into the parking lot where he was found. A finger-stick glucose determination done by paramedics at the scene revealed a blood glucose level too low to be recognized by color on the stick. Treating this patient as a psychiatric emergency would most likely have led to his death. He was strongly counseled to wear a medical identification device in the future.

Chapter 13—Gynecology

1. What is your first priority?

  Although she does not demonstrate any signs of respiratory distress, your first priority is to maintain oxygenation. Initiate high-flow oxygen administration via a nonrebreather mask at 100 percent concentration.

2. What else should you do?

  Your assessment reveals that she is febrile and hypotensive indicating that she is probably septic. You should establish at least one intravenous access with a large bore needle in a large vein and begin fluid resuscitation per protocol. Cardiac monitoring would also be appropriate for this patient. Expedite transport to the hospital.

3. What do you suspect is the likely cause of her signs and symptoms?

  With her history of a recent gynecological procedure and her presentation (fever, abdominal pain, and vaginal discharge) you suspect that she has developed endometritis (an infection of the uterine lining).

4. Since your patient is a minor, do you have any legal requirement to notify her parents or obtain their consent before treating her?

  No. In many states, older teens are able to give consent for medical care. Given that she is living independently in a college setting, she is likely to be considered an emancipated minor and thus is able to give consent. Certainly, her parents should be made of aware that she is going to be hospitalized but that is not your responsibility at this time. Once a definitive decision is made by a physician about the plan of care, she can contact her parents. It's likely that the physician will also want to talk to them.

Chapter 14—Obstetrics

1. What is your first priority?

  Monitor her airway and maintain oxygenation and circulation. Place her in the left lateral recumbent position to promote venous return and to help protect her airway. Remember that you are caring for two patients, so you should check FHTs. Continue to monitor her level of consciousness. Contact medical direction to advise on the situation.

2. What do you suspect is the likely cause of her signs and symptoms?

  The most likely cause for her condition is that she has had an eclamptic seizure.

3. Your patient's husband is very concerned about the well-being of his wife and baby. What should you tell him?

Explain that you think she may have had a seizure due to her high blood pressure. Reassure him that, while this is a potentially serious situation, mother and baby seem to be doing okay at this time (if, in fact, that is your impression). However, it is important that she be taken to the hospital for evaluation immediately.

4. *How should this patient be transported to the hospital?*

Keep her on oxygen and transport in the left lateral recumbent position. Continue to monitor her vital signs and FHTs en route. Handle her gently and keep lighting low. Transport her quickly but without lights and sirens which may trigger another seizure.

Glossary

2,3-diphosphoglycerate (2,3-DPG) chemical in the red blood cells that affects hemoglobin's affinity for oxygen.

aberrant conduction conduction of the electrical impulse through the heart's conductive system in an abnormal fashion.

abortion termination of pregnancy before the 20th week of gestation. The term "abortion" refers to both miscarriage and induced abortion. Commonly, "abortion" is used for elective termination of pregnancy and "miscarriage" for the loss of a fetus by natural means. A miscarriage is sometimes called a "spontaneous abortion."

absence seizure type of generalized seizure with sudden onset, characterized by a brief loss of awareness and rapid recovery.

absolute refractory period the period of the cardiac cycle when the myocardial cells have not completely repolarized and stimulation will not produce any depolarization whatever.

acclimatization the reversible changes in body structure and function by which the body becomes adjusted to a change in environment.

acid a substance that liberates hydrogen ions (H+) when in solution.

acquired immunity immunity that develops over time and results from exposure to an antigen.

action potential the stimulation of myocardial cells, as evidenced by a change in the membrane electrical charge, that subsequently spreads across the myocardium.

activated charcoal a powder, usually pre-mixed with water, that will adsorb (bind) some poisons and help prevent them from being absorbed by the body.

active immunity acquired immunity that occurs following exposure to an antigen and results in the production of antibodies specific for the antigen; immunity developed after birth as a result of a direct exposure to an antigen or disease.

active transport movement of a molecule through a cell membrane from a region of lower concentration to one of higher concentration; movement requires energy consumption within the cell.

acute arterial occlusion the sudden occlusion of arterial blood flow.

acute gastroenteritis sudden onset of inflammation of the stomach and intestines.

acute myocardial infarction (AMI) *see* myocardial infarction.

acute pulmonary embolism blockage that occurs when a blood clot or other particle lodges in a pulmonary artery.

acute renal failure (ARF) the sudden-onset of severely decreased urine production.

acute tubular necrosis a particular syndrome characterized by the sudden death of renal tubular cells.

addiction compulsive and overwhelming dependence a drug; an addiction may be physiological dependence, a psychological dependence, or both.

Addisonian crisis form of shock associated with adrenocortical insufficiency and characterized by profound hypotension and electrolyte imbalances.

Addison's disease endocrine disorder characterized by adrenocortical insufficiency. Symptoms may include weakness, fatigue, weight loss, hyperpigmentation of skin and mucous membranes.

adhesion union of normally separate tissue surfaces by a fibrous band of new tissue.

adult respiratory distress syndrome (ARDS) form of pulmonary edema that is caused by fluid accumulation in the interstitial space within the lungs.

affect visible indicators of mood.

afferent carrying impulses toward the central nervous system. Sensory nerves are afferent nerves.

afterbirth the placenta and accompanying membranes that are expelled from the uterus after the birth of a child.

afterload the resistance against which the heart must pump.

AIDS *see* human immunodeficiency virus (HIV).

airborne transmitted through the air by droplets or particles.

alkali a substance that liberates hydroxyl ions (OH⁻) when in solution; a strong base.

allergen a substance capable of inducing allergy of specific hypersensitivity. Allergens may be protein or non-protein, although most are proteins.

allergic reaction an exaggerated response by the immune system to a foreign substance.

allergy a hypersensitive state acquired through exposure to a particular allergen.

Alzheimer's disease a degenerative brain disorder; the most common cause of dementia in the elderly.

amniotic fluid clear, watery fluid that surrounds and protects the developing fetus.

amniotic sac the membranes that surround and protect the developing fetus throughout the period of intrauterine development.

amyotrophic lateral sclerosis (ALS) progressive degeneration of specific nerve cells that control voluntary movement characterized by weakness, loss of motor control, difficulty speaking, and cramping. Also called *Lou Gehrig's disease*.

anabolism the constructive or "building up" phase of metabolism.

anaphylaxis an unusual or exaggerated allergic reaction to a foreign protein or other substance. Anaphylaxis means the opposite of "phylaxis" or protection.

anastomosis communication between two or more blood vessels.

anemia an inadequate number of red blood cells or inadequate hemoglobin within the red blood cells.

aneurysm the ballooning of an arterial wall, resulting from a defect or weakness in the wall.

anger hostility or rage to compensate for an underlying feeling of anxiety.

angina pectoris chest pain that results when blood supply's oxygen demands exceed the heart's.

angioneurotic edema marked edema of the skin that usually involves the head, neck, face, and upper airway; a common manifestation of severe allergic reactions and anaphylaxis.

anorexia absence of appetite.

anorexia nervosa psychological disorder characterized by voluntary refusal to eat.

antibody a substance that is produced in response to and destroys a particular antigen.

antidiuresis formation and passage of a concentrated urine, preserving blood volume.

antidote a substance that will neutralize a specific toxin or counteract its effect on the body.

antigen protein on the surface of a donor's red blood cells that the patient's body recognizes as "self" or "not self."

anuria no elimination of urine.

anxiety state of uneasiness, discomfort, apprehension, and restlessness.

anxiety disorder condition characterized by dominating apprehension and fear.

apnea absence of breathing.

apneustic respiration breathing characterized by a prolonged inspiration unrelieved by expiration attempts, seen in patients with damage to the upper part of the pons.

appendicitis inflammation of the vermiform appendix at the juncture of the large and small intestines.

arachnoid membrane middle layer of the meninges.

arrhythmia the absence of cardiac electrical activity; often used interchangeably with dysrhythmia.

arterial gas embolism (AGE) an air bubble, or air embolism, that enters the circulatory system from a damaged lung.

arteriosclerosis a thickening, loss of elasticity, and hardening of the walls of the arteries from calcium deposits.

artifact deflection on the ECG produced by factors other than the heart's electrical activity.

ascending loop of Henle the part of the nephron tubule beyond the descending loop of Henle.

asphyxia a decrease in the amount of oxygen and an increase in the amount of carbon dioxide as a result of some interference with respiration.

ataxic respiration poor respirations due to CNS damage, causing ineffective thoracic muscular coordination.

atherosclerosis a progressive, degenerative disease of the medium-sized and large arteries.

atypical angina *see* Prinzmetal's angina.

augmented limb leads another term for unipolar limb leads, reflecting the fact that the ground lead is disconnected, which increases the amplitude of deflection on the ECG tracing.

autoimmune disease condition in which the body makes antibodies against its own tissues.

autoimmunity *see* autoimmune disease.

automaticity pacemaker cells' capability of self-depolarization.

autonomic nervous system part of the nervous system controlling involuntary bodily functions. It is divided into the sympathetic and the parasympathetic systems.

autonomic neuropathy condition that damages the autonomic nervous system, which usually senses changes in core temperature and controls vasodilation and perspiration to dissipate heat.

axis deviation *see* left axis deviation, right axis deviation.

B lymphocytes cells that attack invaders in humoral immune responses.

bacteria microscopic single-celled organisms that range in length from one to twenty micrometers.

bactericidal capable of killing bacteria.

bacteriostatic capable of inhibiting bacterial growth or reproduction.

barotrauma injuries caused by changes in pressure. Barotrauma that occurs from increasing pressure during a diving descent is commonly called "the squeeze."

basal metabolic rate (BMR) rate at which the body consumes energy just to maintain stability; the basic metabolic rate (measured by the rate of oxygen consumption) of an awake, relaxed person 12 to 14 hours after eating and at a comfortable temperature.

basophil type of white blood cell that participates in allergic responses.

behavior a person's observable conduct and activity.

behavioral emergency situation in which a patient's behavior becomes so unusual that it alarms the patient or another person and requires intervention.

Bell's palsy one-sided facial paralysis with an unknown cause characterized by the inability to close the eye, pain, tearing of the eyes, drooling, hypersensitivity to sound, and impairment of taste.

benign prostatic hypertrophy a noncancerous enlargement of the prostate associated with aging.

bereavement death of a loved one.

biological/organic related to disease processes or structural changes.

bipolar disorder condition characterized by one or more manic episodes, with or without periods of depression.

bipolar limb leads electrocardiogram leads applied to the arms and legs that contain two electrodes of opposite (positive and negative) polarity; leads I, II, and III.

bloodborne transmitted by contact with blood or body fluids.

Bohr effect phenomenon in which a decrease in pCO_2/acidity causes an increase in the quantity of oxygen that binds with the hemoglobin and, conversely, an increase in pCO_2/acidity causes the hemoglobin to give up a greater quantity of oxygen.

bowel obstruction blockage of the hollow space within the intestines.

Bowman's capsule the hollow, cup-shaped first part of the nephron tubule.

bradycardia a slow heart rate; a heart rate less than 60 beats per minute.

bradypnea slow respiration.

brain abscess a collection of pus localized in an area of the brain.

brainstem part of the brain connecting the cerebral hemispheres with the spinal cord. It is comprised of the mesencephalon (midbrain), the pons, and the medulla oblongata.

Brudzinkis's sign physical exam finding in which flexion of the neck causes flexion of the hips and knees.

bruit the sound of turbulent blood flow through a vessel; usually associated with atherosclerotic disease.

bulimia nervosa recurrent episodes of binge eating.

bundle branch block a kind of interventricular heart block in which conduction through either the right of left bundle branches is blocked or delayed.

bundle of Kent an accessory AV conduction pathway that is thought to be responsible for the ECG findings of pre-excitation syndrome.

cardiac arrest the absence of ventricular contraction.

cardiac cycle the period of time from the end of one cardiac contraction to the end of the next.

cardiac depolarization a reversal of charges at a cell membrane so that the inside of the cell becomes positive in relation to the outside; the opposite of the cell's resting state in which the inside of the cell is negative in relation to the outside.

cardiac output the amount of blood pumped by the heart in one minute.

cardiac tamponade accumulation of excess fluid inside the pericardium.

cardiogenic shock the inability of the heart to meet the metabolic needs of the body, resulting in inadequate tissue perfusion.

cardiovascular disease (CVD) disease affecting the heart, peripheral blood vessels, or both.

carina the point at which the trachea bifurcates into the right and left mainstem bronchi.

catabolism the destructive or "breaking down" phase of metabolism.

catatonia condition characterized by immobility and stupor, often a sign of schizophrenia.

cell-mediated immunity generalized, temporary defense mechanism against invaders; immunity resulting from a direct attack of a foreign substance by specialized cells of the immune system.

cellular immunity *see* cell-mediated immunity.

central nervous system the brain and the spinal cord.

central neurogenic hyperventilation hyperventilation caused by a lesion in the central nervous system, often characterized by rapid, deep, noisy respirations.

central pain syndrome condition resulting from damage or injury to the brain, brainstem, or spinal cord characterized by intense, steady pain described as burning, aching, tingling, or a "pins and needles" sensation.

cerebellum portion of the brain located dorsally to the pons and medulla oblongata. It plays an important role in the fine motor movement, posture, equilibrium, and muscle tone.

cerebrospinal fluid watery, clear fluid that acts as a cushion, protecting the brain and spinal cord from physical impact. The cerebrospinal fluid also serves as an accessory circulatory system for the central nervous system.

cerebrum largest part of the brain, consisting of two hemispheres. The cerebrum is the seat of consciousness and the center of the higher mental functions such as memory, learning, reasoning, judgement, intelligence, and the emotions.

chancroid highly contagious sexually transmitted ulcer.

chemotaxis the movement of white blood cells in response to chemical signals.

Cheyne-Stokes respiration a breathing pattern characterized by a period of apnea lasting 10-60 seconds, followed by gradually increasing depth and frequency of respirations.

chlamydia group of intracellular parasites that cause sexually transmitted diseases.

chronic obstructive pulmonary disease (COPD) a disease characterized by a decreased ability of the lungs to perform the function of ventilation.

chronic renal failure permanently inadequate renal function due to nephron loss.

chronotropy pertaining to heart rate.

circumcision the surgical removal of the foreskin of the penis.

cirrhosis degenerative disease of the liver.

claudication severe pain in the calf muscle due to inadequate blood supply. It typically occurs with exertion and subsides with rest.

clonic phase phase of a seizure characterized by alternating contraction and relaxation of muscles.

closed pneumothorax *see* pneumothorax.

colic acute pain associated with cramping or spasms in the abdominal organs.

collecting duct the larger structure beyond the distal nephron tubule into which urine drips.

coma a state of unconsciousness from which the patient cannot be aroused.

communicable capable of being transmitted to another host.

communicable period time when a host can transmit an infectious agent to someone else.

community-acquired infection an infection occurring in a nonhospitalized patient who is not undergoing regular medical procedures, including the use of instruments such as catheters.

compensatory pause the pause following an ectopic beat where the SA node is unaffected and the cadence of the heart is uninterrupted.

complex partial seizure type of partial seizure usually originating in the temporal lobe characterized by an aura and focal findings such as alterations in mental status or mood.

conduction moving electrons, ions, heat, or sound waves through a conductor or conducting medium.

conductivity ability of cells to propagate the electrical impulse from one cell to another.

confusion state of being unclear or unable to make a decision easily.

congestive heart failure (CHF) condition in which the heart's reduced stroke volume causes an overload of fluid in the body's other tissues. *See also* heart failure.

contamination presence of an agent only on the surface of the host without penetrating it.

contractility ability of muscle cells to contract, or shorten.

convection transfer of heat via currents in liquids or gases.

cor pulmonale hypertrophy of the right ventricle resulting from disorders of the lung.

core temperature the body temperature of the deep tissues, which usually does not vary more than a degree or so from its normal 37° C (98.6° F).

coronary heart disease (CHD) a type of CVD; the single largest killer of Americans.

cortex the outer tissue of an organ such as the kidney.

coupling interval distance between the preceding beat and a premature ventricular contraction (PVC).

cranial nerves twelve pairs of nerves that extend from the lower surface of the brain.

creatinine a waste product caused by metabolism within muscle cells.

crepitus crackling sounds or grating sensation.

Crohn's disease idiopathic inflammatory bowel disorder associated with the small intestine.

croup viral illness characterized by inspiratory and expiratory stridor and a seal-bark-like cough.

crowning the bulging of the fetal head past the opening of the vagina during a contraction. Crowning is an indication of impending delivery.

Cullen's sign ecchymosis in the periumbilical area.

current of injury (injury current) the flow of current between the pathologically depolarized area of myocardial injury and the normally depolarized areas of the myocardium.

Cushing's reflex a collective change in vital signs (increased blood pressure and temperature and decreased pulse and respirations) associated with increasing intracranial pressure.

Cushing's syndrome pathological condition resulting from excess adrenocortical hormones. Symptoms may include changed body habitus, hypertension, vulnerability to infection.

cyanosis   bluish discoloration of the skin due to an increase in reduced hemoglobin in the blood. The condition is directly related to poor ventilation.

cystic medial necrosis   a death or degeneration of a part of the wall of an artery.

cystitis   an infection and inflammation of the urinary bladder.

decerebrate posture   sustained contraction of extensor muscles of the extremities resulting from a lesion in the brainstem. The patient presents with stiff and extended extremities and retracted head.

decompression illness   development of nitrogen bubbles within the tissues due to a rapid reduction of air pressure when a diver returns to the surface; also called "the bends."

decontaminate   to destroy or remove pathogens.

decontamination   the process of minimizing toxicity by reducing the amount of toxin absorbed into the body.

decorticate posture   characteristic posture associated with a lesion at or above the upper brainstem. The patient presents with the arms flexed, fists clenched, and legs extended.

deep frostbite   freezing involving epidermal and subcutaneous tissues resulting in a white appearance, hard (frozen) feeling on palpation, and loss of sensation.

deep venous thrombosis   a blood clot in a vein.

defibrillation   the process of passing an electrical current through a fibrillating heart to depolarize a "critical mass" of myocardial cells. This allows them to depolarize uniformly, resulting in an organized rhythm.

degenerative neurological disorders   a collection of diseases that selectively affect one or more functional systems of the central nervous system.

delayed hypersensitivity reaction   a hypersensitivity reaction that takes place after the elapse of some time following reexposure to an antigen. Delayed hypersensitivity reactions are usually less severe than immediate reactions.

delirium   condition characterized by relatively rapid onset of widespread disorganized thought.

delirium tremens (DTs)   disorder found in habitual and excessive users of alcoholic beverages after cessation of drinking for 48–72 hours. Patients experience visual, tactile, and auditory disturbances. Death may result in severe cases.

delusions   fixed, false beliefs not widely held within the individual's cultural or religious group.

dementia   condition involving gradual development of memory impairment and cognitive disturbance.

depersonalization   feeling detached from oneself.

depression   profound sadness or feeling of melancholy.

dermatomes   areas of the skin innervated by spinal nerves.

descending loop of Henle   the part of the nephron tubule beyond the proximal tubule.

diabetes insipidus   excessive urine production caused by inadequate production of antidiuretic hormone.

diabetes mellitus   disorder of inadequate insulin activity, due either to inadequate production of insulin or to decreased responsiveness of body cells to insulin.

diabetic ketoacidosis   complication of Type I diabetes due to decreased insulin intake. Marked by high blood glucose, metabolic acidosis, and, in advanced stages, coma. Ketoacidosis is often called diabetic coma.

dialysate   the solution used in dialysis that is hypo-osmolar to many of the wastes and key electrolytes in blood.

dialysis   a procedure that replaces some lost kidney functions.

diaphoresis   sweatiness.

diastole   the period of time when the myocardium is relaxed and cardiac filling and coronary perfusion occur.

diencephalon   portion of the brain lying beneath the cerebrum and above the brainstem. It contains the thalamus, the hypothalamus, and the limbic system.

diffusion   the movement of molecules through a membrane from an area of greater concentration to an area of lesser concentration.

disease period   the duration from the onset of signs and symptoms of disease until the resolution of symptoms or death.

disinfect   to destroy certain forms of microorganisms, but not all.

dissecting aortic aneurysm   aneurysm caused when blood gets between and separates the layers of the arterial wall.

disseminated intravascular coagulation (DIC)   a disorder of coagulation caused by systemic activation of the coagulation cascade.

dissociative disorder   condition in which the individual avoids stress by separating from his core personality.

distal tubule   the part of the tubule beyond the ascending loop of Henle.

diuresis   formation and passage of a dilute urine, decreasing blood volume; secretion of large amounts of urine.

diverticula   small outpouchings in the mucosal lining of the intestinal tract.

diverticulitis   inflammation of diverticula.

diverticulosis   presence of diverticula, with or without associated bleeding.

down time   duration from the beginning of the cardiac arrest until effective CPR is established. *See also* total down time.

dromotropy   pertaining to the speed of cardiac impulse transmission.

drowning   asphyxiation resulting from submersion in liquid with death occurring within 24 hours of submersion.

drug overdose   poisoning from a pharmacological substance in excess of that usually prescribed or that the body can tolerate.

dura mater   tough outermost layer of the meninges.

dysmenorrhea   painful menstruation.

dyspareunia   painful sexual intercourse.

dyspnea   difficult or labored breathing; a sensation of "shortness of breath."

dysrhythmia   any deviation from the normal electrical rhythm of the heart.

dystonias   a group of disorders characterized by muscle contractions that cause twisting and repetitive movements, abnormal postures, or freezing in the middle of an action.

dysuria   painful urination often associated with cystitis.

ectopic beat   cardiac depolarization resulting from depolarization of ectopic focus.

ectopic focus   nonpacemaker heart cell that automatically depolarizes; *pl.* ectopic foci.

ectopic pregnancy   the implantation of a developing fetus outside of the uterus, often in a fallopian tubes.

effacement   the thinning of the cervix during labor.

efferent   carrying impulses away from the brain or spinal cord to the periphery. Motor nerves are efferent nerves.

Einthoven's triangle   the triangle around the heart formed by the bipolar limb leads.

ejection fraction   ratio of blood pumped from the ventricle to the amount remaining at end of diastole.

electrocardiogram (ECG)   the graphic recording of the heart's electrical activity. It may be displayed either on paper or on an oscilloscope.

encephalitis   acute infection of the brain, usually caused by a virus.

endocrine gland   gland that secretes chemical substances directly into the blood; also called a *ductless gland.*

endometriosis   condition in which endometrial tissue grows outside of the uterus.

endometritis   infection of the endometrium.

endometrium   the inner layer of the uterine wall where the fertilized egg implants.

endotoxin   toxic products released when bacteria die and decompose.

end-stage renal failure   an extreme failure of kidney function due to nephron loss.

enterotoxin   an exotoxin that produces gastrointestinal symptoms and diseases such as food poisoning.

environmental emergency   a medical condition caused or exacerbated by the weather, terrain, atmospheric pressure, or other local factors.

epididymis   a saclike duct adjacent to a testis that stores sperm cells.

epiglottitis   infection and inflammation of the epiglottis.

erythrocyte   red blood cell.

erythropoiesis   the process of producing red blood cells.

erythropoietin   a hormone produced by kidney cells that stimulates maturation of red blood cells.

esophageal varix   swollen vein of the esophagus.

estimated date of confinement (EDC)   the approximate day the infant will be born. This date is usually set at 40 weeks after the date of the mother's last menstrual period (LMP).

evaporation   change from liquid to a gaseous state.

excitability   ability of cells to respond to an electrical stimulus.

exertional metabolic rate   rate at which the body consumes energy during activity. It is faster than the basic metabolic rate.

exocrine gland   gland that secretes chemical substances to nearby tissues through a duct; also called a *ducted gland.*

exotoxin   a soluble poisonous substance secreted during growth of a bacterium.

facilitated diffusion   a form of molecular diffusion in which a molecule-specific carrier in a cell membrane speeds the molecule's movement from a region of higher concentration to one of lower concentration.

factitious disorder   condition in which the patient feigns illness in order to assume the sick role.

fear   feeling of alarm and discontentment in the expectation of danger.

fecal-oral route   transmission of organisms picked up from the gastrointestinal tract (e.g., feces) into the mouth.

fibrinolysis   the process through which plasmin dismantles a blood clot.

filtrate   the fluid produced in Bowman's capsule by filtration of blood.

flail chest   one or more ribs fractured in two or more places, creating an unattached rib segment.

flanks   the part of the back below the ribs and above the hip bones.

flat affect   appearance of being disinterested, often lacking facial expression.

food poisoning   nonspecific term often applied to gastroenteritis that occurs suddenly and that is caused by the ingestion of food containing preformed toxins.

frostbite   environmentally induced freezing of body tissues causing destruction of cells.

fugue state condition in which an amnesiac patient physically flees.

fungus plant-like microorganism.

gastric lavage removing an ingested poison by repeatedly filling and emptying the stomach with water or saline via a gastric tube; also known as "pumping the stomach."

gastroenteritis nonacute inflammation of the gastrointestinal mucosa. Generalized disorder involving nausea, vomiting, gastrointestinal cramping or discomfort, and diarrhea. *See also* acute gastroenteritis.

generalized seizures seizures that begin as an electrical discharge in a small area of the brain but spread to involve the entire cerebral cortex, causing widespread malfunction.

genitourinary system the male organ system that includes reproductive and urinary structures.

German measles *see* rubella.

Glasgow Coma Scale (GCS) tool used in evaluating and quantifying the degree of coma by determining the best motor, verbal, and eye-opening response to standardized stimuli.

glomerular filtration the removal from blood of water and other elements, which enter the nephron tubule.

glomerular filtration rate (GFR) the volume per day at which blood is filtered through capillaries of the glomerulus.

glomerulus a tuft of capillaries from which blood is filtered into a nephron.

gluconeogenesis conversion of protein and fat to form glucose.

glucose intolerance the body cells' inability to take up glucose from the bloodstream.

glycogenolysis the breakdown of glycogen to glucose, primarily by liver cells.

glycosuria glucose in urine, which occurs when blood glucose levels exceed the kidney's ability to reabsorb glucose.

gonorrhea sexually transmitted disease caused by a gram-negative bacterium.

Gram stain method of differentiating types of bacteria according to their reaction to a chemical stain process.

Graves' disease endocrine disorder characterized by excess thyroid hormones resulting in body changes associated with increased metabolism; primary cause of thyrotoxicosis.

Grey-Turner's sign ecchymosis in the flank.

gynecology the branch of medicine that deals with the health maintenance and the diseases of women, primarily of the reproductive organs.

half-life time required for half of the nuclei of a radioactive substance to lose activity by undergoing radioactive decay. In biology and pharmacology, the time required by the body to metabolize and inactivate half the amount of a substance taken in.

hallucinations sensory perceptions with no basis in reality.

hantavirus family of viruses that are carried by the deer mouse and transmitted by ticks and other arthropods.

heart failure clinical syndrome in which the heart's mechanical performance is compromised so that cardiac output cannot meet the body's needs. *See also* congestive heart failure.

heat cramps acute painful spasms of the voluntary muscles following strenuous activity in a hot environment without adequate fluid or salt intake.

heat exhaustion a mild heat illness; an acute reaction to heat exposure.

heat illness increased core body temperature due to inadequate thermolysis.

heatstroke acute, dangerous reaction to heat exposure, characterized by a body temperature usually above 105° F (40.6° C) and central nervous system disturbances. The body usually ceases to perspire.

hematemesis bloody vomitus.

hematocrit the packed cell volume of red blood cells per unit of blood.

hematology the study of blood and blood-forming organs.

hematopoiesis the process through which pluripotent stem cells differentiate into various types of blood cells.

hemodialysis a dialysis procedure relying on vascular access to the blood and on an artificial membrane.

hemoglobin oxygen-bearing molecule in the red blood cells. It is made up of iron-rich red pigment called *heme* and a protein called *globin*.

hemolysis destruction of red blood cells.

hemophilia a blood disorder in which one of the proteins necessary for blood clotting is missing or defective.

hemoptysis expectoration of blood from the respiratory tree.

hemorrhoid small mass of swollen veins in the anus or rectum.

hemostasis the mechanisms that work to prevent or control blood loss.

hemothorax a collection of blood in the pleural space.

hepatitis inflammation of the liver characterized by diffuse or patchy tissue necrosis.

hernia protrusion of an organ through its protective sheath.

herpes simplex virus organism that causes infections characterized by fluid-filled vesicles, usually in the oral cavity or on the genitals.

hilum the notched part of the kidney where the ureter and other structures join kidney tissue.

histamine a product of mast cells and basophils that causes vasodilation, capillary permeability, bronchoconstriction, and contraction of the gut.

homeostasis the natural tendency of the body to maintain a steady and normal internal environment.

hookworm parasite that attaches to the host's intestinal lining.

hormone chemical substance released by a gland that controls or affects processes in other glands or body systems.

human immunodeficiency virus (HIV) organism responsible for acquired immune deficiency syndrome.

humoral immunity specialized, permanent defense mechanism that attacks a particular foreign antigen; immunity resulting from attack of an invading substance by antibodies.

Hymenoptera any of an order of highly specialized insects such as bees and wasps.

hyperbaric oxygen chamber recompression chamber used to treat patients suffering from barotrauma.

hyperglycemia excessive blood glucose.

hyperglycemic hyperosmolar nonketotic (HHNK) coma complication of type II diabetes due to inadequate insulin activity. Marked by high blood glucose, marked dehydration, and decreased mental function. Often mistaken for ketoacidosis.

hyperosmolar a solution that has a concentration of the substance greater than that of a second solution.

hypersensitivity an unexpected and exaggerated reaction to a particular antigen. It is used synonymously with the term *allergy*.

hypertensive emergency an acute elevation of blood pressure that requires the blood pressure to be lowered within one hour; characterized by end-organ changes such as hypertensive encephalopathy, renal failure, or blindness.

hypertensive encephalopathy a cerebral disorder of hypertension indicated by severe headache, nausea, vomiting, and altered mental status. Neurological symptoms may include blindness, muscle twitches, inability to speak, weakness, and paralysis.

hyperthermia unusually high core body temperature.

hyperthyroidism excessive secretion of thyroid hormones resulting in an increased metabolic rate.

hypertrophy stretching; enlargement without any additional cells.

hypoglycemia deficiency of blood glucose. Sometimes called *insulin shock*. Hypoglycemia is a medical emergency.

hypoglycemic seizure seizure that occurs when brain cells aren't functioning normally due to low blood glucose.

hypo-osmolar a solution that has a concentration of the substance lower than that of a second solution.

hypoperfusion inadequately low blood perfusion.

hypothalamus portion of the diencephalon producing neurosecretions important in the control of certain metabolic activities, including body temperature regulation.

hypothermia state of low body temperature, particularly low core body temperature.

hypothyroidism inadequate secretion of thyroid hormones resulting in a decreased metabolic rate.

hypoxia state in which insufficient oxygen is available to meet the oxygen requirements of the cells.

immediate hypersensitivity reaction a hypersensitivity reaction that occurs swiftly following reexposure to an antigen. Immediate hypersensitivity reactions are usually more severe than delayed reactions. The swiftest and most severe of such reactions is anaphylaxis.

immune response complex of events within the body that works toward the destruction or inactivation of pathogens, abnormal cells, or foreign molecules.

immune system the body system responsible for combating infection.

immunoglobulin antibody.

impetigo infection of the skin caused by staphylococci or streptococci.

impulse control disorder condition characterized by the patient's failure to control recurrent impulses.

incubation period time between a host's exposure to infectious agent and the appearance of symptoms.

indeterminate axis a calculated axis of the heart's electrical energy from −90 to −180 degrees. (Indeterminate axis is often considered to be extreme right axis deviation.)

index case the individual who first introduced an infectious agent to a population.

induced active immunity immunity achieved through vaccination given to generate an immune response that results in the development of antibodies specific for the injected antigen; also called *artificially acquired immunity*.

infarction area of dead tissue caused by lack of blood.

infection presence of an agent within the host, without necessarily causing disease.

infectious disease illness caused by infestation of the body by biological organisms.

infestation presence of parasites that do not break the host's skin.

inflammatory process a nonspecific defense mechanism that wards off damage from microorganisms or trauma.

influenza disease caused by a group of viruses.

ingestion entry of a substance into the body through the gastrointestinal tract.

inhalation entry of a substance into the body through the respiratory tract.

injection entry of a substance into the body through a break in the skin.

injury current *see* current of injury.

inotropy pertaining to cardiac contractile force.

intercalated discs specialized bands of tissue inserted between myocardial cells that increase the rate in which the action potential is spread from cell to cell.

interpolated beat a premature ventricular contraction (PVC) that falls between two sinus beats without effectively interrupting this rhythm.

interstitial nephritis an inflammation within the tissue surrounding the nephrons.

intrarenal abscess a pocket of infection within kidney tissue.

intussusception condition that occurs when part of an intestine slips into the part just distal to itself.

ionizing radiation electromagnetic radiation (e.g., x-ray) or particulate radiation (e.g., alpha particles, beta particles, and neutrons) that, by direct or secondary processes, ionizes materials that absorb the radiation. Ionizing radiation can penetrate the cells of living organisms, depositing an electrical charge within them. When sufficiently intense, this form of energy kills cells.

isosthenuria the inability to concentrate or dilute urine relative to the osmolarity of blood.

J wave ECG deflection found at the junction of the QRS complex and the ST segment. It is associated with hypothermia and seen at core temperatures below 32° C, most commonly in leads II and V_6; also called an *Osborn wave*.

Kernig's sign inability to fully extend the knee with hips flexed.

ketone bodies compounds produced during the catabolism of fatty acids, including acetoacetic acid, β-hydroxybutyric acid, and acetone.

ketosis the presence of significant quantities of ketone bodies in the blood.

kidney an organ that produces urine and performs other functions related to the urinary system.

kidney transplantation implantation of a kidney into a person without functioning kidneys.

Korsakoff's psychosis psychosis characterized by disorientation, muttering delirium, insomnia, delusions, and hallucinations. Symptoms include painful extremities, bilateral wrist drop (rarely), bilateral foot drop (frequently), and pain on pressure over the long nerves.

Kussmaul's respiration rapid, deep respirations caused by severe metabolic and CNS problems.

labor the time and processes that occur during childbirth; the physiologic and mechanical process in which the baby, placenta, and amniotic sac are expelled through the birth canal.

latent period time when a host cannot transmit an infectious agent to someone else.

left axis deviation a calculated axis of the heart's electrical energy that equals or exceeds −30 degrees (or in a simplified formula, from 0 to −90 degrees).

leukemia a cancer of the hematopoietic cells.

leukocyte white blood cell.

leukocytosis too many white blood cells.

leukopenia too few white blood cells.

leukopoiesis the process through which stem cells differentiate into the white blood cells' immature forms.

lice parasitic infestation of the skin of the scalp, trunk, or pubic area.

ligament of Treitz ligament that supports the duodenojejunal junction.

lower gastrointestinal bleeding bleeding in the gastrointestinal tract distal to the ligament of Treitz.

Lyme disease recurrent inflammatory disorder caused by a tick-borne spirochete.

lymph overflow circulatory fluid in spaces between tissues.

lymphatic system secondary circulatory system that collects overflow fluid from the tissue spaces and filters it before returning it to the circulatory system.

lymphocyte cell that attacks invader in immune response.

lymphoma a cancer of the lymphatic system.

macrophage after neutrophils, the most common phagocytic white blood cell.

major basic protein (MBP) a larvacidal peptide.

Mallory-Weiss tear esophageal laceration, usually secondary to vomiting.

mammalian diving reflex a complex cardiovascular reflex, resulting from submersion of the face and nose in water, that constricts blood flow everywhere except to the brain.

manic characterized by excessive excitement or activity (mania).

mask a device for protecting the face. *See also* respirator.

mast cell specialized cell of the immune system which contains chemicals that assist in the immune response.

McBurney's point common site of pain from appendicitis, one to two inches above the anterior iliac crest in a direct line with the umbilicus.

measles highly contagious, acute viral disease characterized by a reddish rash that appears on the fourth or fifth day of illness.

medulla the inner tissue of an organ such as the kidney.

medulla oblongata lower portion of the brainstem, connecting the pons and the spinal cord. It contains major centers for control of respiratory, cardiac, and vasomotor activity.

melena dark, tarry, foul smelling stool.

menarche the onset of menses, usually occurring between ages 10 and 14.

meninges membranes covering and protecting the brain and spinal cord. They consist of the pia mater, arachnoid membrane, and dura mater.

meningitis inflammation of the meninges, usually caused by an infection.

menopause the cessation of menses and ovarian function due to decreased secretion of estrogen.

menorrhagia excessive menstrual flow.

menstruation sloughing of the uterine lining (endometrium) if a fertilized egg is not implanted. It is controlled by the cyclical release of hormones. Menstruation is also called a *period*.

mental status the state of the patient's cerebral functioning.

mental status examination (MSE) a structured exam designed to quickly evaluate a patient's level of mental functioning.

mesencephalon portion of the brain connecting the pons and cerebellum with the cerebral hemispheres; also called the *midbrain*. It controls motor coordination and eye movement.

metabolism the sum of cellular processes that produce the energy and molecules needed for growth and repair.

microangiopathy a disease affecting the smallest blood vessels.

miscarriage commonly used term to describe a pregnancy which ends before 20 weeks gestation; may also be called spontaneous abortion.

mittelschmerz abdominal pain associated with ovulation.

mononucleosis acute disease caused by the Epstein-Barr virus.

mood disorder pervasive and sustained emotion that colors a person's perception of the world.

multiple myeloma a cancerous disorder of plasma cells.

multiple personality disorder manifestation of two or more complete systems of personality.

multiple sclerosis disease that involves inflammation of certain nerve cells followed by demyelination, or the destruction of the myelin sheath, which is the fatty insulation surrounding nerve fibers.

mumps acute viral disease characterized by painful enlargement of the salivary glands.

muscular dystrophy a group of genetic diseases characterized by progressive muscle weakness and degeneration of the skeletal or voluntary muscle fibers.

myocardial infarction (MI) death and subsequent necrosis of the heart muscle caused by inadequate blood supply; also *acute myocardial infarction (AMI)*.

myocardial injury injury to the myocardium (heart muscle), typically following myocardial ischemia that results from loss of blood and oxygen supply to the tissue. The injured myocardium tends to be partially or completely depolarized.

myocardial ischemia deprivation of oxygen and other nutrients to the myocardium (heart muscle), typically causing abnormalities in repolarization.

myoclonus temporary, involuntary twitching or spasm of a muscle or group of muscles.

myometrium the thick middle layer of the uterine wall made up of smooth muscle fibers.

myxedema condition that reflects long-term exposure to inadequate levels of thyroid hormones with resultant changes in body structure and function.

myxedema coma life-threatening condition associated with advanced myxedema, with profound hypothermia, bradycardia, and electrolyte imbalance.

nasal flaring excessive widening of the nares with respiration.

natural immunity genetically predetermined immunity that is present at birth; also called *innate immunity*.

naturally acquired immunity immunity that begins to develop after birth and is continually enhanced by exposure to new pathogens and antigens throughout life.

near-drowning an incident of potentially fatal submersion in liquid which did not result in death or in which death occurred more than 24 hours after submersion.

negative feedback a mechanism of response that serves to maintain a state of internal constancy, or homeostasis. Changes in the internal environment trigger mechanisms that reverse or negate the change, hence the term "negative feedback."

neonate   newborn infant.

neoplasm   literally meaning "new form"; a new or abnormal formation; a tumor.

nephrology   the medical specialty dealing with the kidneys.

nephron   a microscopic structure within kidney that produces urine.

neuron   nerve cell; the fundamental component of the nervous system.

neurotransmitter   a substance that is released from the axon terminal of a presynaptic neuron upon excitation and that travels across the synaptic cleft to either excite or inhibit the target cell. Examples include acetylcholine, norepinephrine, and dopamine.

neutropenia   a reduction in the number of neutrophils; a low neutrophil count.

neutrophil   the most common phagocytic white blood cell.

nitrogen narcosis   a state of stupor that develops during deep dives due to nitrogen's effect on cerebral function; also called "raptures of the deep."

noncompensatory pause   pause following an ectopic beat where the SA node is depolarized and the underlying cadence of the heart is interrupted.

normal flora   organisms that live inside our bodies without ordinarily causing disease.

nosocomial   acquired while in the hospital.

obligate intracellular parasite   organism that can grow and reproduce only within a host cell.

obstetrics   the branch of medicine that deals with the care of women throughout pregnancy.

oliguria   decreased urine elimination to 400-500 ml or less per day.

open pneumothorax   *see* pneumothorax.

opportunistic pathogen   ordinarily nonharmful bacterium that causes disease only under unusual circumstances.

organic   *see* biological.

organophosphates   phosphorus-containing organic pesticides.

orthopnea   dyspnea while lying supine.

osmolarity   the measure of a substance's concentration in water.

osmosis   the diffusion pattern of water in which molecules move to equalize concentrations on both sides of a membrane.

osmotic diuresis   greatly increased urination and dehydration that results when high levels of glucose cannot be reabsorbed into the blood from the kidney tubules and the osmotic pressure of the glucose in the tubules also prevents water reabsorption.

ovulation   the release of an egg from the ovary.

pallor   paleness.

pancolitis   ulcerative colitis spread throughout the entire colon.

panic attack   extreme period of anxiety resulting in great emotional distress.

papilla   the tip of a pyramid; it juts into the hollow space of the kidney.

parasite   organism that lives in or on another organism.

parasympathetic nervous system   division of the autonomic nervous system that is responsible for controlling vegetative functions. Parasympathetic nervous system actions include decreased heart rate and constriction of the bronchioles and pupils. Its actions are mediated by the neurotransmitter acetylcholine.

Parkinson's disease   chronic and progressive motor system disorder characterized by tremor, rigidity, bradykinesia, and postural instability.

paroxysmal nocturnal dyspnea (PND)   a sudden episode of difficult breathing that occurs after lying down; most commonly caused by left heart failure.

partial seizures   seizures that remain confined to a limited portion of the brain, causing localized malfunction. Partial seizures may spread and become generalized.

passive immunity   acquired immunity that results from administration of antibodies either from mother to the infant across the placental barrier (natural passive immunity) or through vaccination (induced passive immunity).

pathogen   organism capable of causing disease.

pelvic inflammatory disease (PID)   an acute infection of the reproductive organs that can be caused by a bacteria, virus, or fungus.

penis   the male organ of copulation.

peptic ulcer   erosion caused by gastric acid.

perfusion   the circulation of blood through the capillaries.

perimetrium   the serosal peritoneal membrane which forms the outermost layer of the uterine wall.

perinephric abscess   a pocket of infection in the layer of fat surrounding the kidney.

peripheral arterial atherosclerotic disease   a progressive degenerative disease of the medium-sized and large arteries.

peripheral nervous system   part of the nervous system that extends throughout the body and is composed of the cranial nerves arising from the brain and the peripheral nerves arising from the spinal cord. Its subdivisions are the somatic and the autonomic nervous systems.

peripheral neuropathy   any malfunction or damage of the peripheral nerves. Results may include muscle weakness, loss of sensation, impaired reflexes, and internal organ malfunctions.

peritoneal dialysis a dialysis procedure relying on the peritoneal membrane as the semipermeable membrane.

peritonitis inflammation of the peritoneum, which lines the abdominal cavity.

personality disorder condition that results in persistently maladaptive behavior.

pertussis disease characterized by severe, violent coughing.

pH abbreviation for *potential of hydrogen*. A measure of relative acidity or alkalinity. Since the pH scale is inverse to the concentration of acidic hydrogen ions, the lower the pH the greater the acidity and the higher the pH the greater the alkalinity. A normal pH range is 7.35 to 7.45.

phagocytosis process in which white blood cells engulf and destroy an invader.

pharyngitis infection of the pharynx and tonsils.

phobia excessive fear that interferes with functioning.

pia mater delicate innermost layer of the meninges.

pinworm parasite that is 3-10 mm long and lives in the distal colon.

placenta the organ that serves as a lifeline for the developing fetus. The placenta is attached to the wall of the uterus and the umbilical cord.

plasma thick, pale yellow fluid that makes up the liquid part of the blood.

pleuritic sharp or tearing, as a description of pain.

pluripotent stem cell a cell from which the various types of blood cells can form.

pneumomediastinum the presence of air in the mediastinum.

pneumonia acute infection of the lung, including alveolar spaces and interstitial tissue.

pneumothorax a collection of air in the pleural space, causing a loss of the negative pressure that binds the lung to the chest wall. In an *open pneumothorax*, air enters the pleural space through an injury to the chest wall. In a *closed pneumothorax*, air enters the pleural space through an opening in the pleura that covers the lung. A *tension pneumothorax* develops when air in the pleural space cannot escape, causing a build-up of pressure and collapse of the lung. *See also* hemothorax, spontaneous pneumothorax.

Poiseuille's Law a law of physiology stating that blood flow through a vessel is directly proportional to the radius of the vessel to the fourth power.

poliomyelitis (polio) infectious, inflammatory viral disease of the central nervous system that sometimes results in permanent paralysis.

polycythemia an abnormally high hematocrit due to an excess of red blood cells.

pons process of tissue connecting the medulla oblongata and cerebellum with upper portions of the brain.

portal pertaining to the flow of blood into the liver.

positional asphyxia death from positioning that prevents sufficient intake of oxygen.

positive end-expiratory pressure (PEEP) a method of holding the alveoli open by increasing expiratory pressure. Some bag-valve units used in EMS have PEEP attachments. Also EMS personnel sometimes transport patients who are on ventilators with PEEP attachments.

postrenal acute renal failure acute renal failure due to obstruction distal to the kidney.

posttraumatic stress syndrome reaction to an extreme stressor.

posture position, attitude, or bearing of the body.

precordial (chest) leads electrocardiogram leads applied to the chest in a pattern that permits a view of the horizontal plane of the heart; leads V1, V2, V3, V4, V5, and V6.

preload the pressure within the ventricles at the end of diastole; commonly called the end-diastolic volume.

premenstrual syndrome (PMS) a variety of signs and symptoms, such as weight gain, irritability, or specific food cravings associated with the changing hormonal levels that precede menstruation.

prerenal acute renal failure acute renal failure due to decreased blood perfusion of kidneys.

preventive strategy a management plan to minimize further damage to vital tissues.

primary response initial, generalized response to an antigen.

Prinzmetal's angina variant of angina pectoris caused by vasospasm of the coronary arteries; not blockage per se. Also called vasopastic angina or atypical angina.

prions particles of protein, folded in such a way that protease enzymes cannot act upon them.

proctitis ulcerative colitis limited to the rectum.

prolonged QT interval QT interval greater than .44 seconds.

prostate a gland that surrounds the male bladder neck and the first portion of urethra; it produces fluid that mixes with sperm to make semen.

prostatitis infection and inflammation of the prostate gland.

protozoan single-celled parasitic organism with flexible membranes and the ability to move.

proximal tubule the part of the nephron tubule beyond Bowman's capsule.

psychogenic amnesia failure to recall, as opposed to inability to recall.

psychosis extreme response to stress characterized by impaired ability to deal with reality.

psychosocial related to a patient's personality style, dynamics of unresolved conflict, or crisis management methods.

puerperium   the time period surrounding the birth of the fetus.

pulmonary embolism (PE)   blood clot in one of the pulmonary arteries.

pulmonary over-pressure   expansion of air held in the lungs during ascent. If not exhaled, the expanded air may cause injury to the lungs and surrounding structures.

pyelonephritis   an infection and inflammation of the kidney.

pyramid   the visible tissue structures within the medulla of a kidney.

pyrexia   fever, or above-normal body temperature.

pyrogen   any substance causing a fever, such as viruses and bacteria or substances produced within the body in response to infection or inflammation.

QRS axis   reduction of all the heart's electrical forces to a single vector represented by an arrow moving in a single plane. *See also* vector.

QT interval   period from the beginning of the QRS to the end of the T wave.

rabies   viral disorder that affects the nervous system.

radiation   transfer of energy through space or matter. *See also* ionizing radiation.

reabsorption   the movement of a substance from a nephron tubule back into the blood.

reciprocal   in an ECG, a mirror image seen typically on the opposite wall of the injured area.

recompression   resubmission of a person to a greater pressure so that gradual decompression can be achieved; often used in the treatment of diving emergencies.

reduced nephron mass   the decrease in number of functional nephrons that causes chronic renal failure.

reduced renal mass   the decrease in kidney size associated with chronic renal failure.

referred pain   pain that originates in a region other than where it is felt.

refractory period   the period of time when myocardial cells have not yet completely repolarized and cannot be stimulated again. *See also* absolute refractory period, relative refractory period.

relative refractory period   the period of the cardiac cycle when, although the myocardial cells have not completely repolarized, a sufficiently strong stimulus may produce depolarization.

renal   pertaining to the kidneys.

renal acute renal failure   ARF due to pathology within kidney tissue itself.

renal calculi   kidney stones.

renal dialysis   artificial replacement of some critical kidney functions.

renal pelvis   the hollow space of the kidney at the junction with a ureter.

renin   an enzyme produced by kidney cells that plays a key role in controlling arterial blood pressure.

repolarization   return of a muscle cell to its pre-excitation resting state.

reservoir   any living creature or environment (water, soil, etc.) that can harbor an infectious agent.

resistance   a host's ability to fight off infection.

respiration   the exchange of gases between a living organism and its environment.

respirator   an apparatus worn that cleanses or qualifies the air.

respiratory syncytial virus (RSV)   common cause of pneumonia and bronchiolitis in children.

resting potential   the normal electrical state of cardiac cells.

resuscitation   provision of efforts to return a spontaneous pulse and breathing.

reticular activating system   the system responsible for consciousness. A series of nervous tissues keeping the human system in a state of consciousness.

reticuloendothelial system (RES)   the cells involved in the immune response.

return of spontaneous circulation   resuscitation results in the patient's having a spontaneous pulse.

rhythm strip   electrocardiogram printout.

right axis deviation   a calculated axis of the heart's electrical energy that equals or exceeds +105 degrees (or in a simplified formula, from +90 to +180 degrees).

rubella (German measles)   systemic viral disease characterized by a fine pink rash that appears on the face, trunk, and extremities and fades quickly.

Ryan White Act   federal law that outlines the rights and responsibilities of agencies and health care workers when an infectious disease exposure occurs.

scabies   skin disease caused by mite infestation and characterized by intense itching.

schizophrenia   common disorder involving significant change in behavior often including hallucinations, delusions, and depression.

scrotum   a muscular sac outside of the abdominal cavity that contains the testes, epididymi, and vas deferens.

scuba   abbreviation for self-contained underwater breathing apparatus. Portable apparatus that contains compressed air which allows the diver to breathe underwater.

secondary response   response by the immune system that takes place if the body is exposed to the same antigen again; in secondary response, antibodies specific for the offending antigen are released.

secretion   the movement of a substance from the blood into a nephron tubule.

seizure a temporary alteration in behavior due to the massive electrical discharge of one or more groups of neurons in the brain. Seizures can be clinically classified as generalized or partial.

semen male reproductive fluid.

Sengstaken-Blakemore tube three-lumen tube used in treating esophageal bleeding.

sensitization initial exposure of a person to an antigen that results in an immune response.

sequestration the trapping of red blood cells by an organ such as the spleen.

seroconversion creation of antibodies after exposure to a disease.

sexually transmitted disease (STD) illness most commonly transmitted through sexual contact.

sickle cell anemia an inherited disorder of red blood cell production so named because the red blood cells become sickle-shaped when oxygen levels are low. Also called sickle cell disease.

simple diffusion the random motion of molecules from an area of high concentration to an area of lower concentration.

simple partial seizure type of partial seizure that involves local motor, sensory, or autonomic dysfunction of one area of the body. There is no loss of consciousness.

sinusitis inflammation of the paranasal sinuses.

slow-reacting substance of anaphylaxis (SRS-A) substance released from basophils and mast cells that causes spasm of the bronchiole smooth muscle, resulting in an asthma-like attack and occasionally asphyxia.

sociocultural related to the patient's actions and interactions within society.

somatic nervous system part of the nervous system controlling voluntary bodily functions.

somatic pain sharp, localized pain that originates in walls of the body such as skeletal muscles.

somatoform disorder condition characterized by physical symptoms that have no apparent physiological cause and are attributable to psychological factors.

sperm cell male reproductive cell.

spina bifida (SB) a neural defect that results from the failure of one or more of the fetal vertebrae to close properly during the first month of pregnancy.

spontaneous pneumothorax a pneumothorax (collection of air in the pleural space) that occurs spontaneously, in the absence of blunt or penetrating trauma.

Starling's law of the heart law of physiology stating that the more the myocardium is stretched, up to a certain amount, the more forceful the subsequent contraction will be.

status epilepticus series of two or more generalized motor seizures without any intervening periods of consciousness.

sterilize to destroy all microorganisms.

stroke caused by either ischemic or hemorrhagic lesions to a portion of the brain, resulting in damage or destruction of brain tissue. Commonly also called a cerebrovascular accident or a "brain attack."

stroke volume the amount of blood ejected by the heart in one cardiac contraction.

subcutaneous emphysema presence of air in the subcutaneous tissue.

subendocardial infarction myocardial infarction that affects only the deeper levels of the myocardium; also called non-Q-wave infarction because it typically does not result in a significant Q wave in the affected lead.

substance abuse use of a pharmacological substance for purposes other than medically defined reasons.

sudden death death within one hour after the onset of symptoms.

superficial frostbite freezing involving only epidermal tissues resulting in redness followed by blanching and diminished sensation.; also called *frostnip*.

surface absorption entry of a substance into the body directly through the skin or mucous membrane.

surfactant a compound secreted by the lungs that contributes to the elastic properties of the pulmonary tissues.

survival when a patient is resuscitated and survives to be discharged from the hospital.

sympathetic nervous system division of the autonomic nervous system that prepares the body for stressful situations. Sympathetic nervous system actions include increased heart rate and dilation of the bronchioles and pupils. Its actions are mediated by the neurotransmitters epinephrine and norepinephrine.

synchronized cardioversion the passage of an electric current through the heart during a specific part of the cardiac cycle to terminate certain kinds of dysrhythmias.

syncope transient loss of consciousness due to inadequate flow of blood to the brain with rapid recovery of consciousness upon becoming supine; fainting.

syncytium group of cardiac muscle cells that physiologically function as a unit.

syphilis blood-borne sexually transmitted disease caused by the spirochete *Treponema pallidum*.

systole the period of the cardiac cycle when the myocardium is contracting.

T lymphocytes cells that attack invaders in cell-mediated immune responses.

tachycardia rapid heart rate; a heart rate greater than 100 beats per minute.

tachypnea rapid respiration.

tactile fremitus vibratory tremors felt through the chest by palpation.

tension pneumothorax *see* pneumothorax.

testes male sex organs.

tetanus acute bacterial infection of the central nervous system.

therapeutic index the maximum tolerate dose divided by the minimum curative close of a drug; the range between curative and toxic dosages; also called *therapeutic window.*

thermal gradient the difference in temperature between the environment and the body.

thermogenesis the production of heat, especially within the body.

thermoregulation the maintenance or regulation of a particular temperature of the body.

thrombocyte blood platelet.

thrombocytopenia an abnormal decrease in the number of platelets.

thrombocytosis an abnormal increase in the number of platelets.

thrombosis clot formation in coronary arteries or cerebral vasculature.

thyrotoxic crisis toxic condition characterized by hyperthermia, tachycardia, nervous symptoms, and rapid metabolism; also known as *thyroid storm.*

thyrotoxicosis condition that reflects prolonged exposure to excess thyroid hormones with resultant changes in body structure and function.

tocolysis the process of stopping labor.

tolerance the need to progressively increase the dose of a drug to reproduce the effect originally achieved by smaller doses.

tonic-clonic seizure type of generalized seizure characterized by rapid loss of consciousness and motor coordination, muscle spasms, and jerking motions.

tonic phase phase of a seizure characterized by tension or contraction of muscles.

total down time duration from the beginning of the arrest until the patient's delivery to the emergency department.

toxicology study of the detection, chemistry, pharmacological actions, and antidotes of toxic substances.

toxidrome a toxic syndrome; a group of typical signs and symptoms consistently associated with exposure to a particular type of toxin.

toxin any chemical (drug, poison, or other) that causes adverse effects on an organism that is exposed to it; any poisonous chemical secreted by bacteria or released following destruction of the bacteria.

tracheal deviation any position of the trachea other than midline.

tracheal tugging retraction of the tissues of the neck due to airway obstruction or dyspnea.

transient ischemic attack (TIA) temporary interruption of blood supply to the brain.

transmural infarction myocardial infarction that affects the full thickness of the myocardium and almost always results in a pathological Q wave in the affected leads.

trench foot a painful foot disorder resembling frostbite and resulting from exposure to cold and wet, which can eventually result in tissue sloughing or gangrene; also called *immersion foot.*

trichinosis disease resulting from an infestation of *Trichinella spriralis.*

trichomoniasis sexually transmitted disease caused by the protozoan *Trichomonas vaginalis.*

tuberculosis (TB) disease caused by a bacterium known as *Mycobacterium tuberculosis* that primarily affects the respiratory system.

umbilical cord structure containing two arteries and one vein that connects the placenta and the fetus.

unipolar limb leads electrocardiogram leads applied to the arms and legs, consisting of one polarized (positive) electrode and a nonpolarized reference point that is created by the ECG machine combining two additional electrodes; also called augmented limb leads; leads aVR, aVL, and aVF.

upper gastrointestinal bleeding bleeding within the gastrointestinal tract proximal to the ligament of Treitz.

urea waste derived from ammonia produced through protein metabolism.

uremia the syndrome of signs and symptoms associated with chronic renal failure.

ureter a duct that carries urine from kidney to urinary bladder.

urethra the duct that carries urine from the bladder out of the body; in men, it also carries reproductive fluid (semen) to the outside of the body.

urethritis an infection and inflammation of the urethra.

urinary bladder the muscular organ that stores urine before its elimination from the body.

urinary stasis a condition in which the bladder empties incompletely during urination.

urinary system the group of organs that produces urine, maintaining fluid and electrolyte balance for the body.

urinary tract infection (UTI) an infection, usually bacterial, at any site in the urinary tract.

urine the fluid made by the kidney and eliminated from the body.

urology the surgical specialty dealing with the urinary/genitourinary system.

urticaria the raised areas, or wheals, that occur on the skin, associated with vasodilation due to histamine release; commonly called "hives."

varicella viral disease characterized by a rash of fluid-filled vesicles that rupture, forming small ulcers that eventually scab.

varicose veins dilated superficial veins, usually in the lower extremity.

vas deferens the duct that carries sperm cells from epididymis to urethra.

vasculitis inflammation of blood vessels.

vasopastic angina *see* Prinzmetal's angina.

vector a force that has both magnitude and direction. *See also* QRS axis.

ventilation the mechanical process of moving air in and out of the lungs.

virulence an organism's strength or ability to infect or overcome the body's defenses.

virus disease-causing organism that can be seen only with an electron microscope.

visceral pain pain arising in hollow organs such as the ureter and bladder.

visceral pain dull, poorly localized pain that originates in the walls of hollow organs.

volvulus twisting of the intestine on itself.

von Willebrand's disease condition in which the vWF component of factor VIII is deficient.

Wernicke's syndrome condition characterized by loss of memory and disorientation, associated with chronic alcohol intake and a diet deficient in thiamine.

whole bowel irrigation administration of polyethylene glycol continuously at 1–2 L/hr through a nasogastric tube until the effluent is clear or objects are recovered.

window phase time between exposure to a disease and seroconversion.

withdrawal referring to alcohol or drug withdrawal in which the patient's body reacts severely when deprived of the abused substance.

Zollinger-Ellison syndrome condition that causes the stomach to secrete excessive amounts of hydrochloric acid and pepsin.

Index

Abdominal aorta, 75
Abdominal aortic aneurysm, 217–218
Abdominal emergencies. *See* Abdominal
pain; Gastrointestinal diseases and
emergencies; Renal and urologic emergencies
Abdominal exam, 376, 386, 407–408
Abdominal pain. *See also* Gastrointestinal
diseases and emergencies
    classification of, 363
    colicky, 378
    gynecological, 643, 647–649
        management of, 649
    hematological disease and (wood
    alcohol), 490
    management of patients with,
    408, 649
    in toxicological emergencies, 435
    transport and, 408
    urologic emergencies and, 404
Aberrant conduction, 156
Abortion, 669–671
Abruptio placentae, 673–674
Abscesses
    brain, 304
    intrarenal, 422
    perinephric, 422
Absence seizures (petit mal seizures), 296
Absolute refractory period, 94
Accelerated idioventricular rhythm, 141
Accelerated junctional rhythm, 136–137
Acclimatization, hyperthermia and, 511
Acetaminophen, in large doses, 449
Acetazolamide (Diamox), 537
Acetylcholine, 80, 264
Acids, 443
Acini, 322, 388
Acquired immunity, 348–349
Acrocyanosis, 687
Action potential, 82
Activated charcoal, 433
Active immunity, 349, 560
Active labor, 666
Active transport, 399
Acute arterial occlusion, 219
Acute gastroenteritis, 372–373
Acute idiopathic thrombocytopenia
purpura (ITP), 497
Acute mountain sickness (AMS), 538
Acute myocardial infarction. *See*
Myocardial infarction
Acute pulmonary embolism, 218–219
Acute renal failure (ARF), 409–413
Acute tubular necrosis, 410
Adam's apple (thyroid cartilage), 8
Addiction, 461, 620

Addisonian crisis, 341
Addison's disease (adrenal insufficiency),
339, 341
Adenocarcinoma, 51
Adenosine (Adenocard), 117, 139, 176
ADH (antidiuretic hormone), 320
Adhesion, intestinal, 382, 384
Adrenal cortex, 319, 324
Adrenal glands, 324–325
    disorders of, 339–341
Adrenal medulla, 319, 324
Adult respiratory distress syndrome
(ARDS), 36–38, 528
Advanced cardiac life support,
hypothermia and, 522–523
Adventitious sounds, in cardiac patients, 168
Afterbirth, 657
Afterload, 78
Age-related disorders, 624–625
AIDS (acquired immune deficiency
syndrome), 570–573
Airborne route, 555
Air pressure, effects on gases, 528–529
Airway. *See also* Lower airway;
Respiratory diseases; Upper airway;
Upper-airway obstruction
    assessment of, 24
    management of
        anaphylactic reactions, 354
        toxic inhalation, 53
        upper-airway obstruction, 36
Airway resistance, 13
Alcohol abuse, 462, 463–468
    consequences of, 466–467
    general alcoholic profile, 466
    physiological effects of, 463
    withdrawal syndrome, 467–468
Alcoholism, 464
    chronic, 289
Aldosterone, 325
Alkalinizing agents, 180
Alkalis, 443
Allergens, 350
Allergies (allergic reactions), 347,
349–351
    assessment findings in, 356
    in cardiac patients, 165
    case study, 346–347
    management of, 357
    patient education, 357–358
Alpha particles, 540
Alpha receptors, 79–80
Alteplase (Activase; tPA), 179
Altered mental status, 275
    management of, 287

Altitude illnesses, 536–539
Alveolar dead space, 15
Alveoli, 9–11
    diffusion and, 16
Alzheimer's disease, 304
Amiodarone (Cordarone), 176
Amnesia, psychogenic, 621
Amniotic fluid, 658
Amniotic sac, 658
Amphetamines, 463, 465
Amyotrophic lateral sclerosis (ALS), 306
Anabolism, 327
Analgesics, 408
Anaphylaxis (anaphylactic reactions),
350–356
    assessment findings in, 352–354
    management of, 354–356
    patient education, 357–358
Anastomoses, 75
Anatomical dead space, 15
Androgenic hormones, 325
Anemias, 492–494
Aneurysm, 217–218
Anger, 617
Angina pectoris, 191, 194–196
Angioneurotic edema (angioedema), 351
Angiotensin-converting enzyme (ACE),
326
Angiotensin I, 326
Angiotensin II, 326
Angiotensinogen, 326
Anorexia nervosa, 621, 622
Anterior descending artery, 75
Anterior great cardiac vein, 75
Anterior pituitary gland, 317, 318, 320, 321
Antibodies, 347, 557–559
Antidepressants
    newer, 447
    tricyclic, 445–446
Antidiuresis, 400
Antidiuretic hormone (ADH), 320
Antidotes to toxic substances, 433–434
Antidysrhythmics, 175–176
Antigens, 347, 557, 558
    blood transfusion and, 484
Antihistamines
    for anaphylaxis, 355
    hyperthermia and, 510
Antisocial personality disorder, 622
Anuria, 409
Anxiety
    in cardiac patients, 163
    defined, 616
Anxiety disorders, 616
Aorta, 74, 75

APGAR scoring, 687–689
Apnea, 20
Apneustic respirations, 20, 282
Appendicitis, 385–386
Arachnoid membrane, 265
ARDS (adult respiratory distress syndrome), 36–38
Arrhythmia, 97
Arterial blood pressure, renal control of, 401, 414
Arterial gas embolism (AGE), 531, 534
Arterial PCO2, 16
Arterial system, 76
Arteries, 76
    bronchial, 11
    coronary, 75
    pulmonary, 11, 74
Arterioles, 76
Arteriosclerosis, 217
Artifacts, on ECGs, 84–85
Artificial pacemaker rhythm, 152–153
Ascending aorta, 75
Ascending loop of Henle, 397
Asphyxia, 24
Aspirin
    for cardiac ischemia, 179
    overdose of, 448
Asthma, 38, 43–47
    airway resistance in, 13
    assessment of, 44–45
    in children, 45, 48
    pathophysiology of, 43–44
Asystole (cardiac standstill), 150–151
Ataxic respirations, 282
Ataxic (Biot's) respirations, 20
Atherosclerosis, 217
Atherosclerotic disease, peripheral arterial, 219
Atherosclerotic heart disease (ASHD), 196
Atria, 71
    dysrhythmias originating in the, 109–122
        atrial fibrillation, 120–123
        atrial flutter, 118–119
        atrial tachycardia, 108–111
        multifocal atrial tachycardia, 110–111
        paroxysmal supraventricular tachycardia, 114–117
        premature atrial contractions, 113
Atrial fibrillation, 120–123
    in hypothermia, 520
Atrial flutter, 118–119
Atrial natriuretic hormone (ANH), 326
Atrial pathways, internodal, 83–84
Atrial syncytium, 80
Atrial tachycardia, 108–111
    multifocal, 110–111
Atrioventricular blocks. See AV blocks
Atrioventricular (AV) bundle, 81
Atrioventricular valves, 73
Atropine sulfate, 175–176

Atypical angina, 191
Augmented limb leads, 85
Augmented limb leads (unipolar limb leads), 226–227
Aura, 295
Auscultation
    of cardiac patients, 168
    of chest, 28–29
Autoimmune diseases, 480
Autoimmunity, 559
Automaticity of heart cells, 83
Autonomic nervous system, 263, 275. See also Parasympathetic nervous system; Sympathetic nervous system
    disorders of, 277
    hypothalamus and, 317
Autonomic nervous system (ANS), 276
Autonomic neuropathy, 510
AV blocks (atrioventricular blocks), 122–133, 241
    classification of, 123
    first-degree, 124–125
    sites of, 123
    third-degree, 130–131, 245
    Type II (Mobitz II), 128–129
    Type I second-degree (Mobitz I), 126–127, 241
AV junction
    originating within the (AV blocks), 122–131
        first-degree AV block, 124–125
        third-degree AV block, 130–131
        Type II second-degree AV block, 128–129
        Type I second-degree AV block, 126–127
    sustained or originating in the, 132–139
        accelerated junctional rhythm, 136–137
        common ECG features of, 133
        junctional escape complexes and rhythms, 134–135
        premature junctional contractions, 132, 133
Avoidant personality disorder, 622
AV sequential pacemakers, 152
Axis deviation, 229–231
Axons, 264

Back pain, 307–310
Bacteria, 551–552
Bactericidal, 552
Bacteriostatic, 552
Barbiturates, 463, 464
Barotrauma, 530, 532
Barrel chest, in emphysema patients, 40
Basal metabolic rate (BMR), 508
Basophils, 351, 478–479
B cells, 347
Behavior, defined, 608

Behavioral changes, in cardiac patients, 164
Behavioral disorders. See Psychiatric and behavioral disorders
Bell's palsy, 306
Benign prostatic hypertrophy, 396
Benzodiazepines, 465
Benzodiazepines (diazepam), 463
Bereavement, 618
Beta1 receptors, 80
Beta agonists, for anaphylaxis, 355
Beta blockers, 180
    hyperthermia and, 510
Beta particles, 540
Biological psychiatric disorders, 609–610
Bipolar disorder, 619
Bipolar limb leads, 85, 224, 226
Bites, snake, 457–460
Black widow spider bites, 456–457
Bladder, urinary, 402
Blastocyst, 657
Blebs, 39
Bleeding
    lower gastrointestinal, 376–377
    in pregnancy, 669–674
    upper gastrointestinal, 369–370
    vaginal, non-traumatic, 649
        during pregnancy, 666
Blood. See also Circulation; Hematological disorders
    components of, 473–481
        leukocytes (white blood cells), 476–480
        plasma, 473–474
        platelets, 481
        red blood cells, 474–476
    high altitude and, 537
Bloodborne diseases, 555
Blood clots (coagulation), 481–483
Blood glucometer, 286
Blood pressure
    arterial, renal control of, 401, 414
    hypertensive emergencies, 208–209
Blood transfusion, 484–486
Blood typing, 484–485
B lymphocytes, 558–559
Body dysmorphic disorder, 620
Bohr effect, 474
Borderline personality disorder, 622
Bowel irrigation, whole, 433
Bowel obstruction, 382–385
Bowman's capsule, 397
Boyle's Law, 529
Bradycardia, 96
    sinus, 99–101
Bradykinesia, 305
Bradypnea, 32
Brain, 265, 268–270
Brain abscess, 304
Brainstem, 269
Braxton-Hicks contractions, 678
Breathing. See also Respiration(s)
    assessment of, 24–25

Breath sounds. *See also* Respiration(s)
    abnormal, 30
    of cardiac patients, 168
    normal, 29
Bretylium, 176
Bronchi, 8–9
Bronchial arteries, 11
Bronchial veins, 11
Bronchial vessels, 11
Bronchioles, 9
Bronchitis, chronic, 41–43
Bronchospasm, 13, 39
Brown recluse spider, 454–456
Brudzinki's sign, 583
Bruits, 282
Bulimia nervosa, 621–622
Bundle branch blocks, 156, 245–249
Bundle of His, 84, 222
Bundle of Kent, 157

Cafe coronary, 35
Calcitonin, 322
Calcium channel blockers, 180
Calcium stones, 419
Cancer, lung, 51–52
Candida albicans, 551
Capillaries, 76
    pulmonary, 10, 16–18
Capnometry, 33–34
Carbon dioxide
    diffusion and, 16
    gas exchange and, 11
    perfusion and, 18
    ventilation and, 16
Carbon monoxide, 439
    inhalation of, 53–54
Carcinoma
    epidermoid, 51
    large cell, 51
    small cell (oat cell), 51
Cardiac arrest, 212–216
Cardiac conduction (cardiac conductive
system), 83, 222
    abnormalities of, 240–254
        AV blocks, 241–245
        bundle branch blocks,
        245–249
        chamber enlargement,
        249–254
Cardiac cycle, 77–78
Cardiac depolarization, 81–82
Cardiac medication poisoning, 442–443
Cardiac output, 78
Cardiac physiology, 77–84. *See also* Heart
    autonomic nervous system and,
    78–80
    electrophysiology, 80–81
Cardiac plexus, 79
Cardiac standstill (asystole), 150–151
Cardiac tamponade, 206–207
Cardinal positions of gaze, 280
Cardiogenic shock, 209–212
    field assessment of, 210

management of, 210–212
myocardial infarction and, 196,
    197, 210
Cardiology, 62–258
Cardiopulmonary resuscitation (CPR). *See
also* Resuscitation
    hypothermia and, 522
Cardiovascular disease (heart disease), 68.
See also Coronary heart disease
    during pregnancy, 665
Cardiovascular emergencies
    assessment in, 160–170, 220
        allergies, 165
        chest pain, 162–163
        common symptoms,
        162–165
        focused history, 162–166
        physical examination,
        166–170
        scene size-up and initial
        assessment, 161–162
        subtle signs of cardiac
        disease, 167
    case study, 67
    management of, 170–221
        acute arterial occlusion, 219
        acute pulmonary embolism,
        218–219
        advanced life support,
        170–171
        aneurysm, 217–218
        angina pectoris, 191,
        194–196
        atherosclerosis, 217
        basic life support, 170
        cardiac arrest, 212–216
        cardiac tamponade,
        206–207
        cardiogenic shock, 209–212
        carotid sinus massage, 190,
        192–193
        defibrillation, 180–183
        ECG monitoring in the field,
        171–174
        heart failure, 202–206
        hypertensive emergencies,
        208–209
        myocardial infarction (MI),
        196–202
        noncritical peripheral
        vascular conditions, 219–221
        pharmacological
        management, 175–180
        precordial thump, 175
        support and
        communication, 190
        synchronized cardioversion,
        183, 186, 187
        transcutaneous cardiac
        pacing, 186, 188–189
        vagal maneuvers, 174
        vascular disorders, 221
        vasculitis, 219

Cardiovascular system
    anatomy of, 70–77. *See also* Heart,
    anatomy of
        peripheral circulation, 76–77
    high altitude and, 537
    neurological emergencies and, 282
    during pregnancy, 659–661
Carina, 8
Carotid arteries, bruits (murmurs) in, 169
Carotid sinus massage, 190, 192–193
Carotid system, 269
Carpopedal spasm, 30, 57
Catabolism, 327
Catatonia, 615
Catatonic schizophrenia, 616
Caustic substances, 443–444
Cell-mediated immunity, 558
Cellular immunity, 347, 349
Centers for Disease Control and
Prevention (CDC), 550
Central nervous system (CNS), 263. *See
also* Neurologic emergencies
    anatomy and physiology of,
    264–271
        brain, 265, 268–269
        neurons, 264
        protective structures, 265
    disorders of, 275–276
    respiratory diseases and, 58
Central neurogenic hyperventilation,
20, 282
Central pain syndrome, 305
Cephalopelvic disproportion, 693
Cerebellum, 269
Cerebral cortex, 268
Cerebral homeostasis, 276
Cerebral thrombus, 290
Cerebrospinal fluid, 16, 265
Cerebrum, 268
Cesarean section, 673, 682, 689, 692, 695
Chamber enlargement, 249–254
Chancroid, 599–600
Charcoal, activated, 433
Chemical restraint, 631
Chemotaxis, 477
Chest, inspection of, 26–28
Chest cavity, inspiration and, 12
Chest pain
    in cardiovascular patients, 162–163
    gastrointestinal emergencies that
    can cause, 366
    myocardial infarction and,
    197–198, 201
    pleuritic, 50
Chest wall
    diseases that affect, 19
    expiration and, 13
    inspiration and, 12–13
Cheyne-Stokes respirations, 19–20, 281
Chickenpox (varicella), 581–582
Childbirth. *See* Delivery
Chlamydia, 599, 647
Cholecystitis, 386–388

Cholelithiasis, 386
Chordae tendoneae, 73
Chronic bronchitis, 41–43
Chronic obstructive pulmonary disease (COPD), 5, 28, 30, 31, 38
Chronic renal failure (CRF), 413–419
Chronotropy, 80
Cigarette smoking, 8
COPD and, 39
    emphysema and, 39, 40
    lung cancer and, 51
Ciguatera (bony fish) poisoning, 452
Cilia, 7, 8
Circle of Willis, 269, 271
Circulation
    collateral, 75
    coronary, 75
    fetal, 662–663
    peripheral, 76–77
Circumcision, 403
Circumflex artery, 75
Cirrhosis of the liver, 371–372
Claudication, 217
Clitoris, 638
Clonic phase, 295
Clostridium botulinum, 451, 591
Clostridium tetani, 560
Cluster headaches, 300
Clusters, personality disorder, 622
Coagulation, 481–483
    disorders of, 497–498
Cocaine, 462–464
Cognitive disorders, 614–615
Cold disorders, 516–524
    frostbite, 523–524
    hypothermia, 517–523
    pathophysiology of, 506–509
    trench foot, 524
Cold diuresis, 522
Colic, 378
Colitis, ulcerative, 377–378
Collateral circulation, 75
Collecting duct, 397
Collecting tubule, 397
Colloid, 321
Color of patient, respiratory status and, 23
Coma (unconsciousness), 275
    diabetic (diabetic ketoacidosis), 330–332
    hyperglycemic hyperosmolar nonketotic (HHNK), 330–333
    myxedema, 338–340
Common cold (viral rhinitis), 585
Common pathway, 482
Communicable infectious agents and diseases, 556
Communicable period, 557
Community-acquired infections, 422
Complement system, 559
Complex partial seizures, 296
Conception, 661
Concretions, 450–451
Conduction, 506

Conductive disorders, dysrhythmias resulting from, 154–157
Conductivity of heart cells, 83
Confusion, in behavioral emergencies, 611
Congestive heart failure (CHF), 204–206
Consciousness. See also Coma; Mental status
    altered forms of, 275
    level of
        in cardiac patients, 163
        in renal and urologic emergencies, 407
    loss of. See Syncope
Contamination, 556
Contraceptives, 644–645
Contractility of heart cells, 83
Convection, 506
Conversion disorder, 620
COPD (chronic obstructive pulmonary disease), 5, 28, 30, 31, 38
Coral snake bites, 460
Cordarone (amiodarone), 176
Core body temperature (CBT), 507, 510
Coronary arteries, 75
Coronary artery bypass graft (CABG), 202
Coronary heart disease (CHD), 68
Coronary sinus, 75
Cor pulmonale, 39, 202
Corpus callosum, 268
Corticosteroids, for anaphylaxis, 355
Cortisol, 324
Cough
    in asthma, 44
    in cardiac patients, 163
Cough reflex, 8
Counter-current heat exchange, 509
Coupling interval, 142
CPR, 213
Crackles (rales), 30
Cramps, heat (muscle), 511–513
Cranial nerves, 273, 274
    assessment of, 284
Creatinine, 401
Crepitus, 28
    in cardiac patients, 169–170
Crohn's disease, 378–380
Croup, 589
Crowning, 667
Cullen's sign, 367
Current of injury, 232, 234
Cushing's reflex, 285
Cushing's syndrome (hyperadrenalism), 339–341
Cyanide, 438–439
Cyanosis, respiratory status and, 23
Cystic medial necrosis, 218
Cystine stones, 419
Cystitis, 421, 648
Cysts
    ovarian, 648
    spinal, 309

Dalton's Law, 529
Decerebrate posture, 283
Decompression illness, 531, 532–533
Decontamination
    methods and procedures, 566–567
    in toxicological emergencies, 432–433
Decorticate posturing, 283
Deep venous thrombosis, 219–220
Defibrillation, 180–185
Defibrillator paddles, 181–182
Defibrillators, 181
Degenerative neurological disorders, 304–307
Degranulation, 351
Dehydration, heat disorders and, 515
Deja vu, 296
Delayed hypersensitivity, 349
Delirium, 615
Delirium tremens (DTs), 467
Delivery
    abnormal, 689–693
        breech presentation, 689–690
        cephalopelvic disproportion, 693
        limb presentation, 692
        maternal complications, 694–696
        meconium staining, 694
        of multiple births, 693
        occiput posterior position, 692–693
        postpartum hemorrhage, 694–695
        precipitous delivery, 693–694
        prolapsed cord, 691–692
        shoulder dystocia, 694
        uterine inversion, 695–696
        uterine rupture, 695
    by cesarean section, 673, 682, 689, 692, 695
    field, 683–686
Delta wave, 157
Delusions, in schizophrenia, 615
Demand pacemakers, 152
Dementia, 615
Dendrites, 264
Dependence, 620
Dependent personality disorder, 622
Depersonalization, 621
Depolarization, cardiac, 81–82
Depression, 618–619
Dermatomes, 271
Descending loop of Henle, 397
Diabetes
    gestational, 665, 677
    insipidus, 320
    mellitus, 326–330
        Type I, 329
        Type II (non-insulin-dependent), 329–330

Diabetic ketoacidosis (diabetic coma), 330–332
Diagnostic and Statistical Manual of Mental Disorders, Fourth Edition (DSM-IV), 614
Diagnostic testing, of respiratory system, 32–34
Dialysate, 417
Dialysis, 395
    peritoneal, 418–419
    renal, 416–418
Diamox (acetazolamide), 537
Diaphoresis (perspiration)
    in cardiac patients, 163
    respiratory status and, 23
Diaphragm, 12
    diseases that affect, 19
Diastole, 77
Diazepam (Valium), 179
Diencephalon, 268
Diet-induced thermogenesis, 506
Diffusion, 16–17
    diseases that affect, 21
Digitalis (Digoxin, Lanoxin), 180
Dilatation, 680
2,3-diphosphoglycerate (2,3-DPG), 475
Disease period, 557
Disinfection, 566–567
Disk injury, 308
Disorganized schizophrenia, 616
Dissecting aortic aneurysm, 218
Disseminated intravascular coagulation (DIC), 499
Dissociative disorders, 621
Distal tubule, 397
Diuresis, 400
    cold, 522
    osmotic, 329, 401
Diuretics, hyperthermia and, 510
Divers Alert Network (DAN), 535–536
Diverticula, 380
Diverticulitis, 380–381
Diverticulosis, 380
Diving emergencies, 528–536
    arterial gas embolism (AGE), 534
    classification of injuries, 530–531
    general assessment of, 531–532
    nitrogen narcosis, 535
    pathophysiology of, 530
    pneumomediastinum, 535
    pressure disorders, 532
    pulmonary over-pressure accidents, 534
Dobutamine (Dobutrex), 177–178
Dopamine (Intropin), 177
Down time, 213
2,3-DPG (2,3-diphosphoglycerate), 475
DPT (diphtheria/pertussis/tetanus) vaccine, 349
Dromotropy, 80
Drowning, 525–527
Drug overdose, 462
Dry drowning, 525–526

Dual-chambered pacemakers, 152
Ductus arteriosus, 663
Ductus venosus, 663
Dura mater, 265
Dysmenorrhea, 644
Dyspareunia, 644
Dyspnea, 24
    in asthma, 44
    in cardiac patients, 163
Dysrhythmias, 97–157
    atria, originating in the, 109–122
      atrial fibrillation, 120–123
      atrial flutter, 118–119
      atrial tachycardia, 108–111
      multifocal atrial tachycardia, 110–111
      paroxysmal supraventricular tachycardia, 114–117
      premature atrial contractions, 113
    AV junction
      originating within the (AV blocks), 122–131
        first-degree AV block, 124–125
        third-degree AV block, 130–131
        Type II second-degree AV block, 128–129
        Type I second-degree AV block, 126–127
      sustained or originating in the, 132–139
        accelerated junctional rhythm, 136–137
        common ECG features of, 133
        junctional escape complexes and rhythms, 134–135
        premature junctional contractions, 132, 133
    causes of, 97–98
    classification of, 98–99
    conduction disorders, resulting from, 154–157
      pre-excitation syndromes, 157
      ventricular conduction, disturbances of, 156–157
    defined, 97
    electrolyte imbalances and, 157
    mechanism of impulse formation and, 98
    myocardial infarction and, 197–200
    pulseless electrical activity (PEA), 154, 155
    SA node, originating in the, 99–107
      sinus arrest, 106–107
      sinus bradycardia, 99–101
      sinus dysrhythmia, 104–105
      sinus tachycardia, 102–103
    sinus, 104–105

ventricles, originating within the, 140–153
    accelerated idioventricular rhythm, 141
    artificial pacemaker rhythm, 152–153
    asystole (cardiac standstill), 150–151
    premature ventricular contractions (PVCs), 142–144
    ventricular escape complexes and rhythms, 141
    ventricular fibrillation, 148–149
    ventricular tachycardia, 144–147
Dystonias, 305
Dysuria, 648

Eating disorders, 621–622
ECG graph paper, 87–88
ECG leads, 85–87, 224–228
    bipolar, 226
    heart surfaces and, 95
    precordial, 228
    unipolar (augmented), 226–227
ECG monitoring, 86
    in the field, 171–174
    prehospital, 255–258
    single-lead, 221–222
ECG recording, 222–224
ECGs (electrocardiograms), 84–93. *See also* Dysrhythmias
12-lead, 221
      normal, 231–233
    axis deviation, 229–231
    cardiac depolarization and, 81
    cardiac tamponade and, 207
    disease findings, 232–240
    electrical changes in the heart and, 88–95
      lead systems and heart surfaces, 95
      P-R interval (PRI) or P-Q interval (PQI), 93
      P waves, 88
      QRS complex, 88
      QRS interval, 93
      QT interval, 93
      refractory period, 94
      S-T segment, 93, 94–95
      T waves, 89
      U waves, 89, 93
    mean QRS axis determination, 228
    rhythm strips, 84, 95–98
Eclampsia, 675, 676
Ecstasy (MDMA), 463
Ectopic beats, 98
Ectopic foci, 98
Ectopic pregnancy, 649, 671–672
Edema
    angioneurotic, 351
    in cardiac patients, 164, 167

laryngeal, 53
pulmonary, 5
    cardiogenic, 36–37
    congestive heart failure and, 204–206
    high altitude (HAPE), 38
    non-cardiogenic, 36–38
Effacement of the cervix, 678, 680
Egophony, 50
Einthoven, Willem, 224
Einthoven's triangle, 85, 86, 226
Ejection fraction, 77–78
Electrical mechanical dissociation, 154
Electrocardiograms (ECGs). *See* ECGs
Electrolytes
    cardiac function and, 80
    tubular handling of, 399–400
Electrons, 540
Emboli, pulmonary, 5
Embolic strokes, 290
Embolism, pulmonary, 54–56
    acute, 218–219
    pregnancy and, 696
Embryonic stage, 661
Emotional status. *See also* Psychiatric and behavioral disorders
    assessment of, 278–279
Emphysema, 10, 39–41
    subcutaneous, 28
Encephalitis, 592–593
Encephalomyelitis, 593
End-diastolic volume (preload), 78
Endocardium, 71
Endocrine system (endocrine glands), 315
    anatomy and physiology of, 316–326
        adrenal cortex, 319
        adrenal glands, 324–325
        adrenal medulla, 319
        gonads, 325
        hypothalamus, 317, 318
        ovaries, 319, 325
        pancreas, 319, 322–324
        parathyroid glands, 318, 322
        pineal gland, 319, 325–326
        pituitary gland, 317–318, 320–321
        testes, 319, 325
        thymus, 318
        thymus gland, 322
        thyroid gland, 318, 321–322
    case study, 313–315
    disorders and emergencies of, 326–341
        adrenal glands, 339–341
        pancreas, 326–336
        thyroid gland, 336–339
Endocrinology, 312–341
Endometriosis, 648–649
Endometritis, 648
Endometrium, 641
Endotoxins, 552
End-stage renal failure, 395, 413
End-tidal CO2, 34

End-tidal CO2 detector, 286
Entero-hepatic circulation, 450
Enterotoxins, 451
Environmental emergencies, 502–544. *See also* Cold disorders; Diving emergencies; Heat disorders
    case study, 504
    defined, 505
    drowning and near-drowning, 525–527
    high altitude illness, 536–539
    homeostasis and, 505–506
    nuclear radiation, 539–544
Environmental pollutants, respiratory diseases and, 5
Environmental toxins, COPD and, 39
Eosinophils, 478, 479
Epicardium (visceral pericardium), 71
Epidermoid carcinoma, 51
Epididymis, 403
Epigastrium, in cardiac patients, 167, 170
Epiglottitis, 49, 589
Epinephrine (adrenalin), 177, 324
    for allergic reactions, 357
    for anaphylaxis, 354–355
Episiotomy, 637
Erythema migrans (EM), 595
Erythroblastosis fetalis (hemolytic disease of the newborn), 485
Erythrocytes (red blood cells), 401, 414, 474
Erythropoeitin, 473
Erythropoiesis, 476
Erythropoietin, 326, 401
Eschar, 443
Escherichia coli (E. coli), 422, 552, 591–592
Esophageal varices, 370–372
Estimated date of confinement (EDC), 661
Estrogen, 325, 637
Ethylene glycol, 465
Evaporation, 507
Excitability of heart cells, 83
Exertional heatstroke, 514
Exertional metabolic rate, 508
Exocrine glands, 315
Exotoxins, 451, 552
Expiration, 12, 13
Expiratory reserve volume, 14
Expulsion stage, 680–681
External cardiac pacing, 186, 188–189
Extremities, respiratory status and, 30
Extrinsic pathway, 482
Eyes, of neurological patients, 280

Facial expressions, anguished, in cardiac patients, 164
Facial paralysis, 280, 281
Facilitated diffusion, 399
Factitious disorders, 620–621
Fainting. *See* Syncope
Fallopian tubes, 641
False labor, 678

Fatigue, in cardiac patients, 164
Fear, in behavioral emergencies, 611
Fecal-oral route, 555
Female reproductive system, anatomy and physiology of, 637–641
Fetal circulation, 662–663
Fetal development, 661–662
Fetal heart tones (FHTs), 661
Fetal stage, 661
FEV (forced expiratory volume), 15
Fever (pyrexia), 516
Fibrinogen, 481
Fibrinolysis, 482
Field delivery, 683–686
Filtrate, 398
First-degree AV block, 124–125, 241
Fixed-rate pacemakers, 152
Flail chest, 19
Flat affect, in schizophrenia, 615
Flora, normal, 550, 551
Flumazenil, 463
Flunitrazepam (rohypnol), 463
Follicle stimulating hormone (FSH), 641, 642, 656
Food poisoning, 451–452, 591–592
Foramen ovale, 663
Forced expiratory volume (FEV), 15
Forebrain, 268
Fresh-water drowning, 526
Frostbite, 523–524
Fugue state, 621
Functional residual capacity, 14
Fundal height, 666
Fundus, 640
Fungi, 554
Furosemide (Lasix), 179

Gallstones, 386
Gambling, pathological, 623
Gamma rays, 540
Gastric lavage, 433
Gastrin, 326
Gastroenteritis, 373–374, 590–591
    acute, 372–373
Gastrointestinal diseases and emergencies, 360–390
    accessory organ diseases, 385–390
        appendicitis, 385–386
        cholecystitis, 386–388
    assessment of, 365–367
    case study, 361–362
    general pathophysiology, 363–365
    general treatment of, 367–368
    infections, 590–592
    lower GI diseases, 376–385
        bowel obstruction, 382–385
        Crohn's disease, 378–380
        diverticulitis, 380–381
        hemorrhoids, 381–382
        hepatitis, 389–390
        lower gastrointestinal bleeding, 376–377

pancreatitis, 388
ulcerative colitis, 377–378
upper gastrointestinal diseases,
368–376
acute gastroenteritis, 372–373
esophageal varices, 370–372
gastroenteritis, 373–374
peptic ulcers, 374–376
upper gastrointestinal bleeding,
369–370
Gastrointestinal system, during pregnancy,
661
GCS (Glasgow Coma Scale), 284–285
Geiger counter, 541
Generalized seizures, 295
Genitalia
external, female, 637
internal, female, 639–641
Genital warts, 598
Genitourinary system, 395
Geriatric patients, 624–625
German measles (rubella), 586–587
Gestational diabetes, 665, 677
Glasgow Coma Scale (GCS), 284–285
Glomerular filtration, 398
Glomerular filtration rate (GFR), 398
Glomerulus, 397
Glottic opening, 8
Glucagon, 323, 324
Glucocorticoids, 324–325
Gluconeogenesis, 323, 324
Glucose, 323–324
metabolism of, 327–328
Glucose (blood glucose)
determination of, 334–335
low. See Hypoglycemia
regulation of, 328–329
tubular handling of, 400–401
Glucose intolerance, 414
Glucosuria, during pregnancy, 661
Glycogen, 324
Glycogenolysis, 323, 324
Glycosuria, 329
Gonads, 325
Gonorrhea, 596–597
Gonorrhea (Neisseria gonorrhoeae), 647
Gram stain, 551, 552
Grand mal seizures (tonic-clonic
seizures), 295
Granules, 351
Granulocytes, 351, 478
Graves' disease, 336–338
Grey-Turner's sign, 367
Growth hormone (GH), 321
Growth hormone inhibitory hormone
(GHIH), 317
Growth hormone releasing hormone
(GHRH), 317
Guillian-Barré Syndrome (GBS), 59
Gynecological emergencies, 647–652
assessment in, 643–646
case study, 635–636
defined, 637

ectopic pregnancy, 649
endometriosis, 648–649
endometritis, 648
management of, 646–647
mittelschmerz, 648
pelvic inflammatory disease (PID),
647–648
ruptured ovarian cysts, 648
traumatic, 650–652
vaginal bleeding, non-traumatic, 649
Gynecology, 634–652

Habituation, 461
HACE (high altitude cerebral edema), 539
Haldane effect, 18
Half-life, 540
Hallucinations, in schizophrenia, 615
Hallucinogens, 463, 465
Hantavirus, 589, 590
HAPE (high altitude pulmonary edema), 38
Hashimoto's thyroiditis, 480
Havrix, 575
Head, respiratory assessment and, 26
Headache, 300–301
in cardiac patients, 164
Heart
anatomy of, 70–75
blood flow, 74
chambers, 71–72
coronary circulation, 75
tissue layers, 71
valves, 73–74
autonomic nervous system and,
78–80
electrophysiology of, 80–81
physiology of, 77–84
Heart disease. See Cardiovascular disease;
Cardiovascular emergencies
Heart failure, 197, 202–206
congestive (CHF), 204–206
Heart rate, analyzing, 96
Heart rate calculator rulers, 96
Heart rhythm. See also Dysrhythmias
analyzing, 96–97
Heart sounds, in cardiac patients,
168–169
Heat conservation and loss, mechanisms
of, 517
Heat (muscle) cramps, 511–513
Heat disorders, 510–516
dehydration and, 515
fever (pyrexia), 516
heat (muscle) cramps, 511–513
heat exhaustion, 513–514
heatstroke, 514–515
hyperthermia, 510–511
pathophysiology of, 506–509
Heat exhaustion, 513–514
Heat illness, 510
Heatstroke, 514–515
Helicobacter pylori, 373–375
Hematemesis, 369
Hematochezia, 373

Hematocrit, 476
Hematological crises, 494
Hematological disorders, 471–499
case study, 471–472
general assessment and
management of, 486–492
general management,
491–492
initial assessment, 487
physical exam, 488–491
SAMPLE history, 487–488
scene size-up, 487
managing specific problems,
492–499
red blood cell diseases,
492–494
white blood cell diseases,
495–496
Hematology, 470–499
defined, 472
Hematopoiesis, 473
Hematopoietic system, 473. See also
Blood
Hemiblocks, 248–249
Hemodialysis, 417
Hemodilution, 526
Hemoglobin, 474
laboratory evaluation of, 476
perfusion and, 17, 18
Hemolysis, 476
Hemolytic disease of the newborn
(Erythroblastosis fetalis), 485
Hemolytic transfusion reaction, 485–486
Hemophilia, 497–498
Hemoptysis, 25
Hemorrhage. See also Bleeding
intracranial, stroke and, 289–294
postpartum, 694–695
Hemorrhagic strokes, 291–292
Hemorrhoids, 381–382
Hemostasis, 481–483
Hemothorax, 19
Henry's Law, 529
Heparin, 351
Hepatitis, 389–390, 574–577
Hepatitis A, 574–575
Hepatitis B, 575–576
Hepatitis C, 576
Hepatitis D, 576
Hepatitis E, 576–577
Hering-Breuer reflex, 15
Hernia, intestinal, 382, 383
Herpes simplex, 588–589
Type 2, 598–599
HHNK (hyperglycemic hyperosmolar
nonketotic) acidosis, 330–333
High altitude cerebral edema (HACE), 539
High altitude illness, 536–539
High altitude pulmonary edema (HAPE),
38, 538–539
Hilum, 11
of kidney, 397
Hindbrain, 269

Histamine, 351
Histrionic personality disorder, 622
HIV (human immunodeficiency virus), 570–574
Homeostasis, 315
    cerebral, 276
    environmental conditions and, 505–506
Hookworms, 554
Hormones, 315, 316
    hypothalamic, 317
    pancreatic, 323
    pituitary, 317
        anterior pituitary, 321
        posterior pituitary, 320
    thyroid, 321
Host defenses, 551
Host resistance, 557
Human chorionic gonadotropin (hCG), 326
Human immunodeficiency virus (HIV), 570–574
Humoral immunity, 347, 558
Hydrocarbons, toxicity from, 444
Hydrofluoric acid, 444
Hymen, 638
Hymenoptera insects, 351
Hymenoptera stings, 454
Hyperadrenalism (Cushing's syndrome), 339–341
Hyperbaric oxygen chamber, 533
Hypercalcemia, 80
Hypercapnia, 535
Hyperglycemia, 328
Hyperglycemic hyperosmolar nonketotic (HHNK) acidosis, 330–333
Hyperkalemia, 80, 157
Hyperosmolar, 399
Hypersensitivity, 349
    delayed, 349
    immediate, 350
Hypertension, during pregnancy, 665
Hypertensive disorders of pregnancy, 674–676
Hypertensive emergencies, 208–209
Hypertensive encephalopathy, 208
Hyperthermia, 510–511
Hyperthyroidism, 336
Hypertrophy, ventricular, 249
Hyperventilation, central neurogenic, 282
Hyperventilation syndrome, 57–58
Hypochondriasis, 620
Hypoglycemia (insulin shock), 328, 330–331, 333, 336
Hypoglycemic seizure, 336
Hypokalemia, 157
Hypo-osmolar, 399
Hypothalamus, 268, 317, 318, 508
Hypothermia, 157, 517–523
    degrees of, 518
    mechanisms of heat conservation and loss and, 517
    predisposing factors, 517
    preventive measures, 518

signs and symptoms of, 518–520
    treatment for, 520
Hypothyroidism, 336, 338–339
Hypoxemia, 30
Hypoxia, 21, 30, 31, 35
    chronic bronchitis and, 42, 43
Hypoxic ventilatory response (HVR), 536–537

Idiopathic epilepsy, 295
Idiopathic thrombocytopenia purpura (ITP), acute, 497
Immediate hypersensitivity, 350
Immune response, alterations in, 480
Immune system, 347–349, 558–559
Immunity (immune response)
    acquired, 348–349
    active, 560
    cell-mediated, 558
    cellular, 347, 349
    humoral, 347, 558
    induced active (artificially acquired immunity), 348
    lymphocytes and, 479–480
    natural (innate immunity), 348
    naturally acquired, 348
    passive, 560
Immunization
    chickenpox, 581–582
    hepatitis, 575, 576
    meningitis, 583–584
    pneumonia, 581
Immunoglobulins (Igs), 347, 559
Impending doom, feeling of, in cardiac patients, 164
Impetigo, 600
Impulse control disorders, 623
Incomplete bundle branch block, 156
Incubation period, 557
Indeterminate axis, 230
Index case, 549–550
Induced active immunity (artificially acquired immunity), 348
Induced passive immunity, 349
Infarction, bowel, 382
Infectious crises, 494
Infectious diseases, 546–604
    assessment of patients with, 568–570
    body's defenses against, 558–561
    case study, 548
    chancroid, 599–600
    chickenpox (varicella), 581–582
    chlamydia, 599
    common cold (viral rhinitis), 585
    contraction, transmission, and stages of, 555–557
    control of, in prehospital care, 561–568
    croup (laryngotracheobronchitis), 589
    defined, 549, 556
    encephalitis, 592–593
    epiglottitis, 589

    exposures to, 567
    food poisoning, 591–592
    gastroenteritis, 590–591
    gastrointestinal, 590–592
    genital warts, 598
    gonorrhea, 596–597
    hantavirus, 590
    hepatitis, 574–577
    herpes simplex Type 2, 598–599
    herpes simplex virus, 588–589
    HIV (human immunodeficiency virus), 570–574
    impetigo, 600
    influenza, 584–585
    lice, 600–601
    Lyme disease, 595–596
    measles (rubeola), 585–586
    meningitis, 582–584
    microorganisms and, 550–555
    mononucleosis, 588
    mumps, 586
    nervous system, 592–596
    nosocomial, 602
    patient education and, 602
    pertussis (whooping cough), 587–588
    pharyngitis, 589
    pneumonia, 580–581
    preventing transmission of, 603–604
    public health agencies and, 550
    public health principles, 549–550
    rabies, 593–594
    respiratory syncytial virus (RSV), 587
    rubella (German measles), 586–587
    scabies, 601–602
    sexually transmitted diseases (STDs), 596–600
    sinusitis, 589–590
    of the skin, 600–602
    tetanus, 594–595
    trichomoniasis, 599
    tuberculosis, 577–580
    upper respiratory (URI), 48–49
Inferior vena cava, 74
Inflammatory process, 480
Influenza, 584–585
Ingested toxins, 430, 434–436
Inhalation
    of carbon monoxide, 53–54
    of toxic substances, 52–54, 437
Injected toxins, 431, 453–461
Injury current, 232, 234
Inotropy, 80
In SAD CAGES (mnemonic), 618
Insect stings, 454–457
Inspection, of respiratory system, 26–28
Inspiration, 12–13
    medulla and, 15
Inspiratory capacity, 14
Inspiratory reserve volume, 14
Insulin, 323–324

Insulin-dependent diabetes mellitus (IDDM), 329
Insulin shock (hypoglycemia), 328, 330–331, 333, 336
Interatrial septum, 71
Intercalated discs, 80
Intercostal muscles, 12
Intermittent explosive disorder, 623
Internodal atrial pathways, 83–84
Interpolated beat, 142
Interstitial nephritis, 410
Interventricular septum, 71
Intracranial pressure, increased, 289
Intrarenal abscess, 422
Intrinsic pathway, 482
Introitus, 638
Intussusception, intestinal, 382, 383
Ionizing radiation, 540. See Nuclear radiation
Ipecac, syrup of, 433
Iron, toxicity from, 450–451
Ischemic phase, 642
Islets of Langerhans, 322–323
Isoproterenol, 177
Isosthenuria, 414
Isotopes (radioisotopes), 540

Jugular veins, distention of, 26, 27
Jugular venous distention (JVD), 205, 282
Junctional escape complexes and rhythms, 134–135
J waves (Osborn waves), 157, 520

Kernig's sign, 583
Ketoacidosis, diabetic (diabetic coma), 330–332
Ketone bodies, 328
Ketosis, 328
Kidneys. See also Renal and urologic emergencies
  anatomy and physiology of, 396–401
Kidney stones (renal calculi), 395, 419–421
  case study, 394
Kidney transplantation, 395
Kleptomania, 623
Korsakoff's psychosis, 289
Kussmaul's respirations, 20, 282, 331

Labia majora, 637
Labia minora, 637, 638
Labor, 680–683. See also Delivery
  active, 666
  Braxton-Hicks contractions and, 678
  false, 678
  management of a patient in, 681–683
  preterm, 678–679
  stages of, 680
Landsteiner, Karl, 484
Large cell carcinoma, 51
Laryngeal edema, 53
  airway obstruction caused by, 36

Laryngitis, 49
Laryngopharynx, 8
Laryngospasm, 53
Laryngotracheobronchitis (croup), 589
Larynx, 8
Latent period, 557
Lateral marginal veins, 75
Lead II, 86
Lead poisoning, 451
Left anterior hemiblock, 249
Left atrial enlargement (LAE), 249, 250
Left axis deviation, 229, 230
Left bundle branch, 84
Left bundle branch block, 246–248
Left coronary artery, 75
Left posterior hemiblock, 248
Left ventricular failure, 202
Left ventricular hypertrophy (LVH), 249, 250
Leukemias, 495–496
Leukemoid reaction, 495
Leukocytes (white blood cells), 476–480, 558
Leukocytosis, 495
Leukopenia, 495
Leukopoiesis, 477
Lice, 600–601
Lidocaine, 176
Ligament of Treitz, 369
Limbic system, 268
Limb leads, 85
Limb presentation, 692
Lithium, 447–448
Liver
  cirrhosis of, 371–372
  hepatitis, 389–390
Low back pain, 308
Lower airway, anatomy of, 8–11
Lower gastrointestinal bleeding, 376–377
Lower gastrointestinal (GI) diseases, 376–385
  bowel obstruction, 382–385
  Crohn's disease, 378–380
  diverticulitis, 380–381
  hemorrhoids, 381–382
  hepatitis, 389–390
  lower gastrointestinal bleeding, 376–377
  pancreatitis, 388
  ulcerative colitis, 377–378
Lower respiratory tract (lower airway), diseases that affect, 19
Lumen, 76
Lung cancer, 51–52
Lung capacities, 14
Lung compliance, 13–14
Lung diffusion, 16–17
Lung perfusion, 17–18
Lungs, 11. See also Respiratory system
Lung volumes, ventilation and, 14–15
Luteinizing hormone (LH), 641, 642, 656
Lyme disease, 595–596
Lymphatic system, 559–560

Lymphocytes, 479, 558
Lymphomas, 496

McBurney's point, 385, 386
Major basic protein (MBP), 479
Mallory-Weiss syndrome, 369
Mallory-Weiss tear, 369
Mammalian diving reflex, 527
Manic-depressive disorder, 619
Manic episodes, 619
Marginal artery, 75
Marijuana, 465
Marine animal injection, 461
Masks, 579
Mast cells, 351
MCL1 (modified chest lead 1), 86
MDMA (Ecstasy), 463
Measles, German (rubella), 586–587
Measles (rubeola), 585–586
Meatus, 7
Meconium staining, 694
Medications
  antidysrhythmic, 175–176
  of cardiac patients, 165
  sympathomimetic agents, 177–178
Medulla, ventilation and, 15
Medulla oblongata, 269
Megakaryocytes, 481
Melatonin, 325–326
Melena, 369
Menarche, 641
Meninges, 265, 267
Meningitis, 300, 582–584
Menopause, 643
Menorrhagia, 649
Menstrual cycle, 641–643
Menstrual periods (menses), 641
  assessment of, 644
Menstruation, 642–643
Mental status. See also Consciousness
  altered, 275
    management of, 287
  assessment of, 278–279, 284
  in behavioral emergencies, 611, 613
  respiratory status and, 23
Mercury poisoning, 451
Mesencephalon, 269
Metabolic rate, 508–509
Metabolism, 315
  glucose, 327–328
  steady-state, 508
Metals, toxicity from, 450–451
Metastases, 302
Methanol (wood alcohol), 465, 466
Methicillin-resistant Staphylococcus aureus (MRSA), 602
Microangiopathy, 410
Microorganisms, 550–555
Midbrain, 269
Mineralocorticoids, 325
Minute alveolar volume, 15
Minute respiratory volume, 14

Miscarriage (spontaneous abortion), 648, 670
Mitral valve, 73
Mittelschmerz, 648
Mobitz I block. *See* Type I second-degree AV block
Mobitz II block. *See* Type II second-degree AV block
Modified chest lead 1 (MCL1), 86
Monoamine oxidase inhibitors (MAOIs), 446
Monocytes, 479
Mononeuropathy, 276–277
Mononucleosis, 588
Mons pubis, 637
Mood disorders, 617–619
Morphine sulfate, in emergency cardiac care, 178
Motor system status, 283
MRSA (methicillin-resistant *Staphylococcus aureus*), 602
Multifocal atrial tachycardia, 110–111
Multiple births, 693
Multiple myeloma, 499
Multiple personality disorder, 621
Multiple sclerosis, 304
Mumps, 586
Mural emboli, 219
Murphy's sign, 387
Muscle cramps (heat cramps), 511–513
Muscles, intercostal, 12
Muscular dystrophy, 304
Musculoskeletal system, during pregnancy, 661
Mushrooms, poisonous, 452–453
Myeloma, multiple, 499
Myocardial infarction (MI), 196–202, 234, 235
    cardiogenic shock and, 196, 197, 210
ECGs (electrocardiograms) and, 238–240
    evolution of, 235
    field assessment, 197–199
    in-hospital management of, 201–202
    localization of, 235
    precipitating event in, 196
    prehospital management of, 199–201
    subendocardial, 196, 234–235, 237
    transmural, 196, 235
Myocardial injury, 232
Myocardial ischemia, 232
    drugs used for, 178
Myocardium, 71
Myoclonus, 306
Myometrium, 641
Myxedema, 336, 338–339
Myxedema coma, 338, 339

Nalbuphine, in emergency cardiac care, 178
Naloxone, 463
Narcissistic personality disorder, 622
Narcotics, 464

Narcotics/opiates, 463
Nares (nostrils), 5
    flaring of, 24
Nasal cavity, 5–7
Nasal flaring, 24
Nasal septum, 7
Nasopharynx, 8
National Institute for Occupational Safety and Health (NIOSH), 550
Natural immunity (innate immunity), 348
Naturally acquired immunity, 348
Natural passive immunity, 349
Nausea, in cardiac patients, 164
Near-drowning, 525, 527–528
Nebulized medications, administration of, 45–47
Neck, respiratory assessment and, 26
Negative chronotropic agents, 80
Negative feedback, 508
Negative inotropic agents, 80
Neisseria gonorrhoeae (*N. gonorrhoeae*), 596
Neonatal care, 686–689
Neoplasms, brain and spinal cord (neurological), 302–304
Nephritis, interstitial, 410
Nephrology, 395
Nephrons, 396–397
Nervous system. *See also* Autonomic nervous system; Central nervous system; Somatic nervous system
    anatomy and physiology of, 262–275
    infections, 592–596
    ventilation and, 19–21
Neurologic emergencies, 260–310
    assessment and management of, 286–310
        airway and breathing, 287
        altered mental status, 287–289
        circulatory support, 287
        headache, 300–301
        neoplasms, 302–304
        pharmacological interventions, 287
        psychological support, 287
        seizures, 294–299
        stroke and intracranial hemorrhage, 289–294
        syncope (fainting), 299
        transport considerations, 287
        "weak and dizzy" patients, 301–302
    case study, 261–262
    management of
        brain abscess, 304
        degenerative neurological disorders, 304–307
    pathophysiology of nontraumatic, 275–286
        alteration in cognitive systems, 275

autonomic nervous system disorders, 277
central nervous system disorders, 275–276
cerebral homeostasis, 276
focused history, 279–280
general assessment findings, 277–286
geriatric considerations, 286
peripheral nervous system disorders, 276–277
physical examination, 280–285
scene size-up and initial assessment, 277–279
Neuromuscular disorders, during pregnancy, 666
Neurons, 264
Neurotransmitters, 79, 264
Neutrons, 540
Neutropenia, 479, 495
Neutrophils, 478, 479, 558
Nifedipine (Procardia, Adalat), 538
NIOSH (National Institute for Occupational Safety and Health), 550
Nipride (sodium nitroprusside), 179
Nitrogen narcosis, 530–531, 535
Nitroglycerin, in emergency cardiac care, 178
Nitrous oxide (Nitronox), in emergency cardiac care, 178
Noncompensatory pause, 113
Non-insulin-dependent diabetes mellitus (NIDDM), 329–330
Non-Q wave infarction, 196
Non-steroidal anti-inflammatory drugs (NSAIDs), 449–450
Norepinephrine, 79, 177, 264, 324
Normal flora, 550, 551
Nose, 5
Nosocomial infections, 422, 602
NSAIDs (non-steroidal anti-inflammatory drugs), 449–450
Nuclear physics, 539–540
Nuclear radiation (radioactive emergencies), 539–544
    effects on the body, 541
    management of, 543–544
    safety principles, 542–543

Obligate intracellular parasites, 553
Obsessive-compulsive disorder, 622
Obstetrics, 637
Obstetrics (obstetric patients), 654–696
    anatomy and physiology of, 656–661
    case study, 655–656
    general assessment of, 664–667
    general management of, 667
    terminology used in, 664
Obstructive lung diseases, 38–48. *See also* Asthma; Chronic obstructive pulmonary disease (COPD); Emphysema

Occiput posterior position, 692
Occlusive strokes, 290
Occupational Safety and Health
Administration (OSHA), 550
Oliguria, 409
Oncotic pressure, 474
Opiates, 463
Opportunistic pathogens, 551
Oral intake, of cardiac patients, 166
Organic headaches, 300
Organic psychiatric disorders, 609–610
Organophosphates, 431
Oropharynx, 8
Orthopnea, 25
Osborn wave (J wave), 157
Osborn waves (J waves), 520
Osmolarity, 399
Osmosis, 399
Osmotic diuresis, 329, 401
Osmotic pull, 474
Ostia, 75
Otitis media, 49
Ovarian cysts, ruptured, 648
Ovaries, 319, 325, 641
Overdose, drug, 462
    defined, 428
Ovulation, 642, 656–657
Oxygen
    administration of
        in anaphylaxis, 354
        heatstroke and, 515
    in emergency cardiac care, 178
Oxygen dissociation curve, 17
Oxygen saturation, 32, 33
Oxygen transport, red blood cells
and, 474
Oxytocin, 320–321

Pacemakers, artificial pacemaker rhythm,
152–153
Pain
    abdominal. See also
    Gastrointestinal diseases and
    emergencies
        classification of, 363
        colicky, 378
        gynecological, 643, 647–649
        management of, 649
        hematological disease and
        (wood alcohol), 490
        management of patients
        with, 408, 649
        in toxicological
        emergencies, 435
        transport and, 408
        urologic emergencies
        and, 404
    back, 307–310
    chest
        in cardiovascular patients,
        162–163
        gastrointestinal emergencies
        that can cause, 366

        myocardial infarction and,
        197–198, 201
        pleuritic, 50
    during pregnancy, 666
    referred, 404
    in urologic emergencies, 404
    visceral, 363, 404
Pain disorder, 620
Pallor, respiratory status and, 23
Palpation
    abdominal, 407
    of respiratory system, 28
Palpitations, in cardiac patients, 164
Pancolitis, 377
Pancreas, 319, 322–324
    disorders of the, 326–336
        diabetes mellitus, 326–330
        diabetic ketoacidosis
        (diabetic coma), 330–332
        hyperglycemic hyperosmolar
        nonketotic (HHNK)
        acidosis, 330–333
        hypoglycemia (insulin
        shock), 328, 330–331,
        333, 336
Pancreatitis, 388
Panic attacks, 616–617
Papillary muscles, 73
Paralytic shellfish poisoning, 452
Paranasal sinuses, 7
Paranoid personality disorder, 622
Paranoid schizophrenia, 616
Parasites, 554
Parasympathetic nervous system, 263, 275
Parathyroid glands, 318, 322
Parathyroid hormone (PTH), 322
Parietal pericardium, 71
Parietal pleura, 11
Parkinson's disease, 305
Paroxysmal junctional tachycardia (PJT),
137–139
Paroxysmal nocturnal dyspnea (PND), 25,
204–206
Paroxysmal supraventricular tachycardia
(PSVT), 114–117, 137–139
Partial seizures, 295, 296
Passive immunity, 349, 560
Pathogens, 347, 550, 551
    opportunistic, 551
Pathological gambling, 623
Pathological Q wave, 198
Patient education, about infectious
diseases, 602
Peak expiratory flow rate (PEFR), 33, 45
Peak flow, 15, 33
PEEP (positive end expiratory pressure), 38
PEFR (peak expiratory flow rate), 33, 45
Pelvic inflammatory disease (PID),
596–597, 647–648
Penicillinase-producing N. gonorrhoeae
(PPNG), 596
Penis, 403
Peptic ulcers, 374–376

Percussion
    of the abdomen, 407
    of respiratory system, 28, 29
Percutaneous transluminal coronary
angioplasty (PTCA), 201–202
Perfusion, 17–18
    diseases that affect, 21
Pericardiocentesis, 207
Pericardium, 71
Perimetrium, 641
Perinephric abscesses, 422
Perineum, 637, 683, 686, 692
Peripheral arterial atherosclerotic
disease, 219
Peripheral circulation, 76–77
Peripheral cyanosis, respiratory status
and, 23, 30
Peripheral nervous system, 263, 273. See
also Autonomic nervous system; Somatic
nervous system
    disorders of, 276–277
Peripheral neuropathy, 276
Peripheral vascular conditions,
noncritical, 219–221
Peritoneal dialysis, 418–419
Peritonitis, 363
Personality disorders, 622–623
Pertussis, 587–588
Petit mal seizures (absence seizures), 296
PH, 16
Phagocytosis, 477, 558
Pharyngitis, 49, 589
Pharynx, 8
Phenargan (promethazine), 179
Phobias, 617
Physical examination. See also
Auscultation; Inspection; Palpation;
Percussion; specific procedures and types
of disorders
        of cardiac patients, 166–170
        in gastrointestinal emergencies, 367
        of gynecological patients, 645–646
        infectious diseases and, 569–570
        in neurologic emergencies, 280–285
        of obstetric patients, 666
        of respiratory system, 26–34
            abnormal breath sounds, 30
            auscultation, 28–29
            diagnostic testing, 32–34
            head and neck, 26
            inspection, 26–27
            normal breath sounds, 29
            palpation, 28
            percussion, 28
            vital signs, 30–32
        in toxicological emergencies, 432,
        435–436
Physiological dependence, 461
Physiologic shunt, 11
Pia mater, 265
Pineal gland, 319, 325–326
Pinworms, 554
Pituitary gland, 317, 318, 320–321

Pit viper bites, 458–460
Placenta, 326, 657
    previa, 672–673
Placental stage of labor, 681
Plants, poisonous, 452–453
Plasma, 473–474
Plasmin, 482
Plasminogen, 482
Platelets, 481
Pleura, 11
Pleural cavity, inspiration and, 12–13
Pleural friction rub, 30
Pleuritic chest pain, 50
Pluripotent stem cells, 473
Pneumocystis carinii, 551
Pneumomediastinum, 531, 535
Pneumonia, 49–51, 580–581
    VZV, 581
Pneumothorax, 19, 531
    spontaneous, 56–57
Poiseuille's Law, 76
Poison Control Centers, 429–430
Poisoning. *See also* Toxicological
emergencies
    defined, 428
    food, 591–592
Poliomyelitis (polio), 306–307
Polycythemia, 492, 494
    emphysema and, 39–40
Polyneuropathy, 276, 277
Pons, 269
Positional asphyxia, 631
Position of patient, respiratory status and,
22–23
Positive chronotropic agents, 80
Positive end expiratory pressure (PEEP), 38
Positive inotropic agents, 80
Posterior descending artery, 75
Posterior pituitary gland, 317, 318,
320–321
Postpartum hemorrhage, 694–695
Postrenal acute renal failure, 410–411
Posttraumatic stress syndrome, 617
Postural instability, 305
Posture
    in behavioral emergencies, 611
    in renal and urologic
    emergencies, 406
PPD (purified protein derivative) skin test,
562, 577–578
PPNG (penicillinase-producing *N.
gonorrhoeae*), 596
P-Q interval (PQI), 93
Precipitous delivery, 693–694
Precordial leads, 85, 228
Precordial thump, 175
Preeclampsia, 674, 675–676
Pre-excitation syndromes, 157
Pregnancy, 644. *See also* Delivery; Labor;
Obstetrics (obstetric patients); Puerperium
    complications of, 668–679
        abortion, 669–671
        abruptio placentae, 673–674

bleeding, 669–674
Braxton-Hicks
contractions, 678
ectopic pregnancy, 671–672
gestational diabetes, 677
hypertensive disorders,
674–676
medical complications,
674–679
medical conditions, 669
placenta previa, 672
supine-hypotensive
syndrome, 676–677
trauma, 668–669
    ectopic, 649, 671–672
    physiologic changes of, 658–661
    prenatal period, 656–664
Preload (end-diastolic volume), 78
Premature atrial contractions, 113
Premature junctional contractions, 132, 133
Premature ventricular contractions
(PVCs), 142–144
Premenstrual syndrome (PMS), 643
Prenatal period, 656–664
Prepuce, 638
Prerenal acute renal failure, 409–410
Pressure disorders, 532–534
Preterm labor, 678–679
Primary response, 347–348
P-R interval (PRI), 93, 97
Prinzmetal's angina, 191
Prions, 553, 554
Procainamide, 176
Proctitis, 377
Progesterone, 325
Prokaryotes, 551
Prolapsed cord, 667, 691–692
Proliferative phase, 642
Prolonged QT interval, 93
Promethazine (Phenargan), 179
Prostate gland, 403
Prostatic hypertrophy, benign, 396
Prostatitis, 422
Protective custody, suicidal patients
and, 434
Prothrombin, 481, 482
Protons, 540
Protozoa, 554
Proximal tubule, 397
Pseudoseizures, 296
Psychiatric and behavioral disorders,
606–631
    age-related conditions, 624–625
    anxiety and related disorders,
    616–619
    assessment of, 610–614
        focused history and physical
        examination, 611–613
        initial assessment, 611
        mental status examination,
        613
        psychiatric medications, 614
        scene size-up, 610–611

bipolar disorder, 619
case study, 607–608
cognitive disorders, 614–615
dementia, 615
depression, 618–619
dissociative disorders, 621
eating disorders, 621–622
factitious disorders, 620–621
impulse control disorders, 623
management of, 625–627
mood disorders, 617–619
panic attacks, 616–617
pathophysiology of, 609–610
personality disorders, 622–623
phobias, 617
posttraumatic stress syndrome, 617
schizophrenia, 615–616
somatoform disorders, 620
substance related disorders, 620
suicide, 623–624
violent patients and restraint,
627–631
Psychiatric medications, assessment of
psychiatric or behavioral disorders
and, 614
Psychogenic amnesia, 621
Psychological dependence, 461
Psychological support, in allergic or
anaphylactic reactions, 356
Psychosis, 624
    Korsakoff's, 289
Psychosocial (personal) disorders, 610
Pubic symphysis, 637
Puerperium, 679–689
Pulmonary arteries, 11, 74
Pulmonary capillaries, 10, 16–18
    permeability of, 21
Pulmonary edema, 5
    cardiogenic, 36–37
    congestive heart failure and,
    204–206
    high altitude (HAPE), 38
    non-cardiogenic, 36–38
Pulmonary emboli, 5
Pulmonary embolism, 54–56
    acute, 218–219
    pregnancy and, 696
Pulmonary embolism (PE), 202
Pulmonary over-pressure, 531, 534
Pulmonary shunting, 21
Pulmonary veins, 11, 74
Pulmonary vessels, 11
Pulse, of cardiac patients, 169
Pulseless electrical activity (PEA),
154, 155
Pulse oximeter, 286
Pulse oximetry, 32–33
Pulsus alternans, 205
Pulsus paradoxus, 31, 205
Pump failure, 197
Purified protein derivative (PPD) skin test,
577–578
Purkinje system, 84

P waves, 88, 97
    dysrhythmias originating in the AV
        junction and, 133
Pyelonephritis, 422
Pyrexia (fever), 516
Pyrogens, 516
Pyromania, 623

QRS axis, 228
QRS complex, 88, 97
    dysrhythmias originating in the AV
        junction and, 133
    pacemaker rhythms and, 153
QRS interval, 93
QT interval, 93
Quality factor (QF), 541
Q waves, 88
    myocardial infarction and, 196,
        198, 199
    pathological, 198

Rabies, 593–594
Radiation, 506
    nuclear (radioactive emergencies),
        539–544
        effects on the body, 541
        management of, 543–544
        safety principles, 542–543
Radiation absorbed dose (RAD), 541
Radioisotopes (isotopes), 540
Rape, 650–652
Reabsorption, 398
Recompression, 533
Red blood cell diseases, 492–494
Red blood cells, 474–476
Reduced nephron mass, 414
Reduced renal mass, 414
Reentry, 98
Referred pain, 364–365, 404
Reflexes, 271
Refractory period, 94
Relative refractory period, 94
Relaxation phase, 77
Relteplase (Retavase), 179
Renal acute renal failure, 410
Renal and urologic emergencies, 403–423
    acute renal failure, 409–413
    assessment in, 404–408
    chronic renal failure (CRF),
        413–419
    pathophysiologic basis of pain, 404
    urinary tract infection (UTI),
        421–423
Renal calculi (kidney stones), 395,
419–421
    case study, 394
Renal dialysis, 416–418
Renal failure
    acute, 409–413
    chronic (CRF), 413–419
    end-stage, 413
Renal pelvis, 397
Renin, 326

Reperfusion, 195
    myocardial infarction and,
        198–199
Repolarization, 82
Reproductive system, female, 637–641
    during pregnancy, 659
Reservoirs, 555
Residual volume, 14
Resistance, 557
Respiration(s), 18, 507
    apneustic, 282
    ataxic, 282
    Cheyne-Stokes, 19–20, 281
    Kussmaul's, 282, 331
Respirators, 578–579
Respiratory diseases, 5, 18–21, 34–59
    adult respiratory distress syndrome
        (ARDS)/non-cardiogenic
        pulmonary edema, 36–38
    asthma, 43–48
    carbon monoxide inhalation,
        53–54
    central nervous system dysfunction,
        58–59
    chronic bronchitis, 41–43
    extrinsic risk factors, 5
    genetic predisposition to, 5
    hyperventilation syndrome, 57–58
    intrinsic risk factors, 5
    lung cancer, 51
    management of, 34–35
    obstructive lung diseases, 38–41
    pneumonia, 49–51
    pulmonary embolism, 54–56
    spontaneous pneumothorax, 56–57
    toxic inhalation, 52–53
    upper-airway obstruction, 35–36
    upper respiratory infection (URI),
        48–49
Respiratory effort, respiratory status
and, 23
Respiratory emergencies, 4
Respiratory membrane, 10, 21
    diffusion and, 16
Respiratory muscles, dysfunction of, 59
Respiratory rate, 31
Respiratory status, CNS illness or injury
and, 281–282
Respiratory syncytial virus (RSV), 587
Respiratory system, 4–34
    anatomy of, 5–18
        alveoli, 9–11
        bronchi, 8–9
        larynx, 8
        lower airway, 8–11
        nasal cavity, 5–7
        pharynx, 8
        upper airway anatomy, 5–11
    assessment of, 22–34. *See also*
    Physical examination, of
    respiratory system
        ability to speak, 23
        airway, 24

        breathing, 24–25
        color, 23
        general impression, 22–25
        history, 25–26
        initial assessment, 22–25
        mental status, 23
        nasal flaring, 24
        position, 22–23
        respiratory effort, 23
        scene size-up, 22
        tracheal tugging, 24
    pathophysiology of. *See*
    Respiratory diseases
    physiological processes of, 11–18
        diffusion, 16–17
        perfusion, 17–18
        ventilation, 11–16
    during pregnancy, 659
Resting potential, 81–82
Restlessness, in cardiac patients, 163
Restraint of violent patients, 627–631
Resuscitation, 213–214
    of hypothermia victims, 522
    neonatal, 688–689
    withholding and terminating,
        214–216
Reticular activating system (RAS), 269, 270
Reticuloendothelial system (RES), 558
Return of spontaneous circulation
(ROSC), 213
Reverse transcriptase, 570
Rewarming, active, 520
Rewarming shock, 522
Rhinitis, 49
Rhonchi, 30
Rhythm strips, electrocardiographic
(ECG), 84, 95–98
Right atrial enlargement (RAE), 249, 250
Right axis deviation, 229
Right bundle branch, 84
Right bundle branch block, 245–246
Right coronary artery, 75
Right ventricular failure, 202
Right ventricular hypertrophy (RVH),
249, 250
Rigidity, in Parkinson's patients, 305
Roentgen equivalent in man (REM), 541
Rohypnol (Flunitrazepam), 463
R-R interval, 96
RSV (respiratory syncytial virus), 587
Rubella (German measles), 586–587
Rubeola (measles), 585–586
Rupture of the membranes (ROM), 658
R waves, 88
Ryan White Act, 567

Salicylates, 448
Salmonella, 592
Saltwater drowning, 526–527
Scabies, 601–602
Scene size-up
    cardiovascular assessment and,
        161–162

gastrointestinal emergencies, 365
  respiratory system and, 22
Schizoid personality disorder, 622
Schizophrenia, 615–616
Schizotypal personality disorder, 622
Scombroid (histamine) poisoning, 452
Scorpion stings, 457
Scrotum, 403
Seafood poisonings, 452
Sea urchins, 461
Secondary response, 348
Second-degree AV blocks
    Type II (Mobitz II), 128–129, 241
    Type I (Mobitz I), 126–127, 241
Secretin, 326
Secretion, 398
Secretory phase, 642
Sedatives, 465
Seizure disorders, during pregnancy, 665
Seizures, 294–299
    generalized, 295
    hypoglycemic, 336
    partial, 295, 296
Selective serotonin re-uptake inhibitors
(SSRIs), 447
Semen, 403
Semilunar valves, 73
Sengstaken-Blakemore tube, 370
Sensitization, 349
Sensorimotor evaluation, 282–283
Septum
    interatrial, 71
    interventricular, 71
Sequestration of red blood cells, 476
Seroconversion, 557
Serotonin syndrome, 447
Sexual assault, 650–652
Sexually transmitted diseases (STDs),
596–600
    chancroid, 599–600
    chlamydia, 599
    genital warts, 598
    gonorrhea, 596–597
    herpes simplex Type 2, 598–599
    syphilis, 597–598
    trichomoniasis, 599
Sexual purposes, drugs used for, 463
Shock, cardiogenic, 209–212
    field assessment of, 210
    management of, 210–212
    myocardial infarction and, 196,
    197, 210
Shoulder dystocia, 694
Sickle cell disease, 493–494
Simple diffusion, 399
Simple partial seizures, 296
Sinoatrial (SA) node, 83
Sinus arrest, 106–107
Sinus bradycardia, 99–101
Sinus dysrhythmia, 104–105
Sinuses, paranasal, 7
Sinusitis, 49, 589–590
Sinus tachycardia, 102–103

Six-second method, 96
Skin
    of cardiac patients, 167
    infectious diseases of the, 600–602
Skull, 265, 266
Sleep, high altitude and, 537
Slow-reacting substance of anaphylaxis
(SRS-A), 351
Small cell carcinoma, 51
Smell, sense of, 7
Smoking. See Cigarette smoking
Snakebites, 457–460
Snoring, 30
Sociocultural (situational) causes of
behavioral disorders, 610
Sodium nitroprusside (Nipride), 179
Somatic nervous system, 263
Somatic pain, 363–364
Somatization disorder, 620
Somatoform disorders, 620
Somatostatin, 324
Speaking ability, respiratory status and, 23
Sperm cells, 402
Spina bifida (SB), 306
Spinal cord, 269, 271, 272
    nontraumatic disorders, 307–310
    respiratory diseases and, 59
Spirometry, 33
Spontaneous abortion (miscarriage), 670
Spontaneous pneumothorax, 56–57
Sputum, respiratory status and, 26
SRS-A (slow-reacting substance of
anaphylaxis), 351
SSRIs (selective serotonin re-uptake
inhibitors), 447
Stable angina, 191
Starling's Law of the Heart, 78, 204
Status asthmaticus, 45
Status epilepticus, 298–299
Steady-state metabolism, 508
Stem cells, pluripotent, 473
Sterilization, 567
Stingrays, 461
Stings, insect, 454–457
Stretch receptors, 15
Stridor, 30
Strokes, 289–294
    embolic, 290
    hemorrhagic, 291–292
    occlusive, 290
    thrombotic, 290
Stroke volume, 78
Structural lesions, 275
Struvite stones, 419
S-T segment, 93, 94–95
Subcutaneous emphysema, 28
Subendocardial infarction, 196,
234–235, 237
Substance abuse. See also Alcohol abuse
    commonly abused drugs, 462–465
    defined, 461
Substance abuse and overdose, 461–468
Substance related disorders, 620

Sudden death, 212
Suicidal patients, 434
Suicide, 613, 623–624
Superior vena cava, 74
Superior vena cava syndrome, 52
Supine-hypotensive syndrome, 676–677
Surface-absorbed toxins, 437–438
Surface absorption of toxic substances, 431
Surfactant, 10, 526
Surgical menopause, 643
Survival, 213
S waves, 88
Sympathetic nervous system, 263, 275
Sympathomimetic agents, 177–178
Synchronized cardioversion, 183,
186, 187
Syncope, in cardiac patients, 164
Syncope (fainting), 297, 299–300
Syncytium (pl. syncytia), 80
Syphilis, 597–598
Syrup of ipecac, 433
Systemic lupus erythematosis (SLE), 480
Systole, 77

Tachycardia (rapid heart rate), 24, 96
    atrial, 108–111
        multifocal, 110–111
    paroxysmal junctional (PJT),
    137–139
    paroxysmal supraventricular,
    114–117
    respiratory distress and, 30–31
    sinus, 102–103
    ventricular, 144–147
Tachypnea, 32
Tactile fremitus, 28
Tension headaches, 300
Tension pneumothorax, 19, 56–57
Testes, 319, 325, 402
Testosterone, 325
Tetanus, 560–561, 594–595
Thalamus, 268
Theophylline, 450
Therapeutic index, 445
Thermal gradient, 506
Thermogenesis (heat generation), 506
Thermolysis (heat loss), 506–507
Thermoreceptors, 508
Thermoregulation, 507–508
Thermoregulatory thermogenesis, 506
Third-degree AV blocks, 130–131, 245
Thoracic aorta, 75
Thorax, of cardiac patients, 167, 169
Thrombin, 482
Thrombocytes, 481
Thrombocytopenia, 481, 497
Thrombocytosis, 481, 497
Thrombolytic agents, 178–179
Thrombophlebitis, 218
Thrombopoietin, 481
Thrombosis, 483
    deep venous, 219–220
Thrombotic strokes, 290

Thrombus, 196
  cerebral, 290
Thymosin, 322
Thymus, 318
Thymus gland, 322
Thyroid cartilage (Adam's apple), 8
Thyroid gland, 318, 321–322
  disorders of the, 336–339
Thyrotoxic crisis ("thyroid storm"), 338
Thyrotoxicosis, 336
Thyroxine, 321–322
TIAs (transient ischemic attacks), 292
Tic douloureux, 305–306
Tidal volume, 14
Tissue plasminogen activator (tPA), 289
T lymphocytes, 558
Tolerance of drugs, 461
Tonic-clonic seizures (grand mal seizures), 295
Tonic phase, 295
Tonsils, 8
Torsade de pointes, 144–146, 186
Total down time, 213
Total lung capacity, 14
Toxic inhalation, 52–53
Toxic-metabolic states, 276
Toxicological emergencies, 428–461
  acetaminophen, 449
  antidepressants
    newer, 447
    tricyclic, 445–446
  assessment and management of, general principles of, 431–434
  carbon monoxide poisoning, 439
  cardiac medication poisoning, 442–443
  caustic substances, 443–444
  cyanide, 438–439
  epidemiology of, 429
  food poisoning, 451–452
  hydrocarbons, 444–445
  hydrofluoric acid, 444
  ingested toxins, 434–436
  inhaled toxins, 437
  injected toxins, 453–461
    black widow spider bites, 456–457
    brown recluse spider, 454–456
    general principles of management, 453–454
    insect stings, 454–457
    marine animal injection, 461
    pit viper bites, 458–460
    scorpion stings, 457
    snakebites, 457–458
  lithium, 447–448
  metals, 450–451
  monoamine oxidase inhibitors (MAOIs), 446
  non-steroidal anti-inflammatory drugs (NSAIDs), 449–450

Poison Control Centers and, 429–430
  routes of toxic exposure, 430–431
  salicylates, 448
  surface-absorbed toxins, 437–438
  theophylline, 450
Toxicology, 428
Toxidromes, 438
Toxins, 347, 428
Trachea, 8
Tracheal deviation, 28
Tracheal position, in cardiac patients, 166–167
Tracheal tugging, 24
Transcutaneous cardiac pacing, 186, 188–189
Transfusion, blood, 484–486
Transient ischemic attacks (TIAs), 292–294
Transitional fibers, 123
Transmural infarction, 196, 235
Transport
  abdominal pain and, 408
  positioning and restraining violent patients for, 630–631
Tremor, 305
Trench foot, 524
Trichinosis, 554–555
Trichomoniasis, 599
Trichotillomania, 623
Tricuspid valve, 73
Tricyclic antidepressants, 445–446
Triiodothyronine, 321–322
Triplicate method, 96
Tuberculosis, 577–580
Tubular handling
  of glucose and urea, 400–401
  of water and electrolytes, 399–400
Tumors, spinal, 309
Tunica adventitia, 76
Tunica intima, 76
Tunica media, 76
Turbinates, 7
T waves, 89
Type I diabetes mellitus, 329
Type II diabetes mellitus (non-insulin-dependent diabetes mellitus), 329–330
Type II second-degree AV block (Mobitz II), 128–129
Type I second-degree AV block (Mobitz I), 126–127, 241

Ulcerative colitis, 377–378
Ulcers, peptic, 374–376
Umbilical cord, 658
Unconsciousness (coma), 275
Undifferentiated schizophrenia, 616
Unipolar leads, 85
Unipolar limb leads (augmented limb leads), 85, 226–227
Unstable angina, 191

Upper airway (upper respiratory tract), 9
  anatomy of, 5–11
  diseases that affect, 19
Upper-airway obstruction, assessment and management of, 35–36
Upper gastrointestinal bleeding, 369–370
Upper gastrointestinal diseases, 368–376
  acute gastroenteritis, 372–373
  esophageal varices, 370–372
  gastroenteritis, 373–374
  peptic ulcers, 374–376
  upper gastrointestinal bleeding, 369–370
Upper respiratory infection (URI), 48–49. See also Pneumonia
Urea, 395
  tubular handling of, 400–401
Uremia, 414
Uremic syndrome, 415
Ureters, 401
Urethra, 402, 638–639
Urethritis, 421
Uric acid stones, 419
Urinary bladder, 402
Urinary stasis, 421, 422
Urinary system, 395–423. See also Renal and urologic emergencies
  anatomy and physiology of, 396–403
  during pregnancy, 661
  nontraumatic tissue problems, 403
Urinary tract infection (UTI), 421–423
Urination, pain or burning with (dysuria), 648
Urine, 395
Urologic emergencies. See Renal and urologic emergencies
Urology, 395
Urticaria, 353
Uterine atony, 695
Uterine rupture, 695
Uterus, 640
U waves, 89

Vagal maneuvers, 174
Vagina, 639
Vaginal bleeding
  non-traumatic, 649
  during pregnancy, 666, 669–674
Vagus nerve, 80
Valium (diazepam), 179
Valves of heart, 73–74
Vancomycin-resistant enterococcus (VRE), 602
Vaqta, 575
Varicella (chickenpox), 581–582
Varicella-zoster immune globulin (VZIG), 582
Varices, esophageal, 370–372
Varicose veins, 220
Varivax, 581, 582
Vascular disorders, 220

Vascular headaches, 300
Vasculitis, 219
Vas deferens, 403
Vasoocclusive crises, 494
Vasopressin, 466
Vasopressors, for anaphylaxis, 355
Vasospastic angina, 191
Vectors, 228
Veins, 77
　　bronchial, 11
　　pulmonary, 11, 74
Venous system, 77
Ventilation, 11–16
　　airway resistance and, 13
　　defined, 11
　　diseases that affect, 19–21
　　inspiration and expiration, 12–13
　　lung compliance and, 13–14
　　lung volumes and, 14–15
　　obstructive lung diseases and, 39
　　regulation of, 15–16
Ventricles, 71
Ventricular aneurysm, 197
Ventricular conduction, disturbances of,
156–157

Ventricular escape complexes and
rhythms, 141
Ventricular fibrillation, 148–149
　　in hypothermia, 520
Ventricular syncytium, 80
Ventricular tachycardia, 144–147
Venules, 77
Verapamil, 117, 122, 139, 176
Vertebral column, 267
Vertebral injury, 309
Vertebrobasilar system, 269
Vestibule (false vocal cords), 8
Vestibule (mons pubis), 638
Violent patients, 627–631
Viral rhinitis (common cold), 585
Virulence, 556–557
Viruses, 553
Visceral pain, 363, 404
Visceral pericardium (epicardium), 71
Visceral pleura, 11
Vital capacity, 14
Vital signs, respiratory distress and,
30–32
Vocal cords, 8
Volvulus, intestinal, 382, 384

Vomiting
　　in cardiac patients, 164
　　induction of, in toxicological
　　emergencies, 433, 436
Von Willebrand's disease, 498

Warts, genital, 598
Water, tubular handling of, 399–400
"Weak and dizzy" patients, 301–302
Wernicke's syndrome, 289
Wet drowning, 525–526
Wheezing, 30
　　in asthma, 44
White blood cell diseases, 495–496
White blood cells (leukocytes), 476–480
Whole bowel irrigation, 433
Window phase, 557
Withdrawal, 462
Withdrawal syndrome, alcohol, 467–468
Wolff-Parkinson-White (WPW)
syndrome, 157
Work-induced thermogenesis, 506
Wright Spirometer, 33

Zollinger-Ellison syndrome, 375